KU-538-966

To AMW and JMW

With love,
JLC

To ES, MTM, and PGM

With love,
ERM

CONTRIBUTORS

EVE CALIGOR, MD
Associate Clinical Professor of Psychiatry, College of
Physicians & Surgeons of Columbia University, New
York, New York; Faculty, Admitting Psychoanalyst,
Columbia University Psychoanalytic Center for
Training and Research, New York, New York;
Associate Attending Psychiatrist, Presbyterian
Hospital, New York, New York

Psychological Factors Affecting Medical Conditions

FRANCINE COURNOS, MD
Professor of Clinical Psychiatry, College of
Physicians & Surgeons of Columbia University, New
York, New York; Director, Washington Heights Com-
munity Service, New York State Psychiatric Institute,
New York, New York; Research Faculty, Columbia
University Psychoanalytic Center for Training and
Research, New York, New York

Schizophrenia and Other Psychotic Disorders

JANIS L. CUTLER, MD
Associate Clinical Professor of Psychiatry, Co-Director
of Medical Student Education in Psychiatry, College
of Physicians & Surgeons of Columbia University, and New
York State Psychiatric Institute, New York, New York;
Associate Attending Psychiatrist, Presbyterian Hospital,
New York, New York

*Case Formulation: Assessment and Treatment Planning;
Personality Disorders; Life Development; Therapeutic Settings*

MICHAEL J. DEVLIN, MD
Assistant Professor of Clinical Psychiatry, College of
Physicians & Surgeons of Columbia University, New
York, New York; Assistant Attending Psychiatrist,
Presbyterian Hospital, New York, New York

Eating Disorders

ROBERT E. FEINSTEIN, MD
Associate Clinical Professor of Psychiatry, College
of Physicians & Surgeons of Columbia University,
New York, New York; Director, Behavioral Science
in Family Practice Residency Program, St. Joseph
Medical Center, Stamford, Connecticut; Faculty,
Columbia University Psychoanalytic Center for
Training and Research, New York, New York

*Cognitive and Mental Disorders Due to General
Medical Conditions; Suicide and Violence*

EWALD HORWATH, MD
Associate Clinical Professor of Psychiatry, College of
Physicians & Surgeons of Columbia University, New
York, New York; Director, Intensive Care Unit, Wash-
ington Heights Community Service, New York State
Psychiatric Institute, New York, New York

Schizophrenia and Other Psychotic Disorders

STEVEN E. HYLER, MD
Associate Professor of Clinical Psychiatry, College
of Physicians & Surgeons of Columbia University,
New York, New York; Staff Psychiatrist, Inwood
Clinic, Washington Heights Community Service, New
York State Psychiatric Institute, New York, New York;
Associate Attending Psychiatrist, Presbyterian
Hospital, New York, New York

Somatoform and Factitious Disorders

DAVID A. KAHN, MD
Associate Clinical Professor of Psychiatry, College of
Physicians & Surgeons of Columbia University, New
York, New York; Associate Director of Psychiatry
and Associate Attending Psychiatrist, Presbyterian
Hospital, New York, New York

Mood Disorders

HERBERT D. KLEBER, MD
Professor of Psychiatry, College of Physicians
& Surgeons of Columbia University, New York, New
York; Director, Division on Substance Abuse, Columbia
University, New York, New York; Director, Division on
Substance Abuse, New York State Psychiatric Institute,
New York, New York; Attending Psychiatrist,
Presbyterian Hospital, New York, New York

Alcohol and Substance Abuse Disorders

FRANCES R. LEVIN, MD
Assistant Professor of Clinical Psychiatry, College of
Physicians & Surgeons of Columbia University, New
York, New York; Director, Educational Activities for the
Division on Substance Abuse, Columbia University,
New York, New York; Assistant Attending Psychiatrist,
Presbyterian Hospital, New York, New York

Alcohol and Substance Abuse Disorders

ERIC R. MARCUS, MD
Clinical Professor of Psychiatry and Social Medicine
and Director, Behavioral Sciences Curriculum and
Medical Student Education in Psychiatry, College of
Physicians & Surgeons of Columbia University, New
York, New York; New York State Psychiatric Institute,
New York, New York; Training and Supervising
Analyst, Columbia University Psychoanalytic Center
for Training and Research, New York, New York;
Attending Psychiatrist, Presbyterian Hospital, New
York, New York

Personality Disorders

PHILIP R. MUSKIN, MD
Associate Professor of Clinical Psychiatry, College
of Physicians & Surgeons of Columbia University, New
York, New York; Associate Chief of Service Consultation
Liaison Psychiatry and Associate Attending Psychi-
atrist, Presbyterian Hospital, New York, New York

Anxiety Disorders

DAVID D. OLDS, MD
Associate Clinical Professor of Psychiatry, College of
Physicians & Surgeons of Columbia University, New
York, New York; Supervising and Training Analyst,
Columbia University Psychoanalytic Center for
Training and Research, New York, New York;
Associate Attending Psychiatrist, Presbyterian
Hospital, New York, New York

Psychotherapy

LYLE ROSNICK, MD
Assistant Professor of Clinical Psychiatry, College of
Physicians & Surgeons of Columbia University, New
York, New York; Faculty, Columbia University
Psychoanalytic Center for Training and Research, New
York, New York; Assistant Attending Psychiatrist,
Presbyterian Hospital, New York, New York

The Psychiatric Interview

L. MARK RUSSAKOFF, MD
Former Associate Professor of Clinical Psychiatry,
College of Physicians & Surgeons of Columbia
University, New York, New York; former Deputy
Director, New York State Psychiatric Institute, New
York, New York; Director of Psychiatry, Phelps
Memorial Hospital, Sleepy Hollow, New York

Psychopharmacology

JONATHAN A. SLATER, MD
Assistant Clinical Professor of Psychiatry, College of
Physicians & Surgeons of Columbia University, New
York, New York; Faculty, Columbia University
Psychoanalytic Center for Training and Research,
New York, New York; Director of Pediatric
Consultation Liaison, Presbyterian Hospital, New
York, New York

Life Development

MICHAEL H. STONE, MD
Professor of Clinical Psychiatry, College of Physi-
cians & Surgeons of Columbia University, New York,
New York; Staff Psychiatrist, MidHudson Psychiatric
Center, New York, New York; Fellow, New York Hos-
pital Personality Disorders Institute, New York, New
York

Personality Disorders

LESLIE R. VOGEL, MD
Assistant Clinical Professor of Psychiatry, College of
Physicians & Surgeons of Columbia University, New
York, New York; Assistant Attending Psychiatrist,
Presbyterian Hospital, New York, New York

Anxiety Disorders

PREFACE

Psychiatry is the field of medicine that concerns itself with those illnesses that have emotional or behavioral manifestations—in other words, mind/brain disorders. Psychiatric illnesses are extremely common and exact a great personal and social cost in terms of disability, suffering, and even death. This book is intended as an introductory text that prepares medical students, physicians, and other health professionals for the clinical task of working with patients with psychiatric disorders. As such, it focuses on basic issues such as recognition and assessment of psychiatric illness, and not on detailed descriptions of treatment. The text's clinical orientation is equally well-suited for medical students during their third-year rotation in psychiatry, nonpsychiatric physicians, psychiatric residents, and other health professionals who work with patients with psychiatric disorders, including psychologists, social workers, nurses, and occupational therapists.

Patients with emotional and behavioral difficulties are often discouraged from seeking help by the stigma that they, their families, and even physicians tend to attach to psychiatric illnesses. All health care providers should be sensitive to the shame that patients with psychiatric problems may have. Being well-informed about the signs and symptoms of the most common psychiatric disorders improves the physician's chances of recognizing these disorders in patients. Familiarity with the course and prognosis of these conditions enhances the ability to refer patients for appropriate treatment and to complete the first step in the referral process, which is frequently education and reassurance.

The book is divided into three sections. The first section provides a framework for approaching assessment and treatment planning, with chapters on case formulation and the psychiatric interview. These chapters demonstrate how to obtain and synthesize clinical data and to generate an appropriate differential diagnosis and treatment plan. The second section presents the major psychiatric disorders, the special topic of suicide and violence, and an overview of the stages of life development, from infancy to old age, and associated psychopathology. Each of the disorder chapters consists of six major subsections: diagnostic and clinical features, the interview, differential diagnosis, medical evaluation, etiology, and treatment. The third section focuses on treatment in the chapters on psychotherapy and psychopharmacology.

Diagnostic and Clinical Features

The use of diagnostic categories has a particular history in psychiatry and, over the past 25 years, the field has been concerned with improving diagnostic reliability and consistency. Throughout this book, reference is made to the *Diagnostic and Statistical Manual,* 4th edition (DSM-IV), which is published by the American Psychiatric Association, the professional organization of psychiatrists in the United States. In the DSM-IV, the diagnostic criteria for psychiatric disorders are polythetic (i.e., more than one combination of symptoms will qualify for a particular diagnosis) and are intended only as guidelines for physicians who ultimately must use their own judgment in making the best diagnoses. The disorders are presented without one etiological theory being endorsed over another. Relevant tables of DSM-IV criteria are included throughout the disorder chapters.

The DSM-IV is the best and most widely referenced diagnostic system currently available. It is not, however, a perfect system but rather an evolving one. Discussions of the clinical and diagnostic features of the various psychiatric disorders therefore include, whenever relevant, the ways in which the DSM-IV criteria do not necessarily reflect the clinical presentation that is most often observed.

The Interview

In all of medicine, the clinical interview is the basis on which diagnoses are made and therapeutic alliances between patients and physicians are forged. Even in this age of advanced medical technology, no sophisticated test can take the place of a careful, complete history that is empathically obtained. Clinical interviewing as a sophisticated art is perhaps nowhere more apparent than in psychiatry. The central importance of the clinical psychiatric interview is reflected in the positioning of this section early in each disorder chapter and in the Interviewing Guidelines boxes included in each of these chapters.

Etiology

As in the rest of medicine, the description of psychiatric syndromes and their effective treatments has generally preceded an understanding of their pathophysiology and etiology. The past 15 to 20 years has witnessed an explosion in the understanding of some of the neurobiological mechanisms that underlie many psychiatric disorders. Advances in neuroimaging, molecular genetics, and other basic science techniques hold the promise for even more knowledge in the not too distant future. But enthusiasm must be tempered by the sobering realization that the mind and the ways in which it can become disturbed are exceedingly complex—so much so that, for example, researchers struggling to understand the etiology of schizophrenia have compiled many probably significant but currently isolated observations and thus do not seem to be much closer to solving the mystery of how and why 1% of the world's population is afflicted with this devastating illness.

Some in the field have worried that the emphasis on neurobiology has replaced the previous tradition of the biopsychosocial model, which attempts to consider the whole patient, encompassing a biologically endowed human being with a particular psychology and social context. Psychiatrists continue to struggle with the issue of how much of an effect external factors such as family, environment, and psychic trauma have on the onset and course of psychiatric disorders. A fundamental assumption of this book is that, in the "nature versus nature" debate, both sides have validity: Genetic loading and, perhaps, intrauterine exposure play an important role in the etiology of many psychiatric disorders, but interpersonal, developmental, and other "nurture" issues seem to be crucial as well. This is not to say that particular family constellations or developmental events can be directly causally associated with specific disorders. Indeed, psychiatry made a tragic error in making such an association when it assigned blame to "schizophrenogenic mothers" in previous generations. However, certain associations can be noted between life experience and psychiatric understanding of an individual suffering from psychiatric symptoms.

Another, related set of assumptions influencing the presentation of clinical material in this book is the belief that wishes and fantasies outside of people's awareness can

10 03172866

have a profound influence on their emotional state and behavior, and that individuals' current thoughts, feelings, and relationships with others are a product of their past emotional experiences and relationships. While these mental patterns and processes are characteristics of everyone, shaping personality and relationships, they also at times contribute to the development of psychiatric symptoms. This psychodynamic approach is described in detail in the chapter on the psychiatric interview and is applied to emotional development in the chapter on life development. The psychodynamic approach to treatment planning is presented in the chapter on case formulation.

The variability among the etiology sections in the disorder chapters reflects the different levels of knowledge and understanding available for each of the psychiatric disorders, as well as the more or less significant role one variable or another may play for a particular disorder. Thus, recent advances in the neurobiology of panic disorder are described in detail in the anxiety chapter because these findings have come together in a way that seems to explain why and how certain medications are effective in the treatment of panic disorder. The current results regarding the neurobiology of schizophrenia are presented in less detail because they have fewer practical implications at this time. For other disorders such as the mood and personality disorders, much active research has been productive, but their etiologies still remain in the realm of the highly speculative.

Turning from the biological to the psychosocial, the clinical approach to some disorders is more conducive to a detailed consideration of psychodynamic, family, and cultural issues. For example, the clustering of eating disorders in particular socioeconomic groups, as well as recent changes in the incidence of these disorders, suggests that social and cultural factors play a significant role in their etiology. The clinician must be aware of these factors in order to recognize and treat as well as prevent these disorders.

Treatment

Patients come to physicians and other health professionals in order to receive help. In some cases that help is only in the form of information. In other instances specific treatments can be offered as well. Treatment planning requires a collaborative effort between patient and clinician. While detailed descriptions of specific treatments for each psychiatric condition are beyond the scope of this book, the principles of treatment planning and the ways in which those principles need to be modified for particular settings and for particular patients are emphasized.

As medicine approaches the 21st century, physicians are challenged to continue to provide excellent care, scientifically based and compassionately delivered, for patients in the face of many economic and social pressures. Psychiatry's strong clinical tradition should serve its patients and the entire field of medicine well. It is the intent of this book to provide the practicing clinician with a foundation that is biopsychosocially based and psychiatrically informed.

JANIS L. CUTLER
ERIC R. MARCUS

ACKNOWLEDGMENTS

Psychiatry could not have been completed without the support to us, and to medical student education, of our psychiatry department leaders at the College of Physicians & Surgeons of Columbia University and New York State Psychiatric Institute. Dr. Herbert Pardes, Chair of the Department of Psychiatry, Vice President for the Health Sciences, and Dean of the Faculty of Medicine, is himself a national leader in medical education. He understands that educational scholarship and pedagogical programs require commitment from the top and he has provided it. His leadership and encouragement have been inspirational. Dr. John Oldham, Director of New York State Psychiatric Institute, for years supervised us in our development and administration of teaching programs. His calm wisdom, sincere devotion to teaching, and patient perseverance are deeply appreciated. Dr. Ronald Rieder, Associate Chair for Education, has had oversight responsibility for education in our department. His high standards, creativity, and energetic dedication to teaching have made him a valued role model. Dr. Jack Gorman, Deputy Director of New York State Psychiatric Institute, and a graduate of our medical school, has always made it clear that medical students have a "friend in court" when he is needed by us.

The Columbia University Psychoanalytic Center for Training and Research is a rare gem in medical education. It has provided us over many years with teachers, with an intellectual milieu for our research ideas, and with the courage to fight for a broadly based medical education program. Our Department of Psychiatry is one of the leading research departments in the world. The many internationally known researchers here have taught and encouraged us and provided teaching manpower and the exciting intellectual atmosphere from which great teaching springs. Our large voluntary clinical faculty is devoted to clinical work with patients. Our teaching programs could not have survived, let alone prospered, without their generous commitment over many years. We give them all our deep thanks. As a product of our medical student teaching program, *Psychiatry* reflects our daily work over the years with bright medical students who have enriched our professional lives with with their enthusiasm and intellectual curiosity.

This book could not have been completed without the tireless efforts of our dedicated assistant, Edith White. We would like to express our appreciation to Marji Toensing and Martha Cushman for their editorial assistance and William Schmitt and Judith Fletcher of W.B. Saunders for their useful guidance. Anne-Marie Shaw of W.B. Saunders served as developmental editor. Her thoughtful approach to the field of psychiatry and to the task of creating a textbook has shaped *Psychiatry* fundamentally from the outset. It has been a great pleasure to work with her.

CONTENTS

SECTION   III

TREATMENT,   269

NOTICE

Psychiatry is an ever-changing field. Standard safety precautions must be followed, but as new research and clinical experience broaden our knowledge, changes in treatment and drug therapy become necessary or appropriate. Readers are advised to check the product information currently provided by the manufacturer of each drug to be administered to verify the recommended dose, the method and duration of administration, and contraindications. It is the responsibility of the treating physician, relying on experience and knowledge of the patient, to determine dosages and the best treatment for the patient. Neither the publisher nor the editors assume any responsibility for any injury and/or damage to persons or property.

THE PUBLISHER

SECTION I

ASSESSMENT

CHAPTER ONE

CASE FORMULATION:

ASSESSMENT AND TREATMENT

PLANNING

JANIS L. CUTLER, MD

In psychiatry, as in other areas of medicine, the case formulation is the physician's systematic recording and integration of historical information given by the patient and of the physician's observations for the purpose of generating a coherent treatment plan. The case formulation is an essential means of communication among health care professionals who may be involved in the patient's present or future treatment. It serves as documentation of the physician's evaluation. (The physician should remember that patients and other parties, such as insurance companies and the courts, may be able to gain access to the written case formulation, as well as to all other parts of patients' medical records.)

When patients come to physicians with complaints and concerns, they hope to receive help, comfort, and information. They do not necessarily think in terms of diseases or syndromes and frequently do not know what information about themselves and their problems physicians need to have. Patients initially describe and organize their complaints and concerns in a way that makes sense to themselves. The presentation varies a great deal from patient to patient and is affected by many factors, including their medical knowledge, level of anxiety, coping and defense mechanisms, and attitude toward physicians. Physicians should listen to the complaints from the patients' perspective and add their own questions and observations to develop a complete picture of the patients' problems, resources, and strengths, in a way that will facilitate treatment planning. In the case formulation, both the diagnosis (which categorizes patients according to signs and symptoms) and the description of patients' strengths and vulnerabilities (i.e., what makes them unique) play important roles in determining the best treatment approach.

The **written case summary** should reflect the process of case formulation (Fig. 1–1) and involves a number of steps, which also serve to organize the written formulation. The focus varies, depending on the setting in which the patient is being evaluated (see Chapter 14, Therapeutic Settings) and the goals of the interaction (which relate to the chief complaint). The quantity and depth of information in the case formulation also vary. The formulation may be based on a brief emergency room interview, a one-hour outpatient visit, an extensive outpatient evaluation consisting of four weekly sessions, or several weeks of inpatient sessions. In general, the less time physicians spend with patients, the less information they will have for the assessment and the more questions that will be left unanswered in the formulation. The written record may be an admission note to an inpatient unit or day program, an off-service note (summarizing treatment by the previous staff when psychiatrists change), an outpatient evaluation summary, or a discharge summary (a review of completed treatment course, usually of an inpatient). Every institution has its own requirements and vocabularies for case formulations, but the objectives are always the same: The formulation communicates the physician's understanding of patients and their needs to other clinical staff persons and helps the physician and staff crystallize and integrate this information into a treatment plan.

A psychiatric case formulation is recorded in the same format as a medical case formulation, with some modifications. In general, it consists of the chief complaint and identifying information (age, marital status, occupation, ethnicity, and religion), history, findings, impressions, treatment plan, and prognosis. If a patient is seen more than once, an additional section labeled "Hospital Course" or "Summary of the Evaluation" may be added to indicate the course of the patient throughout the evaluation process, including all changes in symptoms and functioning. The components of the case formulation are

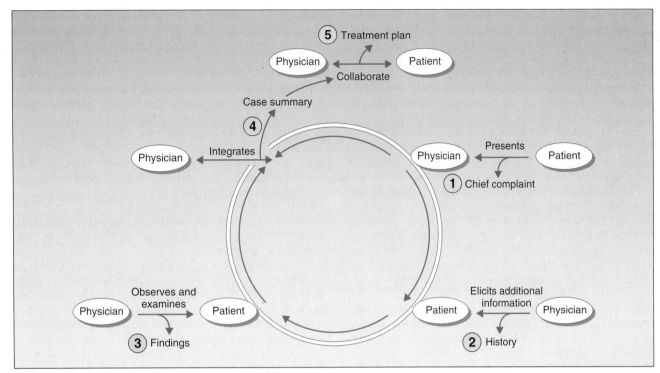

FIGURE 1–1. Steps in creating the case formulation. (1) The patient presents the chief complaint to the physician. (2) As the interview proceeds, the physician elicits additional information from the patient in order to obtain the history of the present illness, the past psychiatric history, medical history, psychosocial history, and family history. The physician also conducts a review of systems. (3) Findings from the physical examination, mental status examination (including how the patient relates to the physician), and laboratory and other test results are collected. (4) The physician then integrates all of the information and generates a descriptive and diagnostic impression. (5) Together, the patient and physician create a theoretically sound and feasible treatment plan.

listed in Table 1–1. The case material is rarely organized in the way the patient presents it in the interview. In fact, beyond the basic headings, it almost invariably is not. The written record more closely reflects the organization and thought processes of the physician as he or she comes to understand and integrate the patient's problems. The interview and the written formulation do, however, begin at the same place: the chief complaint.

TABLE 1–1.   Components of the Case Formulation

Chief Complaint (CC)
History
   History of the present illness (HPI)
   Past psychiatric history
   Past medical history
   Review of systems (ROS)
   Psychosocial history
   Family history
Findings
   Physical examination (PE)
   Mental status examination (MSE)
   Laboratory and other tests
Impression
   Case summary
   Differential diagnosis
   Multiaxial evaluation
   Predisposing and precipitating factors
Treatment plan
Prognosis

CHIEF COMPLAINT

The chief complaint is the reason the patient gives for seeking help. It does not necessarily reflect the problem that the patient needs help with the most—in fact, the chief complaint may be misleading. ⟹ For example, a patient who complains of feeling "nervous," a seemingly innocuous symptom, may be suffering from a number of psychiatric disorders, ranging from depression to psychosis. A male patient whose chief complaint is that he is "losing his mind" is just as likely, if not more so, to be suffering from panic attacks as from psychosis. One elderly man who had little formal education, no history of mental illness, and a tendency to be unaware of his emotional state gave this initial description of what turned out to be a clear-cut case of major depression: "I'm not long for this world—I'm very weak, I have a funny feeling in my stomach, my head is full, I can't eat or sleep. ⟸

Patients with the same disorder may initially give entirely different chief complaints. ⟹ For example, two middle-aged women noticed breast lumps and made appointments with their internists. One woman's chief complaint was fatigue. When she was under stress, she tended to use denial, and she "forgot" the lump until her physician began to examine her. At that time, she mentioned the lump, which was of much more concern to her, and to her physician, than the fatigue, which may have been related to her worry about the lump and may not have had a more specific basis. The second woman's "chief complaint" was the lump, which she talked about in a straightforward manner, complete with her own assessment of the diagnostic possibilities.

Arriving at an overall formulation for these two patients involves quite different processes, although the "differential diagnosis" is the same: cyst, benign tumor, or malignant tumor. For one patient, the true chief complaint is easily identified; for the other, it nearly slips by without mention. Each woman's unique response to her anxiety-provoking symptom is reflected in her presenting complaint and should be included in the case summary and overall formulation: One woman tends to use denial as a coping mechanism; the other, intellectualization. Their different responses will also be reflected in their treatment plans. The denial of the first patient could impede a prompt workup and should be regarded as part of the problem, not necessarily to be changed but certainly to be kept in mind. The intellectualization of the second patient can be regarded as a strength to be used by her and her physician as the evaluation proceeds. If both of these women are eventually diagnosed with invasive cancer with widespread metastases, a defensive character style that had been detrimental could become a strength, and vice versa. In other words, when a patient is facing a terminal illness, denial may be helpful, whereas intellectualization, although it contributes to the patient's understanding of the illness, may block an associated emotional reaction and make the patient more vulnerable to a major depression. ◀▬

HISTORY
History of the Present Illness

Keeping in mind that the chief complaint may be misleading, the physician begins the interview by eliciting the history of the present illness, starting with the chief complaint and working backward. The physician allows the interview to follow any number of different paths, depending on the patient's leads and the physician's intuition, in order to develop a **chronological, systematic outline** of the signs and symptoms of the current episode, which culminated in the patient's decision to come for help. Explanations of why the patient has come for help at this time and why the need for help was presented in the way it was are crucial to the history. Only when this history-taking process is complete does the "present illness" and its chronology become apparent. The best history of the present illness is composed after the differential diagnosis has been generated, because the history should support the differential diagnosis. Physicians sometimes attempt to "write up" an initial assessment while interviewing the patient. This approach usually results in a confused record that lacks the integration and synthesis required, by definition, for a formulation, because the physician has not thought about the information before writing it down.

If the patient's current episode of illness exists within the context of a chronic psychiatric syndrome, the history of the present illness can begin with the symptoms of the first episode of illness ever experienced or with the current exacerbation, leaving the early symptoms and previous episodes to be summarized in the past history. Each approach has advantages and disadvantages. If the diagnosis is unclear or should be modified, a history of the present illness covering the entire course of the illness that summarizes the signs and symptoms may lead to a particular diagnosis. If the diagnosis has been clearly established, previous episodes can be summarized in the past history section. Eliciting a history from patients with personality disorders is often challenging because they frequently do not have egodystonic symptoms and may have great difficulty in articulating their problems (see Chapter 8, Personality Disorders).

The physician must conduct the interview in a way that allows the patient's **interpersonal relationships,** as well as certain aspects of inner life, to be assessed. This information should then be integrated in a way that leads the clinical audience to the diagnostic possibilities. ▬▶ For example, a 25-year-old graduate student complaining of "depression" described, in the initial interview, a confusing mixture of vague symptoms, which she subsequently dismissed. She presented long, overly detailed complaints about people in her life who she was not able to clearly differentiate from one another. During the interview, the physician used his knowledge of psychiatric diagnosis to focus on the patient's distorted perceptions of others, her inability to describe herself in a coherent fashion, her self-destructive behavior, and her chronic feelings of emptiness. A clinical picture of borderline personality disorder gradually emerged. Without adequate knowledge of the psychiatric syndromes and their diagnostic criteria, the physician would not have been able to perform an adequate interview or make an accurate diagnosis. ◀▬

Although the written history of the present illness and the past history will not reflect the confusion of the first half of the interview, the physician may comment upon the patient's circumstantiality and tangentiality in the mental status examination part of the written summary. The following history of the present illness summarizes the findings for the above patient in a succinct manner that facilitates arriving at the appropriate diagnosis:

▬▶ The patient reports a chronic feeling of emptiness. She avoids being alone at all costs and experiences intense anxiety when she is alone. She has repeatedly engaged in self-destructive behavior, including superficially cutting her arm with a razor blade. The patient denies substance abuse and suicide attempts. Her patterns of relationships have been stormy. She rapidly becomes involved in intense relationships and then, just as quickly, becomes disillusioned with and enraged by the same person she had been idealizing. In one instance, she began meeting several times a week with one of her male professors, initially talking about course work and issues relevant to her field of interest but soon confiding in him about her personal concerns. She saw him as warm and supportive, "a treasure." After one occasion when he had to cut a visit short, she became furious and reported, "I thought he was special, but he's just like everyone else—selfish and self-centered." ◀▥

Without directly referring to the DSM-IV criteria, the narrative description of the patient in the history of the present illness points the reader in the general direction of a personality disorder, and specifically to the diagnosis of borderline personality disorder. This **focus** is a conscious editorial decision on the part of the interviewer. In other situations, it would not be necessary or appropriate to include such detailed information about the patient's relationships. This case also demonstrates the benefit of providing **brief specific examples** from the patient's life to illustrate particular problems. For inexperienced clinicians, informed focusing can be difficult. Medical students and residents frequently complete long detailed case formulations that force the reader to find the essential information among the less important information. Although not ideal, overwriting is preferable to cutting indiscriminately. Novice physicians also frequently lack the self-confidence to be less inclusive; with experience, they find that "less is more" (i.e., the more focused and concise the written presentation, the clearer the information). A clearly formulated, well-presented history should lead all readers to generate the same differential diagnosis.

Past Psychiatric History

The past psychiatric history should include descriptions of **previous episodes of psychiatric illnesses** that are unrelated to the present one. In addition to describing past symptoms and syndromes, the past psychiatric history should specify the **treatment** received and the **outcome** of that treatment.

Historical information particularly relevant to the current clinical questions should be included. ▦▶ For example, a patient who had had schizophrenia for 10 years suffered a psychotic exacerbation after the sudden death of her mother. She presented to the emergency room with this chief complaint: "I'm hearing voices telling me to kill myself." The woman had been followed since the onset of her illness by a psychiatrist who was on the staff at the same hospital. Her past history was clearly documented in previous chart entries and could be briefly summarized in the current case formulation, highlighting the information that was most relevant for the decisions to be made: Has the patient been suicidal before? Has she ever had command auditory hallucinations? Has she acted upon them or done anything to hurt herself? Has she had to deal with other losses, and, if so, how did she do so? Is she usually compliant with treatment? This information should be the focus of the past psychiatric history. In other words, this patient's history of difficulty dealing with loss and impulse control is more essential than is a complete review of her previous psychotic symptoms. It is important to remember that the purpose of the written record is to communicate needed information. ◀▥

In many other cases, past symptoms are crucial for confirming or modifying a previous diagnosis. Even subtle changes in the diagnosis can have a significant impact on treatment planning.

Like the history of the present illness, the past psychiatric history should include **pertinent negative findings.** The list of conditions that have not been present should not be all-inclusive. In fact, not all of the information obtained in the interview should be recorded. Instead, positive and negative findings should be of sufficient detail to provide someone reading it with the information necessary to generate a case formulation but should not contain extraneous information. Beginners will obviously find it difficult to know what is important and what is not, what fits a particular clinical pattern and should be highlighted, what fits but is of secondary importance, what does not fit but should be included because it is so significant that it calls the working diagnosis into question, and what does not fit but can be minimized because it is probably a spurious finding.

Past Medical History

The past medical history is an essential part of all psychiatric case formulations. Many medical conditions have direct psychiatric manifestations (see Chapter 5, Cognitive and Mental Disorders Due to General Medical Conditions). Chronic illnesses such as diabetes, asthma, and arthritis, as well as acute and short-lived but stressful medical events such as an emergency appendectomy or severe pneumonia requiring hospitalization, may be significant stresses with which patients must cope. The patient's approach to health and illness and to physicians, including issues such as compliance with prescribed treatments and avoidance of prohibited risk-taking behaviors such as smoking, can be elicited in the context of the past medical history.

Review of Systems

The review of systems, as the name implies, records the **presence or absence of current symptoms** in each **major system of the body,** including the central nervous system. Psychiatric and medical symptoms that appear to be unrelated to the patient's present illness should be recorded in this section of the case formulation. For suggestions on how to elicit a comprehensive psychiatric review of systems, see Chapter 2, The Psychiatric Interview. (For suggestions on how to conduct a medical review of systems, see DeGowin (1994), listed below in Selected Readings, and other textbooks.)

Psychosocial History

The psychosocial history consists of the patient's **personal and family histories.** In medical case formulations, the family history is a discrete category that focuses particularly on the medical conditions of first-degree relatives. In psychiatric case formulations, the same approach can be used, or the family history can be incorporated into the personal history, since other family information, such as birth order and profiles of significant people present in the family during the patient's childhood, is important to the overall formulation and is related to the history of relationships.

The personal history should cover the patient's childhood, adolescence, and adulthood; sexual history; and alcohol and drug use. Whereas the other sections of the case formulation tend to focus on disease and disability, this section should focus on health and areas of strength. The childhood history should include any unusual findings about childbirth, infancy, and the attainment of developmental milestones. The family atmosphere and separations or changes in the status of significant adults should be described, and inquiries must always be made about the possibility of physical and sexual abuse. Performance at school and peer relationships are important. Childhood illnesses and symptoms should be noted. The earliest memories can be useful, particularly in contributing to the psychodynamic formulation. A picture of school and occupational functioning, friendships, and intimate relationships, including marriages, should be provided for adolescence and adulthood.

It can be extremely helpful to note the timing of events in the personal history in parallel with the timing of events in the patient's psychiatric history. While obtaining the personal history, the physician should keep in mind the key psychiatric events in the patient's life and make note of when they occur in relation to life circumstances. Important errors can be made if the physician does not specifically inquire about this sequence. ➠ One patient reported that her depression occurred in March of 1978 and then later stated that her mother died in December of 1978. When the physician double-checked this sequence, the patient corrected the physician, and her own dates, with surprise, saying, "The depression must have been in March of 1979, because it was definitely after my mother's death." ◀ Patients are not necessarily aware of these connections and sequences, but they may be of great importance. ➠ A man in his fifties, who had, at best, an ambivalent relationship with his father, presented with a major depression. While obtaining a parallel psychosocial history, the physician learned that the patient's father was dying of cancer. When the physician raised the possibility that the patient might be "upset" about his father's impending death (but did not suggest that the depression might be causally related), the patient completely denied any reaction. He insisted that he was prepared for his father's death because his father had been ill for several years and was in his eighties. Later in his treatment, it became apparent that the impending loss of his father was, indeed, having a profound impact on him. ◀

The following psychosocial history of a 19-year-old woman who was admitted to an inpatient unit with the diagnosis of bulimia nervosa is an example of the level of detail appropriate for a typical psychosocial history. ➠ The patient is the youngest of three children born to middle-class parents living in an affluent suburb. Her father, who teaches college biology, is a nervous, suspicious man, who gets drunk every night in front of the television set. Her attractive mother dominates the family and participates in an active social life. The patient's two sisters have been successful academically, athletically, and socially and are currently at various stages of completing graduate work at Ivy League schools. Her family is superficially warm and supportive, but the emphasis is apparently on remaining pleasant to the exclusion, as much as possible, of any problems or bad feelings.

The patient describes herself as having been a withdrawn and shy child. She felt excluded from, and inferior to, her peers and frequently stayed home, complaining of "stomachaches." She was a good student, nonetheless, earning grades of B+ and A. During adolescence, with her mother's coaching, she became popular, participating in extracurricular activities with a circle of superficial friends whom she would go out of her way to please. She spent weekends "partying," abusing alcohol, amphetamines, cocaine, and marijuana. She was "never without a boyfriend," molding herself to her latest boyfriend's specifications in order to be the "perfect girlfriend," and she became sexually active. After graduation from high school, she attended a prestigious college several hundred miles away, where she immediately felt lonely and out of place. She left after her first semester and spent the rest of the year isolated at home. ◀

This is not an all-inclusive psychosocial history, because some categories of information are not included or are mentioned only briefly. This lack of completeness further demonstrates the editing process that is necessarily involved in approaching a patient and formulating a case. The history does contain a lot of information that is important for understanding the patient as an individual and that will contribute to a psychodynamic formulation and reasonable treatment plan. Much of the missing information will need to be addressed at some point, and part of the initial treatment plan should be to obtain further information to fill in some of the gaps.

FINDINGS

In addition to the mental status examination, other observational material to be recorded in this portion of the written record are the physical examination, laboratory findings, and the results of other testing modalities. Vital signs and a detailed neurological examination are of particular importance.

Mental Status Examination

The mental status examination is the physician's **objective description** of the patient's **current mental state,** which should be recorded without judgment or conclusion. Table 1–2 lists the main cate-

TABLE 1–2.   Mental Status Examination

Category	Definition	Common "Normal" Descriptors	"Abnormal" Descriptors
Appearance, behavior, and speech	A detailed description of the patient as he or she appears during the clinical encounter, including interactions with the interviewer. Motor behavior and the rate, volume, and modulation of speech should be described as well.	See sample MSEs in Box 1–1 and Box 1–3.	
Mood	Subjective feeling state of the patient sustained over much of the interview	Euthymic	Dysthymic, sad, irritable, expansive, euphoric, nervous, angry
Affect	Objective description of the patient's emotional state as observed by the clinician	Full range	Constricted, blunted, flat, inappropriate, labile
Thought process	The organization of the patient's thoughts as reflected in his or her verbal productions	Coherent and goal directed	Tangential, circumstantial, loosening of associations, flight of ideas, word salad, blocking, neologisms
Thought content	The themes of the patient's thoughts during the interview, including preoccupations and ruminations as well as overt signs and symptoms of psychopathology	No evidence of delusions; denies obsessions, suicidal and homicidal ideation	Presence of delusions (specify type—grandiose, paranoid, somatic, religious), ideas of reference, overvalued ideas, obsessions, ruminations, suicidal and homicidal ideation; paucity of thought—describe and give examples
Perception	Assessment of perceptual symptoms: illusions, depersonalization, derealization, hallucinations	Absent	Describe; specify type of hallucination
Cognitive	Assessment of the patient's abilities with regard to attention and orientation as well as intellectual functions including memory, calculations, fund of knowledge, and capacity for abstract thought	Alert, attentive, and oriented × 3 Describe findings of each test done	
Insight	The patient's understanding of himself or herself in the context of wanting or needing help; also referred to in dynamic terms as "observing ego"	Intact, excellent	Fair, impaired (include explanation)
Judgment	Closely related to insight but refers specifically to actions patient will take based on insight; usually reflects impulse control	Intact, excellent	Fair, impaired (include explanation)

gories of the examination. Like the rest of the physical examination, it does not include historical information, nor does it include subjective complaints (with the exception of mood, see below). This distinction is a source of confusion for many beginning clinicians, who incorrectly report historical data in the mental status examination. For example, an appetite or sleep disturbance might be recorded as part of the emotional state, using the faulty reasoning that those symptoms can be present as part of a mood disorder.

The mental status examination should be recorded in a systematic fashion. Systematic, however, does not necessarily mean cursory. Table 1–3 provides guidelines for recording the mental status examination. Novice physicians make four common mistakes in recording the mental status examination. One mistake is to use an outline format to make a perfunctory checklist that does not convey a clear description of the patient's unique mental status. Although the examination should follow a standard structure with specific headings, it should have de-

TABLE 1–3.   Guidelines for Recording the Mental Status Examination

"Do's"	"Don't's"
Objectively describe the patient's current mental state.	Include subjective complaints (except mood).
Convey a clear description of the patient's unique mental status examination.	Include historical information.
Provide detailed descriptions, including examples and brief patient quotes.	Use uninformative generalities such as "within normal limits" or "well developed and well nourished."
Record information systematically, following a standard structure with specific headings.	Provide either a sparse outline or a disorganized narrative.
Label positive findings and psychopathology.	Include diagnostic conclusions.
Mention pertinent negatives.	Include excessive detail.

tailed descriptions, including examples and brief patient quotes.

A second mistake is to record too little information when the mental status examination is "normal." Positive findings and gross psychopathology tend to be more readily noted than behavior and thoughts that are not obviously "abnormal" (i.e., they do not represent clear-cut signs and symptoms). The quotation marks indicate that the terms "normal" and "abnormal" are relatively useless. Some findings, particularly of psychotic or affective symptoms, can be regarded as abnormal. However, patients can look,

---

BOX 1–1. Mental Status Examinations for Patient A and Patient B

Patient A

Patient A is a 36-year-old woman with obsessive-compulsive disorder.

Appearance

The patient is 5'8" and slender. She is usually neatly attired in a feminine but slightly out-of-date dress, high-heeled shoes, brightly painted fingernails, and jewelry, but never wears a watch. Her thick, wavy, red hair falls below her shoulders and frames her pretty face. She has bright, wide-set, almond-shaped blue eyes, a fair complexion, and a warm smile.

Speech and Behavior

The patient arrives late and walks quickly down the hall to the office, where she knocks and immediately opens the door. She carelessly throws her coat over an adjacent chair, sits down, and smiles nervously, asking how I am. Speaking rapidly, she gazes into space, glancing at me intermittently and then meeting my eyes when she's completed a thought or when I'm speaking. She seductively sweeps her bangs away from her face, peering upward, or nervously twists the ends of her hair, suggesting the vulnerability of a little girl.

Mood

"Nervous."

Affect

Full range, from tearful sadness to good-natured laughter.

Thought Process

Circumstantial and tangential, without loosening of associations. She frequently interrupts herself with qualifications, searching for precisely the appropriate word, or requests to backtrack because an important detail was overlooked. The boring intricacy of her explanations seems to be associated with particularly affect-laden material.

Thought Content

The patient describes several obsessions, many relating to her worry that if she does not read numbers and names over repeatedly, she will make a mistake. For example, she fears that if she reads a label incorrectly at work, she will mix the wrong reagents, resulting in a substance that might harm her or show her to be "incompetent." Her concern with numbers extends to the telephone: When calling her lover, she obsessively worries that she will call another man and have an "intimate conversation" with him, without realizing he is not her lover. No evidence of delusions. Denies suicidal and homicidal ideation.

Perception

Patient denies auditory and visual hallucinations.

Cognitive

Alert and oriented ×3. Recalls 3/3 objects after five minutes (see Chapter 2, The Psychiatric Interview). Digit span 7 forward, 6 reverse. Serial 7s completed painstakingly but with no errors. Fund of knowledge excellent with regard to current events and past presidents to Nixon (no errors). Above average intelligence, as reflected in sophisticated vocabulary. Ability to think abstractly excellent, as demonstrated by patient's use of metaphor and comparisons during the interview.

Insight

Good. The patient finds her symptoms "very strange, irrational," and regards them as a "psychiatric problem."

Judgment

Good. Patient has sought treatment and appears motivated to pursue whatever recommendations are made.

Patient B

Patient B has more striking findings than Patient A. Patient B is a 17-year-old man with a diagnosis of schizophrenia, who was admitted to the hospital three weeks ago after making a suicide attempt.

Appearance, Speech, and Behavior

Patient is a young man with neatly styled, curly blond hair, who makes good eye contact with the interviewer. He has a somewhat wide-eyed, blank, unchanging expression on his face and blinks infrequently. His casual shirt is clean and neat. The patient sits quietly in his seat, rarely shifting position. He occasionally uses his hands to emphasize a point. His speech is clear, at times slightly fast, and remains in a monotone throughout the interview.

Mood

"Good, happy to be alive."

Affect

Blunted.

Thought Process

Coherent and goal-directed, without loosening of associations.

Thought Content

Denies paranoid delusions; "happy to be alive" after suicide attempt; denies current suicidal ideation; no evidence of homicidal ideation but not specifically asked.

Perception

Denies hallucinations.

Cognitive

Oriented ×3; short-term memory good (3/3 objects in two minutes); long-term memory appears good, though dates need to be corroborated; fund of knowledge good (President Bush, candidates); simple calculation with money correct; difficulty with serial 7s; serial 3s slow, with mistakes that the patient immediately caught and corrected.

Insight

Patient appears to have an excellent understanding of having a "mental illness" that has profoundly affected his life: "I've lost so much."

Judgment

Patient appears to be cooperative with his treatment; understands need for follow-up after discharge.

sound, and feel very different and yet fit the description of "within normal limits" or "well developed, well nourished" that is ubiquitously found in medical records. Enough detail should be provided to allow an astute observer to pick out the patient by appearance, behavior, and other mental status findings from a group of people.

Overly inclusive mental status examinations are not particularly useful, either. The third mistake is to include too much information or every possible detail, making it difficult for the reader to sort out the important from the trivial facts.

The final mistake, which sometimes occurs in conjunction with overinclusiveness, is to record the findings in an unorganized narrative form. A narrative format is acceptable, although less preferable, if the physician adheres strictly to a standard order. Frequently, however, the narrative form is used to avoid organizing and categorizing the information. The organization of the material should reflect the thinking of the interviewer and move the reader toward the concluding formulation.

Box 1–1 illustrates the wealth of information that can be conveyed by a well-organized, descriptive, concise mental status examination for two patients. Note that even in categories that do not have many clear-cut positive findings, much of the descriptive detail is still relevant and useful. Pertinent negative findings should be included, as well, just as they were in the history section of the formulation. The formulation for Patient A shows how helpful it can be to include carefully chosen examples or quotations from the patient. The quotations do not need to be lengthy; in fact, each one should be no more than a sentence or two. The most efficient way to use quoted phrases is to intersperse them frequently with unquoted material. A sign of a lazy physician is reams of unedited quotations.

The significance of the phrasing commonly used in the mental status examination (and in Box 1–1) should be understood. A notation that the patient "denies" a particular symptom implies that the patient has been specifically and directly asked about that symptom. A notation that there is "no evidence of" a symptom implies that the interviewer did not observe the symptom and did not specifically inquire about it. This difference is illustrated in the thought content section in Box 1–1. If the presence or absence of symptoms is of particular importance, as it is for Patient B, it is a good idea to state clearly that the physician does not know whether the symptom is present by using the notation "not specifically asked."

Physical Examination

A thorough physical examination should be performed and documented in the case formulation for all psychiatric patients. The physical examination should be thorough because, even though there are no neurological findings, a systemic illness may be present that is producing psychiatric symptoms. Patients with clear-cut psychiatric disorders can also have general medical conditions that can be missed if a thorough physical examination is not performed.

Laboratory Tests

Blood and urine tests are frequently crucial adjunctive data to a thorough history in ruling out general medical conditions as possible causes of psychiatric symptoms or unrelated medical illnesses requiring treatment. In addition to the standard chemistry and hematological panels, toxicology screening should always be considered to rule out substance abuse (see Chapter 7, Alcohol and Substance Abuse). Specialized blood tests and other modalities such as CT scanning, magnetic resonance imaging (MRI), electroencephalography (EEG), and a neuropsychological battery of tests should be used to screen for possible causes of delirium (e.g., fever, cardiovascular instability) or neurological conditions with behavioral manifestations that could be mistaken for a psychiatric disorder (e.g., a patient with a brain tumor located in the frontal lobes might present with symptoms of a mood disorder). All testing should be done with an eye toward balancing costs (both economic costs and health risks to the patient) with possible benefits. This judgment is based on a realistic estimate of the probability of a particular condition given its prevalence and the patient's presentation (see chapters on individual disorders, particularly Chapter 5, Cognitive and Mental Disorders Due to General Medical Conditions, for specific indications).

IMPRESSIONS

Once all of the information has been collected and the physician has made his or her observations, a great deal of integration and planning still needs to be done. The physician's impressions of the patient and the symptoms can be organized into four discrete sections that build on one another: (1) the case summary, (2) the differential diagnosis, (3) the multiaxial evaluation, and (4) the predisposing and precipitating factors.

Case Summary

The first step in this process is descriptive. The findings are summarized and taken a step further from the more patient-focused perspective of the history and the purely observational tone of the mental status examination. A case summary of Patient B in Box 1–1 might read as follows: "Patient is status-post (i.e., has made) a recent suicide attempt in the context of paranoid delusions, command auditory hallucinations, and depressed mood. Mental status examination is significant for blunted affect. Patient is currently not psychotic nor a significant suicide risk."

Although this description alone is not sufficient because it could apply to many patients, it is a step toward identifying which findings in this patient are similar to those found in other patients (i.e., toward making a diagnosis). It is also a step toward completing other aspects of the overall assessment that can be at least as important as the diagnosis: Is the patient a danger to himself or herself or to others? Will the patient be compliant with medication and other treatment recommendations?

Two of the physician's conclusions in the case summary about Patient B deserve highlighting. First, the physician concludes that the patient is not psychotic. This term is at a level of overall assessment that does not belong in the mental status examination itself but should be included in the case summary as the physician begins to reach conclusions. Similarly, while the patient's thoughts, fantasies, and plans regarding suicide are recorded in the mental status examination, the physician's impression of the patient's suicidality should be made in the case summary.

Box 1–2 further illustrates the difference in labeling and integrating information in the history and case summary, or clinical impression. The history is descriptive and detailed, uses fewer psychiatric labels, and presents the facts in such a way that readers can make their own judgments as to the validity of the interviewer's conclusions. It is crucial for less experienced interviewers, particularly medical students and residents, to adhere to this sequence of first presenting the data and then recording their conclusions about the data because they may be too inexperienced to judge whether the patient truly has

the signs and symptoms noted, such as anhedonia or diurnal variation.

The case summary may include statements about the patient's current level of functioning and behavior patterns. The history of the present illness described in detail for the patient above, who was binging and cutting herself, might be paired with the following impressions: "Patient has been withdrawn, with impulsive, angry outbursts, self-destructive behavior, and an identity disturbance."

Differential Diagnosis

Diagnostic labels are useful for summarizing patterns of data, predicting the course of an illness and the recovery from it, and suggesting treatment options. Assigning a diagnostic label identifies common features but tends to blur the more subtle, and not so subtle, distinctions among individual patients with the same diagnosis. The clinical impressions section of the case formulation addresses this shortcoming, although it, too, tends to focus on patterns. Describing a patient from a **biopsychosocial perspective,** including a psychodynamic formulation, should capture the full sense of a complex individual who is not just a "receptacle" for a particular disorder. The biopsychosocial formulation is described in detail below (see Predisposing and Precipitating Factors, below, and Box 1–3); it is mentioned here to point out the limitations of diagnostic labels (i.e., they serve a particular purpose but do not give the whole picture). These limitations can be counterbalanced in a complete case formulation.

In the systematic process of case formulation, the **diagnostic impression** is a separate step that is reached only after the patient's psychopathology has been summarized descriptively. Following this sequence keeps physicians disciplined and helps them consider systematically all appropriate diagnoses. This sequence does not mean that physicians are not thinking about diagnoses until this point. On the contrary, diagnostic possibilities are being entertained, patterns are being sought, and hypotheses considered and discarded all the while the physician is gathering data and making observations. By the time the physician puts pen to paper, the most likely diagnoses should have been identified. The entire formulation is written with those diagnoses in mind. However, following the formal sequence of steps (i.e., first, the history and observations; next, the summary of the psychopathology and other findings; and, finally, the diagnostic impressions) ensures that each section does indeed follow logically from the previous one.

Identifying specific diagnoses should be relatively simple after the psychopathology has been carefully described. The first question to answer is which **general category of psychopathology** does the patient fit into, based on the history of the present illness and the mental status examination. These categories include the psychotic, mood, anxi-

---

BOX 1–2. History of the Present Illness and Case Summary for Patient C

History of the Present Illness

The patient, a 35-year-old woman, has been feeling "down" virtually every day for the past month, with poor concentration at work ("It's like my head is in a fog"), passive suicidal ideation ("I wouldn't mind if I didn't wake up in the morning. I haven't thought about doing anything to hurt myself, though."), and almost constant tiredness. She gets pleasure from none of the activities that she usually enjoys, even when she forces herself to try and participate, such as going to the movies with friends. She has no appetite and has lost 10 pounds. Has difficulty falling asleep (takes at least an hour), wakes up two or three times during the night and has trouble getting back to sleep (usually falls asleep at midnight, is up at 3:00 and 5:00 A.M., although does not need to get out of bed until 7:00 A.M.), and never really feels rested. Has tremendous difficulty getting ready for school in the morning, describing her mood and attitude as being at their lowest points then and gradually lifting over the course of the day.

Case Summary

Patient has one-month history of depressed mood without reactivity, anhedonia, significant weight loss, sleep disturbance with difficulty falling asleep as well as middle night awakening and early morning awakening. Diurnal variation is present, as well as passive suicidal ideation without intent or plan.

TABLE 1–4. Global Assessment of Functioning (GAF) Scale

Consider psychological, social, and occupational functioning on a hypothetical continuum of mental health–illness. Do not include impairment in functioning due to physical (or environmental) limitations.

Code

100 **Superior functioning in a wide range of activities, life's problems never seem to get out of**
 | **hand, is sought out by others because of his or her many positive qualities. No**
91 **symptoms.**

90 **Absent or minimal symptoms** (e.g., mild anxiety before an exam), **good functioning in all areas, interested and involved in a wide range of activities, socially effective, generally satisfied with life, no more than everyday problems or concerns** (e.g., an occasional
81 argument with family members).

80 **If symptoms are present, they are transient and expectable reactions to psychosocial stressors** (e.g., difficulty concentrating after family argument); **no more than slight impairment in social, occupational, or school functioning** (e.g., temporarily falling behind in
71 schoolwork).

70 **Some mild symptoms** (e.g., depressed mood and mild insomnia) **OR some difficulty in social, occupational, or school functioning** (e.g., occasional truancy, or theft within the household),
61 **but generally functioning pretty well, has some meaningful interpersonal relationships.**

60 **Moderate symptoms** (e.g., flat affect and circumstantial speech, occasional panic attacks) **OR moderate difficulty in social, occupational, or school functioning** (e.g., few friends, conflicts
51 with peers or co-workers).

50 **Serious symptoms** (e.g., suicidal ideation, severe obsessional rituals, frequent shoplifting) **OR any serious impairment in social, occupational, or school functioning** (e.g., no friends, un-
41 able to keep a job).

40 **Some impairment in reality testing or communication** (e.g., speech is at times illogical, obscure, or irrelevant) **OR major impairment in several areas, such as work or school, family relations, judgment, thinking, or mood** (e.g., depressed man avoids friends, neglects family, and is unable to work; child frequently beats up younger children, is defiant at home, and is
31 failing at school).

30 **Behavior is considerably influenced by delusions or hallucinations OR serious impairment in communication or judgment** (e.g., sometimes incoherent, acts grossly inappropriately, suicidal preoccupation) **OR inability to function in almost all areas** (e.g., stays in bed all day; no
21 job, home, or friends).

20 **Some danger of hurting self or others** (e.g., suicide attempts without clear expectation of death; frequently violent; manic excitement) **OR occasionally fails to maintain minimal personal hygiene** (e.g., smears feces) **OR gross impairment in communication** (e.g., largely inco-
11 herent or mute).

10 **Persistent danger of severely hurting self or others** (e.g., recurrent violence) **OR persistent inability to maintain minimal personal hygiene OR serious suicidal act with clear expecta-
1 tion of death.**

0   Inadequate information.

The rating of overall psychological functioning on a scale of 0–100 was operationalized by Luborsky in the Health-Sickness Rating Scale (Luborsky L: "Clinicians' Judgments of Mental Health." *Archives of General Psychiatry* 7:407–417, 1962). Spitzer and colleagues developed a revision of the Health-Sickness Rating Scale called the Global Assessment Scale (GAS) (Endicott J, Spitzer RL, Fleiss JL, Cohen J: "The Global Assessment Scale: A Procedure for Measuring Overall Severity of Psychiatric Disturbance." *Archives of General Psychiatry* 33:766–771, 1976). A modified version of the GAS was included in DSM-III-R as the Global Assessment of Functioning (GAF) Scale.

ety, cognitive, and personality disorders. If one of these disorders is present in a patient, the findings will usually be evident in the mental status examination as well as in the history. Once the general category is determined, more specific details must be considered. This is where epidemiological and phenomenological knowledge is most crucial.

For example, a 19-year-old with no prior psychiatric history presents with auditory hallucinations and grandiose delusions, which have been occurring for six months. Because of the frequent onset of schizophrenia during adolescence, this disorder quickly becomes the most likely diagnosis, based on this brief piece of history. Substance abuse and bipolar disorder would be two other possibilities in the differential diagnosis. A 35-year-old woman with the same presentation is much more likely to be suffering from a mood disorder with a manic or mixed episode, while a 65-year-old woman would be given a diagnosis of psychiatric disorder due to a general medical condition until this was proved otherwise. ◀▥ A closer look at more details about the patient's condition will either confirm the initial diagnosis or will suggest other, less obvious diagnoses.

The degree of certainty regarding the diagnosis depends in part on the amount of detailed historical information available. A brief initial evaluation interview will probably generate a long list of possible differential diagnoses, whereas a formulation composed at the end of a lengthy hospital stay should present a fairly definite diagnostic impression.

Multiaxial Evaluation

Mental health professionals involved in the development of the *Diagnostic and Statistical Manual of Mental Disorders* (DSM) have attempted to create a biopsychosocial approach to diagnosis. This approach is reflected in the multiaxial system: **Axis I** covers the psychiatric diagnoses; **Axis II** specifies life-long psychiatric disorders (i.e., personality disorders and mental retardation); **Axis III** identifies nonpsychiatric medical conditions; **Axis IV** notes the presence of contributing psychosocial stressors; and **Axis V** rates the patient's highest level of social and occupational functioning over the previous year (see Table 1–4).

Personality disorders are placed on a separate axis in order to encourage their use to facilitate further research into the clinical utility of those particular diagnoses. Disorders can be present on both Axis I and Axis II, although the clinician should exercise caution in diagnosing a personality disorder in the context of an acute Axis I condition. For example, patients in the midst of a major depressive episode may appear to have symptoms characteristic of a number of personality disorders, such as dependent or avoidant personality disorder, which then resolve when the mood disorder resolves. As the DSM has evolved, more emphasis has been placed on allowing for comorbidity—in other words, more than one Axis I condition can be present at the same time.

Predisposing and Precipitating Factors

The formulation is not complete even after a diagnosis has been reached. The diagnosis reflects only those signs and symptoms that the patient shares with other patients who have the same disorder. This diagnostic labeling is crucial for purposes of communicating with others involved with the patient's care and for beginning to establish a prognosis and develop a treatment plan, but it is not sufficient for describing an individual person who is suffering from an illness. The biopsychosocial approach describes the **patient's strengths and vulner-**

abilities and helps to convey the patient's individuality. Vulnerabilities can also be labeled as possible predisposing or precipitating factors. The psychodynamic formulation is an extremely useful part of the psychiatric case formulation because it summarizes the key psychological issues of the patient.

The following case write-up illustrates the formulation of the four parts of the clinical impressions, based on the history and findings.

▥▶ The patient is a 25-year-old single female law student, who presented for a psychiatric consultation with a chief complaint of being "sad and tearful" for the past three to four weeks. She felt "down" and hopeless nearly all the time and was getting further and further behind in her studies, although examination time was approaching. She cried many times a day and enjoyed virtually nothing. Her sleep was fitful and interrupted, and she woke up exhausted and dragged herself out of bed in the morning with great difficulty. She had no appetite and was forcing herself to eat but so far had lost no weight.

Her symptoms, which had been worsening, had begun in the context of the following psychosocial stressor: For the past two years, the patient had been intimately involved with a fellow law student. In the fall semester of their final year, about four weeks prior to the patient's presentation, her lover had revealed that although he cared about her very much and wanted to continue seeing her while they were classmates, he planned to relocate wherever he found the best job and had no intention of coordinating that choice with her. In other words, he had put her on notice that he was breaking up with her in seven months. Prior to this discussion, she had assumed that they would look for jobs together and perhaps even consider marriage. In response to her lover's news, the patient had become increasingly sad, blaming herself for his lack of interest in making a long-term commitment to the relationship: "There must be something wrong with me, or he'd want to stay." She had not entertained the possibility that there was nothing wrong with her, that she was quite lovable, and that he had a problem with commitment to an intimate relationship. She harbored no feelings of resentment toward him but was angry with herself for being "such a loser." ◀▥ Box 1–3 shows the case formulation for this patient.

TREATMENT PLAN

Having completed a careful description of the patient's problems, their possible origins, and the patient's capacity to deal with those problems, the physician is finally ready to formulate a treatment plan.

First, given the differential diagnosis, the physician should outline the plan for establishing **a firm diagnosis** (e.g., obtain a history from family members; obtain prior treatment records). Second, immediate and long-term goals and concomitant recommendations for treatment should be delineated. One obvious fact needs to be stated here because it is, un-

BOX 1–3.   Case Formulation Using Biopsychosocial Approach for Patient D

History of the Present Illness
Past Psychiatric History

No prior treatment or episodes of depression. Denies history of mania.

Past Medical History

Has been in excellent health. Last physical examination two years ago was completely normal.

Psychosocial History

The patient, an only child, described her early childhood as "happy." When she was 5 years old, her father suddenly left the family, relocating several hundred miles away for about two years, and then returning, without explanation. The patient always excelled in school and had a small circle of close friends. After graduation from high school, she chose a nearby prestigious college, where she did well academically, dated occasionally, and became sexually active with a couple of men. Her move to an urban law school was her first major separation from home, and the relationship that she developed with her boyfriend was her first long-term intimate relationship. Once they began seeing each other, she quickly felt that she was in love. She found him to be "outgoing, serious, sensible, rational," and she felt good when she was with him.

Family History

No overt history of psychiatric problems, although father's "mid-life crisis" when he left the family may have represented a major depressive episode.

Findings
Mental Status Examination

Appearance: The patient is slim and petite, dressed in stylish jeans and sweater. Her dress reinforces her juvenile appearance, as do her below-the-shoulder, blunt-cut blond hair and minimal makeup. Her pretty face is particularly notable for her expressive brown eyes.

Speech and Behavior: The patient walks into the office confidently, but her smile is hesitant as she settles into the chair. She tells her story slowly in a quiet voice, making intermittent eye contact.

Mood: "Depressed."

Affect: Constricted, sad, tearful.

Thought Process: Coherent and goal-directed.

Thought Content: No evidence of delusions; presence of passive suicidal ideation without intent or plan (states she's been feeling so miserable, she wouldn't mind if she didn't wake up in the morning, but she has not thought about doing anything to hurt herself).

Perception: Denies auditory hallucinations.

Cognitive Function: Alert and oriented ×3. Unable to concentrate on object recall or digit span. Intelligence seems above average based on vocabulary.

Insight: Good, feels something is wrong.

Judgment: Also good, wants professional help.

Impressions
Case Summary

Patient with no prior psychiatric history now presents with a three- to four-week history of depressed mood, anhedonia, impaired concentration, loss of appetite, and sleep disturbance, which began after she learned of the impending loss of her first long-term intimate relationship.

Differential Diagnosis

Inexperienced clinicians might be misled to consider an adjustment disorder with depressed mood as the most likely disorder in the differential diagnosis. While there was a clear precipitant in this case, when sufficient symptoms for a major depression are present, that diagnosis takes precedence. Uncomplicated bereavement might also be considered but should be dismissed, since there was no death and in, fact, not even a clear-cut end to the relationship. A "double depression" may now exist, with a major depressive episode superimposed on dysthymia, although there is no particular evidence to support that diagnosis at this time. Her cognitive deficits are most likely accounted for by a pseudodementia accompanying her major depression.

Multiaxial Evaluation

Axis I: Major Depressive Disorder, Single Episode.

Axis II: Deferred.

Axis III: None.

Axis IV: Threatened loss of boyfriend.

Axis V: GAF = 50 (current).

Predisposing and Precipitating Factors

Biological Factors: Possible genetic predisposition, suggested by possible family history.

Psychological Factors: The father abandoned the family when the patient was a child and was probably at a stage of development where she would have had an intense attachment to him. This event clearly had a profound impact on her sense of herself as a lovable person as well as an attractive female. A 5-year-old girl's relationship with her mother tends to be quite ambivalent, as the child struggles with conflicting feelings of loving attachment and competitive aggression. In the case of this patient, developmentally appropriate guilt over these competitive feelings with her mother may have been compounded by the father's sudden disappearance. In the magical cognitive universe of a 5-year-old, his loss may have seemed causally related to the aggressive and tender longings with which she was struggling (i.e., the fantasy that he left to escape from her or to punish her, or both). She made an unconscious compromise to accommodate the conflict between her emotional needs and her excessive guilt: She became inhibited and was reluctant to allow herself to feel anger or dependence, and, in this way, reduced the guilt that she felt. But this inhibition was not without a price: The anger was still present and actually made her more vulnerable to depression because she turned the anger around on herself, which made her feel less guilt-ridden than if she had directed it outward.

Unfortunately, this young woman chose exactly the "wrong" man for herself, a man who would reenact the abandonment that had been so painful the first time around. (Such maladaptive patterns may be played out again and again as patients hope to better master the trauma and conflicts that they could not master as children.)

Social Factors: Isolation from family and friends.

Treatment Plan
Biological Treatment

Physical examination

Thyroid function tests

Antidepressant medication

Psychological Treatment

Supportive psychotherapy

Social Treatment

Expand social network

Prognosis

Excellent

fortunately, sometimes neglected: The **patient's goals** must be given prime importance when a treatment plan is being developed. The recommendations should include not only the ideal treatments but also those that are feasible given the patient's resources. The biopsychosocial perspective is useful in treatment planning because it focuses on all aspects of the patient's problems and their solutions. **Biological factors** might be treated with medication, electroconvulsive therapy, hypnosis, or bright-light phototherapy; **psychological factors** with various forms of psychotherapy; and **social factors** with hospitalization or other environmental changes, such as mobilizing a wider friendship network, joining a self-help group such as Alcoholics Anonymous, or obtaining additional work skills.

Box 1–4 shows how the biopsychosocial approach can be used to tailor a treatment plan to meet the needs of Patient D, who was discussed in the text above and in Box 1–3.

PROGNOSIS

The prognosis is a prediction of the course an illness will take (i.e., it is the physician's educated guess as to how a particular illness will play itself out in a particular patient). This prediction is based on the physician's specific knowledge of the individual patient and general knowledge of diseases (e.g., a major depressive episode tends to resolve with adequate psychopharmacological and psychotherapeutic treatment, whereas schizophrenia tends to be characterized by years of waxing and waning symptoms and progressive impairment). In other words, given the diagnosis, as well as the patient's strengths and vulnerabilities, to what extent will he or she recover and perhaps even achieve better personal adjustment?

➡ The patient in Boxes 1–3 and 1–4, for example, has several strengths: She is highly intelligent, in excellent physical health, persistent in applying herself to academic work, able to form close attachments to others, and quite likable. These qualities bode well for a positive response to treatment. In addition, her disorder is highly treatable and has an excellent response to medication. This patient also has several vulnerabilities: She is socially isolated and confused about how to handle her current relationship. Overall, the prognosis is excellent for her recovery from major depression. How she will fare socially and psy-

---

BOX 1–4.   Treatment Plan Based on Biopsychosocial Approach for Patient D

Biological Factors

To rule out the most likely causes of a general medical condition that might explain the signs and symptoms, the patient should undergo a thorough physical examination, and thyroid function tests should be obtained. Since major depression is quite responsive to medication (see Chapter 3, Mood Disorders), an antidepressant is clearly indicated as part of the treatment plan for this patient, if she is amenable to the idea. In selecting the appropriate antidepressant, it is important to consider the patient's insomnia and the side effects that she might find most and least tolerable (e.g., she was concerned about the possible weight gain associated with tricyclic antidepressants and any sedation that would make her feel "out of control").

In making the diagnosis, the patient should be observed for evidence of a personality disorder as well as a comorbid Axis I disorder as treatment proceeds and the major depression resolves. Obtaining additional history will be helpful as well.

Psychological Factors

After one evaluation session, many questions remain with regard to this patient's underlying conflicts, strengths, and vulnerabilities. The hypothesis regarding the impact that the temporary loss of her father had on her self-esteem and relationships, particularly with men, will require further exploration, clarification, and confirmation. In the initial physician-patient interactions, the emphasis should be on developing a therapeutic alliance that will support and encourage the patient through the initial weeks of depression. In providing support, a balance needs to be struck: Calm and genuine reassurance is necessary and helpful (e.g., telling the patient that "This illness is treatable, and we will work together to make you better"), but overly optimistic guarantees should be avoided.

The second step in this patient's psychological treatment should be psychotherapy. The ideal intensity and duration of the therapy is difficult to predict early in the course of treatment of this mood disorder. When the depression lifts, the following factors will be of crucial importance in formulating a more specific plan for psychotherapy: the patient's psychological mindedness (i.e., her ability to think about or explore underlying motivations and conflicts), her motivation to achieve increased psychological awareness, and her capacity to withstand the stress of intensive psychotherapy, as well as her financial resources and time availability. Keeping in mind the psychological issues that are of most concern at this time, the physician should be particularly attuned to the patient's concerns with regard to separations and abandonment, including those that occur within the treatment setting (e.g., when the psychiatrist takes a vacation).

Social Factors

As in many cases, the psychological and social issues, and the best way to help the patient with them, are interrelated. This patient's lack of a more extensive support system, which is a social problem, is closely related to her insecurity in relating to others, which is a psychological problem. Although it is not easy to make major changes in the social sphere until at least some work is done on psychological problems, change can sometimes occur more readily in one sphere than in another. Thus, this patient needs to expand her social network and find confidantes and friends outside of her relationship with her boyfriend. Specific suggestions might direct her to making such contacts (e.g., encouraging her to become involved in a school organization). Social skills training or group psychotherapy would be other therapeutic recommendations that might be helpful. If the patient fails to pursue these suggestions or has difficulty carrying them out, these problems should be explored in psychotherapy. They can provide a useful source of information about the patient's psychological makeup.

chologically is much more difficult to predict. If she proves to be psychologically minded and amenable to psychotherapy, her prognosis is very good for gaining improved self-esteem and more confidence in herself and for developing more fulfilling personal relationships. ◀▥

Selected Readings

DeGowin, R. L. DeGowin and DeGowin's Diagnostic Examination, 6th ed. New York, McGraw-Hill, 1994.

MacKinnon, R. A., and S. C. Yudofsky. Principles of the Psychiatric Evaluation. Philadelphia, J. B. Lippincott, 1991.

Perry, S., A. M. Cooper, and R. Michels. The psychodynamic formulation: its purpose, structure, and clinical application. American Journal of Psychiatry 144:543–550, 1987.

Practice Guideline for Psychiatric Evaluation of Adults. Work Group of Psychiatric Evaluation of Adults (Fogel, B. S., and R. Shellow, co-chairs). American Journal of Psychiatry 152 (Supplement):64–80, 1995.

Shea, S. C. Psychiatric Interviewing: The Art of Understanding. Philadelphia, W. B. Saunders Company, 1988.

CHAPTER TWO

THE PSYCHIATRIC INTERVIEW

LYLE ROSNICK, MD

The primary purpose of a clinical psychiatric interview is for the physician to obtain enough information about the patient to complete a psychiatric evaluation. (The qualifier *clinical* is added to differentiate this type of psychiatric interview from other psychiatric interviews, usually performed for research purposes, in which structured or semistructured questionnaires are administered by specially trained persons.) A psychiatric evaluation requires that the physician make a diagnostic and prognostic assessment and formulate a treatment plan. In order to make this assessment and formulation, information must be gathered in the interview about the patient's present and past psychiatric symptoms; previous psychiatric treatment; and past and present ability to function in social, personal, academic, and vocational spheres. The second purpose of the clinical psychiatric interview is therapeutic in nature. When the interview is conducted in a supportive and empathic manner, the very act of the physician's seeking information from the patient may help alleviate the patient's suffering.

INTERVIEW MODELS
The Medical Model

The psychiatric interview and other medical interviews share some similarities. In both types, the patient is seeking professional help. Both types of interviews include the patient's subjective account of symptoms and the physician's more objective assessment of how the patient looks, thinks, and feels. In the general medical interview, this more objective assessment is the physical examination; in the psychiatric interview, it is the mental status examination. The physician begins both interviews by considering the patient's chief complaint (i.e., what caused the patient to seek professional help at that particular point in time). In both, the patient is asked about the present illness and the past history. The psychiatric interview includes a general survey of the major realms of psychopathology, which is analogous to the review of systems, an essential component of other medical evaluations. However, because the patient's past and present thoughts, feelings, and behavior are of potential interest in the psychiatric interview, the type of information gathered about the patient is different from that gathered in the medical interview. The psychiatric interviewer is interested not only in the illness but also in the ways the patient experiences and copes with it.

A crucial distinction between the two kinds of interviews is the interviewer's different expectations of the patient. In customary medical interviews, a patient is asked a number of relatively specific questions, to which straightforward and brief answers are expected. But for the psychiatric interview to be most productive, the patient needs to respond to the interviewer's questions more spontaneously and at greater length.

Within the conceptual framework of the medical model, psychiatric symptoms are seen as direct manifestations of an illness, just as, for example, chest pain is seen as a possible symptom of myocardial infarction. In accordance with the medical model, the interviewer is interested in recording the presence or absence of symptoms of pertinent illnesses or syndromes. The physician also tracks the course of symptoms and looks for factors that exacerbate or alleviate them, including the effects of previous treatment. Like other medical symptoms and illnesses, psychiatric symptoms and illnesses have an etiology, which is known or unknown, an onset, course of illness, and treatment response. Panic disorder, obsessive-compulsive disorder, and major depression are examples of psychiatric illnesses that lend themselves particularly well to the medical model concept.

The Psychodynamic Model

The medical illness model of psychopathology provides a necessary but insufficient framework for the psychiatric interviewer. To be most effective, the interviewer must approach the patient's symptoms from a psychodynamic point of view, as well. According to psychodynamic models of the mind, psychiatric symptoms are reflections of **underlying psychological processes**. Object relations theory and ego psychology are two psychodynamic models that are particularly relevant to interviewers who want to understand the patient's thoughts, feelings, and behavior in their full complexity, including his or her interactions with the interviewer.

Object Relations Theory

According to this theory, the building blocks of the mind are memories, particularly memories of emotional interactions with significant others (e.g., parents, siblings, and teachers) during infancy and childhood. Each such memory is stored in the form of a mental image of the person's self, the **self representation,** paired with the mental image of the other person, **object representation,** involved in the emotional interaction. Each pair of self and object representations is recorded as a memory that is accompanied by the strong feelings that prevailed during the original interaction. Table 2–1 gives examples of prototypal pairs, or **dyads,** of self and object representations that are linked by particular affects.

These representational dyads are of special interest to the psychiatric interviewer because they provide an invaluable way of understanding the past's influence on the present. Patients' present interactions activate representations of similar interactions that have been stored in the form of self-object pairs. Memories of such past experiences strongly influence patients' present perceptions and behaviors. It is as though patients' significant emotional experiences from the past become confused with similar important interactions in the present. The stronger the feeling attached to the interaction, the greater the likelihood that a representation will be activated. These feelings frequently surface during physician-patient interviews, which thus serve as a laboratory in which physicians can observe directly manifestations of the types of memories of self-object representations characteristic of their patients. When patients consult physicians, they often are anxious, fearful, or even terrified. They may feel doomed or cursed, angry or resentful, or needy and helpless. They commonly have regressed and, feeling childlike, regard their physicians as parents from whom they are seeking assistance, protection, or deliverance. Patients may experience themselves as hungry, crying children and their doctors as either responsive, omnipotent, gratifying caretakers or unresponsive, depriving, inadequate nurturers. As the example below shows, patients who have felt rejected by caretakers are predisposed to feel rejected by their physicians.

➡ A 23-year-old woman presented at a psychiatric clinic with the chief complaint of having been "dumped" by her boyfriend. Her personal history revealed the particularly relevant fact that her father had died unexpectedly when she was five years of age. She seemed grateful and cooperative during her first psychiatric interview with a male medical student, who was about the same age as her ex-boyfriend. The student was surprised when the patient failed to show up for her second appointment. The following is a hypothetical explanation of her behavior toward the student in terms of object relations. In the first interview, the patient responded so positively to the student because his behavior reminded her of her ex-boyfriend's behavior on past occasions when he had been caring and supportive. However, she experienced the termination of the interview as a loss that recapitulated the breakup with her boyfriend and the death of her father. The separation from the medical student between interviews also left her feeling bereft and abandoned, as if she had been deprived of her boyfriend and her father all over again. Resolving to avoid another "rejection," the patient turned the tables on the student and preemptively "stood him up" for the second appointment. In the first interview, the patient experienced herself as well cared for (self image) and the medical student as concerned and nurturing (object representation). After the interview, she perceived herself to be the abandoned one (self representation) and the absent student to be the one who had "dumped" her (object image). By deliberately failing to show up for the second appointment, she was able to regard herself as the one in control and the heartbreaker (self image), who had abandoned the student and rendered him the helpless, jilted victim (object image). ⬅

TABLE 2–1. Prototypal Dyads of Self and Object Representations

Self Representation	Object Representation	Prevailing Affect
Hungry, crying child	Absent, unresponsive caregiver	Anger, feeling of deprivation
Hungry, crying child	Responsive, gratifying caregiver	Feelings of gratification, love
Grandiose, entirely self-sufficient child	Unneeded, irrelevant caregiver	Feelings of triumph, contempt, or indifference

The psychiatric interviewer must be an active participant and collaborator. Interviewers question patients and listen to what they report; they also observe patients and analyze what they see. The implications of this difference in perspective from the conventional medical perspective are vast and worthy of emphasis. In the object relations model, patients and interviewers jointly observe and reflect upon what they mutually experience in the interview.

Interviewers learn to monitor and use their own mental and emotional reactions to patients as another source of information. The thoughts, feelings, and fantasies they experience during and after the interview may reveal a great deal about their patients' thoughts, feelings, and ways of interacting with others. Informed by object relations theory, the physician keeps in mind the following questions:

How is the patient experiencing me?
How is the patient portraying himself or herself to me?
How does the patient want me to experience and view him or her?
Why is the patient talking to me about this subject now?

Virgil leading Dante on a tour of the Underworld in *The Inferno* may provide a more useful image for the interviewer to keep in mind than the image of a physician performing a procedure on a compliant but passive patient. Another helpful way to think of the interviewer is as a safari guide leading someone through a jungle. The guide has "tracking skills," as it were, and the patient's psyche is the "uncharted, un-explored" territory that must be traversed. The patient must grant the interviewer "access" to his or her mind. The skilled interviewer has the techniques to persuade the patient to do so, as well as enable the patient to learn from what they jointly encounter.

Ego Psychology

In this psychodynamic conceptualization, the mind is the site of psychological conflicts between an individual's basic wishes and fears. The specific nature of these wishes and fears varies in accordance with a person's stage of development and predominant level of psychological functioning. Freud's four stages of psychosexual development (the oral, anal, phallic, and oedipal stages) still afford an invaluable way of categorizing the prototypal constellations of human wishes and fears.

Psychosexual Development. According to Freud, each stage of an individual's psychosexual development is characterized by a particular wish and a corresponding fear. The wish associated with the oral stage is to gratify dependency yearnings, and the prototypal fear is of losing the mother or mother surrogate. The anal phase is marked by a conflict between compliance and defiance. The wish is to assert one's individuality (e.g., by saying "no"), and the related fear is of losing the approval of the significant caretaker. The wish characteristic of the phallic phase is to exhibit one's superiority (e.g., by being the strongest, most beautiful or intelligent, or fastest) and to be admired and acknowledged as "number one." The attendant fear is of defeat, humiliation, and exposure as inadequate or inferior. The oedipal wish is to win a competition with the parent of the same sex for the affection of the opposite-sex parent. The fear is of retaliation by the rival parent, which typically is experienced consciously or unconsciously as a fear of bodily damage (i.e., literal or figurative castration). See Table 2–2 for a summary of these constellations.

The conflicts characteristic of each level of psychosexual development are never completely resolved. Rather, they persist throughout life and exert an ongoing influence upon an individual's thoughts, feelings, and behavior.

TABLE 2–2.   Freud's Phases of Psychosexual Development

Stage	Predominant Wish	Predominant Fear
Oral	Dependency gratification	Loss of object (e.g., mother)
Anal	Assertion of autonomy; defiance versus compliance	Loss of love of parent or caretaker
Phallic	Admiration for one's prowess and superiority; triumph	Inadequacy, humiliation, defeat, inferiority
Oedipal	Rivalry with same-sex parent for affection of opposite-sex parent	Attack from same-sex parent (e.g., castration)

In this theoretical model, the hypothetical psychic agency that serves as the repository of sexual and aggressive drives is the **id.** The **superego** encompasses a person's conscience and ego ideal, which is the idealized mental representation of the kind of person an individual feels he or she should be. The superego is the source of guilt and fears of retribution (e.g., in the form of abandonment, subjugation, or castration) that the person anticipates as punishment for forbidden oral, anal, phallic, and oedipal wishes. Therefore, the wish-fear conflicts can also be conceptualized as struggles between the id and the superego.

The third psychic agency of the mental apparatus is the **ego,** the "executive branch" of the mind, which performs many functions, including the resolution of wish-fear conflicts. According to ego psychology, psychiatric symptoms are manifestations of compromises, resulting from the ego's efforts to mediate between conflicting wishes and fears (i.e., to mediate between the id and the superego), as the following case illustrates:

➡ A 23-year-old unemployed man, who lived with his parents, was suffering from a psychogenic paralysis of his right arm. Psychiatric evaluation revealed that he was harboring urges to hit his father, who, the patient said, frequently humiliated and "lorded it over" him. The young man felt guilty about his forbidden desire, which he unconsciously experienced as patricidal, and worried that he might seriously injure his father if he were to attack him. He admitted that he often wished that his father would die, so that he could live alone with his mother, to whom he felt very close. The patient anticipated that his father, the police, or God would administer the punishment that the patient felt he deserved in retaliation for these forbidden wishes, according to the dictates of his superego (i.e., castration or death).

A physician using the ego psychology model could construct the following psychodynamic formulation to facilitate further inquiry into and understanding of this patient's psychopathology. The young man's desire to attack his father had anal, phallic, and oedipal roots. He desperately wanted to escape from his controlling father and triumph over him in a struggle that he experienced as a matter of life or death. However, he felt guilty about his desire to challenge his father's authority and, indeed, to dethrone and kill him and be left alone with his mother. His paralyzed arm was the means by which his ego resolved the conflict between his desires and his guilty fears. This conversion reaction rendered him physically unable to attack his father. The useless limb also represented a punishment that the young man's ego had unconsciously inflicted upon him for his patricidal wishes. He gratified his id by expressing aggression, but the aggression was directed toward himself and not his father. He placated his superego by sparing his father and by retaliating against himself for his own forbidden desires. However, this attempt at conflict resolution was maladaptive because the patient had forfeited the use of his arm in the process. ⬅

Defense Mechanisms. Defense mechanisms such as the conversion reaction are employed by the ego to assist the psyche in its attempts to avoid experiencing painful thoughts and feelings generated by wish-fear conflicts. Box 2–1 provides definitions of

---

BOX 2–1. Defense Mechanisms

Primitive Defense Mechanisms

   Denial is the refusal to perceive or register as significant external events (e.g., the destructive consequences of one's own behavior).

   Dissociation is the splitting off of thoughts and associated feelings from conscious awareness, as if to place them in a separate mental compartment. This occurs in amnesia, fugue states, multiple personality disorder, and splitting.

   Splitting is seeing things as all or nothing (e.g., all good or all bad). It occurs when contradictory sets of thoughts and feelings are dissociated from each other. At any given time, the individual is under the influence of only one of the contradictory mental sets.

   Idealization, which is related to splitting, is seeing another person as perfect and ignoring the faults of that individual.

   Devaluation, which is also related to splitting, is maintaining an entirely negative view of another person by ignoring the person's virtues.

   Projection is attributing one's own thoughts, feelings, or impulses to another individual. Person A is sexually attracted to person B, but person A's ego blocks the desire from entering his or her own conscious awareness because of guilt. Person A tries to disavow the sexual desire by projecting it onto person B (i.e., by imagining that person B is attracted to him or her).

   Acting out is expressing thoughts and feelings in actions rather than words (e.g., missing an appointment because one is afraid of becoming too dependent on the physician rather than keeping the appointment and discussing this fear with the physician).

   Projective identification is a complex operation that involves projection and acting out and has multiple steps. Person C imagines that person D is regarding and treating person C in a particular way (e.g., contemptuously). Person C is actually feeling and behaving toward person D as he imagines person D is regarding and treating him. Person C's behavior frequently provokes person D into doing unto person C what person C already imagines is happening. In other words, person C unwittingly brings about the very reaction he or she dreads (i.e., contemptuous treatment).

Mature Defense Mechanisms

   Suppression is a partly conscious mechanism by which the individual wishes to put something unpleasant out of his or her own awareness and does so.

   Repression is blocking a thought, feeling, or memory from conscious awareness (e.g., forgetting a painful experience).

   Reaction formation is acting opposite to one's own desires, which one wants to disavow (e.g., a person who is conflicted over his or her own dependency yearnings who spends all of his or her time taking care of others).

   Intellectualization is thinking or talking about an emotion-laden subject in an unemotional way (i.e., while experiencing and expressing no feelings).

   Rationalization is attributing one's behavior to a cause that one finds more acceptable than the actual cause when one does not want to face or admit the real reason (e.g., a man who says that he lives with his mother because she needs him when the true reason is that he fears being separated from her).

---

defense mechanisms that are often observed during psychiatric interviews.

   Transference and Resistance.   The interviewer should be familiar with these two concepts of ego psychology because nearly every patient will experience them to some degree during a psychiatric interview. **Transference** occurs when an individual unconsciously perceives an imagined or exaggerated similarity between people in the present and significant childhood caretakers. Under the influence of transference, patients' responses are inappropriate to the current interactions.

   ➡ For example, a boy who had been beaten repeatedly by his father refused to be seen by a male physician when he was brought to the emergency room. His previous experiences of an older male authority figure, namely, his father, had been so horrendous that he was unable to feel safe with a male physician, regardless of how kind and caring he appeared to be. ◀

   Resistance, which may be conscious or unconscious in nature, is anything that prevents a patient from being aware of certain thoughts and feelings or from communicating them spontaneously and openly to the interviewer. **Unconscious resistance** results from the ego's employment of defense mechanisms to block out awareness of painful thoughts or feelings. For example, a patient who cannot think of anything to say during an interview is exhibiting resistance secondary to repression. Absenteeism and lateness that could be avoided are common examples of acting out (e.g., expressing anger, fear, or ambivalence by not showing up for an appointment instead of talking about these feelings with the physician).

   Conscious resistance occurs when patients intentionally oppose the interviewer (e.g., refuse to answer questions or provide vital information). Such resistance frequently stems from the patient's transference to the physician (e.g., the patient experiences the physician as uncaring and threatening or as a rival to be defeated). With this knowledge in mind, physicians should ask themselves the following questions as they conduct the interview:

What are the patient's principal wishes and fears?
Which defense mechanism is the patient relying on to avoid facing and discussing painful issues?
How is the patient experiencing the physician in the transference (i.e., with which important person from the past is the patient equating the physician)?
Of what is the patient guilty?
What punishment does the patient anticipate for these real or imagined transgressions?
What kind of person does the patient aspire to be?
In what ways does the patient fall short of this ideal?

CONDUCTING THE INTERVIEW

   Conducting an informative and therapeutic interview requires that the physician carefully consider a variety of issues that range from the seemingly mundane, such as scheduling appointments and arranging the setting, to the subtle and sophisticated, such as how to question a patient about intimate, painful thoughts and feelings in a manner that will alleviate distress and thereby facilitate the discussion. Such an interview not only affords the patient immediate relief from suffering but also provides the physician with the information required for definitive, long-range treatment planning.

To perform this type of interview, the physician should keep in mind that (1) most patients are eager to talk with physicians, especially when they are in pain and incapacitated and (2) a **therapeutic alliance** is achieved when patients sense that the physician is treating them with respect, is interested in what they have to say, and has the knowledge and skills required to help them (i.e., that the interviewer is caring and competent). To develop and maintain a therapeutic alliance, the interviewer should strive to be thoughtful and empathic during every interaction with the patient. Respect and consideration of the patient's needs and concerns should be shown even before the interview begins.

Scheduling the Interview

Interviews should be scheduled in advance whenever possible. This is sometimes difficult for harried physicians in certain settings (e.g., inpatient units), but the benefits are significant. Patients feel more important when they have a definite meeting time rather than when they are expected to just "hang around" until the interviewer has time to talk with them. Such consideration enhances the development of rapport between the patient and interviewer. Scheduling meetings at fixed times also affords the interviewer the opportunity to observe the patient's behavior with regard to the appointment (e.g., if the patient is late, it may be because of anxiety, anger, or a wish to be in control).

The Interview Setting

Medical students and physicians in clinics, emergency rooms, and inpatient units often have little control over the setting of the psychiatric interview. The place available for such a meeting is not likely to be a private office replete with comfortable furniture, books, and works of art. It is more likely to be a sparsely furnished, windowless room or even a hallway. Regardless of the locale, the interviewer should try to focus complete attention on the patient and attempt to make him or her as comfortable as possible. The interviewer can ask if the patient is satisfied with the room temperature, inviting input into whether a window should be opened or the air conditioner turned off. Such a request indicates that the interviewer wants the patient to collaborate actively in the interview. There should be no physical barriers, such as a desk, between the interviewer and the patient that could impede the establishment of rapport.

Most importantly, the interviewer should also feel comfortable and endeavor to make the patient feel emotionally and physically secure. A frightened, preoccupied interviewer cannot conduct a successful interview, and a fearful, distracted patient cannot do his or her part. Certain measures can be taken if either person is frightened. For example, the presence of a security guard in the room might make a paranoid patient feel more comfortable. The interviewer of a potentially assaultive patient might choose to conduct the interview in a patient lounge or waiting room, where a guard or other staff member would be nearby and where the participants could sit farther apart and not feel cornered. The interviewer's fears should never be ignored, even if they seem irrational or exaggerated. Instead, the interviewer should seek advice and direction from someone with more knowledge and experience. Patients should be interviewed only under conditions in which everyone involved feels safe.

Beginning the Interview

The patient should not be kept in the dark (i.e., made to guess who the interviewer is and what is happening). The physician should greet the patient by shaking hands, saying, "Hello," and addressing the patient by his or her last name, unless the patient is a child. The physician should state his or her name, title, the capacity in which he or she will be relating to the patient, for how long, and the goals for the interview. The following introductions show how this can be accomplished in only a few brief sentences.

"Hello, Mrs. Hughes, I am Sally Smith, a third-year medical student. I will be working on this Unit for 5 weeks. I will be meeting with you twice per week, in addition to your sessions with Dr. Jones (the psychiatric resident). The primary purpose of our meetings will be to help me to learn how to interview patients in a more helpful way. Hopefully you also will find them to be beneficial."

"Mr. Williams, hello. I'm Edgar Thompson, a fourth-year medical student. I and my fellow students will be doing your psychiatric evaluation for admission to this clinic. I and Dr. Evans, my supervisor, will be meeting with you for three 45-minute sessions. After our evaluation has been completed we will discuss our findings with you, and we will refer you for ongoing treatment, if it is indicated."

From the very beginning, it is crucial to treat the patient as an active collaborator, rather than a passive subject. In enlisting the patient's assistance as a fellow explorer of his or her own mind, it may be helpful to explain how he or she can function to make the interview most useful. Such candor maximizes the likelihood that the patient will trust the interviewer and feel safe. The interviewer should emphasize that unedited, spontaneous thoughts and feelings are of primary importance to the success of the interview and should encourage the patient to relate as many details and specific examples as possible. It may be helpful to acknowledge that this approach to history-taking is different from those used in other types of interviews.

Chief Complaint and History of Present Illness

The immediate focus of the interview should be the chief complaint and the history of the present illness. The interviewer may commence with an open-ended question, such as, "How can I be of help?" or "What brought you to the clinic?" Some patients require little prompting to answer such questions in great detail. When this happens, the interviewer should sit back and listen attentively to the story as it unfolds, making note of issues that should be explored further and resisting the temptation to interrupt.

A patient who readily reveals thoughts, feelings, and experiences to the interviewer usually has a lot to say and wants the interviewer to know how he or she is feeling and what his or her concerns are. Such a patient will derive considerable benefit from sharing this information with the physician. In the process, crucial information is provided. While listening, the physician should be assessing the patient's capacity for goal-directed thinking, the ways in which thoughts are organized and the content and flow of ideas (e.g., the subjects that the patient chooses to discuss, those that are avoided, and the order in which they are discussed). The physician also obtains important information about the patient's mental process by observing nonverbal behavior, including appearance (e.g., personal hygiene, grooming, facial expression, posture, and mannerisms) and mode of speaking (e.g., amount, rate, and tone of speech).

While narrating, the patient communicates feelings, thoughts, and behaviors that he or she finds problematic, undesirable, or even unbearable. The nature of the patient's subjective distress or maladaptive behaviors is an indispensable clue that directs the interviewer to areas requiring further exploration. The interviewer listens for the patient's spontaneous report of symptoms that indicate psychiatric illnesses. When enough symptoms have surfaced to suggest a differential diagnosis, the interviewer should begin to look for points of entry at which the patient can be questioned in detail about the chief complaint and other possibly related symptoms. This section of the interview is characterized by numerous closed-ended, yes-or-no questions and answers, much like a focused medical history. For example, a person who says "I feel depressed or anxious," and reports having felt sad and blue for several weeks can be questioned about the other symptoms of major depression, including suicidal ideation; changes in weight, appetite, energy level, and sleeping patterns; and a decreased interest in life. The chief complaint and history of the present illness can be explored further with inquiries about the onset, course, and severity of symptoms and factors that ameliorate and exacerbate the symptoms. The interviewer can ask about syndromes or illnesses that may be associated with the present illness. For instance, a patient complaining of frequent full-blown panic attacks should be questioned about past and present consumption of alcohol or minor tranquilizers because these substances are often used to alleviate the anticipatory anxiety, fear of sudden death or loss of control, or sense of terror that accompanies panic attacks.

This technique produces an up-to-date, relevant database, which can be recorded as a chronological account of symptoms, characterized according to time of onset, quality, intensity, duration, presence or absence of associated symptoms, and the like. The symptoms can then be categorized as illnesses, whenever possible. This approach is best suited for DSM Axis I illnesses, such as obsessive-compulsive disorder or major depression, which readily lend themselves to conceptualization via the symptom-based medical model.

Other points at which the interviewer should intervene are when the patient seems to be running out of material to relate, begins to repeat things, goes off on tangents, or becomes vague, overly general, or even incomprehensible. These behaviors often signify resistance (i.e., the patient is in the midst or on the verge of discussing an emotion-laden or conflictual topic). In order to help the patient overcome the resistance, the interviewer should intervene by (1) closely observing and exploring the resistant behavior, (2) ascertaining the source of the resistance, (3) determining whether it is conscious or unconscious in nature, and (4) presenting this information to the patient (Fig. 2–1). For example, it is frequently sufficient for the interviewer to comment upon the nature of the resistance and the possible motives behind it: "I noticed that you became silent after mentioning your father's death. Perhaps it's difficult for you to continue talking about such a painful matter." When such a resistance interpretation is effective, the patient will resume the discussion of the affect-laden subject.

Past Psychiatric History

After a patient's present psychiatric illness has been explored, the interviewer must inquire about past psychiatric problems and treatment. The following questions show one approach to obtaining the past psychiatric history:

Have you ever been depressed (been anxious, had panic attacks, heard voices) in the past? When? What were your symptoms? How did you feel or behave that makes you now think that you were depressed (anxious, etc.)? Were your symptoms different from the ones you're experiencing now?
Did you consult a doctor or therapist at that time? What did the doctor or therapist say? Did you take medication? Were you in therapy?
Have you ever seen a psychiatrist or therapist before? Has there been a time when you thought that you should have?

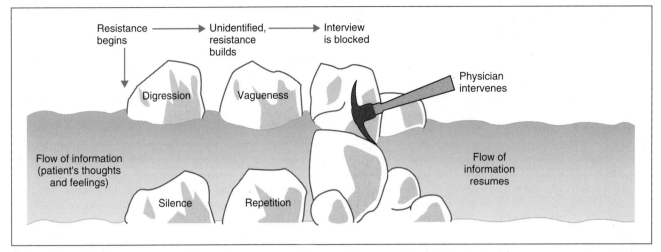

FIGURE 2–1. Resistance and intervention in the interview. Resistance may be met at any point in the interview process. Resistance occurs when the patient "runs out" of material or becomes repetitive, digressive, or vague about his or her thoughts and feelings and the flow of information decreases or stops. If this resistance is not identified by the physician, the interview gets stuck. To help the patient overcome resistance and restore the flow of information, the physician must intervene by first determining whether the source of the patient's resistance is conscious or unconscious and then presenting this determination to the patient. Through observation and exploration of the resistance, the continued flow of information will be facilitated.

Was there ever a time when you couldn't function at school, at work, or in social relationships? Tell me about it.

Have you ever tried to kill yourself? What thoughts have you had about suicide over the course of your lifetime?

Have you ever been hospitalized for psychiatric reasons?

Past Medical History

Next, it is crucial that the physician explore certain aspects of the patient's medical history. Does the patient have medical illnesses that may be associated with or be causes of certain types of psychiatric illnesses? Several examples readily come to mind, such as hypothyroidism and depression, hyperthyroidism and panic attacks, and seizure disorders and aggressive outbursts. Is the patient taking a medication that can produce psychiatric symptoms as a side effect (e.g., a beta blocker may cause depression)? Is the patient taking a medication that could interact adversely with a psychotropic agent (e.g., as meperidine may interact with a monoamine oxidase inhibitor)? Has the patient ever had a seizure or head injury (e.g., fractured skull, concussion, or subdural hematoma) that could predispose the patient to seizures if the patient is given psychotropic medications that lower the seizure threshold (e.g., antidepressants, antipsychotics)? Questions that may be useful in eliciting the past medical history are as follows:

Have you ever taken a medication regularly for any chronic, nonpsychiatric medical problem, such as insulin for diabetes or a medication for high blood pressure? Have you ever suffered from any such conditions?

Have you ever had an operation?

Have you ever had a convulsion, skull fracture, or any serious head injury?

Give me a complete list of all the drugs that you take currently, including vitamins, over-the-counter drugs, and substances obtained at health food stores.

Have you ever been in a serious accident?

Do any medical illnesses run in your family?

Do you have an internist or family doctor? When was your most recent checkup? Did you have blood tests, an electrocardiogram, or other tests?

Have you ever had a life-threatening illness?

Have you ever been hospitalized or taken to an emergency room?

Are you allergic to any medications or to anything else?

Review of Major Realms of Psychopathology
General Screening Questions

No exploration of present and past psychiatric illnesses is complete without questioning the patient about the major categories of psychiatric symptoms, or realms of psychopathology. The **psychiatric review of systems** involves a general survey of past and present mental health to determine whether or not the patient suffers from a psychotic disorder, mood disorder, anxiety disorder, substance-related disorder, cognitive disorder, or personality disorder. These disorders, in particular, should be kept in mind because they comprise the majority of illnesses with which psychiatric patients present. A patient may report one problem but not another, either because it occurred in the past, is happening in the present with minor symptoms, or is happening in the present and the patient does not realize it. Almost always, however, hints of any major illnesses are revealed by the present illness and cue the interviewer to specifically focus on the possible presence of these illnesses if they are not spontaneously elaborated upon by patients.

It is neither desirable nor possible to question every patient about every category, however. It would be absurd to query a 35-year-old nuclear physicist who has been functioning well at work about cognitive impairment when no evidence of memory loss or an altered sensorium has been found during the exploration of the present illness. However, the interviewer should omit only those screening questions that are obviously irrelevant or that have been answered during the preceding part of the interview.

The following questions illustrate how a survey of the realms of psychopathology can be conducted in a reasonable amount of time:

Have you ever had a problem with depression? Have you ever felt sad and blue much of the time for more than a few hours? Do you tend to see the glass as half empty rather than half full?

Have you ever felt euphoric, as if you were in more than a normal good mood—almost like being high on a drug—talking a mile a minute, needing very little sleep to feel rested, and going on spending sprees or being sexually indiscreet?

Have you ever been unusually irritable—snapping at people without provocation, with a shorter fuse than usual—for more than a few hours or days at a time?

Has anxiety ever been a problem for you? Has it ever affected your functioning at work, at home, or in social relationships? Have you ever had a panic attack, where your heart was pounding, you were gasping for breath, and you thought you were dying, losing control, or losing your mind?

Have you ever intentionally starved yourself to lose weight? Have you ever abused laxatives? Have you ever made yourself vomit or given yourself enemas to lose weight?

Have you or anybody important to you ever thought that you have a problem with alcohol or other drugs?

Have you or anybody close to you ever felt that you had or have a problem with your memory or with remaining alert and knowing where you were, why you were there, or whom you were with? Have you been losing things more frequently than usual? Have you ever had difficulty counting change or performing other simple tasks that usually are easy for you? Has anyone told you that you've been different lately? In what ways?

Some people who are depressed (anxious, manic) find that their minds play tricks on them. They may have thoughts that later do not make sense to them, such as that they have a brain tumor even though neurological tests were negative, or that they have special powers. Have you ever experienced such thoughts while depressed (euphoric, using cocaine, under stress)? Have you ever heard voices or seen things that were not there when you were under the influence of a drug, feeling hopeless, or feeling under stress?

When you were depressed (anxious, fearful, hopeless, panicky), have you ever felt like ending your own life? Have ever tried to kill yourself? Have you ever wished that you were dead? (All patients should be asked about suicide at some point during the initial interview.)

How would you or others close to you describe yourself as a person? Who is important to you? Describe them to me. Describe for me in detail a typical day in your life. What do you do for fun? Have you ever had a problem with temper, driving recklessly, gambling, going on spending sprees, or binge eating or drinking? Have you ever been arrested or done anything for which you would have been arrested if you had been caught? What kinds of problems do you have at work or in other relationships? Have you ever cut, burned, or hit yourself to alleviate painful feelings? Do you tend to act impulsively?

If the patient's answers to these inquiries suggest certain disorders, the patient can be questioned at greater length about them. Sample questions for the realms of psychopathology are given below.

Mood Disorders

An important goal of every psychiatric evaluation is to determine whether a patient is currently suffering from or has ever suffered from major depression, dysthymia, mania, or hypomania.

Depression and Dysthymia

Have you felt sad, blue, or down in the dumps most of the time on most days recently?

Have you found yourself worrying more than usual or more than is warranted (e.g., about health or finances)? For how long?

Have you ever felt that way for weeks at a time? How many?

How old were you when you first felt that way?

If a patient responds affirmatively to these questions, he or she can be asked in detail about present or past neurovegetative symptoms of depression:

Tell me what your depression is like.

How were your thoughts, feelings, and behavior different when you were depressed from when you were feeling your best?

Have you been feeling depressed recently?

What has your mood been like?

Have you had crying spells?

Have you noticed any change in your appetite?

Have you either lost or gained weight?

Have you experienced a craving for junk food, chocolate, or carbohydrates?

Have you found it harder to wake up in the morning?

Do you find yourself sleeping more than usual?

Do you have trouble falling asleep or staying asleep?

Do you ever wake up a couple of hours before the alarm clock is set to go off and find yourself unable to get back to sleep?

Have you recently experienced less pleasure from activities that ordinarily give you pleasure?

Are you less interested in things that usually interest you?

Do you find yourself less energetic than usual?

Does everything feel like more of a burden?

Do you have trouble concentrating?

Have others noticed a change in you?

Do you find that you are less efficient at work or less creative, even if others have not noticed any difference in your performance? Have you found yourself letting things go around the house and neglecting your personal appearance?

Have you felt hopeless?

Have you been sitting around more, watching more TV? Or have you felt agitated and restless, pacing or picking at yourself?

Have you been talking less or moving more slowly than usual?

Suicide

How close have you come to trying to kill yourself? What stopped you?

Have you ever done anything potentially life-threatening even if you did not consciously want to die at the time?

Has anyone in your family ever committed suicide to your knowledge?

Has anyone close to you ever committed suicide?

Have you ever wished you would get cancer, be run over by a car, or die in your sleep so that you could perish without having to kill yourself?

How hopeless have you felt?

Have you ever heard a voice telling you to kill yourself?

Have you ever had a specific plan for how you would kill yourself? Did you take any steps to implement the plan?

Mania and Hypomania

Have you ever felt euphoric, by which I mean in better than a normal good mood, almost like on a drug high? For how long? For days or weeks at a time?

Have you ever experienced periods of increased irritability, during which your fuse is shorter than usual and you snap at people more easily? At whom? Have you sometimes done more than verbally snap at others? Have you thrown things, broken furniture, or gotten into fistfights? Has your temper ever gotten you into trouble at work or interfered with your relationships?

During these euphoric or irritable periods, have you always been under the influence of drugs such as cocaine or alcohol? Or have you been euphoric or irritable even when you were drug-free?

During such periods of time, have you experienced any of the following symptoms?

Insomnia: Have you needed much less sleep than usual to feel rested?

Hyperactivity: Have you been much more active or moving more rapidly than usual? Have you been drinking more alcohol recently to try to calm yourself down?

Spending sprees: Have you gone on any unusual shopping sprees? Have you spent money more freely than usual in a way that's out of character for you?

Pressured speech: Have you been more talkative than usual? Has your speech been more rapid than usual? Has it been so rapid that people at times have had difficulty understanding you?

Grandiosity: Have you ever felt that you have extraordinary abilities? At times, have you felt that whatever you do would turn out well, even when you did not have a basis for your optimism (e.g., embarking on an expensive business venture in a line of work of which you are ignorant)?

Distractibility: Have you found it more difficult than usual to stay focused on a particular subject or activity?

Poor judgment: Have you found yourself behaving in foolish, self-destructive, or provocative ways that are out of character for you, such as giving away money, being inappropriately sexually seductive, or becoming involved in shouting matches or fistfights?

Anxiety Disorders

Each psychiatric evaluation should include an assessment of whether the patient has or has had generalized anxiety, panic attacks (partial or full-blown), obsessive-compulsive symptoms, or phobic symptoms.

Generalized Anxiety

Has anxiety ever been a problem for you? Tell me about it.

Have you ever been much more anxious than usual for a significant period of time? For how long?

Are you more anxious than most people?

Everybody experiences anxiety differently. What does it feel like for you?

What physical symptoms do you experience when you are anxious?

Panic Attack or Disorder

Have you ever had a panic attack or an anxiety attack? What was it like?

People use these terms differently. By a panic attack, I mean the following. A panic attack has a definite beginning and end. It is marked by a subjective feeling of absolute terror. People having panic attacks frequently imagine that they are having heart attacks or say that they feel like they are about to drop dead, lose control, or "lose their minds." A true panic attack always includes prominent physical symptoms, such as pounding of the heart; gasping for breath; feeling short of breath, lightheaded, or as if you are about to faint; "pins and needles" in your hands, feet, or face; perspiring heavily; feeling hot or flushed, tremulous, or as if you have "butterflies" in your stomach.

Have you ever had such an attack? Tell me about it.

Which symptoms did you experience?

What did you do about it? How many such attacks have you had?

How frequently? When and where do they tend to occur?

How long do they last?

Obsessive-Compulsive Symptoms or Disorder

Have you ever been troubled by thoughts, feelings, or impulses that repeatedly pop into your mind, unbidden, and that resist your efforts to put them out of awareness? The thoughts, feelings, or urges may be embarrassing or make no sense. Tell me about them.

How do they affect you?

What have you done to combat the problem?

Have you ever had to perform counting, checking, or cleaning rituals to avoid feeling anxious? Some common examples are checking the clock to ensure that the alarm is set, checking the stove to be certain that the gas is turned off, or double-checking that a door or window is locked. Tell me about it.

Has the need to perform these rituals interfered with your functioning?

In what ways?

Have you ever been unable to leave your home without returning to check on something?

Are you unusually fearful of contaminating others or of being contaminated by them?

Do you tend to horde things? Are you unable to throw things out, even when they have no sentimental value?

When do you feel compelled to count, check, or clean?

Phobias

Have there ever been any places, activities, or situations that you avoid or dread because you experience unbearable anxiety when you are in those places or situations or doing those activities?

Have you ever been afraid to leave your home or apartment by yourself?

Are you able to drive alone, through tunnels, or across suspension bridges?

Do you avoid or dread public speaking for fear that you will humiliate yourself or make a fool of yourself?

Has eating in public ever been a problem for you?

Are you reluctant or unable to use public lavatories?

Are you reluctant or unable to ride subways or elevators?

What makes those situations especially difficult for you?

Have you ever had or feared having a panic attack in any of those places or situations?

Substance-Related Disorders

Have you or anybody close to you ever felt that you have had a problem with drugs or alcohol? Tell me about it.

Has the use of alcohol or drugs ever interfered with your functioning at school, at work, or in relationships?

Tell me about your drinking habits. When do you drink? Every day? What do you tend to drink? How much? Do you ever get drunk? How often? Have you ever had blackouts? Do you ever drink in the morning? Have you ever woken up with the shakes (hand tremors)? Have you ever found yourself unable to stop drinking? Has drinking ever gotten you into trouble with the law?

Do you use recreational drugs other than alcohol? Have you ever? What? When? How much? What effect did it (they) have on you? Has anybody in your family ever had a problem with alcohol or drugs?

See Chapter 7, Alcohol and Substance Abuse Disorders, for additional examples.

Cognitive Disorders

Patients with significant cognitive impairment frequently demonstrate their difficulties with orientation or memory early in the evaluation. The patients, their relatives, or their friends may have cited loss of memory or disorientation in the chief complaint. Milder degrees of impairment are more difficult to detect without a formal neuropsychological assessment. The initial manifestation of cognitive brain dysfunction may be a "personality change." When the history or mental status suggests a cognitive brain disorder, the interviewer can use questions such as the following to identify patients who should be referred for neuropsychological testing:

Have you noticed or have others told you that you've not been yourself lately, that you've been acting strangely or out of character? Tell me about it. What have they said?

Have you recently had any problem with your memory?

Have you been misplacing or losing things more frequently?

Have you been forgetting appointments lately?

Have you gone places and then found yourself unable to remember why you were there?

Have you found yourself losing track of the time of day or the date?

Have you found yourself somewhere but were unable to identify where you were?

If the answers to the above questions suggest that a cognitive brain dysfunction is present, the following questions should be asked to obtain additional information:

You (or "Your spouse" or "I") have been concerned about your memory. Let me ask you some questions to clarify whether there is a problem. I am going to ask you to recall three things for me after five minutes. First, I will tell them to you. Then I want you to immediately repeat them to me, so that we can be sure that you heard them correctly. After five minutes, we'll see how many you remember. (The novice psychiatric interviewer will find it useful to remember that this assessment will be more demanding and meaningful if the patient is asked to recall three different types of items, such as Philadelphia, red chair, and the number 10, rather than three items of the same type.)

Subtract 7 from 100 and continue to subtract 7 from whatever number is left ($100 - 7 = 93 - 7 = 86 - 7 = 79$, etc.). Repeat the following numbers forward: e.g., 1749, then 28391, then 618492, etc. (A person should be able to repeat seven numbers forward.) Repeat the following numbers backward: e.g., 1826 becomes 6281. (A person should be able to repeat four or five digits backward.)

What is similar about an apple and an orange? What is similar about a table and a chair? (These are tests of the capacity for generalizing.)

What do the following proverbs mean? A rolling stone gathers no moss. People who live in glass houses shouldn't throw stones. (These are tests of the capacity for abstraction, but their utility is limited by factors of intelligence and cultural background.)

All of these tests of cognitive function may be affected by many factors, including a decreased level of concentration, poor motivation, a high level of anxiety, poor proficiency in English, or a wish to thwart the interviewer. They can provide only presumptive evidence of cognitive dysfunction, and this suspicion must be confirmed by additional formal testing. It should be noted that many patients without cognitive brain dysfunction complain of memory loss (e.g., patients who are depressed or are taking antidepressants). Such patients are greatly relieved when they do well on the above questions.

Psychosis

Patients are considered psychotic if they are hallucinating or manifesting evidence of delusional thinking or a formal thought disorder (i.e., loosening of associations, neologisms, blocking, or word salad) (see also Chapter 4, Schizophrenia and Other Psychotic Disorders). By the end of the interview, a psychotic patient with a thought disorder will usually have demonstrated it, especially during discussions of emotion-laden subjects. Some delusions will surface spontaneously or in response to open-ended, nonspecific inquiries, especially the bizarre and acute delusions suffered by patients with impaired insight or judgment. However, in many instances, delusional thinking becomes apparent only in response to specific questions. If it is appropriate, the patient can be asked about delusions directly:

When you've been under pressure, has your mind ever played tricks on you?

At such times, have you found yourself having ideas or thinking things that later did not make sense to you, such as that somebody was trying to harm you or that you had an illness even when doctors had told you that you didn't?

Have you ever felt that you had unusual, almost magical powers or that you could perform virtually superhuman feats?

For some other patients, it is best to elicit evidence of delusional thinking indirectly (i.e., by means of a series of increasingly pointed questions): Has anyone been talking about you behind your back? Anyone whom you know? What have they been saying? Have they or anybody else been out to get you?

If a patient reports difficulties with others: These people seem to be giving you a very hard time. Have you ever felt that anyone was trying to harm you?

Questioning with regard to hallucinations requires judgment and tact. Patients who have reported using psychedelic drugs can be asked if they have ever had auditory or visual hallucinations while using drugs. It is a natural point of entry then to ask if they have ever experienced auditory or visual hallucinations at any other time. Another way of asking about hallucinations is to say, "Have you ever found yourself, under stress, having odd or unusual experiences that you don't have at other times?" Some patients, especially those who have reported hallucinations in the past, can be asked directly about such symptoms.

Eating Disorders

Has your weight ever dropped so low that you required hospitalization or that your health was affected?

What was your lowest weight?

Describe a typical binge for you.

When do you tend to binge?

Have you ever taken ipecac to make yourself vomit?

How do you induce vomiting?

How frequently do you vomit?

Have you ever vomited or had diarrhea to the point where your potassium level was low?

How many enemas do you give yourself per day?

How many laxatives do you take per day?

Personality and Personality Disorders

Personality can be defined as an individual's characteristic ways of feeling, thinking, and behaving. During a psychiatric evaluation, all of a patient's behavior forms the basis for assessing personality. The following two questions are particularly helpful in affording the interviewer insight into a personality: (1) How would you describe yourself as a person? (2) How would you describe the people who are most important to you? The way in which patients answer these questions may indicate whether they function on a neurotic, borderline, or psychotic level of personality organization. Psychotic patients, for example, may become disorganized in the face of such a personal question, which requires capacities for self-reflection and abstract thinking. Borderline patients, who extensively employ denial and splitting as defense mechanisms, will provide "all good" or "all bad" descriptions of themselves and others. On the other hand, neurotic patients characteristically employ more "mature" defense mechanisms, such as repression, intellectualization, and reaction formation. They are able to describe themselves and others as real people who have positive, negative, and potentially contradictory personality features.

The following questions should shed further light on a patient's personality:

What do you do for fun?
Describe for me in great detail a typical day in your life, including not only your actions but your thoughts and feelings.
What in life is most important to you?
Of what about yourself are you most proud?
What would you most like to change about yourself?
How would others describe you (people who know you well, casual acquaintances)?
Tell me about your relationships.
Of what are you most ashamed?
What are your hopes and aspirations?
What are your greatest fears?
Who are your enemies?
Tell me about how you handle your finances.

A crucial aspect of personality is **impulse control.** The following questions will provide information for reaching meaningful conclusions about this most important realm of behavior:

Do you have a problem with your temper?
Do you ever drive recklessly?
What do you do when you lose your temper?
Have you ever gotten into fistfights?
When you get angry, how do you express it? Physically? Verbally? Have you ever thrown things or broken furniture? What's the most damage you've ever done?
Have you ever attacked another human being? With fists? Fists open or closed? With a weapon? A knife or a gun? Do you own any weapons?
Have you ever been arrested?
What have you ever done that would or could get you into trouble with the law if it were to be discovered? (Of course, the answer to this question reflects on an individual's conscience or lack thereof, as well as on his or her level of impulsivity.)

Psychosocial History

No history is complete without the patient's account of his or her life story, which includes not only the sequential facts but also the plot that connects those facts. The interviewer is interested in who the main characters have been, what has motivated the

patient to do what he or she has done, and what conflicts, crises, or tragedies have been encountered by the patient.

Another important component of the patient's life history is the emotional history, which focuses on emotional reaction patterns and associated object relations. Information about basic object relations tendencies will enable the physician to predict the characteristic ways in which the patient will respond to physicians and treatment. It will most easily yield the Axis II personality disorder diagnosis.

The most useful technique for eliciting the psychosocial history is for the interviewer to say, "Tell me about your life" and then quietly listen, speaking only to encourage the patient to continue talking or to address resistances that the patient cannot overcome alone. The relevant life history is that which most clearly elucidates the patient's story. Because the interviewer does not know the patient's story or even the most relevant points of it, he or she cannot anticipate the direction it will take and should avoid closed-ended questions. With some encouragement, most patients find a way to tell their stories in their own words. In doing so, they reveal their characteristic modes of emotional adaptation, information that is necessary for planning treatment.

Another reason for disturbing the natural flow of the story telling as little as possible is that the form and organization of the story are important aspects of the patient's mental functioning and of the story itself. Many psychiatric illnesses affect not only the content of the story but the organization of the story, and this can be readily revealed in the telling if it is spontaneous.

With practice, obtaining the psychosocial history will become as comfortable for the physician as the more structured part. Even when time must be carefully rationed, the experienced physician can still elicit a tremendous amount of information with this technique and come to some sound conclusions. This is possible, in part, because the interview experience often increases the intensity of a patient's characteristic emotional processes, which become, therefore, more available to the patient's report and may even intrude on the patient's behavior. At various times, the interviewer must ask closed-ended questions to help the patient elaborate on certain crucial aspects of the story. The following questions can be used by the interviewer when it is necessary to supplement the patient's narrative.

What is your earliest memory?
Tell me about your childhood.
Where did you grow up, go to school, and so on?
Who lived at home? Parents? Siblings? Grandparents? What was your position in the birth order?
Were you ever separated from a parent for any length of time?
Did you have any operations or serious illnesses or accidents as a child?
How did you do in school (elementary school, junior high school, high school, college)? Were you

ever truant, expelled, or suspended? Any awards? Any difficulties? How were your grades? What your best and worst subjects?

Tell me about your friendships (in grade school, adolescence, college; in recent years).

Did you participate in sports or other extracurricular activities or organizations?

What past experiences do you recall with the most pleasure (most dread, etc.)?

What did your parents do for a living? How were things for your family financially?

Family History

It is imperative that the interviewer obtain the patient's family history because many psychiatric illnesses occur in several members of a family; therefore, the family history can be of prognostic and diagnostic significance (e.g., a patient whose same-sex parent committed suicide has a more serious risk for suicide than a patient whose family has no history of suicide, all other factors being equal). The following questions demonstrate one approach:

Has anybody else in your family ever been depressed (suicidal, had panic attacks, etc.), even if they were never diagnosed or treated as such?

Have any of your relatives ever taken tranquilizers, antidepressants, or other psychiatric medications?

To your knowledge, has anybody in your family ever committed suicide (had a breakdown, been hospitalized for psychiatric reasons)?

Has anybody in your family ever had a problem with drugs or alcohol?

Has anybody in your family ever been arrested or done things that would have gotten them into trouble with the law if they had been caught?

Has anybody in your family ever had a problem with his or her temper (driving recklessly, gambling, going on spending sprees, binge eating)?

Mental Status Examination

The interviewer will be able to collect much of the information required for a mental status examination while eliciting the history and observing the patient. Many of the questions described above in realms of psychopathology are equally useful in assessing current signs (the verb tense needs to be adjusted, e.g., "Are you currently hearing voices?"). Inexperienced interviewers will often regard the mental status examination as a completely discrete part of the interview. With experience, the physician is able to integrate the collection of information from the mental status examination with the history of the present illness, which relates most directly to the patient's current mental state. The one portion of the mental status examination that does generally require a separate introduction is cognitive testing. This part of the interview can be introduced with a neutral statement, such as, "Now I'm going to ask you

some questions to assess your memory and concentration." Cognitive testing and the mental status examination are discussed in Chapter 5, Cognitive and Mental Disorders Due to General Medical Conditions, and in Chapter 1, Case Formulation.

SAMPLE INTERVIEWS

The following excerpts are from interviews in which resistances arose from the beginning and proved to be major obstacles for the interviewers, who responded in different ways.

Interview One

Interviewer: "What brought you to the hospital? What was happening?"

Patient: "Well, my daughter died last winter, and she would have been 6 years old next week, and I began having flashbacks of memories of an incident that occurred at my neighbor's during my childhood. This morning, I was having that flashback. I felt as if I were almost reliving the experience and becoming a little girl." (The patient was visibly distraught and on the verge of tears.)

Interviewer: "Did the memory come after that?"

Patient: "I can't remember when I first remembered it."

Interviewer: "Did your daughter's upcoming birthday stir up these thoughts?"

Patient: "I don't know."

The interviewer began with characteristic, classic open-ended questions: "What brought you to the hospital? What was happening?" In response, the patient provided an emotion-laden answer about the death of her child and about flashbacks of traumatic memories, including an experience she had the morning of the interview, in which she felt almost as if she were a little girl reexperiencing a trauma. The patient's answer was a confusing hodgepodge about two subjects (i.e., thoughts of her daughter and flashbacks of traumatic memories). The nature and intensity of her feelings undoubtedly interfered with her ability to think and speak clearly.

It is logical that the interviewer would be puzzled and want to make sense of her initial reply. However, the interviewer inadvertently adopted a line of questioning that closed off the discussion. First, he asked who, what, when, where, and how questions, as a journalist would. This gave the patient the impression that the most important thing to the interviewer was finding out which came first, the flashbacks or the thoughts about her daughter. Then the interviewer asked the patient if thoughts of her daughter had triggered the flashbacks. He (rightly) suspected this connection. Yet the question elicited only an "I don't know." It would have been more empathic and productive for the physician to have shown an interest in what the patient was feeling. At this point, it was evident that the interview was going nowhere.

If the interviewer had considered his interaction with the patient from an object relations point of view, he may have been able to "diagnose" the cause of the stalemate. At the beginning of the interchange, the patient poured out an emotion-laden jumble of traumatic memories and flashbacks of tragedies she had experienced, including her daughter's death. The interviewer felt horrified, overwhelmed, or confused. He was either afraid to invite her to share her feelings with him, or he did not realize that her unexpressed feelings would prevent her from providing complete, meaningful answers to his questions.

Instead of exploring her feelings, he chose to sidestep them by asking a detail-oriented question about what came first: "Did the memory come after that?" This question was as unclear as the patient's answer to the preceding question, possibly because the interviewer was feeling so uncomfortable. The patient answered, "I can't remember." She was unable or unwilling to clarify the chronology for him. The interviewer's next query was an effort to create order out of chaos by trying to determine what had triggered her flashbacks. He shifted his focus from chronology to etiology: "Did your daughter's birthday stir up these thoughts?" She responded, "I don't know." The patient intentionally or unintentionally refused to answer the questions. She did not experience the interviewer's agenda of trying to determine the chronology and etiology as being the same as her agenda. Her priorities were to feel better by discussing her thoughts and feelings about her dead child and the flashbacks.

The patient's view of the interaction in terms of object relations is shown in Table 2–3. The patient seemed to be saying, through her nonanswers, that she did not want to assist the interviewer if he would not meet her needs.

The stalemate can also be viewed from the vantage point of ego psychology. In the patient's transference, she experienced the interviewer as an aloof, unempathic, unsympathetic, distant, unhelpful caretaker (i.e., like her father). She did not spontaneously and directly express her anger and resentment toward the interviewer when he failed to inquire about or empathize with her pain and suffering. Rather, her anger and resentment were expressed indirectly by her refusal or inability to answer his questions. This constituted a massive resistance to the progress of the interview (e.g., toward developing rapport, relieving suffering, and providing the interviewer with the required diagnostic information).

Interview Two

Interviewer: "Could you tell me a little bit about yourself? How old are you?"
    Patient: "Nineteen years old."
Interviewer: "You live where?"
    Patient: "Connecticut."
Interviewer: "Who do you live with?"
    Patient: "My mom and my sister and my three cats."
Interviewer: "Where is your father?"
    Patient: "He lives in Alabama."
Interviewer: "Your parents are divorced, then."
    Patient: "Yes."
Interviewer: "How long have they been divorced?"
    Patient: "About four years."
Interviewer: "How far have you gone in school?"
    Patient: "Freshman year of college."
Interviewer: "Have you ever been married?"
    Patient: "No."
Interviewer: "So you've always lived at home?"
    Patient: "Yes."

The physician began this interview with a brief attempt at asking an open-ended question: "Could you tell me a little bit about yourself?" But before she allowed the patient to answer, the interviewer added, "How old are you?" At that point, the interview took the form of a series of direct questions that required specific, factual answers.

In the first eight questions, the interviewer sought only demographic information about the patient and her family members (e.g., where they lived, with whom they lived, whether they were married or divorced). It is understandable that the physician wanted to know something about the details of the patient's life. Perhaps this interviewer initially felt more comfortable asking questions with predictable, unemotional answers. The interview deteriorated into one in which the patient compliantly provided brief answers to numerous "survey" questions. The questions effectively inhibited the patient from sharing what was on her mind, namely, her thoughts, feelings, fantasies, wishes, and fears.

At that point, the interviewer realized what had happened and "switched gears," reverting to an open-ended question about the chief complaint:

Interviewer: "Can you tell me what brought you to the clinic?"
    Patient: "For this clinic I've been on the waiting list six months."

The patient did not even actually answer the question. Nevertheless, the question and the reply

TABLE 2–3. Object Relations in Interview One: Patient's View

Patient (Self Representation)	Interviewer (Object Representation)	Prevailing Affect
Misunderstood, deprived of comfort	Aloof, unempathic	Hurt, disappointed
Withholding from interviewer in retaliation	Unsympathetic, intellectualized	Angry, sad

represented a turning point in the interview, because, at that juncture, the interview and the patient came to life. The patient rose to the challenge and accepted the invitation to open up by sharing her most pressing feelings. It was as if the patient (accurately) interpreted the open-ended question as an invitation to reveal what mattered to her and as a signal that the interviewer was now willing and able to let her talk and have some control over the topics discussed.

The interviewer immediately realized that the patient had let her in on her feelings toward the clinic (and, by extension, toward the therapist herself). The interviewer wisely continued to manifest interest by asking the patient to elaborate:

Interviewer: "You want to tell me about that?"
Patient: "I don't know. Maybe you can tell me. Six months is a mighty long time."
Interviewer: "So you clearly have a lot of feelings about it. Please tell me about them."

With this intervention, the interviewer took another giant step toward establishing a therapeutic alliance by explicitly inviting the patient to share her feelings.

These interviews illustrate two basic principles of psychiatric interviewing: (1) When experiencing strong feelings during an interview, the patient will "stonewall" (i.e., resist) the interviewer unless he or she is given an opportunity to express those feelings. (2) When a significant resistance to the progress of an interview manifests itself, it must be addressed before the interview can proceed productively.

CONCLUDING THE INTERVIEW

The interviewer should allow as much time as necessary to accomplish the goals of a particular interview. This depends on a number of factors, such as whether there will be other interviews, whether the situation is an emergency, and whether the patient requires hospitalization. How an interview should be concluded depends on the nature and purpose of the interview.

During the final portion of a **one-time interview** and in the **final interview of an evaluation**, the interviewer should ask the patient to provide any additional information that might help the interviewer to better understand the patient's situation. Even after a lengthy interview, a patient may make surprising revelations. The interviewer should then present a summary of the findings and treatment recommendations and give the patient time to react to what has transpired. If necessary, the interviewer should address any fears or alleviate any distress the patient might have so that the patient will be composed enough to leave with dignity. The interviewer should ask additional questions if the patient appears to be confused or angry. The patient should be encouraged to implement follow-up treatment plans and to call the interviewer if further questions arise.

In the **emergency room,** an interview cannot be terminated until these crucial questions have been answered:

Does the patient require an emergency medical workup?
Does the patient require hospitalization?
Is constant observation required because the patient is dangerous to himself or herself or others?
Does the patient require immediate treatment with medication?
Must family members, friends, or significant others be contacted or interviewed before the patient can leave?
What kind of follow-up treatment, if any, is required?

After the interviewer has obtained the necessary information, made the diagnostic and prognostic conclusions, and formulated a treatment plan, the interviewer should share the impressions and treatment recommendations with the patient and the patient's relatives and significant others, if appropriate. This should be done in a sensitive manner, employing language and concepts that the patient and other laypersons can comprehend. After allowing time for questions concerning diagnosis, prognosis, and treatment recommendations, the interviewer should conclude by reiterating the importance of follow-up evaluations and treatment, when indicated.

Physicians working in **outpatient settings** customarily are charged with the task of performing psychiatric evaluations that usually take two to five appointments of a specified length (e.g., 45–60 minutes). During the first appointment, the interviewer must obtain the following information:

Is the patient a danger to himself or herself or others?
Does the patient require hospitalization?
Can the patient be allowed to leave unescorted?
Can or should the patient be given medication on the spot or before the second session?

The way in which the interview will be concluded depends on the answers to these and other questions, as the following examples illustrate. To a patient requiring hospitalization, the interviewer might say: "Mr. Smith, Dr. Fisher and I want you to go into the hospital today. The antidepressant medication will help you but not for a few weeks. In the meantime, you need the support of hospital staff around the clock to help you resist those urges to kill yourself. We are in the process of notifying your family and contacting hospitals to see which one has a bed for you."

To a patient not requiring hospitalization: "Mrs. Jones, we've covered a lot of ground today, getting filled in about what you've been going through. But we'll need to know more about you and your problems before we can make our final treatment recommendations. So, why don't you come back next Tuesday at the same time for a second appointment?

After that visit, we'll have a better idea about how many additional times we'll need to meet. In the meantime, have you ever taken a sleeping pill? It is very safe if taken as directed and should help you feel better while we decide what other medication to prescribe, if any."

Selected Readings

Halleck, S. L. Evaluation of the Psychiatric Patient: A Primer. New York, Plenum Medical, 1991.

Kernberg, O. F. Early ego integration and object relations. Annals of the New York Academy of Science 193:233–247, 1972.

MacKinnon, R. A., R. Michels. The Psychiatric Interview in Clinical Practice. Philadelphia, W. B. Saunders Publishing Company, 1971.

MacKinnon, R. A., S. C. Yudofsky. Principles of the Psychiatric Evaluation. Philadelphia, J. B. Lippincott Company, 1991.

Nemiah, J. C. Foundations of Psychopathology. New York, Oxford University Press, 1961.

Shea, S. C. Psychiatric Interviewing: The Art of Understanding. Philadelphia, W. B. Saunders, 1988.

Trzepacz, P. T., R. W. Baker. The Psychiatric Mental Status. New York, Oxford University Press, 1993.

Ogden, T. H. On projective identification. International Journal of Psycho-Analysis 60:357–373, 1979.

Wallace, E. R. Dynamic Psychiatry in Theory and Practice. Philadelphia, Lea and Febiger, 1983.

SECTION II

PSYCHOPATHOLOGY

CHAPTER THREE

MOOD DISORDERS

DAVID A. KAHN, MD

Mood, or affective, disorders pose a significant public health problem because they are relatively common and their recurrent nature profoundly disrupts patients' lives. Depression alone afflicts one in eight Americans during their lifetimes and costs the U.S. economy more than $43 billion annually in medical treatment and lost productivity. Affective symptoms are frequently seen in general medical patients and cause increased use of medical services as well as increased rates of morbidity and mortality.

Fifteen percent of patients with severe mood disorders die from suicide. Overall, patients with mood disorders die at a younger age, especially from cardiovascular disease, than the general population. As a group, they also show impairment on numerous measures of social functioning, including measures of marital and occupational functioning. Mood disorders are associated with high rates of substance abuse, which may be a form of self-medication. About one-fourth of depressed patients and up to one-half of bipolar patients abuse alcohol or illegal drugs, percentages that are far higher than the general population rate of 8%. The rate of occupational, social, and physical disabilities of patients with mood disorders is equal to or greater than that for patients with other major chronic illnesses, including hypertension, diabetes, coronary artery disease, lung disease, gastrointestinal disease, and arthritis. Depressed patients spend more days in bed than patients in all of these categories, except for those with coronary artery disease. They become medically ill more often and show greater physical disability and sometimes higher death rates when ill. For example, the death rate six months after acute myocardial infarction is increased fivefold in depressed patients. Even patients with mild depression or just a few symptoms, who fall short of a formal diagnosis, tend to overuse general medical services.

It is essential for physicians to understand that mood disorders are neither normal variations in mood nor appropriate reactions to severe stress. These disorders are distinguished from normal moods and reactions by the duration and intensity of the patient's suffering and the degree of his or her functional impairment. It is also crucial for physicians, and the general public, to realize that mood disorders do not represent a failure of "will power" or some other form of moral weakness. Fortunately, there is a growing recognition that mood disorders are medical illnesses that require much more aggressive diagnosis and treatment by physicians. The publication of *Depression in Primary Care: Clinical Practice Guidelines* by the U.S. Agency for Health Care Policy and Research (1993) is testament to this awareness.

Door-to-door surveys conducted in the 1980s in many cities in the United States and in other countries yielded relatively uniform findings regarding the lifetime prevalence of mood disorders in the industrialized world (Table 3–1). The Epidemiologic Catchment Area (ECA) survey sponsored by the National Institute of Mental Health used structured interviews with trained interviewers to determine the prevalence rates of various DSM-III disorders in five U.S. communities. The point prevalence of depressive disorders in primary care practice settings is about double that of the general population. This may reflect the increased help-seeking behavior in depressed patients.

Despite the seriousness of mood disorders, only one-third of individuals with these disorders are properly diagnosed or treated. A recent study showed that although 20% of patients in primary care clinics were clinically depressed, only one-half had been diagnosed as such by a physician. Several factors might account for this underrecognition. First, in general medical settings, many patients with mood disorders present with unexplained somatic complaints, especially pain and insomnia, rather than a clearly stated emotional complaint. Second, it is sometimes difficult to distinguish mild mood disorders from the normal emotional ups and downs of life. Third, and perhaps most importantly for persons with severe mood disorders, is the stigma associated with mental illness. Most people—and sometimes even physicians—tend to fear, criticize, or ignore mental illness. In order to avoid the risk of being seen as weak, in their own eyes or the eyes of others, many individuals with mood disorders choose not to get professional help, preferring to "tough it out." This sometimes results in dire consequences for themselves and their families.

Most experts view the mood disorders as an etiologically diverse group of illnesses with symptoms appearing as the expressions of final common pathways. In time, it is hoped that researchers will

TABLE 3–1. Epidemiology of Mood Disorders

	Depressive Disorders	Bipolar Disorders
Prevalence	Major depression point: Men: 2.3–3.2% Women: 4.5–9.3% Major depression lifetime: Men: 7–12% Women: 20–25% More common in divorced or separated individuals Dysthymia lifetime: Men: 4.1% Women: 2.2%	Bipolar I lifetime: 0.4–1.6% Bipolar II lifetime: 0.5% More common in upper socio-economic classes Equal in sex and race High rates of divorce Cyclothymia lifetime: 0.4–1%
Age of Onset	Late 20s or 30s; childhood possible* May have much later onset† Individuals born after 1940 have greater rates and earlier onset than those born earlier.‡	Late teens or early 20s; childhood possible* Cyclothymia may precede late onset of overt mania or depression.
Family and Genetic Studies	Unipolar patients tend to have relatives with major depressive and dysthymic disorders and fewer with bipolar disorders. Early onset, recurrent course, and psychotic depression appear to be heritable.	Bipolar patients have many relatives with bipolar disorder, cyclothymia, unipolar depression, and schizoaffective disorder.
Twin Studies	Concordance in monozygotic twins: 59% for recurrent depression 33% for single episode only The concordance rates for monozygotic twins are 4 times greater than those found in fraternal (dizygotic) twins.**	Concordance in monozygotic twins: 65–80%

*Childhood symptoms may not always be the same as adult symptoms; children may exhibit greater behavioral disturbance (e.g., as seen in family and school settings) and less expression of emotional symptoms.

†Careful evaluation may reveal special psychosocial factors, contributing medical conditions, or subtle earlier mood disturbances that escaped diagnosis and treatment.

‡In a phenomenon known as the "cohort effect," individuals born after 1940 are developing unipolar and possibly bipolar disorders at greater rates and with earlier ages of onset than those born prior to 1940. This is not an artifact of diagnostic trends but seems to represent a genuine epidemiological change that might reflect effects of the post–World War II social or physical environment on the expression of these disorders.

**Limited data on twins reared apart from each other (and from their parents) tend to show comparable results, strengthening the interpretation that familial illness is from shared genes, not only shared environment. However, molecular genetic studies of chromosomal material from large families with affective illness have not yielded replicable findings of markers. Researchers have not yet been able to implicate specific chromosomes or markers or to choose between single or multiple gene models.

identify the specific metabolic and molecular genetic abnormalities that interact with psychosocial risk factors to produce mood disorders, as is currently being done for other diseases, such as cancer and heart disease. Such information would greatly increase the physician's ability to specify diagnosis and treatment. In the meantime, the physician must rely on wisdom and judgment in designing the treatment of individual patients, taking into account the many possible biological, psychological, and social factors.

NORMAL AND ABNORMAL MOODS

Mood can be understood as the amalgam of emotions that a person feels over a period of time. **Affect** is the way the mood is displayed. The effects of mood on a person's behavior are complex and widespread. A person's mood shapes his or her conscious attention, interest, and motivation and alters his or her unconscious autonomic functions, such as those related to vagal tone and sleep physiology. Many physical sensations, such as energy, pain, muscle tension, hunger, satiety, and sexual pleasure, have strong emotional components that influence the production and intensity of these sensations; thus, changes in a person's mood state can effect changes in his or her energy and behavior. Also, it is normal for seemingly conflicting emotions to coexist. For example, a medical student cramming late at night for an examination may feel worried, angry, and proud simultaneously or within a span of minutes; a person who undertakes an altruistic act such as jumping into an icy pond to rescue a child may feel a blend of love, terror, pain, and joyful relief.

Emotions interact to motivate a person to take action toward important goals. However, when certain emotions predominate and persist beyond their usefulness in motivating appropriate behavior, they become pathological. This is what happens in patients with mood disorders. For instance, if the medical student described above became persistently depressed after failing an earlier test and began to view himself as worthless and hopeless, was unable to eat, sleep, or concentrate, and felt suicidal, he would not be able to study effectively. Similarly, mood has a profound influence on **interpersonal behavior.** The extreme high or low moods of an individual often disrupt his or her relationships with others; in addition, such a person commonly finds it difficult to maintain constructive relationships, whether through bad luck or lack of skill, which adds to his or her emotional pain. For instance, the struggling student who can unwind with friends or join a study group has coping skills that may prevent frustration from becoming overt depression, whereas a student who does not have these skills and relationships may be at risk for sinking further into his or her depressed feelings.

Another feature of a mood disorder, in contrast with normal emotional experience, is **constricted emotional range.** Patients with mood disorders are emotionally stuck. Because one or more emotions persist more intensely and for a much longer time than circumstances warrant, these patients lose much of their emotional flexibility and, therefore, their ability to adapt to changing circumstances; they have trouble "shifting gears" within a normal repertoire of complex emotions. Normally, after a loss or victory, a person has intense feelings of sadness or elation for a time, which gradually give way to new responses to life's events. After the loss of a romantic attachment, for example, some depressed individuals repeatedly experience symptoms so severe that they are unable to get out of bed for weeks. In contrast, some persons experience a manic "high" and become so euphorically obsessed with a speculative investment strategy that they are unable to experience warning signs, such as self-doubt, and eventually suffer financial harm.

Mood is also closely linked to **cognition.** For example, research into memory physiology suggests that perceptions and thoughts (i.e., "what happened") are best retained when they are linked with strong emotional memories (i.e., "how it felt"). In persons with mood disorders, a filter is introduced that distorts normal perceptions and memories or subjects them to selective recall. This distorting process can dramatically affect a central aspect of mood, self-worth. **Self-worth** is one component of a person's permanent self-image that stretches over time and includes perceptions of past experiences, current abilities, and future plans. In patients with mood disorders, the perception of self-worth goes through unstable gyrations. Typically, a depressed patient views past events with undue criticism and guilt, feels worthless, and finds the world an unpromising place. In contrast, the manic patient glorifies his or her abilities and finds the world a stimulating place. Understanding the concept of self-worth and the distortions a person makes in his or her record are important when diagnosing and treating patients with mood disorders.

DIAGNOSTIC AND CLINICAL FEATURES

The mood disorders consist of the **depressive** and **bipolar disorders.** These disorders are recognized as distinct groups because they share both specific symptoms and features of longitudinal course. The predominant symptom of any mood disorder is **a distinct period of abnormally and persistently altered mood.** Bipolar disorder, also known as **manic-depressive illness,** is distinguished from depressive disorders by the occurrence of manic or hypomanic (i.e., mildly manic) episodes in addition to depressive episodes. Figure 3–1 schematizes these categories. Most depressed patients feel sad or "low," and most manic patients feel euphoric, irritable, or "high." Patients with mood disorders also experience **behavioral, cognitive, and psychomotor changes,** which may constitute their presenting complaints. The key feature of the longitudinal course of mood disorders is a tendency toward cycles of recurrence. Although some patients have only a single episode during their lives, most have multiple episodes, or recurrences, interspersed with periods of remission, known as **euthymia,** or normal mood. Some patients have chronic symptoms and never achieve full recovery. As with many other major medical illnesses, the prevention of relapse and the recognition of persistent low-grade symptoms between episodes are critical elements in the long-term treatment of patients with mood disorders.

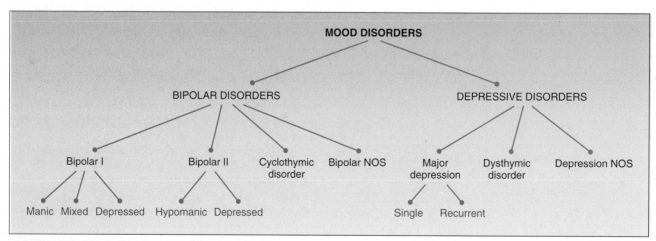

FIGURE 3–1. Mood disorders listed in the DSM-IV. Patients with bipolar disorders have had at least one episode of mania or hypomania. Bipolar I disorder consists of recurrences of mania and major depression or mixed states. Bipolar II disorder consists of recurrences of major depression and hypomania (mild mania). Cyclothymic disorder consists of recurrent brief episodes of hypomania and mild depression. Bipolar disorder not otherwise specified (NOS) is for partial syndromes, such as recurrent hypomania without depression. Depressive disorders include major depression, which is usually recurrent but sometimes happens as a single lifetime episode, and dysthymic disorder, which is mild depression lasting at least two years. Depressive disorder NOS is the diagnostic term for partial syndromes, such as patients who are depressed but have too few criteria for major depression and whose depression has been too brief for dysthymic disorder. (Adapted and reproduced, with permission, from Goodwin, F. K., and K. R. Jamison. Manic-Depressive Illness. New York, Oxford University Press, 1990.)

Major Depression

Psychological Symptoms and Signs

The DSM-IV criteria for major depression stipulate that a patient have a persistent, distinct feeling of depression or loss of pleasure or interest in usual activities that lasts for at least two weeks. In order to complete the diagnosis, at least four associated symptoms must also be present (Table 3–2). When describing a **depressed mood,** patients often say they feel sad or "blue," are "down in the dumps," have an ache or an empty feeling in their heart or in the pit of their stomachs, or feel the need to cry. **Sad feelings** are often accompanied by persistent lowered self-esteem or self-criticism. These are two features generally not observed in persons who are responding to external losses. In his classic paper "Mourning and Melancholia," Sigmund Freud noted that mourners feel sad over the loss of a loved one but any feelings of guilt or self-blame generally pass after several weeks. In contrast, depressed patients often feel sad because they experience a personal **sense of guilt or inadequacy.** Feelings of guilt or de-

fectiveness may not be related to a specific external loss and may be so irrational that they develop into a specific delusion. Typical examples are found in persons who believe that they have committed horrible crimes or are emitting foul odors that offend others. These feelings of guilt and shame may be quite subtle. Mood disorders occur in some people near retirement age. For example, someone who is facing the loss of the structure and social reinforcement provided by the workplace may begin to feel that his or her personal qualities (e.g., talents, vigor) and opportunities are actually declining.

Another aspect of sadness is intense pessimism and hopelessness. ➠ Depressed patients tend to discount the past, feel that the future has been destroyed, and find it hard to imagine they will ever feel well again. One graduate student, for example, became depressed about, and felt ashamed of, the difficulty she was having mastering a new field of study and withdrew from friends and pleasurable activities. Wondering whether she had deserved the Phi Beta Kappa award she received in college and feeling that she fraudulently presented herself to the world

---

TABLE 3–2. DSM-IV Diagnostic Criteria for Major Depressive Episode and Specifiers for Recurrent Major Depressive Disorder

Criteria for Major Depressive Episode

A. Five (or more) of the following symptoms have been present during the same 2-week period and represent a change from previous functioning; at least one of the symptoms is either (1) depressed mood or (2) loss of interest or pleasure. **Note:** Do not include symptoms that are clearly due to a general medical condition, or mood-incongruent delusions or hallucinations.

  (1) depressed mood most of the day, nearly every day, as indicated by either subjective report (e.g., feels sad or empty) or observation made by others (e.g., appears tearful). **Note:** In children and adolescents, can be irritable mood
  (2) markedly diminished interest or pleasure in all, or almost all, activities most of the day, nearly every day (as indicated by either subjective account or observation made by others)
  (3) significant weight loss when not dieting or weight gain (e.g., a change of more than 5% of body weight in a month), or decrease or increase in appetite nearly every day. **Note:** In children, consider failure to make expected weight gains
  (4) insomnia or hypersomnia nearly every day
  (5) psychomotor agitation or retardation nearly every day (observable by others, not merely subjective feelings of restlessness or being slowed down)
  (6) fatigue or loss of energy nearly every day
  (7) feelings of worthlessness or excessive or inappropriate guilt (which may be delusional) nearly every day (not merely self-reproach or guilt about being sick)
  (8) diminished ability to think or concentrate, or indecisiveness, nearly every day (either by subjective account or as observed by others)
  (9) recurrent thoughts of death (not just fear of dying), recurrent suicidal ideation without a specific plan, or a suicide attempt or a specific plan for committing suicide
B. The symptoms do not meet criteria for a Mixed Episode.
C. The symptoms cause clinically significant distress or impairment in social, occupational, or other important areas of functioning.
D. The symptoms are not due to the direct physiological effects of a substance (e.g., a drug of abuse, a medication) or a general medical condition (e.g., hypothyroidism).
E. The symptoms are not better accounted for by bereavement (i.e., after the loss of a loved one, the symptoms persist for longer than 2 months or are characterized by marked functional impairment), morbid preoccupation with worthlessness, suicidal ideation, psychotic symptoms, or psychomotor retardation.

Specifiers for Major Depressive Disorder, Recurrent

Specify (for current or most recent episode):
  Severity/Psychotic/Remission Specifiers
  Chronic
  With Catatonic Features
  With Melancholic Features
  With Atypical Features
  With Postpartum Onset
Specify:
  Longitudinal Course Specifiers (With and Without Interepisode Recovery)
  With Seasonal Pattern

as a promising scholar, she feared that her inadequacies would be exposed, at long last, in graduate school and that she would be unable to complete her degree. ◄■ **Anxiety** in the form of worry or outright panic often accompanies pessimistic thoughts. Fears of being alone and unable to cope are common. A triad of helplessness, hopelessness, and worthlessness often summarizes the feelings of sadness.

Depressed patients also lose interest and pleasure in things, people, or activities they normally enjoy (the second item in category A of the DSM-IV criteria). When the loss of pleasure is nearly total, it is referred to as **anhedonia.** Patients with anhedonia cannot be cheered by activities they normally enjoy, such as playing with their children or watching television. They feel apathetic and unenthusiastic; their interest in physical pleasures, such as food or sex, seems dull, flat, or deadened. In severe anhedonia, patients lose interest in their most important emotional ties to other people. ■► For example, a normally vibrant woman with a family and an active career became extremely withdrawn and unable to function when depressed. She stayed in bed as much as possible in a half-waking, half-sleeping state. Initially, she worried about getting her children to school on time and sharing household chores with her husband. Eventually, she became indifferent to these concerns and even stopped feeling anxious. In other words, she gave up. She left her job and felt that it was hopeless to maintain ties that might enable her to return later. Although she seemed to be emotionally dead, she was anything but indifferent to her inner state. She felt acute pain because of the distance she felt from the people who she knew she loved. Her growing sense of burdening them caused her to think constantly about suicide. Thus, the very relationships that had previously given her pleasure now gave her unbearable pain because she could not maintain them. ◄■

The DSM-IV criteria distinguish sadness from loss of interest, in part because some patients do not sense or articulate the former and focus more on the latter. In extreme cases, patients are unable to express sadness even though they have all of the other objective symptoms of depression. Patients with this condition, known as **alexithymia** (meaning without words for feelings) typically present with fatigue or other vague medical complaints. They say that they are distressed and have lost interest in their normal activities, which they often attribute to their physical problems, but also say that they do not feel sad or worthless. The presence of other symptoms of depression, such as sleep disturbance, confirms the diagnosis. Patients with **masked depression** may present with severe pain (often head, pelvic, abdominal, or low back pain) and deny that they feel sad although they suffer from loss of interest and other symptoms of depression.

Behavioral Symptoms and Signs

Behavioral, cognitive, and psychomotor symptoms may occur with depression. The **behavioral symptoms** are changes in appetite, sleep patterns,

energy levels, and sex drive. They are often referred to as "vegetative" symptoms because they reflect dysregulation of the simplest survival activities and are generally thought to be tied to endocrine, autonomic, and circadian functions of the hypothalamus. Patients with these symptoms usually experience decreased appetite, often with significant weight loss, and have trouble falling or staying asleep. **Terminal insomnia,** or waking early in the morning, is a classic symptom of depression. A patient with terminal insomnia typically falls asleep at the usual hour and then wakes up at 3:00 or 4:00 A.M. with a feeling of deep sadness, dread, or anxiety. In contrast, about 30% of depressed patients have "atypical," or "reversed," vegetative signs; they tend to sleep more than usual and have increased appetites. Physical fatigue or loss of energy occurs independently of sleep and nutritional problems and may occur equally as often with either insomnia or hypersomnia. A common symptom that patients may be embarrassed to report is a loss of interest in sex, which can be a source of frustration to them and their partners. Occasional menstrual changes and gastrointestinal complaints, such as nausea or constipation, are other symptoms of possible endocrine or autonomic dysfunction (they are not mentioned in the DSM-IV).

Cognitive dysfunction is another way in which patients are affected by depression. Patients may describe reading the same page over and over again or watching television without comprehending what they have read or seen. For example, a habitual reader of novels may be unable to read anything longer than a light magazine article, a student may find it hard to write a term paper, a homemaker may be unable to organize a shopping list, or a factory worker may continually make assembly line errors. Such patients may say that their minds are just not "working properly." This cognitive deficiency is usually not a simple matter of having distracting thoughts and, in some cases, is more serious than an inability to concentrate on the immediate task at hand. Patients may forget recent events or become disoriented as to the time of day. Some patients exhibit frank confusion and do not recognize people they know or are unable to find their way around. Severe confusion of this sort is called **pseudodementia,** although there is nothing "pseudo" about it. Rather, it is a transient dementia that resolves when the depression is treated. Elderly patients and patients with baseline central nervous system disease are more likely than others to suffer from transient dementia. In fact, depression is important in the differential diagnosis of any patient presenting with dementia characterized by withdrawal, apathy, or irritability.

Psychomotor activity is usually diminished in depressed patients. Their thoughts, speech, and motor movements are often subjectively experienced and objectively observed to be slowed down or retarded, sometimes to the point of muteness and virtual immobilization, which is known as **psychomotor**

retardation. Patients feel that their minds and bodies are "trapped in molasses." Basic social behavior, such as looking up at someone entering the room, may disappear; it may be difficult to get out of bed, get dressed, take medicine, attend to personal hygiene, see a doctor, or even make a telephone call to ask for help. Decisions as simple as which foods to buy at the grocery store can be overwhelming. If psychomotor retardation is combined with severe apathy, loss of appetite, and overall self-neglect, it can lead to medical emergencies, such as malnutrition, dehydration, electrolyte imbalance, and infections from decubitus ulcers or uncleaned urine and feces. Some patients exhibit **psychomotor agitation,** in which they have rapid, repetitive thoughts and speech and frenzied movements, such as unstoppable crying, pacing, or hand wringing. These patients often feel very anxious and hopeless, complaining sometimes of nearly constant panic. They may physically cling to others and unintentionally provoke angry responses in families and caregivers. When severe agitation and insomnia are present, it is important to consider the possibility of a mixed affective state, in which patients present with simultaneous symptoms of mania and depression (see Bipolar Disorder, below).

A patient's behavioral, cognitive, and psychomotor symptoms may vary considerably throughout the course of a day. Two special patterns of this variation are diurnal variation and mood reactivity, each of which is an important diagnostic feature of depression. With **diurnal variation,** the patient consistently feels worst at one particular time of the day (often, the morning). For example, a patient wakes up early, feels terribly low, and is unable to concentrate, eat, or talk to anyone. Gradually, he or she begins to feel better and, by evening, may feel almost normal. On the next day, however, the pattern repeats itself. With **mood reactivity,** the patient can be cheered up briefly or brought out of the depression by a "good" event, such as being praised by another person, eating a favorite meal, having a visit from a grandchild, or receiving romantic attention. Patients with true anhedonia are, by definition, unable to have a reactive mood. However, relative anhedonia is often seen in a patient with marked diurnal variation; although nothing can cheer the person up during the first part of the day, by evening, some glimmers of old interests and pleasures emerge.

Subtypes of Major Depression

Three subtypes of major depression—melancholia, atypical depression, and depression with psychotic features—are distinguished on the basis of additional symptoms. Two other subtypes—seasonal affective disorder and postpartum depression—are defined by particular precipitants in the course of the illness.

Melancholia is often seen in patients with severe depression. Historically known as the classic form of the illness, melancholia has sometimes been called endogenous because, more than other forms of depression, it tends to appear spontaneously without psychological precipitants. It is associated with significant neurobiological abnormalities that are thought to reflect a genetic or biological cause. Antidepressant medications are essential for patients with melancholia.

The diagnostic criteria for melancholia stipulate that the patient must exhibit severe anhedonia, a lack of reactivity to usually pleasurable stimuli, and three of the following features: a distinct quality of depressed mood that the patient says is different from feelings of disappointment or loss at other times, diurnal variation with a worse state in the morning, early morning insomnia, psychomotor retardation or agitation, and decreased appetite with weight loss.

Up to one-third of depressed patients suffer from **atypical depression,** having the atypical symptoms of increased sleep and appetite (reversed vegetative signs), extreme fatigue, and, sometimes, mood reactivity. Proper diagnosis of patients with atypical depression is important because of its preferential response to the selective serotonin reuptake inhibitor (SSRI) and monoamine oxidase inhibitor (MAOI) classes of antidepressant drugs over the tricyclic antidepressants (TCAs). Atypical depression can be every bit as severe and recurrent as melancholic or "typical" depression, and there is no reason to think it has any less association with neurobiological dysfunction than these forms. Reversed vegetative signs are also relatively common in bipolar depression (i.e., major depression that occurs during the course of bipolar disorder; see Bipolar Disorder, below).

Fifteen percent of depressed patients, including 25% of those admitted to hospitals, have the serious syndrome of **psychotic depression,** in which they experience psychotic symptoms such as delusions and (less commonly) hallucinations, in addition to the other symptoms of major depression. These psychotic symptoms occur only during periods of depression and not at other times in their lives. Psychotic depression tends to occur repeatedly in some patients, is more common in bipolar than unipolar depression, and is a major risk for suicide. Special treatment with a combination of antidepressant and antipsychotic drugs or with electroconvulsive therapy (ECT) is required. The delusions or hallucinations are mood-congruent or mood-incongruent, depending on whether or not the focus of the psychosis has a depressive theme such as guilt, pessimism, disease, or deserved punishment. Acute treatment is the same regardless of mood-congruency, although patients with mood-incongruent symptoms have a worse prognosis for resuming functioning. The delusions of these patients dramatically illustrate guilt, hopelessness, and a sense that one's self or the world has deteriorated beyond repair.

➠For example, one man, an accountant, believed that a minor addition error he had made 10 years earlier was responsible for the demise of his firm. Another man believed that he was "evil incarnate" and that his family would "pay the price for his misdeeds." A woman believed that she was literally burning in hell and had tactile hallucinations of feeling the flames. A man was convinced that he was unable to speak because he thought he had not spoken for a long time while he was depressed, even though he was able to speak loudly and clearly. A man thought his bowels were obstructed and that no food was able to pass through them. He was also convinced that he was going blind because an examination two years earlier had revealed a microembolus. He tried, therefore, to save his vision by not "using it up," believing that only a finite amount existed. He also believed that his landlord had infused his mind with toxic fumes, which caused his thinking to slow down.

An example of a mood-incongruent delusion is a woman who believed that she heard neighbors talking about her through the wall of her apartment, criticizing her diet and clothing. She felt angry and frightened but did not feel that she deserved this criticism or had done anything wrong to provoke it. ◄▬

One-tenth to one-third of patients with major depression experience **seasonal affective disorder,** which is a pattern of symptoms that emerge predictably in the fall or winter months. Lethargy and fatigue are common symptoms. Atypical features of hypersomnia and overeating are frequent but not universal. (Seasonal patterns may be seen in bipolar disorder, as well, especially in bipolar II disorder with hypomania in the spring or summer following a depressive episode during the winter.) Experiments have shown that the pattern is usually related to light deprivation and is more common in northern latitudes. In addition to the standard treatments for depression, phototherapy using bright lights that mimic the wavelengths of natural light, or trips to southerly locales, are uniquely effective in patients with seasonal depression. The disorder is thought to be caused by specific abnormalities of melatonin secretion and other biochemical aspects of the sleep-wake cycle and not by seasonal psychosocial stresses, such as the Christmastime "blues." ▬► One patient with this disorder, a 39-year-old novelist, presented in October with fatigue and writer's block. She described recent cravings for carbohydrates, weight gain, and an inability to cope with laundry, cleaning, and other household chores. Her history revealed a pattern of such difficulties occurring since college. Her symptoms had usually been evaluated as physical ailments, although tests for viral or endocrine disorders had been negative. She responded quickly to treatment with a bright bedside lamp set on a timer to go on early in the morning. ◄▬

In the weeks after they deliver a child, 10% of women experience mood disorders, most often a form of major depression called **postpartum depression.** Psychotic features rarely occur but are of grave concern. This condition is distinct from the transient "baby blues" that 50% of women experience for a few days immediately after giving birth. The enormous psychological and physical changes, including massive new responsibilities for both the mother and father, sleep deprivation, and hormonal fluctuation

have all been considered as possible causes of postpartum depression, but none has been definitively linked to it. Women with a personal or family history of affective disorders are at greater risk, which suggests an underlying vulnerability. The symptoms and treatment of postpartum depression (or mania) are basically the same as for other mood disorders, although special support may be needed for the mother and the family. Mothers with postpartum depression may feel especially guilty about not being able to fully respond to the needs of the newborn infant. In women thought to be at risk, antidepressants can be given or psychotherapy can be started immediately after the birth as a preventive measure. Hormonal treatments are ineffective. Postpartum depression often recurs after subsequent pregnancies and often heralds bipolar disorder.

The DSM-IV criteria for **dysthymic disorder** are shown in Table 3–3. Dysthymic disorder is a milder form of chronic depression, lasting for at least two

---

TABLE 3–3. DSM-IV Diagnostic Criteria for Dysthymic Disorder

A. Depressed mood for most of the day, for more days than not, as indicated either by subjective account or observation by others, for at least 2 years. **Note:** In children and adolescents, mood can be irritable and duration must be at least 1 year.
B. Presence, while depressed, of two (or more) of the following:
   (1) poor appetite or overeating
   (2) insomnia or hypersomnia
   (3) low energy or fatigue
   (4) low self-esteem
   (5) poor concentration or difficulty making decisions
   (6) feelings of hopelessness
C. During the 2-year period (1 year for children or adolescents) of the disturbance, the person has never been without the symptoms in Criteria A and B for more than 2 months at a time.
D. No Major Depressive Episode has been present during the first 2 years of the disturbance (1 year for children and adolescents), i.e., the disturbance is not better accounted for by chronic Major Depressive Disorder, or Major Depressive Disorder, In Partial Remission. **Note:** There may have been a previous Major Depressive Episode provided there was a full remission (no significant signs or symptoms for 2 months) before development of the Dysthymic Disorder. In addition, after the initial 2 years (1 year in children or adolescents) of Dysthymic Disorder, there may be episodes of Major Depressive Disorder, in which case both diagnoses may be given when the criteria are met for a Major Depressive Episode.
E. There has never been a Manic Episode, a Mixed Episode, or a Hypomanic Episode, and criteria have never been met for Cyclothymic Disorder.
F. The disturbance does not occur exclusively during the course of a chronic Psychotic Disorder, such as Schizophrenia or Delusional Disorder.
G. The symptoms are not due to the direct physiologic effects of a substance (e.g., a drug of abuse, a medication) or a general medical condition (e.g., hypothyroidism).
H. The symptoms cause clinically significant distress or impairment in social, occupational, or other important areas of functioning.
Specify if:
   Early Onset: if onset is before age 21 years
   Late Onset: if onset is age 21 years or older
Specify (for most recent 2 years of Dysthymic Disorder):
   With Atypical Features

years, with little or no remission during that time. A major change in psychiatry has been to view chronic, mild depression as a mood disorder. Traditionally, people with these symptoms have been viewed as having personality conflicts or frustrations leading to dissatisfaction with life. It is now clear that mild depression has many similarities with major depression in terms of family history, biological findings, and, probably, treatment response. Patients with dysthymic disorder (even those with just a few symptoms, who do not meet the full diagnostic criteria) have higher rates of medical problems and future episodes of major depression than do individuals with no depressive symptoms at all.

Patients with mild depression fall roughly into two groups: (1) those who have had depressive symptoms since childhood or late adolescence and are likely to develop major depression and never fully recover and (2) those who appear healthy when young but experience major losses, such as the death of a spouse or child, divorce, financial setback, or medical disability at some point in their adult lives and fall into a chronic state of demoralization that may meet the criteria for dysthymic disorder. A phenomenon traditionally called **depressive character** may be seen in individuals with chronic mild depression. Such patients may have long-standing personality difficulties, such as problems in maintaining consistent relationships or in living up to their full academic or occupational potential. They may be irritable, gloomy, and difficult to get along with, especially if they complain to those around them that their "glass is always half empty." Alternatively, they may be hardworking, eager to please, and apparently cheerful but also fearful of making mistakes and never satisfied with themselves.

Traditionally, dysthymic disorder has been treated with long-term psychotherapy or psychoanalysis. Currently, treatment studies are under way to determine whether the medication and short-term psychotherapies used in major depression would be helpful for dysthymic disorder. The newer antidepressant drugs, which do not have the serious side effects of earlier drugs, are being widely used in patients for whom drugs would not have been prescribed in past decades. This use of drugs for mild depression has increased among psychiatrists practicing long-term psychotherapy as well as among primary care providers who previously may not have been comfortable in diagnosing or treating depression.

Suicidal Thoughts and Behaviors

Suicidal thoughts and behaviors are the most lethal complications of depression (Box 3–1). They occur for many reasons, such as the wish to end the pain of the depressive illness or the need to communicate that pain to other people. In psychotic depres-

---

BOX 3–1. Determining the Risk of Suicide

Fifteen to twenty percent of patients with affective disorders severe enough to require hospitalization eventually die from suicide. There are other causes of suicide, but the most important predictor is a diagnosis of depression, which is present in 45–70% of individuals who kill themselves. A number of associated clinical features of depression increase the risk of suicide: melancholia, psychosis, extreme hopelessness, mixed or transitional bipolar states, substance abuse, marked impulsivity, a poor response to medication, definite plans for committing suicide, a history of prior attempts, and a family history of suicide.

Doctors and laypersons sometimes fear that asking about suicide will make it happen. In fact, the opposite is true. Patients may lose trust if they perceive doctors' reticence to discuss suicide as a sign of anxiety, much as they would not trust a surgeon afraid of blood. Talking about suicide, especially in detail with a new patient, can help defuse the intensity of the wish to act on it. Verbalizing the fantasy may bring some emotional relief, substituting for the act if suicide is seen as a way to communicate feelings patients believe are unappreciated by others. Patients test doctors to find out if they are willing to listen to the patients' most disturbed feelings. The best rule is to ask the patient calmly and directly: Do you have thoughts of hurting yourself? or Are you suicidal? are much better phrases than You wouldn't try hurting yourself, would you? or You're not suicidal, are you?

Some patients with underlying personality disorders use suicide threats in order to blackmail or manipulate others in their lives, including doctors. These tendencies become worse during depression and pose special problems that invite power struggles. Doctors must remember that such behavior is not personally directed at them but rooted in patients' chronic low self-esteem and transference expectation or wish of being punished by others. Doctors must therefore use caution in taking any steps that might gratify patients by showing anger or anxiety. For example, the doctor who is fed up with suicide threats and in turn threatens a patient with a punitive hospitalization may precipitate actual attempts because the patient now feels powerful at being able to control the doctor's feelings. Such a patient is also gratified by the message that such behavior elicits greater caretaking. In patients who characteristically use suicide as a means of interpersonal control, threats can sometimes best be defused if doctors say something almost paradoxical, such as the following: "The decision to live or die is yours; I realize that the control is in your hands. If you want my help, I can work with you on your problems." If the doctor is right, it is not unusual for the patient to say later that he felt he was being treated with empathy, like an adult instead of a child, and that this increased his trust.

Such statements cannot be made lightly, without a careful assessment that patients truly can exercise control. With melancholic or psychotic patients for whom suicide seems to be more a determined means to end intrapsychic suffering rather than a means of communication, the most empathic approach might be: "Right now, you feel that your life is not worth continuing. My view is that your illness has greatly impaired your capacity to judge accurately your own self-worth and the external circumstances of your life. I will do everything I can to insure your safety until the illness has been treated, because I think you will view your situation differently when you are well."

Techniques for interviewing and managing suicidal patients are discussed in more detail in Chapter 11, Suicide and Violence.

sion, the patient may believe that death is the punishment he or she deserves for being a bad person. Suicidal thoughts are common and are accompanied by varying degrees of intent. Many patients transiently wish that they would somehow disappear, not wake up from sleep, or be killed in an accident. Such feelings are referred to as **passive suicidality.** Others consider ending their lives more actively but feel restrained by attachments to loved ones or hopes of recovery. A more serious step than suicidal thoughts is a **suicidal gesture,** in which a patient takes potentially lethal actions to communicate despair to others, even though he or she does not definitively plan to die. Suicide gestures are often impulsive, such as swallowing pills after an argument in a setting that makes discovery likely in time for others to call an ambulance. The possibility of lethal miscalculation makes these gestures serious, however. Of greatest concern is the patient who absolutely wants to die and makes plans to do so. Although the patient's functioning may be impaired in most other areas of life, he or she may be able to make detailed plans for committing suicide, which may include consulting medical references on lethal drugs and making plans to obtain a horde of such drugs or making arrangements, for example, to carry out carbon monoxide poisoning. Selecting a date, such as an anniversary, or writing a suicide note is a clear warning of serious intent. In patients with recurrent depressions, a history of suicide attempts is a strong predictor of future attempts. Serious attempts are usually preceded by thoughts and plans for suicide. The physician must ask all depressed patients about past and present suicidal ideas, attempts, and plans (see Box 3–1, The Interview, p. 48, and Chapter 11, Suicide and Violence).

Bipolar Disorder

Patients with bipolar disorder have episodes of mania, hypomania, or mixed states and episodes of depression. The diagnosis of bipolar disorder is made as soon as a patient has one manic episode, even if that person has never had a depressive episode. Almost all patients who become manic will eventually experience depression; about 10% of patients diagnosed with bipolar disorder seem to have only manic episodes. The diagnostic criteria for major depressive episodes are the same for major depressive disorder (also referred to as unipolar depression) and bipolar disorder. The actual diagnostic term is bipolar disorder, current episode depressed. It is interesting to note that atypical depression and psychotic depression are seen more often in patients with bipolar disorder than with major depressive disorder. Two major subtypes of bipolar disorder are bipolar I disorder and bipolar II disorder. Bipolar I disorder refers to patients with mania and a depressive disorder, while bipolar II disorder refers to patients with hypomania and, specifically, major depression (Fig. 3–2). Cyclothymia is a milder illness in which patients have hypomania and mild depressive symptoms that are not sufficiently severe to warrant the diagnosis of major depression. Two other important DSM-IV subtypes, mania with psychotic features and bipolar disorder with rapid cycling, are reviewed below.

Mania

The mood in mania is characterized by **abnormal euphoria or irritability**. The DSM-IV criteria require one week's duration of mania (unless the patient requires hospitalization) (Table 3–4). Brief episodes of mania (e.g., lasting one or two days and erupting just before or after a major depression) may be important clues in diagnosing bipolar disorder and planning appropriate treatment. In manic states, patients have **inflated self-esteem** and heightened interest and pleasure in their surroundings. The world seems to exist for their gratification, and they grandiosely believe that nothing can or should stop them from obtaining what they want. Manic elation quickly blends with irritability if their desires are frustrated. Indeed, anger is often the dominant emotion. Along with the **grandiosity**, there is denial that anything is wrong. **Denial**, which is ubiquitous in most manic patients, is probably caused by the disease itself and represents a nearly delusional state. With some patients, it also seems to protect against a feeling of emptiness that lies below the grandiose visions.

The physical, or vegetative, signs in manic patients include **insomnia**, but unlike in depression, the need for sleep is decreased. Patients feel rested after fewer hours of sleep than they usually require. Unless the physician ascertains how much sleep patients normally need, they may deny having any trouble sleeping. Only with nearly total insomnia does exhaustion become a problem and, therefore, a cause for complaint. Patients often have **increased energy** for all kinds of activities, such as exercising, working late hours, and socializing. The busy pace may become unpleasant. Patients sometimes say this feeling is similar to a motor that is going too fast. Increased sexual drive and potency together with poor judgment may lead to grossly indiscreet behavior, which can become a source of extreme embarrassment later on. Manic patients, unlike depressed patients, have no specific appetite disorder. Some eat robustly and gain weight, whereas others neglect themselves generally, which may lead to weight loss and dehydration.

Manic patients have significant **cognitive changes**. They have racing thoughts, which are expressed as soon as they enter their minds; are easily distracted; and have difficulty focusing on tasks requiring prolonged attention. Typically, they exhibit a rapid or pressured speech pattern, frequently interrupt others, and have difficulty listening to others. One of the first indications that a patient is becoming manic may be a family member's observation (e.g., "She just won't shut up! Even when I go out of the room, she keeps blabbering on to herself. No one else can get a word in edgewise."). In order to get

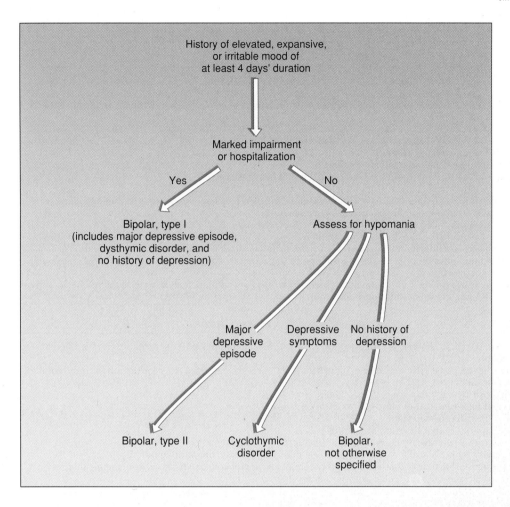

FIGURE 3–2. Assessing for mania and hypomania.

other people to listen to them, such patients may make excessive use of the telephone, and their monthly phone bills may double or triple. Although manic patients are often humorous, their humor tends to bore listeners after a while. They can also erupt into anger, especially if people attempt to ignore them or argue with the points they are trying to make. As the illness becomes severe, the thoughts of manic patients become disorganized and skip rapidly among topics that often have little relationship to each other. This decreased logical connection between thoughts is termed **flight of ideas** (e.g., "Sure, I'm not sleeping. The cars and taxis blew their damn horns all night. You know, I was even late to work because all the cabs were backed up again."). Two other types of speech—clang association and word salad—are characteristic of manic patients. **Clang association** (which gets its name from the German word for "sound") occurs when words are used only for their phonetic sound and not their meaning (e.g., "I got on the bus, I got busted, musted, rusted, like it was Russia!"). **Word salad** is bizarre, incoherent, fragmented speech that is indistinguishable from the speech produced by the thought disorder seen in acute schizophrenia (see Chapter 4, Schizophrenia and Other Psychotic Disorders).

Increased motor activity and agitation that are visible to observers are also characteristic of manic patients. Although motor activity may be purposeful at first (e.g., cleaning the house or getting to places in a hurry), it deteriorates into inappropriate or disorganized actions, such as pacing, fighting, and other behavior. **Manic delirium** occurs when extreme cognitive and psychomotor agitation are accompanied by disorientation, garbled speech, and chaotic behavior. In this condition, which may be thought of as the counterpart to the pseudodementia found in depression, patients may not be able to care for themselves. Their self-neglect can lead to exhaustion, dehydration, and even death.

Many manic patients behave in impulsive ways: Spending sprees, extravagant traveling, sexual affairs, risky business ventures, and so on are the hallmarks of their social dysfunction. Catastrophic ruin may result from the combination of patients' disordered mental attributes (e.g., grandiose plans, rapid thinking, markedly increased sex drive, and denial) and their high level of physical energy that translates ideas into action. Marriages, jobs, lifetime savings, and reputations may be lost. When evaluating manic behavior, it is crucial to obtain a baseline history of the patient's usual patterns of social, sexual, and financial behavior. This information is necessary because the patient may deny that he or she is behaving abnormally. Also, recognition of a mood disorder may be delayed in some patients who have the re-

TABLE 3–4. DSM-IV Diagnostic Criteria for Mania and Hypomania

Criteria for Manic Episode

A. A distinct period of abnormally and persistently elevated, expansive, or irritable mood, lasting 1 week (or any duration if hospitalization is necessary).
B. During the period of mood disturbance, three (or more) of the following symptoms have persisted (four if the mood is only irritable) and have been present to a significant degree:
   (1) inflated self-esteem or grandiosity
   (2) decreased need for sleep (e.g., feels rested after only 3 hours of sleep)
   (3) more talkative than usual or pressure to keep talking
   (4) flight of ideas or subjective experience that thoughts are racing
   (5) distractibility (i.e., attention too easily drawn to unimportant or irrelevant external stimuli)
   (6) increase in goal-directed activity (either socially, at work or school, or sexually) or psychomotor agitation
   (7) excessive involvement in pleasurable activities that have a high potential for painful consequences (e.g., engaging in unrestrained buying sprees, sexual indiscretions, or foolish business investments)
C. The symptoms do not meet the criteria for a Mixed Episode.
D. The mood disturbance is sufficiently severe to cause marked impairment in occupational functioning or in usual social activities or relationships with others, or to necessitate hospitalization to prevent harm to self or others, or there are psychotic features.
E. The symptoms are not due to the direct physiological effects of a substance (e.g., a drug of abuse, a medication, or other treatment) or a general medical condition (e.g., hyperthyroidism).
   Note: Manic-like episodes that are clearly caused by somatic antidepressant treatment (e.g., medication, electroconvulsive therapy, light therapy) should not count toward a diagnosis of Bipolar I Disorder.

Criteria for Hypomanic Episode

A. A distinct period of persistently elevated, expansive, or irritable mood, lasting throughout at least 4 days, that is clearly different from the usual nondepressed mood.
B. During the period of mood disturbance, three (or more) of the following symptoms have persisted (four if the mood is only irritable) and have been present to a significant degree:
   (1) inflated self-esteem or grandiosity
   (2) decreased need for sleep (e.g., feels rested after only 3 hours of sleep)
   (3) more talkative than usual or pressure to keep talking
   (4) flight of ideas or subjective experience that thoughts are racing
   (5) distractibility (i.e., attention too easily drawn to unimportant or irrelevant external stimuli)
   (6) increase in goal-directed activity (either socially, at work or school, or sexually) or psychomotor agitation
   (7) excessive involvement in pleasurable activities that have a high potential for painful consequences (e.g., engaging in unrestrained buying sprees, sexual indiscretions, or foolish business investments)
C. The episode is associated with an unequivocal change in functioning that is uncharacteristic of the person when not symptomatic.
D. The disturbance in mood and the change in functioning are observable by others.
E. The episode is not severe enough to cause marked impairment in social or occupational functioning, or to necessitate hospitalization, and there are no psychotic features.
F. The symptoms are not due to the direct physiological effects of a substance (e.g., a drug of abuse, a medication, or other treatment) or a general medical condition (e.g., hyperthyroidism).
   Note: Manic-like episodes that are clearly caused by somatic antidepressant treatment (e.g., medication, electroconvulsive therapy, light therapy) should not count toward a diagnosis of Bipolar II Disorder.

sources to compensate for any financial damage. Family and friends often "bail out" manic patients whose indiscretions are mild. ⇒ For example, a divorced woman who was living on her savings planned an affordable vacation within the United States. She became manic shortly before her departure date. When her flight was canceled for mechanical reasons, she exchanged and upgraded her ticket for one to Paris, arrived there with no hotel reservations, spent $5,000 in a few days, and had to call her distraught but wealthy brother to wire money for a return flight. The woman's doctor knew nothing of this until the woman's worried son called after seeing his mother a few weeks later. ⇐

Mania With Psychosis

About one-third of manic patients are psychotic. As in depression, the psychosis is classified as **mood-congruent or mood-incongruent** based on whether it focuses on themes that are consistent with the manic state. Psychosis usually develops after earlier manic symptoms have begun to escalate, but it may precede the full manic syndrome by one or two weeks, serving as a warning sign. For example, whenever he was about to enter a manic phase, a patient who had a recurrent delusion that he was Jesus Christ would start to grow a beard; it was a sign that he was transforming into the Messiah.

The most typical mood-congruent manic themes are related to grandiosity, which may take a euphoric form (e.g., a patient imagining that a celebrity is going to marry him or her or believing that he or she possesses answers to the great problems afflicting humanity). For example, during the Persian Gulf War of 1990, many manic patients attempted to contact President Bush with their military plans for a rapid victory. Such grandiose delusions of being on a special mission are classic in manic patients, and it is important to inquire about them specifically. Grandiosity can also take an extremely hostile, paranoid form in patients who think others envy them or want to kill them because of their greatness. This grandiosity is in marked contrast to psychotic depression, in which the patient fears punishment for being bad. The euphoric and paranoid forms of manic grandiosity are often combined. One man believed he was the "godfather," that he had been hospitalized for his own safety, that the movie *Godfather Part 3* was about him, and that, when the movie was released, the Mafia would pick him up at the hospital in a limousine so he could attend the gala benefit premiere.

The behavior of psychotic manic patients can be extremely bizarre and violent toward others, whereas in suicidal psychotic depressive patients, the destructive behavior is directed toward the self. One psychotic manic patient, thinking she was a messenger of God, threw her cat out of a fifth floor window in order to observe the biblical injunction to "sacrifice one small beast" to the Lord. Mood-incongruent delusions are also seen, as in the case of a woman who believed that the colors of traffic lights had been altered from the usual red, green, and yellow. As with depression, patients with mood-incongruent delusions have poorer outcomes in terms of ability to function socially even after the psychotic and mood disorder symptoms have resolved.

Rapid Cycling Subtype

Rapid cycling refers to distinct, sustained periods of mania, hypomania, or depression occurring at least four times a year. The cycles may be alternating sequences of highs and lows or frequent brief bouts of repeated depressions or manias, with only occasional excursions into the opposite pole. Rapid cycling bipolar II disorder is a common pattern. Between episodes, rapid cycling patients may have full, partial, or no recovery. Patients with no intervening recovery are said to be in **continuous cycling** and are very ill indeed. Rapid cycling is disabling because patients find it hard to carry out sustained activities. It is difficult to treat and may be initiated or made worse by antidepressants. Rapid cycling is more common in women and in patients who previously have had multiple bipolar episodes. Patients who experience mood changes over the course of hours or a day are usually considered to have mixed disorders, although the term **ultrafast rapid cycling** has also been used. Whether mixed and rapid cycling states are part of a continuum or are distinct states is unclear.

Mixed States

Mixed states are confusing mixtures of mood and behavior that appear to be "out of synch" with one another. These states can be defined in two ways. According to the DSM-IV, a diagnosis of a mixed mood disorder can be made only if the patient meets all of the diagnostic criteria for mania and major depression simultaneously. By this strict definition, only about 10% of hospitalized patients with mood disorders have mixed states. Less strict definitions specify that only some of the criteria for depression and mania must be met; with such definitions, as many as 50% of hospitalized bipolar patients could receive the diagnosis of a mixed state.

Patients in this broader group tend to have a condition called **dysphoric mania,** which is characterized by a sad, tearful mood, often with suicidality, and motor and cognitive signs of mania, such as irritability, pressured speech, racing thoughts, insomnia, and excessive energy (described by patients as an unpleasant "wired" feeling). Psychosis is also common in mixed states.

Recognition of mixed states is especially important because patients with this condition respond more slowly to standard treatments for pure mania and tend to become worse if treated with antidepressants. Mixed states may occur at various times during a patient's mood cycle. They may be discrete episodes that occur as the predominant type of mood cycle that an individual experiences; they may be a particular stage during a manic episode, usually occurring after the episode has been going on for a while and the patient's functioning has deteriorated; or they may be a transitional phase in a cycle that is going from depression to mania or vice versa. Mixed states are associated with a high risk of suicide, perhaps because they often combine a depressed mood with a high capacity for physical activity.

Hypomania

Hypomania requires fewer of the DSM-IV diagnostic criteria than mania (see Table 3–4). The difference is a matter of degree, especially in regard to the level of functional impairment. Patients with hypomania are usually able to carry out their daily tasks at work or home and are generally not ill enough to require hospitalization. People around them notice that they are behaving differently than usual, however. The unusual behavior is sometimes rather likable, especially if the mood is upbeat. Hypomanic people are energetic and can be goal-directed and well organized in their performance at work and at home. Enhanced creativity, sexual capacity, and leadership ability are not unusual. If all activity is pleasurable, the condition does not come to the attention of a doctor. Many bipolar patients view hypomania as a silver lining and resent its being taken away through treatment. Their heightened cognitive and sensual alertness combined with the increased energy creates a feeling of being superhuman. Phrases like "I've never felt so good before in my life" are typical and should raise the physician's concerns, because, as the syndrome escalates, social and occupational catastrophes may occur. The silver lining usually gives way to depression or escalates to a destructive "high." Typically, the patient's expression of grandiosity combined with increasingly unrealistic ideas leads others to begin questioning the judgment of the hypomanic person. Euphoria soon changes to argumentativeness; social or financial failures begin to occur; and the patient either crashes into despair and depression or pushes the level of denial upward into full-blown mania.

Hypomania may last for months or for only a few days before a full-blown manic episode develops. Patients with repeated cycles often exhibit peculiar changes in behavior, or the so-called **hypomanic alert,** at the start of an episode. ➡ For example, a schoolteacher who was usually depressed, extremely shy, and scrupulously honest, secretly shoplifted shoes over several weeks with no other change in her behavior. She was eventually arrested and then developed a full-blown manic syndrome. A judge dismissed the charges when her psychiatrist testified that the woman had also shoplifted in an isolated period during a manic episode 20 years earlier. ⬅ Psychosis is rare in hypomania but may be seen as a preliminary phase, before the full manic syndrome has developed (as in the case of the patient above who thought he was the Messiah), and is occasionally seen in chronic hypomania.

Cyclothymia

Patients with cyclothymia alternate between mild depressions that are similar to dysthymia, but of short duration, and hypomania. The cycles are continuous and last for several weeks to several months. Rarely do these patients complain specifically about the highs and lows they experience. More commonly, patients will complain only of being depressed at times, not realizing that they have been hypomanic at other times. Spouses or relatives may be aware of the pattern, but they are rarely consulted because the patient's symptoms are generally mild. The physician often makes the diagnosis after observing patients for a period of time and discovering that the "well" periods are, in fact, highs. Another reason that cyclothymics seek treatment is for help with personality or social problems. They often have trouble maintaining relationships, get into arguments when they are hypomanic, and perform inconsistently at school or work. Mild mixed states may also be a part of this illness. In these patients, the predominant complaint is chronic depression with fluctuating sleep patterns, and agitation and irritability. Cyclothymia is sometimes a precursor to the more classic form of bipolar I or bipolar II illness. States resembling cyclothymia can also be seen during incomplete recovery from these more severe disorders.

Course of Illness

Patients with bipolar disorder and the more recurrent forms of unipolar depression have a striking pattern of **decreasing cycle lengths** or increasing frequency of episodes over time. The average well period between the first and second episodes is three to five years. The cycle becomes progressively shorter, reaching a mean of less than one year after the sixth cycle (Fig. 3–3). Some patients develop classic **rapid cycling** (i.e., four or more episodes per year) as the illness progresses over time, entering a prolonged downhill course. This deterioration is not inevitable, however. There is also a group of patients who have a pattern of rapid cycling in which

episodes cluster for a period of time and then diminish in frequency. The shortening of clusters may reflect neurobiological alterations in the brain caused by each successive episode, which result in a lowering of the threshold for illness (see Sensitization and Kindling Theory, below).

Patients with mood disorders are more sensitive to emotional stress. The major life events with which most people are able to cope may precipitate episodes of illness in vulnerable patients. Psychosocial stress is especially likely to trigger episodes early in the course of the illness. These disorders often begin when patients first assume adult responsibilities, such as leaving home, going to college, getting married, or starting to work. While this association may be a coincidence, there is good evidence that these events are **precipitating stresses** for early episodes. After several recurrences, episodes are more likely to occur spontaneously, "out of the blue," with no apparent precipitants. These are autonomous, or endogenous, episodes (Fig. 3–4). Seasonal patterns that are not related to psychosocial stress may be apparent (e.g., wintertime depressions related to decreased light exposure). Precipitated and autonomous episodes are symptomatically indistinguishable, and individuals may, of course, suffer both.

Major Depression

Episodes of major depression usually begin gradually. If untreated, they last an average of six months. Chronicity is a problem: About 20% of depressed patients remain depressed for up to a year or more and 12% for as long as five years. Risk factors for **chronicity** include a strong family history of depression, older age, longer length of illness before treatment is sought, alcoholism, medical illness, disability of spouse, or multiple recent deaths of family members. Fifty to seventy percent of patients with major depression have recurrent episodes in their lifetimes. In those who have more than one episode, the average number is five to six. There is some tendency for individuals to have a recurrence of similar symptoms during each episode, such as melancholia, atypical symptoms, or psychosis, but there are many exceptions. Dysthymic disorder may be a prodrome to major depression, and it is likely to be associated with a less complete recovery after the major depression is over.

Mood disorders beginning after approximately age 50 years are considered **late-onset disorders** and may have causes that are different from those beginning earlier. Recent studies with magnetic resonance imaging (MRI) suggest that many patients with late-onset mood disorder may have early subcortical cerebrovascular disease. Special psychosocial factors, such as loneliness, poverty, and general medical debilitation, may be contributing factors. Physicians should remember, however, that depression is not a normal or commonplace reaction to the events associated with aging but instead is an illness requiring appropriate diagnosis and treatment. Similarly,

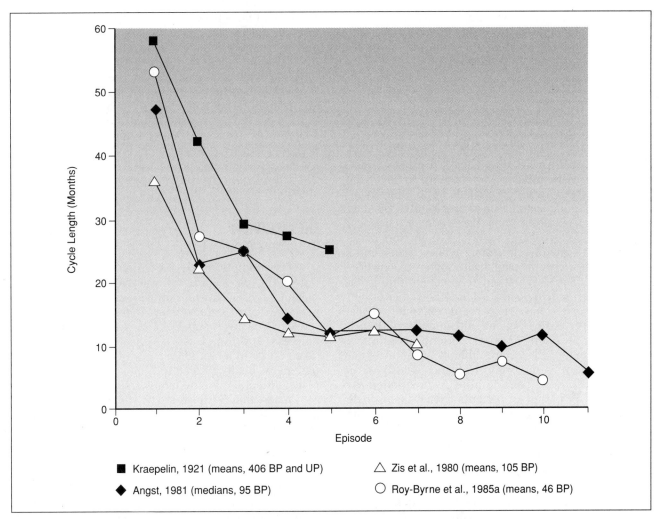

FIGURE 3–3. Relationship between cycle length and episode number. Episodes in recurrent mood disorders occur closer together over time. The first and second episodes are often several years apart. By the fifth episode, the average cycle is less than one year. References are to studies that collected data in unmedicated patients over long periods of time. BP = bipolar; UP = unipolar. (Reproduced, with permission, from Goodwin, F. K., and K. R. Jamison. Manic-Depressive Illness. New York, Oxford University Press, 1990.)

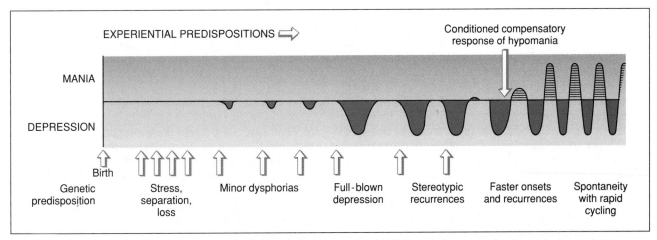

FIGURE 3–4. Natural history of recurrent mood disorders: integrated model. Genetic factors and early environmental stress may predispose an individual to develop a mood disorder. Early episodes are likely to be precipitated by environmental stress, while later episodes are more likely to occur closer together and occur spontaneously, without precipitants. (Reproduced, with permission, from Post, R. M., D. R. Rubinow, and J. C. Ballenger. Conditioning, sensitization, and kindling: implications for the course of affective illness. *In* Post, R. M., and J. C. Ballenger, eds. Neurobiology of Mood Disorders. Baltimore, Williams and Wilkins, 1984.)

adolescents with suicidal thoughts are often suffering from major depression rather than experiencing an understandable reaction to social pressures felt from parents, friends, and schools.

Bipolar Disorder

Patients with bipolar disorder are more likely than those with unipolar depression to have an abrupt "switch" of mood overnight or over a few days. This change is very striking when it occurs: Patients behave normally one day and wake up the next day with rapid speech, altered behavior, and other symptoms. An episode is sometimes precipitated by sleep deprivation, resulting from travel or psychosocial stress, but it often occurs without explanation. Manic episodes are usually shorter in length than depressive episodes. Chronic mania, although rare, has been described. (The first patient to receive lithium had been manic for five years.) Almost all patients with bipolar disorder have **recurrent episodes**. These episodes are more frequent and numerous than in unipolar depression. In some patients, continuous major and milder cycles are difficult to separate and count. Variation in the proportion and severity of the types of episodes is considerable. As mentioned earlier, about 10% of bipolar patients have little or no depression and can be considered to have unipolar mania. Patients with cyclothymia may remain stable or develop a full-blown bipolar disorder.

The degree of recovery between bipolar episodes varies. While many patients are able to resume normal activities within several weeks to months, approximately 40% of patients have significant social dysfunction for up to two years after an episode. Earlier in this century, before drug treatment became available, it was estimated that about one-third of bipolar patients had chronic, mild mood disturbances (i.e., dysthymia, hypomania, cyclothymia, or irritability). Current estimates of chronic symptoms are lower, although undertreatment of mild symptoms is widespread. Patients with mixed states, rapid cycling, mood-incongruent psychosis, or schizoaffective disorder (persistence of psychosis after resolution of mood symptoms; see Differential Diagnosis, below); substance abuse; or poor family support have an increased risk of **chronicity**. Even when they are apparently free of chronic symptoms, many patients have difficulty in functioning in work and family roles for long periods of time after episodes. ➡ For example, one woman recovered fully from a two-year stretch of rapid cycling with frequent mood-incongruent paranoid delusions. She repeatedly failed makeup college courses, however, and could not sustain friendships because of persistent shyness and a vague tendency to make other people feel awkward around her. She remained slightly odd. It took her several years to regain enough cognitive capacity, social skill, and general self-confidence to complete her degree and begin dating. ⬅ Neurobiological deterioration from repeated episodes may play a role in this phenomenon. Another factor is the demoralization

the patient feels from having his or her life constantly interrupted by the illness, which derails friendships and interrupts education, work, and other activities.

Even so, most patients with bipolar disorder function well, especially when they are taking the proper medication. Individuals with bipolar disorder are thought to be overrepresented among successful individuals in the arts and other professions. This association is often attributed to mild, productive hypomanic characteristics, such as increased sociability, energy, and imagination, but it could be a result of the enhanced creativity or perceptiveness associated with an inherently greater range of moods.

THE INTERVIEW
Depressive Disorders

The depletion felt by a depressed patient requires the physician to be active in the interview, making greater efforts than with most other kinds of psychiatric patients to draw them out and show interest. Because the patient may feel so indecisive, helpless, and hopeless, the physician also needs to take charge in a tactfully firm way, urging a doubting patient to begin medication, making clear follow-up plans, and enlisting the family's support.

When taking the history, the physician should ask the patient about normal patterns as well as variations, in order to **establish a baseline** and to accurately assess persistent changes. For example, it is helpful to ask patients with insomnia what time they usually get into bed, how long it takes to fall asleep, and the time at which they usually wake up and then get out of bed. It may emerge, for example, that a man who says he still gets up at his usual time of 7:00 A.M. in fact wakes an hour or two earlier than usual and lies in bed trying to fall back asleep until the alarm goes off. It is also important to note physical illnesses, the taking of sleeping pills and other medicines, and intentional weight loss diets that might mask or mimic vegetative signs.

Depressed patients are more trusting and cooperative when they feel that other people are accepting, and not criticizing, them. Because these patients tend to feel blame from themselves and others, creating an atmosphere that feels accepting to them takes special skill on the part of the physician. Encouragement, however, can be a two-edged sword; while common sense might lead a physician to point out the positive aspects of the patient's life, for example, the patient may interpret this optimism as a belittlement of his or her perceptions. Simplistic reassurances (e.g., "Don't worry. There's nothing to be that upset over.") cause the patient to feel misunderstood and rejected. An empathic way to provide encouragement is to show appreciation of the patient's position by saying, for example, "I understand how bleak everything seems now. It must be very hard for you to believe that you once felt capable of functioning as well as you must have, judging from everything you have accomplished in the past."

Several factors cause a depressed patient to provide an **incomplete or inaccurate history**. First, the cognitive or physiological aspects of depression may interfere: Poor memory and concentration prevent recall or organization of historical material, and psychomotor retardation may make it difficult to convey information within the time allotted for the interview.

Second, the psychological aspects of depression can alter communication. The individual may have distorted perceptions of reality on either a subtle level or at the more overt level of psychosis. For example, a patient whose depression is causing him to perform poorly at work may falsely assume that the boss has always disliked him. The physician may learn from a spouse, however, that the patient is a well-liked, hard-working employee whose lowered performance and failure to appreciate his normal strengths are in fact distinct features of the current depressive episode. Another psychological reason for misreporting is shame, which may cause patients to conceal their true concerns. ➡ In a severe case, it took a ward staff several weeks to discover that an isolated patient was having an olfactory hallucination that he smelled bad and the related delusion that he was therefore being shunned by the other patients. In a more subtle example of shame, an elderly man said he was depressed because he felt guilty about continuing to socialize after his wife became ill. In an interview with the couple, it was clear that his wife was relieved that her husband was staying active. The interviewer then focused more profitably on the man's own fears of aging and loss, brought on by seeing his wife deteriorate. He had thought at first it would have been selfish to bring up his own concerns. ⬅

In overcoming these conscious and unconscious sources of distortion in the interview, it may be useful to invite **family members** to attend. As a rule, the patient should be present when the family gives the history. Occasionally, however, a relative may want to speak privately with the physician, especially when the patient has told the relative a "secret," such as a suicidal or psychotic thought. The physician should meet alone with the relative and listen to what he or she has to say and then encourage the relative to meet with the patient and physician and express his or her concerns openly to them. This open communication usually reassures the patient of the family's concern and helps avoid infantilization of the patient. This joint meeting can also be a time for the physician to help the family understand that urging the patient to cheer up, even when it is done with the best of intentions, may have the opposite effect, especially if the patient already feels like a burden to the family.

The depressed patient's feelings of hopelessness, helplessness, and worthlessness tend to produce **characteristic responses to the physician**. The patient's initial reaction to the physician is based upon the guilt he or she feels about the depression and the expectation of being criticized or even punished for being depressed. One defense mechanism is to try to please the physician by underreporting symptoms so as not to seem like a complainer. Another reaction is to feel rejected and become inwardly angry. Some chronically depressed patients are paranoid just below the surface and are prone to struggle against expected punishment or other mistreatment. The physician who listens carefully may hear a subtle litany of disappointment toward previous physicians who have failed to cure symptoms, especially somatic ones such as unexplained pain or insomnia. The patient may use words of praise and thanks while at the same time using body language to criticize (e.g., saying, with raised eyebrows and a sigh, "All the doctors were very nice, but they were always in a rush to get me out, and, after all those pills, I still have stomach cramps.").

Helplessness and hopelessness may drive the patient to become very dependent on the physician, simultaneously expecting to be rescued while fearing that the physician, like the patient, is powerless to turn the tide. This conflict is often helped by discussing the contradiction openly; to begin such a discussion, the physician might say, "I realize how much you want me to help you feel better and how scary it feels to hear me say it may take several weeks to gauge the effectiveness of the medicine. I can assure you that these are normal reactions in depression and that when it is all over, you'll look back on it like a bad dream." Another aspect of this reaction is the patient's fear that any expression of anger will cause the physician to think the patient is bad.

Physician responses often reflect the symptoms and defenses of particular patients. Compliant or excessively polite patients may make the physician feel omnipotent and elicit rescue fantasies, while more pessimistic or angry patients may cause the physician to feel threatened or helpless. The physician's awareness that such reactions are a defense against opposing feelings helps to form a more complete picture of the patient's problems. ➡ For example, a 54-year-old woman came to the office and readily described the recent onset of classic symptoms of major depression. She was extremely well-groomed, polite, cooperative, and apologetic for crying. She repeatedly leaned toward the doctor and asked, "Do you think you can help me?" and complimented him on his understanding and sympathy. She began to describe a number of deprivations she had experienced in her life, beginning with child abuse and culminating in the recent refusal of her husband to pay for her to complete the college degree that she had foregone early in their marriage. Only when the physician began to probe her feelings of disappointment in important caretakers did she describe detailed plans to asphyxiate herself in the family garage, stating that "No one really cares what becomes of me." Had the physician assumed that the history was complete because of the patient's ingratiating, eager-to-please manner, he might have prematurely reassured her that everything would be all right. His initial pleasure in the patient's superficial faith in him would have prevented his discovery of her concealed, enraged wish for a vengeful suicide. ⬅

This example also illustrates the reactions of a patient who is deeply ashamed of her angry feelings. The anger of depressed patients is often unconscious and is sometimes based on actual past life experiences of being punished or hated for expressing it. Prematurely urging patients to admit they are angry often makes them feel even more guilty and depressed. Usually, a better interview technique is to gradually explore situations in which assertive behavior is appropriate, using actual examples from the patient's current life or even his or her behavior with the physician. For example, once when the physician was late for a session, the patient described above smiled and actually apologized for making him rush. It proved fruitful for the physician to ask her in a sympathetic way if she had trouble acknowledging annoyance whenever she was inconvenienced.

Bipolar Disorder

The relationship between the patient with bipolar disorder and the physician can easily become adversarial for a number of reasons. One reason is that manic or hypomanic patients often seek treatment at the insistence of others, not because they feel that they are suffering. A history from family and friends is usually necessary.

Mania

The psychopathology of mania blocks communication, and patients seem to exert control through such means as humor, uninterruptible speech, sexual seductiveness, or flashes of intimidating anger. The physician may be able to breach this "wall" by exploring problems associated more with depression, such as underlying low self-esteem. This approach allows the patient to express pain and ask for help without feeling embarrassed. ➡ For example, a manic businessman was spending excessive time and money working on a home computer writing a program he thought would finally make him rich. He became enraged whenever his wife questioned the wisdom of buying more and more expensive equipment and staying up all night, disrupting the entire family. He finally admitted to his physician that he was terrified of losing a major account and was desperate to find a realistic way to embark on a different career. He was then able to see the danger of his current behavior and agreed to take medication and work seriously on the problems facing him. ⬅

Having a conversation with a patient who is suffering from severe psychotic or thought-disordered mania is virtually impossible. It is usually counterproductive for the physician to spend time arguing with or countering the illogical thinking of the patient. A manic patient will try to **manipulate** the physician by bargaining to avoid limits or by forcing the physician to agree with any shred of truth in the patient's stories, in order to reinforce denial of his or her illness. Giving in to these manipulations only harms the pa-

tient and prolongs the destructiveness of the episode. The interview should be ended abruptly if the frustrated manic patient explodes into rage. For safety reasons, another person should be present when a patient with severe mania is being interviewed. It is dangerous to believe that one can "talk down" an agitated manic patient. Medication or involuntary hospitalization is often necessary. Studies show that many recovered manic patients retrospectively agree with such steps to restrict their freedom.

The manic patient's reaction to the physician is often the reverse of the reaction found in depressed patients. Depressed patients want help and they fear that the physician may not give it, whereas manic patients want to be left to their own devices and are afraid the physician will interfere. Objection to treatment is the rule, with the exception of the grandiose patient who wants to have the physician listen to and admiringly or sympathetically agree with him or her. The physician's responses to the patient may be marked by ambivalence. With hypomanic patients, it is often tempting to believe the patient's version of a situation, especially if the patient is in the coherent, euphoric, self-confident stage of the upswing. The physician may even vicariously enjoy the patient's enhanced energy and optimism. At the same time, the physician may respond to the patient's controlling and even frightening behavior with anger, fear, or frustration. It is understandably common to feel annoyed with severely resistant manic patients and to wish that they would get into deeper trouble, as though to teach them a lesson. Such a reaction should not, of course, be acted upon. The frustrated physician should remember that the patient has an illness and should not be blamed but helped, even if treatment must begin involuntarily.

The following techniques may engage patients more readily. It is helpful to find some aspect of patients' subjective inner worlds with which the physician can feel agreement and sympathy. The physician should listen to patients tell their side of the story, without interrupting too much, and should avoid challenging the patients' delusions or inconsequential distortions of history or common sense. Confrontations should be chosen extremely carefully (e.g., when it is important to determine if thoughts are delusional by offering possible alternatives). The physician should try to find areas in which patients' perceptions are reasonably accurate (e.g., understanding significant precipitants, such as family problems, serious losses, or life changes like leaving home for the first time). Any hints of depression or low self-esteem can help open the door. For some patients, it may be appropriate to ask whether they are "trying to reach for the stars" because they are unhappy with life as it exists. Another area of **common ground** can be psychophysiological symptoms. Insomnia, racing thoughts, and overactivity eventually lead to feelings of exhaustion, and patients often admit to wishing that they could get some rest or "slow down the motor."

These guidelines are not needed in all cases. Many patients who have experienced previous bipolar episodes learn to recognize mania as dangerous to their well-being and form lasting partnerships with their physicians. Occasionally, first-time patients who are particularly self-observant and appreciative of stable, organized life patterns become frightened by the changes brought on by mania and actively seek help. (See Interviewing Guidelines Box.)

Hypomania

Mild, productive hypomania deserves special comment. A small number of bipolar patients feel their best and function optimally during hypomanic states. They sometimes prefer to receive no medication and would rather keep the physician on "standby." They are willing to pay the price of episodic dysfunction in exchange for enhanced energy, sociability, sexuality, and creativity. The response of the physician is complex. He or she may feel envy or frustration, which may lead to power struggles with the patient, or may vicariously enjoy the patient's exploits and seek to prolong the symptomatological state. Physicians who treat such patients flexibly (perhaps undermedicating them, according to some standards) need to pay careful attention to their own feelings in order to act in the best interests of their patients. The physician who gets a "charge" out of a superenergetic patient may not act quickly enough to recommend an increased dosage of medication, for example. On the other hand, when a patient knows that the physician understands how enjoyable hypomania can be, the patient may accept help more readily and may be willing to collaborate with an "early warning system" (which often involves the family), in order to prevent extreme mood swings.

Interviewing Guidelines

- Be active and directive with a depressed patient.
- Try to strike an empathic balance with a depressed patient, using encouragement but avoiding simplistic reassurance.
- Avoid premature exploration of a depressed patient's unconscious anger.
- Avoid unnecessary confrontations with a manic patient.
- Try to elicit from the manic patient a complaint about some symptom or subjective experience with which the patient wants help.
- Ask all mood disorder patients about usual patterns in order to establish a baseline.
- Family members of patients with mood disorders can be useful sources of information and support.

DIFFERENTIAL DIAGNOSIS

During **normal bereavement** following the death of a loved one, symptoms may be as severe as those found in major depression, with two important exceptions: Low self-esteem is not pervasive (although there may be guilt about the relationship with the deceased person), and symptoms begin to resolve naturally within two to three months. Psychosis is absent, except for culturally influenced symptoms, such as briefly seeing the image or hearing the voice of the deceased.

Mood symptoms occur in most psychiatric illnesses and must be differentiated from the symptoms of the mood disorders.

Signs of depression are seen in patients with **adjustment disorder with depressed mood** after an identifiable psychosocial stress has occurred. These patients experience a spell of depression too mild or brief to be considered either major depression or dysthymia.

Although patients with **mood disorder due to a general medical condition** (previously called organic mood disorder) may appear to be suffering from depression or bipolar disorder, they have, instead, a neurological or medical condition (not including those caused by substance abuse) that directly alters brain function (see Chapter 5, Cognitive and Mental Disorders Due to General Medical Conditions). In general, patients with such disorders tend to lack the sustained changes in self-esteem that are seen in depression and mania, such as extreme feelings of worthlessness or overconfidence, and may show evidence of subtle confusion or dementia. Common structural and physiological medical conditions that alter mood are summarized in Table 3–5. When evaluating a new patient, the physician's primary task is to exclude an organic etiology by obtaining a thorough medical history and, if necessary, by conducting a physical examination and ordering laboratory tests. (The meaning of the word *organic* is an important semantic issue. Many patients with idiopathic mood disorders are thought to have neurophysiological defects that cannot be demonstrated at this time.)

Patients suffering from **dementias,** such as those caused by Alzheimer's disease, may also present with maniclike agitation or with depression. Cognitive and behavioral changes mimicking depression, such as apathy and loss of concentration, are more common than those that mimic mania, such as restlessness and combativeness. The medical evaluation is most important in elderly patients because they are at the greatest risk of having another illness. Although **"pseudodementia"** may be a sign of depression in elderly persons, this assumption should be regarded as a diagnosis of exclusion. The appearance of a late-life affective disorder, especially in patients with no family history of such a condition, suggests a medical etiology.

Schizoaffective disorder is a condition in which a patient is psychotic during an episode of a mood

TABLE 3–5. General Medical Conditions That Can Present With Mood Symptoms

Medical Conditions	Mania	Depression
Endocrine disorders		
Hypothyroidism		+
Hyperthyroidism	+	
Hypercalcemia		+
Addison's disease	+	
Cushing's disease	+	
Heart failure		+
Neurological disorders		
Multiple sclerosis	+	+
Alzheimer's disease	+	+
Stroke	+	+
Tumor	+	+
Temporal lobe epilepsy	+	+
Collagen vascular disease	+	+
Vitamin deficiencies		
B_{12}		+
Folate	+	
Malignant disease (especially of the lung and gastrointestinal tract)		+
Medications		
Sympatholytic antihypertensives	+	
Estrogen and progesterone		+
Excess thyroid hormone	+	
Adrenal steroids	+	+
Antineoplastics		+
Antiparkinson's	+	+

disorder but continues to have psychotic symptoms (i.e., hallucinations or delusions) for at least two weeks after the mood disorder has resolved. This persistence of psychosis during periods of more normal moods characterizes the disorder. Researchers debate whether schizoaffective disorder is actually a combination of two separate diseases, schizophrenia and a mood disorder; a severe form of a mood disorder; or a different disease altogether. In any case, this syndrome is often disabling and difficult to treat.

Generalized anxiety disorder and **panic disorder** can mimic depression. Patients show signs of worry, agitation, demoralization, and social withdrawal. Suicidal thoughts are also common in panic disorder. Depressed patients often have severe anxiety and sometimes panic attacks as part of their illness. There is a high rate of comorbidity with depression and all of the anxiety disorders.

In patients with **personality disorders,** feelings of sadness, despair, hopelessness, and low self-esteem are often apparent. Patients with borderline, histrionic, or narcissistic personality disorders are especially prone to acute bouts of depressed mood and suicidal threats or gestures. Maniclike, irritable hyperactivity and increased libido are also common. Episodes can usually be traced to psychosocial stressors and tend to resolve when external factors change. Patients with borderline personality disorder may use the word *emptiness* to describe their depressed feelings.

In contrast, a patient with a mood disorder may have healthy personality traits at the onset of the disorder, but these may seem to deteriorate as the mood disorder progresses. For this reason, the patient may appear to have a personality disorder when he or she is first seen by the physician. For example, a depressed person may become unusually dependent, or a hypomanic patient may become extremely manipulative or antisocial. To make the diagnosis, the physician must take a careful history to learn as much as possible about what the patient's personality was like before the onset of the affective symptoms. The physician should ask how the patient has dealt in the past with important stresses and developmental stages and how he or she interacted with other people. In general, personality disorders are characterized by long-standing, consistent features of social functioning, fantasy life, and patterns in relationships and attitudes, while mood disorders are characterized by a more abrupt change in mental and social functioning at the time the illness begins. Patients with mood disorders may report that they are no longer themselves. Research suggests that patients with mood disorders are no more likely to have a personality disorder than any person in the general population. Some patients have comorbid mood disorders and personality disorders and require treatment for both.

Patients with long-standing, mild mood symptoms, such as depression or irritability, which were thought to be caused by a personality disorder, may undergo a dramatic change in personality after treatment with antidepressant or mood-stabilizing drugs. These changes raise fascinating questions about the relationship between affective disorders and personality disorders and are of great interest to the general public. Physicians are often asked whether psychotherapy is necessary for certain kinds of ongoing life problems when medications such as fluoxetine (Prozac) can change so many aspects of the personality. Conversely, some patients feel that if antidepressants are pushed upon them too aggressively, areas of personal concern will be ignored. It is valuable to acknowledge some of the uncertainties and to discuss these issues openly when patients raise them.

Schizophrenia can resemble psychotic depression when patients have "negative symptoms" such as social withdrawal and cognitive decline and can resemble mania when patients exhibit grandiose delusions and florid agitation. Thus, the diagnosis of an affective disorder or schizophrenia may not be accurate if it is based on the symptoms present during a single cross-sectional period of an acute psychotic illness. A diagnosis based on a longitudinal evaluation is more reliable. A history of periodic psychotic illnesses with good return to functioning between episodes is more suggestive of an affective disorder, while a history of chronic or deteriorating functioning is more suggestive of schizophrenia. The family history can also help clarify the diagnosis. Finally, the diagnosis is sometimes based on the treatment response, either retroactively or pending the results of a "diagnostic" medication trial. For example, patients who respond well to lithium or who respond better to lithium than to antipsychotics are more likely to have bipolar disorder than schizophrenia.

Other psychotic syndromes, such as **delusional disorder, brief reactive psychosis, or schizophreniform disorder,** may resemble mania or psychotic depression. The main distinguishing factor between these disorders and mood disorders is that the patient's mood symptoms are not the most prominent feature of their illness. The physician must make a somewhat subjective judgment about this. The possibility of a mood disorder may be worth considering in patients with unexplained bouts of psychosis and good recovery between episodes, especially when there is a family history of mood disorder.

Substance abuse, which is a major problem in patients with mood disorders, affects about one-fourth of depressed patients and one-half of bipolar patients. Most patients view substance abuse as "self-medication" (e.g., they use alcohol to quell agitation or insomnia). However, substance abuse can cause or exacerbate affective symptoms. Acute intoxication with stimulants, such as cocaine, "crack" cocaine, or amphetamines, produces a "high" that is indistinguishable from hypomania, except that it lasts from only a few hours to a few days and is followed by exhaustion and, sometimes, depression. Chronic stimulant abuse or intoxication with phencyclidine (PCP, angel dust) may produce a continuous state that mimics mania with paranoid psychosis. Hospitalization is often needed to stop the patient from using the drug long enough for the physician to make a diagnosis. Use of such drugs by individuals with underlying affective disorders or schizophrenia may result in a prolonged exacerbation that does not readily abate after the drugs are stopped. Chronic alcohol abuse can cause feelings of depression, which may improve after several weeks of abstinence. Alcohol may also cause disinhibited behavior that resembles hypomania. Although this state is limited to the period of intoxication, if intoxication occurs frequently, it may produce diagnostic uncertainty. The patient's prolonged abstinence is necessary for the physician to make an accurate diagnosis. A person who is abusing alcohol and drugs may not comply with a regimen of prescription drugs, and this noncompliance may also precipitate depression or mania. Patients who abuse both alcohol and drugs are more difficult to treat and have a high rate of suicide. Alcohol is often used in suicide attempts and may be the factor that triggers impulsive, self-destructive behavior or that enhances the effects of an overdose of pills.

Children and adolescents with mood disorders pose special differential diagnostic problems because they may present primarily with behavioral problems at home and in school rather than with a clear, verbal description of their moods. Problem behaviors include withdrawal, sullenness, truancy, getting poor grades, and tantrums. Similar symptoms may occur in persons with learning disabilities, attention-deficit disorder, antisocial personality disorder, and substance abuse. Psychotic symptoms resembling schizophrenia are often prominent in early-onset bipolar disorder. It is often difficult to distinguish nonpsychotic symptoms from the extreme mood shifts and rebelliousness seen in teenagers or from children's reactions to parental conflicts. Expert assessment by specially trained child psychiatrists, which usually includes interviews with parents and teachers, is essential.

MEDICAL EVALUATION

The medical evaluation of patients with mood disorders includes obtaining a family history, conducting a physical examination, and ordering laboratory tests. The goals are to exclude mood disorders that are caused by a general medical condition and to ensure the safety of treatment with medications. The history and physical examination usually uncover any major systemic illnesses. For patients with depression or mania, the standard laboratory tests are screening for hepatic and thyroid function (including thyroid-stimulating hormone, or TSH); studies of electrolytes, calcium, and blood urea nitrogen and creatinine; a complete blood count; and a urinalysis. Urinary toxicological tests are done to screen for drug abuse. An electrocardiogram may be obtained in patients over age 40 years because of the cardiovascular effects of some psychotropic drugs. The following tests are not part of routine screenings but may be useful under certain circumstances: electroencephalography, brain imaging by magnetic resonance imaging or computed tomography, assays of cobalamin (vitamin B_{12}) and ceruloplasmin, and screening for collagen vascular disease. Ideally, the medical workup should be completed before treatment is initiated, but the clinical condition of the patient often requires that treatment begin as soon as possible. In younger patients who appear to be physically well based on the history and physical examination, it is usually unnecessary to wait for laboratory results before starting treatment.

ETIOLOGY

The biopsychosocial model is useful for understanding the etiology of mood disorders, as it is for other psychiatric and medical disorders. One of the main assumptions of this model is that both normal and abnormal human functioning are produced by complex interactions between a number of biological, psychological, and sociological factors. The psychological and sociological (psychosocial) factors include deprivations or losses experienced in childhood, overwhelming stresses or losses encountered in adulthood, poor social functioning, and distortions in thinking. Abnormalities in brain structure and functioning, which can be of genetic origin or result from trauma or disease, are biological factors that may be involved in the mood disorders by producing abnormal processing of the neurotransmitters as well as by affecting the neuroendocrine and chronobiological systems.

It is likely that the causes of mood disorders are multifactorial and heterogeneous. This conclusion is based on observations of diverse patterns of heredity, symptoms, course, and precipitating stresses. Furthermore, it has been difficult to match completely any biological or psychosocial variable proposed as causal with a distinct clinical group of patients. Instead, a variety of partial risk factors and correlations have emerged. There is another limitation in theories of etiology: When biological and psychosocial abnormalities are discovered, it is not always possible to tell whether they are the causes or the effects of affective illness. Furthermore, "downstream" or secondary effects may be either further contributors to pathological conditions or compensatory efforts of the body and mind to reestablish homeostasis. The reader should keep these caveats in mind as some of the causal theories are reviewed below.

Neurobiological Theories

According to neurobiological theories, mood disorders can be explained by fundamental disorders of the chemical and physiological functions of the brain. Until recently, neurobiologists have largely assumed that apparent relationships of psychosocial stress to mood disorders could be explained by biological vulnerability, much as osteoporosis predisposes to bone fractures. Indeed, it is exciting to anticipate that molecular genetics may eventually identify specific defects in cellular function that cause either spontaneous disturbances of mood or a vulnerability to decompensate under stress. At the same time, it is now recognized that neurobiology may offer crucial insights into the mechanisms whereby psychosocial experiences actually alter the brain at the cellular level in situations of early development and in adult life when there is neuronal plasticity. This enhanced biological model is thought to offer the best integration of epidemiological, social, and psychological data with modern theories of brain functioning, without oversimplifying the equation.

Neurotransmitter Hypotheses

Early biochemical theories of mood dysregulation focused on the neurotransmitter norepinephrine. Several decades ago, it was observed that some patients became severely depressed while taking reserpine, an antihypertensive drug known to deplete norepinephrine. Tricyclic antidepressants (TCAs) coming into use at that time were found to increase the concentrations of **norepinephrine** and another neurotransmitter, **serotonin**. It was hypothesized that decreased levels of these two neurotransmitters in the brain caused depression and that excess amounts caused mania. Efforts to prove this theory by measuring the amounts of these substances or their metabolites in cerebrospinal fluid, urine, blood, and brain tissues (at autopsy) have yielded inconsistent results. In addition, the effects of TCAs and other drugs on synaptic reuptake are almost immediate, while therapeutic effects take weeks to develop. While there is no doubt that these transmitters are related to mood disorders, research now focuses on their interactions with a variety of other brain systems as well as on abnormalities in the function or quantity of receptors for the transmitters. Currently, chronic abnormalities of neurotransmission are thought to result in compensatory but maladaptive changes in the brain's regulation of itself, both at the level of **presynaptic autoreceptors** that provide feedback and possibly in the synaptic structure itself. Antidepressant drugs begin a process in which cells readapt as their exposure to neurotransmitters changes. The readaptation requires altered synthesis of receptor proteins, which may take several weeks to have effects. Also of recent interest is the discovery that norepinephrine may be increased initially in severe depression, mimicking a pathologically prolonged "fight or flight" stress reaction. There is also recognition that certain clinical subtypes of patients may have different abnormalities. For example, there appears to be a fairly specific decrease in serotonin concentration and a compensatory increase in serotonin receptors in the brains of people who have committed suicide by violent means. There is also evidence of decreased serotonin in the cerebrospinal fluid of certain violent criminals. This observation has given rise to the notion that serotonin may play a role in impulsive or violent behaviors, as one piece of the larger puzzle of depression.

Neuroendocrine Hypotheses

The hypothalamic-pituitary axis has been of research interest because it provides a potential window through which higher regulatory centers can be viewed and because peptides in this region are also active in cortical areas and may affect mood directly. Thyrotropin release of thyroid-stimulating hormone has been one such area of focus, but the meaning of the abnormalities discovered is uncertain. The most striking neuroendocrine finding has been of **elevated serum cortisol** with loss of normal diurnal variation in its secretion. This finding has prompted some researchers to suggest a model in which depression is seen as the result of a stress reaction that has gone on for too long. Normally, cortisol rises transiently during stress, producing a state of hyperarousal that is temporarily useful to the organism. Hypercortisolemia can be traced to centrally increased corticotropin-releasing factor (CRF) and corticotropin (ACTH). There is also evidence of an increased adrenal mass in chronically depressed patients. Some researchers now speculate that elevated levels of CRF and ACTH, which were originally thought to represent a merely incidental effect of norepinephrine dysregulation, may be direct sources of depressive symptoms because they have receptors widely distributed in nonhypothalamic areas. Unfortunately, serum tests for hypercortisolemia are not sensitive or specific enough to be of clinical value in treating depression.

Chronobiological Theories

Sleep disturbance is an important aspect of depression and mania. Sleep patterns appear to be regulated by an internal biological clock or chronobiological center in the hypothalamus, hence the name. Studies of the sleep physiology of depression show specific **disruption of rapid eye movement (REM) sleep.** Artificially induced sleep deprivation is known to alleviate depression or precipitate mania in some bipolar patients. Because a number of neurotransmitter and hormone levels follow circadian patterns of activity, it has been suggested that the brain's control of these may be related to brain events in sleep that, if disrupted, lead to biochemical abnormalities, which affect mood. Such disruptions in sleep have also been linked to seasonal affective disorders and to light exposure. Seasonal changes in light exposure also trigger affective episodes in some patients, typically depression in the winter and hypomania in the summer in the Northern Hemisphere. The mechanism for this may involve retinal connections to hypothalamic nuclei that play a role in circadian regulation. It is generally useful to regulate sleep in manic patients; in fact, it now appears to have direct therapeutic effects.

Sensitization and Kindling Theory

Sensitization and the related phenomenon of kindling refer to animal models of recurrent affective disorders. In these models, repeated chemical or electrical stimulation of certain regions of the brain produces stereotypical behavioral responses or seizures. The amount of the chemical or electricity required to evoke the response or seizure decreases with each experience. When this reaction occurs with chemical stimuli, it is called sensitization; when it results from electrical seizure induction, it is known as kindling. In **kindling,** periodic spontaneous seizures occur after sufficient induction. These phenomena have been used as models to explain why, over time, affective episodes, particularly those seen in patients with bipolar disorder, recur in shorter and shorter cycles and more autonomously (i.e., with less relation to environmental precipitants). They suggest that the threshold for certain types of abnormal brain activity drops progressively with repeated experiences of that activity. The potential strength of these theories was first seen when researchers accurately predicted that the anticonvulsant drugs carbamazepine and valproic acid, which interfere with kindling, would have antimanic effects. More recently, it has been shown in animals that kindling causes permanent synaptic changes mediated by altered genetic transcription of important neuronal proteins. It is hypothesized that repeated affective episodes may similarly be accompanied by progressive alteration of brain synapses that lower the threshold for future episodes and increase the likelihood of illness.

The mechanism of **sensitization** may also be genetic encoding, the lasting alteration of gene expression as a result of a stimulus to the organism. Sections of the genome relevant to brain function are activated both by the sensitizing stress and by the animal's response to the stress. The result is learning, in the sense that long-term chemical and microanatomical changes in the brain cause lasting changes in behavior. Sensitization bears a key similarity to recurrent affective illness: infrequent, stress-precipitated episodes gradually change to more frequent, spontaneous episodes. Heritable factors in stress sensitivity and mood disorders could relate to the susceptibility of the gene to altered transcription of relevant proteins. Early life experience might play an important sensitizing role at a time in development when the brain is known to be more plastic; adult experiences that invoke conscious or unconscious memories of earlier stress could activate dormant neural pathways. Mirroring psychodynamic explanations, sensitization theory also suggests that mania may develop as a biologically overcompensated effort to regain equilibrium after depression, eventually becoming a conditioned response that may occur in the absence of depression.

Genetic Factors

Modern genetic studies using epidemiological samples validate the long-standing clinical impression that recurrent affective disorders tend to cluster in families. Relatives of patients with affective disorders are two to three times more likely to be ill than persons in the general population. Although families tend to aggregate in specific disorders along diagnostic lines (e.g., bipolar versus unipolar disorders), the overlap is considerable. Children of affectively ill parents are at especially high risk of developing several psychiatric problems. Up to 27% of children with one affectively ill parent become ill themselves, and many more develop personality or substance abuse problems. If both parents are ill, the rate of major affective illness in their children increases to 50–75%. Early identification of children at risk is an important research topic. The epidemiological evidence indicates that genetic vulnerability to mood disorders is somewhat greater with bipolar disorders than with unipolar depression. Studies of identical and fraternal twins also show impressive genetic links, which are somewhat greater for bipolar disorder than for unipolar depression (see Table 3–1). However, these studies do not show complete concordance in monozygotic twins, which indicates that environmental factors are involved in the expression of the disease. The pattern of inheritance is not mendelian, and genetic or chromosomal markers have yet to be discovered. When couples with strong family histories of mood disorders seek genetic counseling before having children, it is important to point out the difficulty of making accurate predictions.

Genetic factors clearly play a role in some, but not all, patients with mood disorders. The presence of a **genetic predisposition** alone is not sufficient to cause a mood disorder, however, as is evidenced by the **incomplete concordance** between identical twins. The occurrence of mood disorders in patients with no family history of them suggests that an acquired biological deficiency (e.g., genetic mutation, perinatal insult, viral or vascular disease of the brain) is involved, but it is not yet known exactly how important such a deficiency is to the development of mood disorders, especially in comparison to the effects that overwhelming psychosocial factors (e.g., psychological trauma in childhood, severe stress in adulthood) have upon a person's life. The general assumption is that inherited or acquired biological vulnerabilities exist in most patients with recurrent or chronic mood disorders and that social and other environmental factors play various roles in triggering the onset of the disorders.

A debate that runs throughout the search for the etiology is whether any particular **marker** is the cause or the result of the disorder. For example, is pessimism a learned behavior that results in depression, or does it reflect a specific effect of abnormal chemical activity in the area of the brain that controls mood? Similarly, does a biological finding such as elevated corticotropin levels merely reflect a primary defect in norepinephrine function, a defect that can both cause depressed feelings and produce alterations in the hypothalamus, or is the elevated corticotropin level itself toxic to the brain and therefore responsible for depressive symptoms? Another theme is to discover the links between specific clinical groups of patients and specific etiologies or markers. For example, would the results of a specific biological test (e.g., serotonin receptor density) have predictive value in determining whether or not a patient will attempt suicide, or whether or not a particular drug will produce the best response in a particular patient? Preliminary results in some of these areas have emerged in research laboratories, but for the most part the answers to such questions remain speculative.

Psychosocial Theories

Most psychological and sociological theories of mood disorders focus on loss as the cause of depression in vulnerable individuals. Mania receives much less attention because it is considered more of a biologically rooted condition. Even when viewed from a psychological perspective, mania is usually regarded as a condition secondary to depression that arises from an attempt to overcompensate for depressed feelings rather than a disorder in its own right.

Psychoanalytical Theory

Psychoanalytical theory, in general, posits the existence of unconscious mental conflicts and incomplete psychological maturation as important factors in the cause of some mental disorders, including depression. According to this theory, conflicts and maturational difficulties stem from **early life depri-vations** such as severe trauma and parental loss. Unempathic or abusive interactions with caretakers may eventually become internalized (i.e., part of the way in which people think of themselves as adults), believing, for example, that they are bad and unlovable, or that assertiveness can result in punishment. Mastering conflicts, feeling comfortable about asserting one's needs, and achieving a secure sense of self-esteem are major tasks of maturation. Without the adequate gratification of basic needs, a person grows up feeling empty and defective, needing to cling to others for security, and being constantly afraid that other people hate and will abandon him or her. The person may also feel very angry over this sense of deprivation, and afraid that the anger will further alienate other people. It is easy to imagine how a tendency toward depression might result from the simmering of such feelings below the surface of everyday life.

Freud's classic treatise, "Mourning and Melancholia," was a seminal effort to explain why some individuals handle loss appropriately (mourning) while others go on to become depressed (melancholia). He suggested that disturbed individuals who feel incomplete due to early deprivation latch onto other people as if to psychologically incorporate them into themselves and make up for their internal deficit. If the other person leaves, even in a symbolic way (e.g., by making a criticism that feels like an abandonment), the disturbed person feels that a part of himself or herself has gone away. The depressed person is angry at the person who left but, because the other person feels like a part of the depressed person's self, the depressed person experiences this as anger at the self. Anger at the self, unconsciously deflected from the other person, creates the conscious feelings of inadequacy and depression. If made aware of the anger at the other person, the depressed person then fears shame or punishment. Subsequent psychoanalytical theorists refined this complex model, focusing on all the ways in which depression reflects feelings of loss mingled with **dependency, anger** at the dependency, **shame** over the anger, and a personal sense of inadequacy. The concept of loss has also been extended to include the lost hope of attaining personal ideals that were imagined while a person was growing up but were not achieved when the person became an adult. Again, this is a common experience that does not usually cause clinical depression, although some people with deficient early parenting may feel worthless if they fail to attain harshly unrealistic goals.

These variations in psychoanalytical theory share the common idea that experiences echoing earlier losses (i.e., physical loss, loss of love from others, or loss of self-esteem) can precipitate depression in people who are vulnerable because of their psychological immaturity or because of ongoing conflicts over anger and dependency. Modern research has underscored the role that early life experiences play in the formation and the vulnerability to depression. Research ranges from studies of children who were separated from parents in World War II to studies of primates reared in isolation. Whether aggression turned inward is a cause or an effect of depression is still open to debate. Also, many adults develop mood disorders with no discernible childhood trauma, or suffer traumas without becoming overtly depressed as adults. Psychoanalytical theories of treatment recommend focusing on both past and present relationships, including the patient's relationship with the therapist (transference), as a template for understanding the depression.

Interpersonal Theory

Interpersonal theory maintains that social losses in a patient's current life contribute to depression and that improved interpersonal relations may alleviate the symptoms of depression. Sociological theories, amplified by modern epidemiological data of social risk factors for depression and bipolar disorder, are the basis of interpersonal theory. This theory's chief departure from psychoanalytical theory is its deemphasis on internal mental processes, such as conflict and low self-esteem, and its greater emphasis on the importance of **present relationships and coping skills.** The past is important because it reveals the ways in which a patient coped with earlier stresses and what social resources were available during those periods. A note of caution regarding this theory is that sometimes poor social relations are more the result of affective illness than the cause (e.g., a marriage collapses because a depressed spouse cannot meet the partner's needs).

Cognitive Theory

Cognitive theory, which developed from behavioral psychology, proposes that the primary defect in depressive illness is not a matter of mood but of incorrect cognition: Depression results from **distorted thinking,** which causes unrealistically pessimistic and negative views of oneself and the world. The distorted thinking has three central maladaptive elements: negative views of oneself, the world in general, and the future; distorted perceptions of new information and experiences; and logical errors that pervade the processing of new information. While cognitive theorists once thought that all of these distorted patterns were learned behaviors, they now allow for an etiological model that integrates biological, social, and psychological influences.

TREATMENT
Psychotherapy

Many of the research studies that form the basis for recommendations in this section report that some treatments vary in their effectiveness depending on the severity of depression. Researchers use standardized numerical rating scales (e.g., the Hamilton Rating Scale for Depression, Beck Depression Inventory). Each symptom of depression and each area of impaired functioning is rated on a scale of severity, and the total is added. Practicing physicians usually make this assessment less formally but use the same idea. Moderately severe depression might be characterized by feelings of sadness that occur off and on throughout the day but not an overwhelming feeling of gloom; some disturbance of sleep but not complete exhaustion; minimal weight change; no serious suicidal ideation; and enough concentration to allow patients to continue working or attending school. Severe depression is often equated with melancholia or psychotic depression. These features are not always present, however (e.g., in severe atypical depression).

For patients with **severe depression** pharmacological treatment is necessary. Psychotherapy alone, without medication, is usually ineffective. Although severely depressed patients may find it difficult to become engaged in psychotherapy, they may gain some much-needed emotional "breathing room" by meeting a caring, optimistic physician and seeing that their family has been mobilized to take care of them. A number of interventions should be considered, including a temporary respite from routine responsibilities. Major undertakings and decisions should be postponed because the patient's judgment and other psychosocial skills may be impaired. If the physician gives the order, the patient may feel less guilty about postponing plans or taking temporary sick leave. It may be helpful to gently talk over precipitating events and soften self-blame and hopelessness. Family therapy to defuse crises and support a household in stress may be helpful. A careful balance between the patient's initiative and the physician's encouragement allows the patient to return to normal activities even before he or she is completely well.

Hospitalization is sometimes necessary. In addition to providing physical protection, it may provide a welcome sense of being taken care of and relief from responsibility. About 10–20% of severely depressed inpatients improve without medication during the first or second week in the hospital. The physician must be wary of this improvement, however. The **milieu response** rarely lasts and should not preclude aggressive use of appropriate medication. In the hospital, measures to support physical health are important, as are gentle efforts to enhance patients' self-esteem by providing structured activities, such as creative arts, in which success is possible despite impaired cognitive functioning. Morale can also be boosted by the social support that patients receive in group therapy from those who are further along in recovery.

In patients with **moderate or mild depression,** psychotherapy can be quite useful, especially if it is a supportive form in which the therapist plays an active role in shoring up the patient's coping skills and makes suggestions for areas to work on. Patients suffering from the mildest forms of depression, especially if the episode has begun recently and is related to a specific stressor, may improve quite a bit with one or two months of regular sessions for advice, support, and encouragement delivered in a common-sense manner. For patients with somewhat greater difficulties in the mild-to-moderate range of severity, more specific psychotherapy is needed, often in combination with medication.

There are several well-defined approaches to psychotherapy for depression that can be quite helpful. **Psychodynamic psychotherapy,** which is based on the psychoanalytical theory of depression, is the least researched form but the most widely and traditionally used. Two other forms of psychotherapy, **cognitive therapy** and **interpersonal psychotherapy,** have been extensively evaluated in well-designed studies of efficacy in depressed patients and have been codified in concisely written manuals.

Despite their differences in emphasis and technique, all three therapies are similar in their examination of the patient's inner mental life (i.e., perceptions, cognitions, and feelings); reliance upon a warm, empathic relationship between the patient and therapist; and education of the patient by making explicit diagnoses, explaining the etiological theories of mood disorders, and discussing the patient's optimistic prognosis. Many therapists find it helpful to draw eclectically from all three models to address the particular needs and aptitudes of individual patients.

Psychodynamic Psychotherapy

One of the main goals of psychodynamic psychotherapy is to link the patient's past experiences of loss or guilt to current life conflicts that recreate the earlier feelings of abandonment or unworthiness. In this form of psychotherapy, the therapist focuses on the patient's underlying character and any life-long habits of thought, feeling, and behavior that become magnified during depression. The technique is more gratifying and supportive than that used with nondepressed patients, particularly in the early, acute stages of illness, and might include the physician giving advice and avoiding silences. (Depressed patients quickly flounder in a more traditional setting in which the therapist remains quiet and lets the patient set the agenda.) During early treatment (generally, the first few months), the therapist tries to **minimize the patient's guilt** (e.g., by helping him or her to accept feelings of ambivalence or anger about frustrating situations or relationships), identifies a distorted and harsh self-image as the basis for the patient's reactions, and emphasizes the patient's areas of personal strength.

➠ For example, a 40-year-old businessman became depressed after receiving a promotion to head a division of his company. He had trouble eating and sleeping, began drinking more heavily, could not enjoy weekends with his wife and children, and felt sad and anxious most of the time. He reported that he "came to life" only when he made a sales presentation to a new client and could enjoy the client's positive response. It emerged that his father had been an angry and critical man and that the patient had always been frightened of speaking up against him. His parents had divorced when the patient was young, and he had always been more sympathetic toward his mother, who would reward him emotionally for good performances at school. Currently, in his new job, he often had to discipline recalcitrant coworkers and mediate disputes. He found this situation very unpleasant and realized it reminded him of the losing battles he had fought with his father and of his general feelings of intimidation around successful peers. He was afraid that his coworkers would hate him if he took a stand against anyone. He much preferred the sales talks because they were never confrontational. His therapist suggested that his managerial job would become easier if he tried to assert himself more consistently. The coworkers might start to respect him if he could successfully address their problems by making firm decisions. This strategy worked. He began to enjoy his position after he was admired for getting results. ◄

Cognitive Therapy

Cognitive therapy is based on the theory that incorrect cognitions (i.e., negative misperceptions of oneself and the surrounding environment) cause depression. Cognitive therapy is usually conducted weekly for three to four months and consists of stages, which take the form of specific therapeutic goals for the patient to meet. In the beginning, the therapist explains the theory behind cognitive psychotherapy and how it works. He or she then teaches the patient how to systematically monitor the thoughts that accompany depressing feelings and situations. The patient is asked to create a diary of automatic thoughts (given as written homework assignments), which the patient and therapist review together, looking for patterns of negative ideation. They then discuss ways in which these thoughts represent inaccurate self-appraisals. The therapist teaches the patient to question his or her own logic and has the patient try out **new cognitive strategies.** An improvement in the patient's mood results when his or her inaccurate, negative perception of the self has been altered.

For example, a patient's fear of not being able to finish a task may be overcome by completing a series of small subtasks, one at a time; if successful, the patient gradually reverses the conviction that the entire task is impossible. ➠ A case in point is a single female patient who was depressed because she was unable to meet men. An examination of her automatic thoughts revealed that she felt unattractive, was afraid she would say something offensive, and expected to be rejected. Her first subtask was to simply say hello to male and female coworkers when she met them at the copying machine. After she discovered that doing so did not result in a catastrophe, she was told to ask a coworker to lunch. Soon she was going to lunch with a regular group at the office and began to feel better about herself. Although she was unable to set up a string of ideal dates during the 12 weeks of cognitive therapy, she had a marked improvement in her overall outlook. ◄▥

To help people overcome depression, many self-help groups and popular books use cognitive and behavioral approaches to urge them to change the way they see themselves (e.g., passive, defective, victimized, or helpless).

Interpersonal Psychotherapy

The premise of interpersonal psychotherapy is that patients' painful social experiences and troubled interpersonal relationships contribute to their depression. In this form of therapy, physicians help depressed patients deal more effectively with their current social and interpersonal problems. Interpersonal psychotherapy does not attempt to alter long-standing personality traits; instead, it addresses the current context in which the patients' symptoms developed. The goal of treatment is to help patients develop better mechanisms for coping with their particular problems, including developing a better understanding of their emotions and improving their interpersonal skills. Although early life experiences are discussed as influences on adult behavior and personality, the treatment of depression focuses on the patients' current issues rather than looking extensively into their pasts.

As with cognitive therapy, interpersonal psychotherapy generally takes 12–16 weekly sessions. The first few sessions are devoted to identifying the patient's primary problem area, which is drawn from four possibilities: grief, role disputes, role transitions, and lack of interpersonal bonds. During this time, the therapist also educates the patient about the nature of depression and temporarily allows the patient to assume the sick role without guilt so as to facilitate his or her receptivity to help. During the middle stage, a strategy is worked out, using a standardized approach, for resolving the central problem. For example, if the problem involves interpersonal role disputes within a marriage or work setting, the therapist helps to define the stages of the dispute (i.e., complete dissolution, temporary impasse, or possibility of renegotiation). The patient is encouraged to view the situation from all possible perspectives (i.e., miscommunication, faulty perception, unrealistic expectations). The therapist then helps the patient consider alternative explanations or develop **new communication or negotiation skills.** The therapist also provides feedback to the patient about how he or she may be perceived by others. In the final stage, the patient deals directly with the impending loss of the therapeutic relationship and the need to consolidate the lessons learned in treatment.

Long-Term Psychotherapy and Preventive Treatment

After remission of the acute symptoms is achieved, psychotherapy may help to prevent relapse and recurrence. The use of monthly follow-up, or booster, sessions in interpersonal therapy has proved to be a successful tool in preventing relapse. For patients with more severe depression who were treated initially with aggressive pharmacotherapy and who have not been able to participate in meaningful psychotherapy, the continuation period can provide a first opportunity to consider the psychodynamic effects of life stresses and personality issues. For example, when a divorce precipitates a patient's major depression, a longer period of psychotherapy after the acute stage may be valuable in changing some personality flaws, so that the patient is able to establish a more successful relationship in the future. Dwelling on such factors during the acute period of recovery is not always helpful, however. Some patients benefit from raising their psychological defenses and avoiding too much exploration. Psychotherapy can also help patients cope with the consequences of their illnesses, such as time lost from family and work, weakened social ties, and damaged self-esteem.

Psychotherapy in Combination With Pharmacological Treatment

Physicians often combine medication and psychotherapy in treating depression. Research and clinical experience suggest that the benefits are additive. Somatic symptoms such as poor concentration, insomnia, and decreased appetite respond best to medication, whereas social impairment and feelings of guilt or suicidality respond more favorably to psychotherapy. Some patients in certain situations may respond best to only one treatment mode, however. Drug treatment alone may be best when the patient's time or finances are significantly limited or the history indicates that, in earlier depressive episodes, the patient has responded extremely well to medication. Psychotherapy alone is the best treatment if antidepressants are poorly tolerated or medically contraindicated or if earlier episodes resolved quickly without medication.

The personality styles of patients and their attitudes toward treatment modalities also affect the choice of treatment. Some patients, for example, are very interested in their inner psychological conflicts or the psychological meaning of external life events. Some feel that taking a medication is a "crutch" or an intrusion into their autonomous self. Patients who are disturbed at the prospect of opening up too much to a therapist are comforted by the notion that their depression may result from a "chemical imbalance" for which they are not to blame. These commonly expressed concerns reflect the various theories about the etiology of depression (i.e., the role of nurture versus nature). Although a physician cannot always define the cause accurately, it may be possible to do so for an individual patient after getting to know him or her in depth. Each viewpoint also reveals a personal meaning: Patients want treatments that help them maintain a certain ideal image of themselves. For instance, to some people, medication means dependence and psychotherapy means independence, whereas to others, the reverse is true. It is usually appropriate to **respect the patient's choice** if he or she has strong feelings because, for many patients with milder depressions, either drug treatment or a specific psychotherapy may, by itself, be effective. If the patient does not improve, the therapist can later suggest an alternative type of treatment. Combining medication and psychotherapy may also have additive benefits in preventing recurrence. During preventive treatment, the physician must regularly review the patient's compliance with medication, any psychosocial stresses that have developed, and fluctuations in symptoms or functioning that indicate relapse. Breakthrough episodes often require a change in medication or a renewal of active psychotherapy.

Patients who have had recurrent depressions often want to know if they can ever stop taking medication. The physician can approach this concern in several ways. The combination of long-term intensive psychotherapy and antidepressants appears to allow some individuals to improve to the point where their personalities are stronger, more resilient, and less vulnerable to depression. This effect may be especially true for patients with depressions that clearly resulted from unique life stresses, which are now safely past. If these patients are truly resituated (e.g., in an improved marriage or more stable career), it may be reasonable to **discontinue medications.** Careful attention must, however, be paid to any signs of recurrence. Other patients feel so much better when taking medication and tolerate it so well that they are willing to take it for life. These individuals should be encouraged to do so as warranted by the seriousness and frequency of the depressions they have suffered.

Bipolar Disorder

For patients with bipolar disorder, psychotherapy is always combined with medication, both during the acute episodes and for long-term prevention. Patients with acute mania find it difficult to engage in psychotherapy before the medication has taken effect; until it does, the therapist can apply the principles of psychotherapy to understand and manage the patient. Bipolar depression may be treated with the techniques for unipolar depressive disorders presented above, although little research has been conducted as to the efficacy of such treatment. Nonetheless, it can be helpful to attempt psychotherapy as an alternative to antidepressants for individuals who switch easily into mania.

For patients with bipolar disorder, the major goal of psychotherapy is not so much to relieve acute symptoms as it is to **enhance long-term psychosocial stability.** A practical focus on maintaining healthy interpersonal relationships, managing stress, and following healthy habits of sleeping regularly, eating nutritious food, and exercising may promote in patients an overall stability of life-style that is thought to decrease their chances of full-blown relapses. Research

into this treatment, called interpersonal biorhythm psychotherapy, is currently under way.

Teaching patients about the importance of complying with the medication schedule and recognizing early signs of relapse are central tasks. Bipolar patients tend to deny their illness more than patients with depression because they enjoy the enhanced energy, sociability, sexuality, and creativity that they believe they experience in the manic state. For some patients, these enhancements are objectively true as well, at least early in the course of hypomania. Complaints about the side effects of medication (e.g., patients often complain of feeling dull) pose a complex problem. It is important for the physician to find out whether the patient's true "complaint" is that he or she misses feeling "high" and is having trouble accepting the need for medication.

Because of its earlier age of onset, erratic symptoms, frequent recurrences, and tendency to cluster in families, bipolar disorder has different effects on the patient's life than recurrent depression. Particularly if the illness begins during the adolescent years, interruption of developmental tasks may occur, such as solidifying a sense of identity, forming lasting relationships outside the family, and establishing a career path. Learning to discriminate normal from abnormal moods may present problems. Patients may fear strong emotions and believe them to be abnormal; this fear may cause them to avoid emotionally charged or intimate life experiences. In addition, recurrent episodes take an exhausting, cumulative toll on the patient, resulting in prolonged demoralization.

Bipolar disorder also affects the patient's family, spouse, and others. Patients feel guilty and lose relationships because of what they do during manic episodes and what they do not do during depressive episodes. They may also feel angry and guilty about, or identify too closely with, affected parents, siblings, or offspring. Patients may have concerns about genetic transmission and may face the painful decision of whether or not to have children.

Finally, patients often suffer losses during treatment. For those patients who truly are more creative or productive during hypomanic episodes or who experience significant cognitive and physical side effects from lithium, the losses are genuine. For others, the losses are symbolic. Having a chronic illness and needing lifelong medication can lead to lowered self-esteem and feelings of defectiveness. Patients may blame the physician or the medication for their failures in life (e.g., blaming the loss of a job on a tremor caused by medication rather than their erratic, manic behavior).

Psychopharmacological Treatment
Major Depression
Antidepressant Drugs

Numerous well-controlled studies have shown that patients with severe major depression, especially melancholia, are best treated with antidepressant drugs (see also Chapter 16, Psychopharmacology). Sixty to seventy percent of patients respond to antidepressants, whereas only 10–20% of severely depressed patients improve when given placebo. The **tricyclic antidepressants** (TCAs) and **monoamine oxidase inhibitors** (MAOIs), which are the so-called first-generation drugs, have been used since the 1950s and 1960s. Although the efficacy of these medications is the best established in terms of empirical evidence gathered from controlled double-blind studies, they have many unpleasant, dangerous side effects and may be lethal if used in a suicide attempt. The side effects of TCAs include anticholinergic effects, weight gain, orthostatic hypotension, and slowing of cardiac conduction. The side effects of MAOIs are insomnia, orthostatic hypotension, weight gain, hypertensive crisis (when the drug is taken with foods containing tyramine), and numerous interactions with other drugs. Since the late 1980s, many new antidepressants have been introduced that are far safer and have fewer side effects. These include the **selective serotonin reuptake inhibitors** (SSRIs) and other drugs that have various effects on neurotransmitters (e.g., bupropion, venlafaxine, and nefazodone). The newer drugs are as effective as the TCAs and MAOIs in mild-to-moderate depression but have not been as definitively tested in relatively severe depression or melancholia. The new drugs, especially the SSRIs, are the usual first-line choice because of their safety and tolerability. The first-generation drugs are used mainly in patients who do not respond to one or more of the newer medications.

Patients with **atypical depression** have a better response rate to MAOIs and SSRIs (55–75%) than to TCAs (35–50%). Because side effects are a drawback with both TCAs and MAOIs, many patients with atypical depression are now treated first with SSRIs. MAOIs may be used later in the sequence provided sufficient time is allowed to eliminate the SSRI because lethal interactions may occur between these classes of drugs. Patients with **psychotic depression** rarely respond to antidepressants alone and require either the addition of an antipsychotic drug or a course of ECT.

Although studies of the effects of medications in patients with **dysthymia** have not been as thorough as those for major depression, they suggest that antidepressants help most dysthymic patients to a significant degree. Although dysthymia is a mild form of depression, patients suffering from it deserve no less than a careful, systematic sequence of drug trials when the first drug tried does not work. As with mild-to-moderate major depression, it is now common to begin treatment of dysthymia with one of the newer antidepressants, such as an SSRI. Tapering of the medication is often attempted after 6–12 months of treatment, although many patients find it preferable to continue the medication indefinitely when its benefit has proved significant.

Antidepressants must be taken for four to six weeks at the full therapeutic dosage before their complete effect is felt. A full response, however, may occur only after 8–12 weeks because it sometimes takes several weeks for a patient's dosage to reach the therapeutic level. Therefore, unless the patient has severe side effects, the drug should not be stopped until it has been given at an adequate dosage for an adequate length of time. Only then can a patient be considered a nonresponder or partial responder. In general, nonresponders or partial responders suffering from any degree or subtype of depression will benefit from a different type of antidepressant. About 50% of melancholic nonresponders to TCAs achieve remission when they are given MAOIs instead. (These adjustments can bring the overall response rate to 80–90%.) It is common to try a sequence of antidepressants from **different classes** or to **combine two antidepressants,** such as a TCA and an SSRI. Another technique is to augment antidepressants with lithium, stimulants (e.g., dextroamphetamine or methylphenidate), or thyroid hormone (levothyroxine or triiodothyronine). By themselves these **augmenting agents** are not very helpful in treating depression, but seem to enhance the effects of standard antidepressants. Thyroid hormone deserves special consideration as an augmenting agent in patients with low normal thyroid function and should, of course, be used at the beginning of treatment in patients with unequivocal hypothyroidism as indicated by an elevated TSH level.

After 1–2 months of treatment, which is the acute phase, remission occurs. **Continuation treatment**—at the full dosage that was used to resolve the depression—should be maintained for at least **six months** after the acute phase in order to prevent relapse. It has been shown that for patients who have discontinued treatment after their depression has gone into remission, relapse rates are at their highest level in the six months immediately following and then decrease. After 6–12 months of continuation treatment, the dosage should be gradually tapered and the patient should be observed for signs of relapse. When the medication should be stopped depends on individual factors. For example, it would be unwise to stop a college student's medication just before final examinations. If relapse occurs, the same medication is usually, but not always, effective; therefore, it is sometimes necessary to try other medications.

If the patient has been depressed for a long time before receiving treatment or has a history of three or more recurrent episodes, the physician can assume that, without treatment, relapse is inevitable. Therefore, treatment may need to be continued for many years or life. Such long-term use of medication thus becomes a preventive, or prophylactic, phase of treatment. In deciding whether this **prophylaxis** is necessary, the physician needs to consider factors such as the degree of response to and side effects of the medication, the patient's life situation, and the severity and duration of previous episodes. The physician should explain to the patient that although his or her depression is effectively relieved by the taking of antidepressants, these drugs do not cure depression or eliminate the tendency for depression to recur when the medication is stopped. In this sense, the preventive treatment of depression follows the same chronic disease model used for the treatment of hypertension and diabetes.

Electroconvulsive Therapy

Electroconvulsive therapy (ECT) is used for patients who are psychotic, extremely suicidal, or medically ill because of dehydration due to severely decreased oral intake (see Chapter 15, Psychotherapy). It is also useful for other patients who have not responded to sequential trials of medication or who cannot tolerate the side effects of medications. Most patients with melancholic depression who have not responded to medication improve with ECT, particularly when it is administered earlier rather than later in the course of an episode. For patients with delusional depression, studies have shown that ECT is especially effective, making it the treatment of choice for some patients with this life-threatening condition.

With the use of modern anesthesia, ECT has no major medical complications and is often safer than medication for medically ill patients. It produces transient disorientation and short-term retrograde memory loss. The loss of memory is generally limited to the period of time (several weeks) during which ECT is given. Long-term memory gaps, such as forgetting a few facts from the past, are rare.

Adjunctive Drugs

Because antidepressant drugs usually take several weeks to begin working, they are often used in combination with other medications at the beginning of a patient's therapy to provide immediate relief from insomnia, anxiety, or agitation. Short-acting **benzodiazepines,** which may be taken during the day or at night in small divided doses (e.g., lorazepam, 0.5 mg three times daily or 0.5–1 mg at bedtime), help alleviate all of these problems. However, physical dependency may occur if they are used for more than a few weeks. Trazodone, given in a small dose (50–100 mg at bedtime), may be used as an alternative to benzodiazepines for the treatment of insomnia. (Trazodone was first used in this country as an antidepressant, but it tends to be overly sedating when used in full dosages for that purpose.) Some antidepressants, especially the SSRIs and MAOIs, may cause insomnia, which is often alleviated by trazodone or the benzodiazepines. Antipsychotics are useful for severely agitated patients, but tardive dyskinesia may develop if they are continued for more than a few weeks.

Bipolar Disorder

Lithium and Other Mood-Stabilizing Drugs

Drug therapy is essential in bipolar disorder to achieve two goals: rapid control of symptoms in acute episodes of mania and depression, and prevention of future episodes or, at least, reduction in their severity and frequency (see also Chapter 16, Psychopharmacology). The mainstays of somatic therapy are the mood-stabilizing drugs, or bimodal agents, that generally act on both mania and depression. The three drugs in this category are the lithium ion and the anticonvulsants valproate and carbamazepine.

Lithium, in the form of **lithium carbonate,** is the most widely used mood stabilizer. It has potent effects in acute mania, allowing 60–70% of patients to achieve remission within several weeks. Lithium is most helpful in patients with euphoric mania and in those who have relatively few or infrequent episodes. When lithium is ineffective, or when medical problems prevent its use, the anticonvulsants are used. The **anticonvulsants** appear to be more effective than lithium in patients with dysphoric or mixed mania, in rapid cyclers, and possibly in patients who have had multiple episodes. Lithium and anticonvulsants may also be used in combination, in which they are sometimes more effective synergistically than alone.

A mood-stabilizing drug has certain limitations if it is used as the sole medication in acute mania. It may take a week or more before its effects are felt; it does not have sedative effects; and it cannot be given parenterally to uncooperative patients. Therefore, for the first few weeks of treatment, mood stabilizers are usually combined with antipsychotics or benzodiazepines for sedation. The sedative medications also have the advantage of being injectable when necessary. It is extremely important to sedate a manic patient because this helps ensure the safety of the patient and others and because sleep is therapeutic against mania. Conventional **antipsychotics** such as chlorpromazine or haloperidol are rapidly effective in slowing down motor hyperactivity and in treating hallucinations and delusions in psychotic mania. The newer atypical antipsychotics, such as risperidone and olanzapine, may also be helpful and have fewer side effects. Improvements in grandiosity, thought disorders, and psychotic symptoms usually occur within several days and are resolved within a few weeks. **Benzodiazepines,** such as lorazepam or clonazepam, are often used as the sole sedative in patients with milder symptoms or in combination with antipsychotics in those with more severe symptoms. They are not effective when used alone for severe or psychotic mania. When they are combined with antipsychotics, however, lower doses of the antipsychotics can be given, which helps reduce the potentially dangerous anticholinergic, hypotensive, and extrapyramidal side effects of the conventional antipsychotics.

Patients who are taking mood stabilizers require special medical monitoring. Blood levels of lithium must be measured regularly, especially in extremely agitated or medically compromised patients, because this drug can be severely toxic at levels only slightly higher than the usual therapeutic range (0.7–1.2 mEq/L). At therapeutic dosages, common side effects are tremor, weight gain, polyuria, and hypothyroidism. Lithium-induced hypothyroidism should be treated with thyroid replacement because it may mimic or exacerbate depression. Patients sometimes complain of cognitive dullness. Toxic levels of lithium, which may result from dehydration, can produce confusion, ataxia, and death. Patients with heart or kidney disease, including many elderly individuals, cannot take lithium safely.

The side effects of anticonvulsants are usually more benign than those of lithium. Valproate may cause upset stomach, tremor, and weight gain. Carbamazepine may cause sedation, headache, double vision, rash, and benign leukopenia. Very rarely, carbamazepine has caused agranulocytosis and is contraindicated in patients with bone marrow disease.

Electroconvulsive Therapy

Electroconvulsive therapy has powerful, rapid antimanic effects. It should be considered in life-threatening cases of manic violence, delirium, or exhaustion. It is also appropriate in patients who do not respond to medications after many weeks.

Antidepressants

Acute bipolar depression has received little scientific study in comparison with unipolar depression. If antidepressant drugs are given for bipolar depression, they may cause either a switch to mania or a mixed state or may induce rapid cycling. Lithium and the anticonvulsants, which of course do not cause mania, are therefore safer for acute bipolar depression. Unfortunately, they are not as powerful against depression as they are against mania. In a few patients, lithium or anticonvulsants can be used alone with good antidepressant effects. However, the most common treatment for bipolar depression is an antidepressant combined with a mood stabilizer to prevent a manic switch. The antidepressant drugs are the same as those used in unipolar illness, although they are sometimes given in lower dosages and for shorter periods of time as a precaution. Many experts begin with bupropion or the SSRIs. The MAOIs may be the most effective but also have the most side effects. The TCAs may be more likely to cause mania than other antidepressants.

Patients with the rapid cycling subtype, the acute mixed states, and dysphoric mania are difficult to treat. They may respond somewhat better to anticonvulsants or ECT than to lithium. Antidepressants tend to worsen these conditions. In fact, if a patient reports feeling worse after given an antidepressant, this suggests that the apparent agitated depression may actually be a mixed state. Antidepressants should never be given to a patient who is manic.

Preventive Pharmacological Treatment

After an initial manic episode, patients are usually treated for one to two years before consideration is given to tapering off the medication and monitoring them closely for future relapses. After patients have had two or three episodes of bipolar disorder, including depressive episodes, they are usually treated indefinitely because of the near certainty of relapse. Long-term therapy may begin after a single manic episode if the episode is extremely severe and if the family history is positive.

Prevention targets both manic and depressive episodes. Lithium has been the treatment of choice in four decades of international experience. Valproate and carbamazepine, given alone or in combination with lithium, are also often effective, although they have been less well studied. Patient responses fall along a spectrum: approximately one-third have no further episodes and are essentially cured; one-third have less frequent or less severe episodes and function reasonably well; and one-third continue to have relatively frequent and severe episodes, with ongoing disability. **Predictors of poor response** are mixed symptoms, rapid cycling, and multiple previous episodes. In the group with a poor response, it is especially important to try innovative treatments, including aggressive use of anticonvulsants.

Patients who experience breakthrough episodes of mania while they are taking mood stabilizers should be given an antipsychotic drug temporarily. Individuals who suffer breakthrough episodes of depression benefit from antidepressants. Patients with a tendency toward frequent or chronic breakthroughs are treated with a combination of multiple mood stabilizers, long-term antipsychotics, and antidepressants, as needed.

Selected Readings

American Psychiatric Association. Practice guideline for major depressive disorder in adults. American Journal of Psychiatry 150 (No. 4, Supplement):1–26, 1992.

American Psychiatric Association. Practice guidelines for the treatment of patients with bipolar disorder. American Journal of Psychiatry 151 (No. 12, Supplement):1–36, 1994.

Goodwin, F. K., and K. R. Jamison. Manic-Depressive Illness. New York, Oxford University Press, 1990.

Jamison, K. R. An Unquiet Mind: A Memoir of Moods and Madness. New York, Alfred A. Knopf, 1995.

Karasu, T. B. Psychotherapy for Depression. Northvale, New Jersey, Jason Aronson, 1990.

Kendler, K. S., et al. Stressful life events, genetic liability, and onset of an episode of major depression in women. American Journal of Psychiatry 152:833–842, 1995.

Kessler, R. C., et al. Lifetime and 12-month prevalence of DSM-III-R psychiatric disorders in the United States: results from the National Comorbidity Survey. Archives of General Psychiatry 51:8–19, 1994.

MacKinnon, R. A., and R. Michels. The depressed patient. In The Psychiatric Interview in Clinical Practice. Philadelphia, W. B. Saunders, 1971.

Post, R. M. Transduction of psychosocial stress into the neurobiology of recurrent affective disorder. American Journal of Psychiatry 149:999–1010, 1992.

Post, R. M., D. R. Rubinow, and J. C. Ballenger. Conditioning, sensitization, and kindling: implications for the course of affective illness. In Post, R. M., and J. C. Ballenger, eds. Neurobiology of Mood Disorders. Baltimore, Williams & Wilkins, 1984.

Rosenthal, N. E. Diagnosis and treatment of seasonal affective disorder. Journal of the American Medical Association 270:2717–2720, 1993.

Rush, A. J., et al. Depression in Primary Care: Clinical Practice Guidelines. Vols. 1 and 2. U.S. Department of Health and Human Services, Public Health Service, Agency for Health Care Policy and Research. AHCPR Publication Nos. 93-0550 and 93-0551. Rockville, Maryland, April 1993.

Weissman, M. M., et al. Affective disorders. In Psychiatric Disorders in America. Robins, L., and D. Reiger, eds. New York, Free Press, 1990.

CHAPTER FOUR

SCHIZOPHRENIA AND OTHER

PSYCHOTIC DISORDERS

EWALD HORWATH, MD AND
FRANCINE COURNOS, MD

Schizophrenia is characterized by disordered thinking, inappropriate emotional responses, hallucinations, delusions, and bizarre behavior. It affects approximately 1% of the population, and patients with schizophrenia occupy more hospital beds— 25% of all hospital beds and 40% of hospital beds reserved for long-term care—than any other patients with psychiatric illnesses. Schizophrenia is the most well described and studied of the psychotic disorders. The clinical approach to schizophrenia in its acute presentation is similar to the assessment and treatment of patients with brief psychotic disorder and schizophreniform disorder (see Other Psychotic Disorders, below). Schizophrenia is distinct from these disorders, however, in its much more chronic and debilitating course. This aspect of the illness must be understood and addressed by physicians.

Schizophrenia strikes people in the prime of their lives, usually in late adolescence or young adulthood (see Table 4–1 for more epidemiological information). It interferes with school, work, marriage, and parenthood and generally shatters patients' expectations of leading normal lives. One mother of a son with schizophrenia described his anhedonia, or loss of pleasure, as the disorder took hold: "Nothing I can say will express the sheer horror of watching anhedonia creep in and claim the person who once laughed with you, who once hugged you, who once loved to be first on the hill to catch the new powder snow. The lights go out one by one. It is the death of the spirit."

Although schizophrenia is a devastating psychiatric illness that often causes profound impairment in patients' social and occupational functioning, the outcome for many patients with persistent symptoms is not completely bleak; they can be rehabilitated to some degree. Certain treatments, especially psychopharmacological therapy, can improve the quality of life for patients and their families.

DIAGNOSTIC AND CLINICAL FEATURES

Historically, the term *psychotic* was used to describe conditions with a high degree of severity that grossly interfered with patients' functioning. This definition is too nonspecific and has fallen out of use (see Box 4–1, Historical Perspectives on Schizophrenia). Currently in psychiatry, **psychotic** is used to indicate a person's loss of reality testing, which is manifested by delusions, hallucinations, or a formal thought disorder. The presence of these symptoms requires a diagnosis, since, by definition, such symptoms are not part of normal mental functioning (see Chapter 1, Case Formulation). An analogy can be found in general medical practice with, for example, the symptom of fever, which requires a diagnosis of pneumonia, endocarditis, strep throat, or another disorder. Merely describing a patient's symptoms as psychotic does not confer a specific diagnosis upon the patient. The differential diagnosis of psychosis includes schizophrenia and other closely related disorders (i.e., schizophreniform and schizoaffective disorders) as well as the mood disorders, substance-induced disorders, and psychotic disorders due to a general medical condition (see Differential Diagnosis, below).

According to the DSM-IV definition, schizophrenia can be diagnosed in patients who have two or more of the following symptoms for at least one month: hallucinations, delusions, disorganized speech and behavior, affective flattening, alogia, or avolition (Table 4–2). In addition, patients' social or occupational functioning must have deteriorated. Continuous signs of illness, which may include symptoms from the prodromal and residual phases of the illness that are not psychotic, must be present for at least six months (see Course of Illness, below).

Schizophrenic patients may exhibit thought, perceptual, emotional, and behavioral disturbances simultaneously. Catatonic patients, for example, may hear voices commanding them to assume bizarre bodily postures, which they then assume for hours. Patients' symptoms usually wax and wane. Some patients have florid hallucinations early in the course of the illness and develop progressive emotional blunting at a later stage. Symptoms may occur in clusters and interact in complex ways, as in the case of one young man who hallucinated that he heard his mother's persecuting voice and gradually became convinced that his real mother had been replaced by an impostor.

Some psychiatrists suggest that two schizophrenic syndromes exist. The type I syndrome is characterized by positive symptoms (i.e., hallucinations, delusions, and disorganized thinking) and the type II syndrome by negative symptoms (i.e., blunted affect, apathy, and avolition). Hypothetically, these two groups of symptoms relate to different aspects of the underlying disease process. Positive symptoms are most overtly evident during acute exacerbations of schizophrenia, while negative symptoms tend to chronically impair the social and occupational functioning of the patient. The positive symptoms in and of themselves are not sufficient to constitute a diagnosis of schizophrenia; they simply represent a syndrome of psychosis (see Other Psychotic Disorders, below).

Thought Disturbances

People suffering from schizophrenia have two kinds of thought disturbances: formal thought disorder and disorder of thought content. Formal thought disorders affect the relationships and associations among the words used to express thought (i.e., the verbal form the thought takes). Disorders of thought content involve the development of delusions.

Formal Thought Disorder

Many people with schizophrenia have disturbances in conceptual thinking that make their ideas difficult to follow. Their thoughts tend to be strung together by incidental associations, and the connection between one idea and the next may not be readily apparent. Certain types of associations seem to be peculiar to schizophrenia; such disorders of association may lead to increasingly autistic thinking. For example, when asked why he was in the hospital, one patient replied that his mother had "clogged up" his kitchen sinks, which made his thoughts flow out of his head. The most characteristic type of formal thought disorder exhibited by schizophrenic patients is **loosening of associations,** in which thoughts seem completely unrelated, or only obliquely related, to each other. When asked what had brought him to the hospital, one patient with schizophrenia replied, "I was home when a drum began beating. I flew too low." Another type of formal thought disorder is **clanging,** in which conceptual connections between words or thoughts are replaced by sound associations (e.g., cycle and psycho; Pepto-Bismol, peptobismuth, and petrobismuth). Patients with the most severe form of loosening of associations express themselves in a **word salad** (i.e., incoherent patterns of words with no apparent connection or meaning that are strung together). In one case, a young woman approached a nurse and asked for "the thing that goes, the nails who made me barf."

Schizophrenic patients may use words in peculiar ways. These **disturbances in word choice** are another sign of a formal thought disorder. When a woman, for instance, was asked why she was in the hospital, she replied, "Being unhealthy. In my head I feel like I'm a bleed." The use of **neologisms,** which are made-up words with meanings known only to the patient, is common. For example, a man with schizophrenia used the term "fumebook," which he defined as "a special temple to protect you."

Psychotic patients may also experience **thought blocking,** which is a sudden derailment of their train of thought with a complete interruption in the flow of ideas. A young woman trying to explain her school history said that she "took courses . . ." but she could not proceed any further with her thought. Thought blocking may leave patients quite perplexed or embarrassed.

TABLE 4–1.   Epidemiology of Schizophrenia

Disorder	Lifetime Prevalence	Age of Onset	Course of Illness
Schizophrenia	1%	Late adolescence to young adulthood	Chronic with waxing and waning
Schizophreniform disorder	0.2%	Late adolescence to young adulthood	One-third recover within 6 months; two-thirds have final diagnosis of schizophrenia or schizoaffective disorder at end of 6 months.
Schizoaffective disorder*	<1%	Typically, early adulthood; ranges from adolescence to late adulthood	Better prognosis than schizophrenia but significantly worse than mood disorder
Delusional disorder	0.05–0.1%	Typically adulthood, middle age and later	Ranges from remission without relapse to remission alternating with relapse to chronic waxing and waning
Brief psychotic disorder	Uncommon	Late 20s to early 30s	Can resolve within a few days

*More common in women than in men; all other psychotic disorders are equally prevalent among males and females.

BOX 4–1. Historical Perspectives on Schizophrenia

Various psychiatrists have contributed to the current definition of schizophrenia used in the United States. Morel, a European psychiatrist, first used the term *demence precoce* in 1856 to refer to an illness with severe intellectual deterioration beginning in late adolescence. Later, several other psychiatrists described specific variations in presentation or course. In 1871, Hecker delineated a hebephrenic type with a "silly" affect and a deteriorating course, and in 1874, Kahlbaum described catatonia as a mental illness characterized by stupor in the absence of gross neurological disease.

In his landmark textbook of 1896, Emil Kraepelin, a distinguished German psychiatrist, used the term *dementia praecox* to unify these disorders, which were previously considered separate diseases. He specifically referred to a disabling, often deteriorating condition with an onset in young persons. In the most severe cases, it resulted in a dementialike outcome. He emphasized the distinction between dementia praecox, which resulted in deterioration, and manic-depressive psychosis, which had a more favorable outcome, in his view. Neo-kraepelinian revivals of his ideas (e.g., in the DSM-III and DSM-IV) have emphasized the deteriorating course and poor outcome. Schneider considered specific psychotic symptoms, such as delusions of thought control, thought broadcasting, and thought insertion, to be pathognomonic. Although these symptoms are still considered characteristic of schizophrenia, they are also observed in other psychotic disorders.

In 1911, Eugen Bleuler named the disorder *schizophrenia* and described what he believed were specific psychological features: loosening of associations, blunting of affect, autism, and ambivalence (i.e., indecisiveness). Bleuler viewed schizophrenia as having a variable outcome, being either chronic or intermittent in its course, and resulting always in a defect in personality, however slight.

Bleuler's ideas were widely taught in schools of psychiatry in the United States and contributed to a fairly broad, perhaps overinclusive, concept of the illness. It should be noted that even narrow, specific definitions of schizophrenia are likely to include a group of disorders with similarities in symptomatic presentation and response to current psychopharmacological therapies. Disagreements about the nature of the core psychopathology have been significant barriers to determining the true prevalence, predictors of outcome, core neurobiological disturbance, and genetic pattern of inheritance of schizophrenia.

TABLE 4–2. DSM-IV Diagnostic Criteria for Schizophrenia

A. *Characteristic symptoms:* Two (or more) of the following, each present for a significant portion of time during a 1-month period (or less if successfully treated):
  (1) delusions
  (2) hallucinations
  (3) disorganized speech (e.g., frequent derailment or incoherence)
  (4) grossly disorganized or catatonic behavior
  (5) negative symptoms, i.e., affective flattening, alogia, or avolition
  Note: Only one Criterion A symptom is required if delusions are bizarre or hallucinations consist of a voice keeping up a running commentary on the person's behavior or thoughts, or two or more voices conversing with each other.
B. *Social/occupational dysfunction:* For a significant portion of the time since the onset of the disturbance, one or more major areas of functioning such as work, interpersonal relations, or self-care are markedly below the level achieved prior to the onset (or when the onset is in childhood or adolescence, failure to achieve expected level of interpersonal, academic, or occupational achievement).
C. *Duration:* Continuous signs of the disturbance persist for at least 6 months. This 6-month period must include at least 1 month of symptoms (or less if successfully treated) that meet Criterion A (i.e., active-phase symptoms) and may include periods of prodromal or residual symptoms. During these prodromal or residual periods, the signs of the disturbance may be manifested by only negative symptoms or two or more symptoms listed in Criterion A present in an attenuated form (e.g., odd beliefs, unusual perceptive experiences).
D. *Schizoaffective and Mood Disorder exclusion:* Schizoaffective Disorder and Mood Disorder With Psychotic Features have been ruled out because either (1) no Major Depressive, Manic, or Mixed Episodes have occurred concurrently with the active-phase symptoms; or (2) if mood episodes have occurred during active-phase symptoms, their total duration has been brief relative to the duration of the active and residual periods.
E. *Substance/general medical condition exclusion:* The disturbance is not due to the direct physiological effects of a substance (e.g., a drug of abuse, a medication) or a general medical condition.
F. *Relationship to a Pervasive Developmental Disorder:* If there is a history of Autistic Disorder or another Pervasive Developmental Disorder, the additional diagnosis of Schizophrenia is made only if prominent delusions or hallucinations are also present for at least a month (or less if successfully treated).
  Classification of longitudinal course (can be applied only after at least 1 year has elapsed since the initial onset of active-phase symptoms):
  Episodic With Interepisode Residual Symptoms (episodes are defined by the reemergence of prominent psychotic symptoms); *also specify if:* **With Prominent Negative Symptoms**
  Episodic With No Interepisode Residual Symptoms Continuous (prominent psychotic symptoms are present throughout the period of observation); *also specify if:* **With Prominent Negative Symptoms**
  Single Episode In Partial Remission; *also specify if:* **With Prominent Negative Symptoms**
  Single Episode in Full Remission
  Other or Unspecified Pattern

When formal thought disorder occurs in patients who have no demonstrable structural brain damage, it is often considered pathognomonic of schizophrenia. Individuals with a formal thought disorder often have good vocabularies and other evidence of an intellectual capability that is more advanced than their low level of conceptual organization would suggest. A schizophrenic college student may use sophisticated technical terms, for example, to express a completely confusing, disorganized idea.

Disturbances of Thought Content

Patients with schizophrenia typically have **delusions,** which are disorders of thought content. **Delusions** are fixed ideas based on incorrect perceptions of reality that do not stem from a shared system of cultural beliefs, such as religious convictions. Delusions are commonly **paranoid** or **persecutory** and may also be **bizarre, somatic, grandiose,** or **referential** (i.e., referring to events in the environment that the patient believes have special significance for him or her).

The following examples illustrate these different types of delusions, which often occur in combinations. ➡ A young man believed that he was the son of a famous popular singer (grandiose) and thought that his mother was lying to him about his paternity (paranoid). At one point, he saw a limousine driving through his neighborhood, and he became convinced that the singer had sent someone to keep an eye on him (referential). A Dominican woman believed that she was the daughter of the deceased former President of the Dominican Republic and that he would come and rescue her from the hospital (grandiose). A man who was convinced that his brain was leaking out of his head wore a tight cap that he refused to remove because he was sure that it kept his brain in place (bizarre somatic). ⬅

Some delusional beliefs, which are commonly referred to as **Schneider's first-rank symptoms of schizophrenia,** were once considered pathognomonic of schizophrenia. However, recent studies have shown that these symptoms may also occur in other psychotic disorders, such as psychotic mood disorders. They include thought broadcasting, thought insertion, and thought withdrawal. Patients with **thought broadcasting** believe that their thoughts can be perceived by others (i.e., as though the thoughts are being broadcast aloud). One such patient insisted on leaving the hospital because he was convinced that everyone knew his thoughts and that he could have no privacy. Patients with **thought insertion** believe that their thoughts are not their own but are instead the thoughts of another person who has inserted them into their heads. A young male patient, for example, was convinced that his brother transmitted to him a thought telling him to kill their mother. In **thought withdrawal,** patients believe that their thoughts are somehow being removed from their heads.

Perceptual Disturbances

Schizophrenic patients often have unusual perceptual experiences and may develop delusional interpretations of these experiences. **Auditory hallucinations,** in which sounds are heard in the absence of any real auditory stimulus, are the most common type of perceptual disorder in these patients. They may hear the sounds of bells, whistles, whispers, rustlings, and other noises, but, most often, the sounds are of voices talking. Patients commonly hear several voices talking to each other in a critical or disparaging way about themselves or a single voice making threatening or other persecutory comments. One adolescent girl constantly heard the voices of several women calling her a "dirty bitch" and making other nasty remarks about her; one young man heard a voice telling him that he was going to be killed. He was so convinced of this that he ran away from his home and hid in abandoned buildings for weeks.

Schizophrenic patients may have hallucinations that involve other sensory modalities, as well, but these are less common. **Visual hallucinations** are more indicative of delirium or a general medical condition than of schizophrenia. They indicate that a workup is necessary to exclude an acute medical disorder. When visual hallucinations occur in schizophrenia, they are often accompanied by delusional ideas and other sensory perceptions. For example, a religiously preoccupied woman reported that she heard a voice calling and then saw "the Virgin Mary beckoning to me."

Schizophrenic patients may have **tactile hallucinations** (involving sensations of touch or pain) that may be accompanied by paranoid interpretations of perception: One woman with schizophrenia often wailed loudly in pain because she felt a cutting sensation in her head; she was convinced that a group of social workers was hacking at her brain with knives. **Olfactory and gustatory hallucinations** (of taste or smell) have also been described in schizophrenia: A middle-aged man reported that he smelled a foul order and was convinced that his organs were rotting because a neighbor had slipped a white powder under his door.

Emotional Disturbances

The most common emotional change in schizophrenia is a **general "blunting" or "flattening" of affective expression.** Patients seem to be emotionally detached or distant, and their expression of feelings may be limited both in terms of vocal intonation and facial movement. They may describe extremely disturbing experiences with little apparent emotional reaction. They often appear quite wooden and robotlike, and they lack warmth or spontaneity. The emotional blunting may be accompanied by a change in the patient's sense of self. One man reported that he had no feelings whatsoever and that he felt "dead" inside. It is important to recognize that symptoms such as these may be the side effects of antipsychotics, particularly in patients who present with a shuffling gait, tremor, or cogwheel rigidity (see Psychopharmacological Treatment, below).

Paranoid patients feel frightened or enraged in response to a perceived threat or a delusion of persecution. They can be extremely **hostile and guarded** or exquisitely sensitive to any perceived slight. These patients may feel smug in the conviction that they have discovered the source of their persecution and have "caught on" to their persecutors, as in the case of one man who felt clever when he saw a fellow worker winking at someone else because he was sure that this was proof of a plot against him. Grandiose patients may be quite indignant if they feel that they are not receiving the level of respect that is in keeping with their inflated sense of personal status. Some patients feel **perplexed and distressed** about their strange perceptual experiences. Such patients experience emotional relief when they have formed a delusional explanation for their perceptions. ➡ For instance, a woman felt quite perplexed and worried by a sense that her apartment had somehow changed. As her symptoms evolved, she became convinced that the superintendent of her apartment building was entering her apartment and deliberately moving the furniture to retaliate against her for a complaint she had lodged. The delusional conviction was accompanied by both a sense of relief that she now understood the problem and by feelings of rage at the superintendent. ◀▥

Hebephrenic (disorganized) schizophrenia is characterized by an **inappropriate or incongruous affect** in which the emotions that are expressed are inappropriate to the situation or content of thought. Patients, for example, may describe truly frightening experiences while giggling hilariously.

Behavioral Disturbances

Schizophrenic patients may have profound psychomotor retardation or excitement, engage in bizarre acts, or have a gradual diminution of volitional activity. **Catatonic schizophrenia,** in particular, is marked by episodes of bizarre behavior in which patients assume and maintain strange postures and are unresponsive to questions or other stimuli. One man sat fixedly staring at his hand, which he held almost directly over his head. Such patients may have a peculiar rigidity. They may allow their limbs to be moved but may then hold them in the position in which they are placed **(waxy flexibility).** Such bizarre posturing may alternate with extreme psychomotor agitation.

Catatonic posturing is sometimes accompanied by delusions that relate to the behavior. For example, in describing his thoughts, one young man who had been admitted to the hospital with catatonic posturing reported that a remark he made to someone on the street had caused a commercial airplane crash in which many people had died. He was afraid to move or talk because he was convinced that he would cause another crash.

Bizarre behavior in schizophrenic patients is often influenced by delusional fears. In one case, an immigrant who was found running naked down the street later explained that he was being chased by the KGB and the FBI. In another case, a man jumped from a window because he was convinced that he was being pursued by people who wanted to kill him.

A gradual **loss of volition,** accompanied by **apathy** and emotional blunting, is a core symptom in many schizophrenic patients. They often have a history of remaining at home and doing little except watching television. In the most severe cases, patients seem to lose interest in all activities and progressively withdraw into an isolated, inactive, almost vegetative state. These patients usually deny feeling depressed, however. One young man who was brought to the hospital by his mother had remained in his room for the previous six months, urinating and defecating in a bucket.

Subtypes of Schizophrenia

Several subtypes of schizophrenia have been identified in the DSM-IV because they are useful clinical descriptors; however, their validity or stability over time remains to be established. In **paranoid schizophrenia,** systematized delusions or hallucinations involve a single theme, without prominent symptoms of disorganization or a flattened or inappropriate affect. Patients with **disorganized schizophrenia** present with disorganized speech and behavior and a flat or inappropriate affect. **Catatonic schizophrenia** is characterized by disturbed psychomotor behavior, such as rigidity, bizarre posturing, mutism, extreme excitement, or negativism. **Undifferentiated schizophrenia** is associated with hallucinations, delusions, or incoherence but does not meet the criteria for the catatonic, disorganized, or paranoid subtype. Patients with **residual schizophrenia** have persistent residual symptoms, such as emotional blunting, avolition, or odd beliefs, in the absence of gross psychotic symptoms or behaviors.

Other Psychotic Disorders

The signs and symptoms of **schizophreniform disorder** are essentially the same as those of schizophrenia, with two key differences. In schizophreniform disorder, the duration of illness must be at least one month but less than six months. Although impaired social and occupational functioning may be present, it is not required for the diagnosis. For example, a man was able to continue to work for two months after he began having auditory hallucinations accusing him of wrongdoing. It was not until he had a heated argument with a fellow worker who he believed was persecuting him that his occupational functioning was impaired.

The key feature of **schizoaffective disorder** is a major depressive, manic, or mixed episode occurring simultaneously with the characteristic criterion A symptoms of schizophrenia that are described in the DSM-IV (see Table 4–2). During the episode, delusions or hallucinations must be present without any prominent mood symptoms for at least two weeks. For example, one young man was hospitalized twice for acute episodes of mania. After the second episode resolved, he had a persistent delusion that his mother was lying to him about the identity of his true father.

The essential feature of **delusional disorder** is a nonbizarre delusion of at least one month's duration that is not accompanied by hallucinations, disorganized speech, catatonic behavior, negative symptoms, markedly impaired functioning, or bizarre behavior. ▤▶ For example, a 28-year-old single female teacher met a married college professor during a visit to New York City and had a brief affair with him. She then returned to her home and job in Paris. Although she had no further contact with the man, she began to believe that he loved her and wanted her to join him in New York. She impulsively bought a plane ticket and showed up on his doorstep, oblivious to the fact that he lived with his wife and children. She refused to believe his protests that he did not want her there. The patient had a circumscribed delusion in the absence of hallucinations, disorganization, or social and occupational deterioration. A diagnosis of delusional disorder, erotomanic type, was made. ◀▥

In patients with **brief psychotic disorder,** delusions, hallucinations, or disorganized speech or behavior must be present for at least one day but for less than one month. After this brief period, patients return to full premorbid functioning. In one case, an adolescent girl began to have auditory hallucinations in which she heard a voice calling her a "sinner" after one of her brothers had murdered another brother. The hallucinations, as well as agitation, continued for several weeks, but the symptoms then resolved.

The diagnosis of **psychotic disorder due to a general medical condition** is made when hallucinations or delusions are caused by the direct effects of a medical illness. Medical illnesses that can cause psychotic symptoms include, but are not limited to, neurological disorders (e.g., brain tumors, cerebrovascular disease, Huntington's disease, meningitis, encephalitis), endocrine disorders (e.g., thyroid or parathyroid disease, Addison's disease), metabolic disturbances (e.g., hypoglycemia, hypoxia), hepatic encephalopathy, renal failure, autoimmune disease involving the central nervous system, and fluid and electrolyte disturbances. Some medications used for medical illnesses can also induce psychosis (e.g., adrenocorticosteroids, atropine, anticholinergics, ketamine). In one case of psychotic disorder due to a general medical condition, a lawyer was admitted to the hospital with persecutory auditory hallucinations and the delusion that his law partners wanted to kill him. A physical examination showed that he was tachycardic and restless, and laboratory studies confirmed that he had thyrotoxicosis.

The diagnosis of **substance-induced psychotic disorder** is made when hallucinations or delusions are the result of substance intoxication or withdrawal. Substances associated with psychotic symptoms include alcohol, amphetamines, cannabis, cocaine, hallucinogens, inhalants, opioids, phencyclidine, and sedatives. For example, an adolescent boy was brought to the emergency room in a wildly agitated state, screaming that devils were trying to mutilate him. His friends reported that they had attended a party where he was smoking crack cocaine.

Course of Illness

The DSM-IV criteria for schizophrenia include prodromal and residual phases in addition to the active phase of psychotic symptoms. Prodromal and residual symptoms consist of negative symptoms or "near-psychotic" experiences and thoughts such as those observed in patients with schizotypal personality disorder (see Chapter 8, Personality Disorders). By definition, **prodromal symptoms** occur at the onset of the disorder. Usually, the label of prodromal symptoms is applied retrospectively, after the patient has developed florid signs of psychosis. While the DSM-IV criteria require that the symptoms last only six months, the prodrome can persist for several years. **Residual symptoms** tend to last as long as the disorder is present. Acute exacerbations of psychotic symptoms may occur periodically, particularly when patients do not take their antipsychotic medications, and are superimposed on the residual symptoms.

The long-term course of illness is variable. Longitudinal studies obtaining long-term follow-up in Europe and North America found that about one-fourth of schizophrenic patients have **full remission** of symptoms, about one-fourth have **mild residual** symptoms, and about one-half have **moderate to severe symptoms.** Many patients experience a **progressive worsening** of symptoms and functional impairment during the early phase of the illness, which is often manifested as a failure to return to previous levels of functioning. A college student, for example, may have his or her studies interrupted by the illness and then be unable to resume the studies successfully. Most patients, however, have an initial period of deterioration and then reach a plateau in the level of functioning. A long-term follow-up study of patients released from the Vermont State Hospital found that 5–20 years after the onset of the illness, many patients had made a significant recovery in social functioning.

Long-term studies of schizophrenia have identified several predictors of the disorder's outcome. Women tend to have a somewhat better outcome than men with respect to social and marital functioning. When patients are divided into paranoid and nonparanoid subtypes, the paranoid subtype has a somewhat better outcome. **Premorbid factors** such as poor social functioning and schizoid personality predict a worse social outcome, while premorbid factors such as being married and having higher intelligence (as measured by standardized intelligence tests) predict a more favorable outcome. Several studies have found that a **family history** of affective disorder is associated with a better outcome, while a family history of schizophrenia is associated with a worse outcome.

Two prospective multinational studies conducted by the World Health Organization have found that schizophrenic patients in nonindustrialized developing countries tend to have better outcomes than those in developed countries. This observation has led to speculation about how the outcome may be affected by the social differences between developing and industrialized societies, such as the degree of social isolation or support, nature of employment, family milieu, social stigma of mental illness, and survival rates of individuals with perinatal or neonatal brain damage.

THE INTERVIEW

Inexperienced physicians may feel uncomfortable when they first meet with psychotic patients. Several specific guidelines may be helpful in the initial approach to these patients (see Interviewing Guidelines box). In acute treatment settings, patients may be agitated, pacing, or speaking loudly and angrily; physicians should therefore interview patients with another staff member present or in an area where the nursing staff can observe the interaction and provide help if necessary. The interview should be terminated if the physician believes that he or she is in danger. Behavioral signs to watch for include the patient's inability to remain seated, failure to respond to verbal limits, or tendency to talk in a raised or angry tone of voice or make threatening gestures (e.g., make a fist) or accusatory remarks toward the physician.

The first goal in interviewing psychotic patients is to establish an **alliance**. In psychotic disorders, paranoid symptoms may hamper the formation of a trusting relationship. Physicians should listen attentively and respectfully to these patients. Psychotic patients often feel alienated, misunderstood, and unappreciated. They are aware that most people react to them with disbelief, and they benefit from acceptance and empathy for their distress. Physicians should be professional in their interactions. They should introduce themselves, using their full names and titles, and explain what their role is and what they would like to do for the patient. The physician should not sit too close to the patient but remain at least beyond arm's reach. Psychotic patients easily feel intruded upon and require some additional space to feel comfortable.

Physicians should meet with patients only for as long as the patient can tolerate it. For hospitalized patients, brief contacts once or twice a day may be better tolerated than fewer lengthier meetings (e.g., several 45-minute sessions per week). The patient's reaction to the interview should be used as a guide to the length and frequency of the sessions.

Interviewing Guidelines

- Listen attentively and respectfully to the patient in order to establish an alliance.
- Provide structure, keep interactions brief, and steer the interview toward neutral subjects when caring for a disorganized and severely delusional patient.
- Avoid arguing with a patient about delusional beliefs but, at the same time, do not agree with or encourage them.
- Take an educational approach and label psychotic symptoms as reactions to stress.
- Do not remain in a situation that feels dangerous.

Providing a **structure** for the interview is also important. Open-ended questions such as "What problems do you think you are having?" often do not produce informative answers. Simple questions that require simple answers, such as "How old are you? Whom do you live with? Were you seeing a psychiatrist before this hospitalization?" usually help put patients and the physician at ease and make it easier to progress to questions about patients' symptoms. Although the patient may say bizarre things that will make the physician feel uneasy, some areas of patients' intact reality testing will almost always be revealed. This becomes apparent if the physician steers the interview toward neutral subjects.

The physician should be direct without being confrontational. It is helpful to listen respectfully to what patients have to say without agreeing or disagreeing with their unrealistic beliefs. Many schizophrenic patients claim that they are fine and that others are persecuting them. These psychological defenses of denial and projection, which are prominent in psychotic patients, help them reduce feelings of anxiety and low self-esteem. These ideas cannot be changed by contradicting them. On the other hand, it is helpful for physicians to inform patients about their assessment of the reasons for hospitalization, the diagnosis, the purpose of medication, and the treatment plan, even if patients are unlikely to agree with everything. ➡ In one case, when asked what had brought him to the hospital, a paranoid man stated that it was a big mistake caused by his father's overreaction to him. The physician replied that he understood the patient's feeling but that it would be best for the patient to take medication to help him control his anger and that a meeting would be arranged with his father to try and resolve their differences. The meeting revealed that the son had felt persecuted by neighbors and had attempted to smash their door with a hammer. ⬅ Resistance to accepting an illness and medical advice about it is common in all patients, not just psychiatric patients, and it helps to be tolerant when it surfaces.

Psychotic patients have perceptual experiences, such as auditory hallucinations, that are outside the realm of common human experience and can be anxiety-provoking for both patients and interviewers. It is often helpful to take an **educational approach** and help patients recognize that the experience is a symptom of the illness and label it as such. The physician might suggest that the hallucinations are a symptom of stress and that medication may help the patient to cope more effectively. Paranoid patients may not feel reassured at first but are often able to respond to reassurance gradually as their reality testing improves.

Learning to work with psychotic patients can be an intense, emotionally overwhelming experience. Patients may be only partially aware that interviewers are health professionals and see them as intrusive, seductive, hostile, or dangerous. This misperception is symptomatic of the paranoid psychological process, in which patients attribute their own aggressive or sexual impulses to those around them, including the physician. ➡ For example, a young schizophrenic woman became convinced that her physician was making a sexual advance when he came to her hospital room to see if she was free to meet with him. This belief occurred despite his waiting for a response after knocking on her door and asking her to come out of the room. In another case, a man accused a psychiatry resident of being in league with the FBI to lock him up and force him to divulge certain information. ⬅ In such situations, physicians' appropriate response is to reassure patients that they are health professionals and that they and the other staff members want to be helpful and have no intention of harming them.

The physician's initial response to a psychotic patient may be one of anxiety, fear, bewilderment, or amusement. Extremely paranoid and hostile patients may be quite frightening. The degree of fear that the physician feels is an important measure of the hostility that the patient may be feeling and expressing nonverbally. A common error for the physician is to try to overcome or deny being afraid, which may cause the physician to miss the patient's hostility or to continue the interview even after the patient has become increasingly upset or threatening. One resident was struck by a patient when he continued to interview the patient who had started pacing in circles around the resident's chair and making wild gestures.

When a patient is acting in an extremely disorganized or bizarre way, the physician may feel bewildered and not know how to proceed. Asking a structured set of simple, direct questions may restore a sense of order and control to the interview. The physician may ask the patient to describe his or her work history, education, or place of residence: "When is the last time you were working?" "How far did you go in school?" "Where do you live?" A disorganized patient may become sidetracked and pursue bizarre or irrelevant topics. The physician can **refocus the interview** by simply telling the patient that it is time to move on to another subject. For example, when a grandiose patient described her close connection to the British royal family and provided a litany of their lineage, the physician thanked her and then inquired about the people who were living with the patient in her apartment.

A psychotic patient may tell strange stories that strike the physician as funny. These strange tales are a symptom of the illness, and the physician should control the impulse to laugh inappropriately because such a response may be interpreted by the patient as mockery. A physician's emotional responses to a patient can provide important clues as to any unstated feelings the patient may be communicating. The impulse to laugh may be the interviewer's attempt to feel superior and distant from disturbing primitive impulses that a psychotic patient can stir up within the physician. Fear on the part of the physician usually indicates that the patient feels angry and hostile. If the physician feels perplexed, this reaction usually

indicates that the patient's thought processes are disorganized. With increasing experience, a physician can learn to gather important information by being aware of his or her own emotional responses but not overwhelmed by them.

DIFFERENTIAL DIAGNOSIS

The differential diagnosis of schizophrenia includes a long list of other psychiatric disorders that have psychosis, disorganized thinking, inappropriate or blunted emotional responses, or catatonia as symptoms: major depression, mania, delusional disorders, brief psychotic disorder, schizophreniform disorder, schizotypal personality disorder, dissociative disorders, mental retardation, drug-induced psychosis, delirium, hallucinosis, intoxication, dementia with psychosis, alcohol and other drug withdrawal syndromes, and a host of other disorders due to a general medical condition (e.g., those caused by metabolic or central nervous system disturbances).

Although the following symptoms are sometimes seen in schizophrenic patients, they are more characteristic of patients who have a **psychotic disorder due to a general medical condition:** a fluctuating level of consciousness; poor motor coordination; incontinence; inability to perform simple mental tasks (e.g., following commands, naming objects, doing arithmetic, or copying simple geometric designs); disorientation as to person, place, or time; confusion; and memory impairment. If a general medical condition has been ruled out, the other primary mental disorders mentioned earlier should be considered (see Chapter 5, Cognitive and Mental Disorders Due to General Medical Conditions).

In a medical setting, physicians must always assume that patients who are acting abnormally have serious medical disorders. ➡ In one instance, a 53-year-old woman appeared in the emergency room crying and confused. She stated that she was unable to find her way home and gave a history of taking a psychiatric medication. A medical intern completed a physical assessment and reported no abnormal findings. The case was referred to a psychiatrist, with the intern stating, "This woman is a schizophrenic if ever I saw one." The psychiatrist learned that the patient had been working as an accountant until recently and that her symptoms had been present only for several months. She had been feeling depressed and forgetful, and her internist had given her an antidepressant. In addition to getting lost in her own neighborhood, the patient reported urinary incontinence, which is usually a sign of nonpsychiatric illness. A neurologist who subsequently evaluated the patient discovered that she had papilledema, and, eventually, the diagnosis of glioblastoma was made. The psychiatrist reviewed the emergency room intern's report to see if he had examined the patient's fundi. He had done so and had noted that the margins of the optic disks were sharp. Although it seems remarkable, the intern's prejudicial belief that this woman had schizophrenia and was, therefore, not medically ill apparently caused him to miss the papilledema. In addition, he knew little about the diagnostic criteria for schizophrenia, which is unlikely to onset at age 53 years and is usually not associated with urinary incontinence or disorientation as to place. ◄▦

A psychotic illness of brief duration (i.e., lasting more than one day but less than one month) without prodromal or residual symptoms suggests a **brief psychotic disorder.** ▦► Such a disorder was present in a maintenance man who was separated from his wife, had waited in line for gasoline for three hours during an oil shortage, and was told, when his turn came, that the gasoline had just run out. He became agitated and shouted at the attendant. He also became physically threatening, and the police brought him to the emergency room. The man was incoherent, spat at the staff, cursed, and paced wildly. He failed to respond to haloperidol given intramuscularly and was admitted to the acute inpatient unit. In a few days, he had completely recovered his normal behavior and was apologetic for his agitated behavior. The man's prior history of good social and occupational functioning and the brief duration of symptoms with complete resolution suggest that he was suffering from a brief psychotic disorder. ◄▦

Mental retardation usually is associated with a limited capacity for verbal expression. It can often be confirmed by inquiring about the patient's school history and psychometric test results, which will document long-standing intellectual impairment. An onset of illness in early childhood or later adult life should also raise the index of suspicion for a disorder other than schizophrenia. The absence of a history of impairment in social or occupational functioning weighs against the diagnosis of schizophrenia.

A prominent mood disturbance suggests **depression or mania.** However, the differentiation of schizophrenia, schizoaffective disorder, and **bipolar disorder** may be difficult. Patients may have psychotic symptoms that are not accompanied by prominent mood disturbances. ▦► In one case, a 38-year-old man had been given a diagnosis of bipolar disorder. He was hospitalized several times for acute manic episodes, with symptoms of elated mood, incessant talking, energetic pacing, and loud singing of operatic arias. The staff found his mood to be infectious and endearing. During his worst episodes, he had the delusion that he was a close friend of a famous operatic tenor and had to be released from the hospital in order to join him on a world tour. After approximately 10 years of intermittent manic episodes, the psychotic symptoms became more persistent and often remained after the mood disturbance had resolved. At that point, the diagnosis was reevaluated and changed to schizoaffective disorder. ◄▦

Delusional disorder is suggested by the presence of a persistent but relatively circumscribed delusion in the absence of other symptoms typical of schizophrenia. For instance, a young assistant television producer, who was convinced that a cameraman was in love with her, was surreptitiously watching her with his camera, and was following her, had no other symptoms of schizophrenia and was able to continue working.

A history of substance use should alert one to the possibility of **substance-induced psychosis.** ▦► A 26-year-old man with a history of cocaine use, for example, began to smoke crack daily. Two days before he was admitted to the hospital, he began to read the Bible constantly and hear the voice of God speaking to him. He believed that his mother and brother were out to hurt him and became agitated. After he was admitted to the hospital, his urine was tested and found to be positive for cocaine. His psychotic symptoms resolved within several days. ◄▦ Psychotic symptoms may be caused by the use of cocaine, amphetamines, phencyclidine (PCP, angel dust), and other substances. An acute onset of and rapid improvement in symptoms, a history of recent substance use, and a positive urine toxicology screening test suggest a substance-induced disorder. Patients will often deny their substance use, and family members or friends may need to be contacted for additional information (see Chapter 7, Alcohol and Substance Abuse Disorders).

Once all of the historical and physical data have been obtained, a careful review of the criteria in the DSM-IV is needed to establish the most appropriate diagnosis. Even so, observing the patient at a single point in the course of the illness may not clarify the diagnosis fully. Physicians should keep in mind that the diagnosis of schizophrenia requires the patient to be ill for 6 months. The differentiation of schizophrenia from other psychotic disorders may remain unclear until the patient has been observed and followed for an extended period of time.

MEDICAL EVALUATION

When a patient presents with an acute problem or when the duration of illness cannot be established, it is essential to obtain a thorough account of the psychiatric symptoms, their duration, recent life events, substance abuse, physical symptoms, and medical history, including any use of prescription or over-the-counter medications. It may be necessary to speak to family members or others to obtain such information.

In addition, a thorough physical examination and appropriate laboratory tests are needed to rule out general medical conditions. The following tests should be performed as soon as possible: routine blood tests (e.g., complete blood count, electrolytes, blood urea nitrogen, and creatinine), toxicology screening, thyroid and liver function tests, vitamin B_{12} and folate levels, VDRL test, and others, as appropriate. When the neurological examination reveals a focal abnormality, CT scanning of the head is also indicated. Olfactory hallucinations are often clinically associated with temporal lobe epilepsy; an electroencephalogram (EEG) may be necessary to rule out this disorder.

Patients with schizophrenia may have serious physical illnesses that are overlooked. ➡ One 35-year-old woman came to a clinic appointment and became severely agitated. She was brought to the emergency room, where she became totally out of control and was placed in restraints on a stretcher. The examining medical resident learned that she was registered as a patient at the psychiatry clinic and assumed that her agitation was a nonmedical problem. The psychiatry resident examined her, found her to be agitated and disoriented, contacted her clinic, and learned that she had a history of diabetes mellitus. Blood was quickly drawn and the serum glucose level tested, and an ampule of 50% dextrose solution was given intravenously. Within a few minutes, the patient calmed down completely and became reoriented. Laboratory results later showed a serum glucose level of 27 mg/dL, which confirmed the diagnosis of hypoglycemia-induced delirium (see also Differential Diagnosis, above). ⬅

ETIOLOGY

At this time, the etiology of schizophrenia is not known. However, several avenues of investigation have shown promise in revealing the cause of this illness.

Genetic Factors

Evidence for a genetic contribution to the etiology of schizophrenia comes from family, twin, and adoption studies. Family studies have shown that the risk of developing schizophrenia is 10% in siblings of schizophrenic patients and 13% in children with one parent with schizophrenia. In children with two schizophrenic parents, the risk rises dramatically to 46%. The overwhelming majority of relatives of people with schizophrenia do not develop the disorder, however.

Twin studies have found that the **concordance** for schizophrenia in monozygotic twins of a schizophrenic proband is approximately 46%, compared with a concordance of 14% in dizygotic twins. These studies provide strong evidence for a genetic contribution to the predisposition for schizophrenia. However, the fact that the concordance between monozygotic twins, who are genetically identical, is only about 46% is also convincing evidence for a significant environmental role, the nature of which has yet to be determined.

Adoption studies support the broad genetic hypothesis of a predisposition to schizophrenia, but their main contribution has been to show that sharing an environment with someone who has schizophrenia does not account for the familial aggregation of cases (Gottesman, 1982). Although environmental factors undoubtedly contribute in some way to the etiology of schizophrenia, these studies rule out the possibility that schizophrenia in the rearing family is a primary environmental cause.

Recent advances in molecular genetics have raised hopes that segregation and linkage studies may produce definitive evidence of a genetic process and lead to the location and identification of a specific gene that is causally linked to schizophrenia. Efforts toward this end have proved unsuccessful so far.

Neurochemical Factors

The predominant biological hypothesis for a neurophysiological defect in schizophrenia has been the **dopamine hypothesis,** which holds that the psychopathology found in schizophrenia is caused, in part, by a disturbance in the dopamine-mediated neuronal pathways in the brain (Fig. 4–1). This theory is supported by the blocking effect that most antipsychotic drugs have on the postsynaptic dopamine receptors and by the increase in dopamine activity in the dopamine-mediated pathways that psychotomimetic agents (e.g., amphetamines) usually cause.

The dopamine hypothesis is the main argument for a neurophysiological defect in schizophrenia. The human brain has four principal dopamine tracts: the nigrostriatal, mesolimbic, mesocortical, and tuberoinfundibular tracts.

The nigrostriatal tract is involved in the regulation of extrapyramidal motor activity. Excess dopamine activity in this tract is responsible for certain stereotypic behaviors seen in animals who are given dopamine-stimulating agents, such as amphetamine or apomorphine. Deficient dopamine activity in this tract is responsible for the characteristic motor symptoms of Parkinson's disease; the post-synaptic dopamine blockade in this tract accounts for the extrapyramidal side effects of antipsychotic drugs. The role of the nigrostriatal tract in the pathophysiology of schizophrenic symptoms is not clearly understood. This system may play a role in mediating various appetitive behaviors and responses to environmental stimuli, which are often impaired in schizophrenia.

Disturbances in the dopamine functioning of the mesolimbic and mesocortical tracts are hypothesized to play a central role in mediating the disorders of thought, affect, and symbolic processes seen in schizophrenia. Weinberger (1987) has proposed a complex model involving a primary deficiency of dopamine activity in the mesocortical tracts, which results in loss of feedback inhibition and a secondary increase in dopamine activity in the mesolimbic tracts. Weinberger's model suggests that **hypodopaminergic cortical activity** accounts for some of the negative symptoms of schizophrenia (e.g., avolition), while **hyperdopaminergic mesolimbic activity** accounts for the positive symptoms, such as hallucinations and delusions.

The tuberoinfundibular dopamine tract has its cell bodies in the hypothalamus and exerts an inhibitory effect on prolactin secretion from the posterior pituitary gland. It is not known whether this tract plays a role in the pathophysiology of schizophrenia. The dopamine blockade of this pathway is

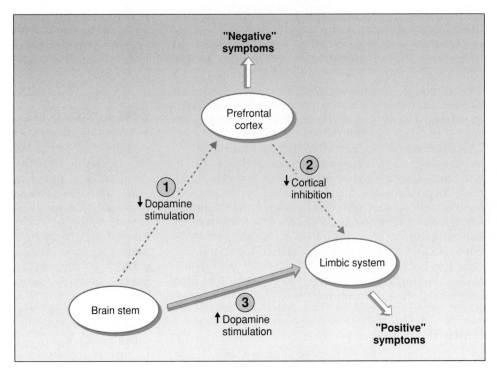

FIGURE 4–1. Neurobiology of schizophrenia. Current evidence suggests that diminished dopaminergic stimulation of the prefrontal cortex (1) may be responsible for the "negative" symptoms of schizophrenia, while the limbic system may produce "positive" symptoms in response to decreased cortical inhibition (2) and increased dopaminergic stimulation (3).

responsible for several important neuroendocrine side effects of antipsychotic drugs, however.

Neurodevelopmental Factors

Recent research has suggested evidence that patients who develop schizophrenia have delayed development as infants. A small subgroup of such offspring has been identified in whom the most severe motor deficits were related to obstetric complications, pandysmaturation, and low birth weight. Findings such as these have stimulated interest in the possibility that schizophrenia may result from a primary developmental lesion that occurs during fetal life, results in subtle developmental delays in infants, and is manifested as frank psychotic symptoms in late adolescence.

Weinberger (1987) has formulated a neurodevelopmental theory of schizophrenia, in which he proposes "a subtle, static structural brain lesion that involves a diffuse system of periventricular limbic and diencephalic nuclei and their connections to the dorsolateral prefrontal cortex . . . which is presumed to have occurred early in development."

Stevens (1992) has more recently hypothesized that schizophrenia may be the consequence of abnormal synaptic reorganization in damaged portions of the hippocampus and other regions of the brain. She proposes that early lesions may have different outcomes based upon the variable, genetically mediated capacity for axonal sprouting that is expressed in adolescence, when a surge of adrenal and gonadal hormones acts as a stimulating factor.

Genetic researchers have proposed that a significant proportion of the development of the brain is under genetic control and that certain genetic defects may be manifested as abnormalities in the central nervous system cell proliferation, cell migration, cell differentiation and death, or connectivity between neuronal networks. Such abnormalities may predispose a person to schizophrenia.

Seasonal Birth Patterns

A number of studies have described a seasonal pattern in the birth rates of people who develop schizophrenia. More patients with schizophrenia were born during the winter and spring months than at other times of the year. In the United States, people with schizophrenia were more likely to be born between December and May. Seasonal differences are most marked in the northeastern and midwestern states and less marked in the southern states. At this time, there is no widespread consensus among investigators as to whether this seasonal birth pattern is a genuine etiological phenomenon or simply an artifact of reporting.

A variety of theories, including nutritional, genetic, and infectious theories, have attempted to relate the birth pattern to the etiology of schizophrenia. Perhaps the most widely disseminated theory is that a viral infection occurring in the mother during gestation may cause schizophrenia in the offspring.

Psychosocial Factors

Psychosocial factors may play a role in the etiology of schizophrenia, but it remains unclear as to what that role might be. The family and social environment of patients with schizophrenia has been examined by researchers hoping to identify any characteristics that might contribute to the development of this disorder. Previously held theories that pointed to the impact of a "schizophrenogenic mother," "double bind" situations, or the presence of grossly deficient early emotional development in schizophrenic patients were seriously flawed by the retrospective, unsystematic observations upon which they were based. Such theories have been largely discarded. Ongoing prospective studies of individuals who are genetically at higher risk for schizophrenia may reveal valid psychosocial factors that influence whether or not a particular person will develop the disorder.

Clinical observations and research data do seem to suggest that **stressful life events** can adversely affect the long-term course of patients with schizophrenia and that family and social factors can influence the prognosis as well (see Psychosocial Treatment, including the discussion of expressed emotion, below). Sometimes patients will suffer an exacerbation of their psychotic symptoms in response to an isolated event, such as the death of a caretaking parent. Other patients' unremitting course of chronically severe symptoms may be caused, in part, by a consistently chaotic psychosocial environment.

Schizophrenia is more common among persons in the **lower socioeconomic classes.** Although a debate continues as to whether this phenomenon is due to social causation (i.e., that specific risk factors in persons of the lowest social class precipitate the illness) or "social drift" (i.e., that people with schizophrenia "drift" into the lowest social class because of the disability caused by the illness), the evidence seems to favor the "social drift" hypothesis. A separate risk factor is the chronic stress of poverty, which may have an adverse effect on the outcome of the illness.

TREATMENT

Pschopharmacology has made the most dramatic contribution to controlling the symptoms and improving the quality of life of patients with schizophrenia and other psychotic disorders. Psychotherapy and other psychosocial treatments, however, are also important because they provide patients with the human connection that helps them develop social skills, educates them about their illness and what to expect, and offers support throughout a long, arduous course of illness. Today, most patients with schizophrenia who need hospitalization stay for only brief periods of time (see Hospitalization, below).

Psychopharmacological Treatment

Beginning in the early 1950s, a number of medications became available that had significant efficacy in treating the hallucinations, delusions, thought disorders, and behavioral agitation associated with schizophrenia; in some respects, the success of these agents revolutionized the management of this disorder. Before they became available, a diagnosis of schizophrenia often resulted in the chronic institutionalization of the patient. With the advent of antipsychotic medications, the symptoms of many patients significantly improved, which allowed them to live outside the confines of mental hospitals.

Standard Antipsychotics

The treatment of choice for the psychotic symptoms (e.g., hallucinations and delusions) of schizophrenia and the other psychotic disorders is a group of medications variously referred to as antipsychotics, neuroleptics, or major tranquilizers (see also Chapter 16, Psychopharmacology). Besides their beneficial effects, these agents also cause certain neurological, or extrapyramidal, side effects, and, because of this, are also called neuroleptics. Although the antipsychotics have sedating and tranquilizing effects, they are not indicated for use as general tranquilizers or sedatives in people who are not psychotic because of the risk of developing neurological side effects, including tardive dyskinesia.

The first widely used antipsychotic in the United States was chlorpromazine, a phenothiazine that was released in 1955. Since then, a variety of other antipsychotics have been used in the treatment of schizophrenia. The standard, or typical, antipsychotics include several chemical classes of drugs. The phenothiazines, developed first, were used almost exclusively for many years and continue to be used widely today. Changes in the core structure of phenothiazine have produced other commonly prescribed agents, such as thioridazine, trifluoperazine, perphenazine, and fluphenazine. Other antipsychotic drugs frequently used are haloperidol, thiothixene, molindone, loxapine, and pimozide.

Although the standard antipsychotics are similarly efficacious in treating schizophrenia, the range of therapeutically effective dosages is quite broad (see Chapter 16, Psychopharmacology). The clinical potencies of the antipsychotics vary in relation to their affinity for blocking D_2 dopamine receptors. The **potency** of each drug is compared with that of chlorpromazine, which is usually viewed as the "standard" for the antipsychotics. The therapeutic dosage for chlorpromazine is 300–800 mg/d. Most patients with acute psychotic symptoms respond to this dosage within six weeks. Improvement in agitation and hallucinations may occur within a few days, whereas improvement in thought disorder and delusions often requires several weeks. Nonresponse is defined as the patient's failure to improve following a six-week course of a given medication at an adequate dosage when there is documentation that the patient has complied in taking the medication.

In clinical practice, higher dosages of chlorpromazine and other antipsychotics are sometimes used for patients with agitated psychosis or for patients who do not respond to lower dosages. In patients with severe agitation or other dangerous, disabling symptoms that fail to respond to standard dosages, the risks involved in increasing the dosage are sometimes justified in order to attempt to relieve the symptoms.

A growing alternative to high dosages of antipsychotics is the use of safe **adjunctive sedatives** (e.g., lorazepam). For agitated psychotic patients whose behavior continues to be difficult to manage when they are taking standard dosages of antipsychotics, adding lorazepam, 2–10 mg/d given in divided doses, is a safe, practical way to provide sedation until the patient responds to an antipsychotic.

A number of studies have attempted to establish a relationship between the serum blood levels of a drug and the clinical response to the drug. A clear correlation has not been shown for most antipsychotics. The most consistent data are for haloperidol. Several studies have suggested that the "therapeutic window" for haloperidol is a blood level of 5–15 ng/mL. Dosages resulting in higher or lower blood levels may not be as effective. For other antipsychotic medications, consistent, reproducible ranges for therapeutic blood levels are not well established. Therefore, blood levels do not play a clear role in managing patients who are taking most antipsychotics.

Antipsychotics have a variety of side effects (see Chapter 16, Psychopharmacology). Among the most common are **anticholinergic side effects,** which consist of dry mouth, blurred vision (i.e., impaired accommodation), urinary hesitation or retention, constipation, and delirium. The most powerful anticholinergic action occurs with the low-potency agents, such as chlorpromazine, thioridazine, and clozapine. For some patients, these effects may present a real danger. This is particularly true for older patients, who are more sensitive to the serious medical complications that may result. Older men with prostatic hypertrophy are at risk for developing urinary retention. All older patients are at risk for serious obstipation or ileus. Deaths have been reported secondary to this complication. Patients at highest risk are those who are taking several different drugs with significant anticholinergic action, such as low-potency antipsychotics plus anticholinergics or tricyclic antidepressants (TCAs).

Another potentially serious side effect is **orthostatic hypotension**. Again, this is most common with the low-potency agents. Dehydrated patients are at greatest risk.

All of the antipsychotics except clozapine have significant risks for **extrapyramidal side effects.** These are seen most commonly with the high-potency agents, such as fluphenazine, trifluoperazine, thiothixene, and haloperidol. Extrapyramidal side effects may be divided into those that appear early and those that appear late in the course of the illness. The side effects with an acute onset include acute dystonia, parkinsonian effects, and akathisia. The side effects that appear late include tardive dyskinesia and tardive dystonia.

Acute dystonia is a sudden muscle spasm that most commonly occurs in the muscles of the tongue, mouth, and neck and, sometimes, in those of the trunk. A patient may say that "My tongue is sticking out and I can't get it back in." Patients may also say that their tongues feel numb, that they cannot talk, or that their faces feel frozen. Other patients develop torticollis, which is sudden torsion of the head and neck to the side. Acute dystonia should be treated as quickly as possible with anticholinergic agents.

Neuroleptic-induced parkinsonism occurs within the first 1–2 weeks of treatment. It usually presents with the characteristic resting hand tremor of 3–5 beats per second. Bradykinesia, which is extremely slow motor movement, and ratchetlike stiffness are common. These side effects respond well to anticholinergic agents.

Akathisia, or motor restlessness, usually begins within the first few weeks of treatment. Many patients say that they "feel like jumping out of their skin." They may not be able to sit still, may pace the hallway continuously, or may constantly shuffle their feet or cross and recross them.

Tardive dyskinesia is the most common late side effect. It usually presents after antipsychotic medications have been used for several years. The chief sign is involuntary movements of the lips, tongue, mouth, jaw, upper and lower extremities, or trunk. Chewing and sucking movements of the mouth and jaw, darting and writhing tongue movements, and facial grimacing are among the most common presentations. Flicking, twisting, or writhing movements of the fingers, hands, toes, or feet are also seen frequently. These movements are irregular, unlike those of a parkinsonian tremor.

Unfortunately, effective treatments for tardive dyskinesia have yet to be developed. If the antipsychotic medication can be stopped, many patients will have a gradual remission of the involuntary movements, although there is often an initial exacerbation of them immediately after the medication is discontinued. For many patients with chronic schizophrenia, however, discontinuing the antipsychotic is not an option, because this may result in an acute exacerbation of the illness. Some patients benefit from vitamin E, 800–1600 IU/d.

An unusual but life-threatening side effect of antipsychotic drugs is **neuroleptic malignant syndrome.** This syndrome consists of the triad of hyperthermia, stiffness or tremor, and sudden changes in mental status. Associated signs include autonomic instability (e.g., hypertension, hypotension, tachycardia, tachypnea, or diaphoresis). In cases of intense, prolonged muscular rigidity, rhabdomyolysis may occur, along with extremely high serum creatine phosphokinase levels, myoglobinuria, and acute renal failure. The mortality rate of neuroleptic malignant syndrome is significant (5–10%). When the diagnosis has been made or is suspected, emergency medical evaluation and supportive measures are mandatory. Rapid cooling of the patient with ice, cold water, or a cooling blanket is indicated, along with an intravenous line to give fluids and maintain the blood pressure.

An increased mortality rate has been reported in cases of neuroleptic malignant syndrome associated with depot neuroleptics, but this potentially fatal syndrome also seems to occur with a broad range of neuroleptic medications, including the low-potency agents. Although the syndrome has some clinical similarity to the malignant hyperthermia syndrome associated with anesthesia, altered calcium transport has not been reported in the skeletal muscle of patients with neuroleptic malignant syndrome.

Several **ophthalmological complications** may result from antipsychotic treatment. The most serious is a pigmentary retinopathy that is associated with the use of thioridazine in dosages of more than 800 mg/d. Such dosages are, therefore, contraindicated. It should be noted that concomitant treatment with propranolol and thioridazine has been shown to increase serum levels of thioridazine. This combination should be avoided, since it may increase the risk for visual impairment due to retinal pigmentation. Prolonged and high-dosage treatment with chlorpromazine has been associated with pigmentary deposits in the cornea and lens; decreasing the dosage or discontinuing the drug is usually effective in alleviating this problem and preventing significant impairment of the vision.

Atypical Antipsychotics

The atypical antipsychotic **clozapine** represents an exception to the pattern of efficacy of the standard antipsychotics. Clozapine is "atypical" for two reasons: It usually does not cause the extrapyramidal side effects associated with the other antipsychotic drugs, and it is effective in some schizophrenic patients who do not respond to standard antipsychotic drugs. Approximately half of such patients improve with this atypical medication. Unfortunately, the use of clozapine is limited because it is associated with a substantial risk of agranulocytosis. The white blood cell count must be followed regularly during the course of treatment.

Within the past several years, three other atypical antipsychotics, risperidone, olanzapine, and quetiapine, have been approved and introduced into the clinical treatment of schizophrenia. These drugs are atypical in that they are associated with a lower affinity for binding to D_2 receptors and a lower risk for extrapyramidal side effects, when they are given at low dosages, than are the standard antipsychotics. Unfortunately, these drugs have not proved to have superior efficacy in the treatment of positive symptoms, such as hallucinations and delusions. Some studies have suggested that these newer drugs may be more effective in the management of negative symptoms, such as lack of volition and motivation, but further study is needed in this area. At the time of this writing, other soon-to-be-released atypical antipsychotics include sertindole and ziprasidone.

Psychopharmacological Treatment for Acute Episodes

Antipsychotic medications are the pharmacological treatment of choice for acute exacerbations of schizophrenia. Acute episodes usually involve new or exacerbated psychotic symptoms, such as hallucinations and delusions, and are often accompanied by a severe thought disorder and disturbances of behavior.

The choice of antipsychotic is governed chiefly by the history of the response to a particular agent or by the **side effect profile** of the drug. With the exception of clozapine, group studies have not demonstrated that one drug has superior efficacy. Generally, one or two standard drugs from different chemical classes are tried initially, and a trial of clozapine may be indicated for patients who fail to respond adequately to a standard medication.

Factors such as the presence of other medical and neurological problems and the patient's age, hydration status, history of side effects, and degree of agitation may also influence the choice of agent. For patients who are older or dehydrated, the low-potency agents, such as chlorpromazine and thioridazine, pose a substantial risk of orthostatic hypotension and injury from falls and probably should be avoided. The low-potency agents are also more likely to cause the anticholinergic side effects described above. Patients with brain damage, dementia, or other cognitive disorders may be more likely to develop delirium or other exacerbations of cognitive impairment.

Because of their sedating effects, the low-potency antipsychotics are often given to schizophrenic patients with severe agitation. Group studies have not demonstrated that the low-potency agents are more effective than the other agents, but experience has shown them to be highly useful in the clinical management of agitation. An alternative strategy is the use of a high-potency antipsychotic along with an adjunctive sedative agent, such as a benzodiazepine or a barbiturate. The benzodiazepine lorazepam, which is a short-acting, well-absorbed intramuscular preparation, may be combined with a high-potency antipsychotic. This combination is a highly effective, safe, widely used treatment for agitated, acutely psychotic patients.

Although a number of studies have shown that typical antipsychotics are effective in the treatment of acute psychotic symptoms, such as hallucinations, delusions, and thought disorder, their effectiveness in treating the negative symptoms, such as blunted affect, social withdrawal, and autism, is less well established. Early studies indicated that some patients showed improvement in some negative symptoms such as social withdrawal, but this may have resulted from the decrease in paranoid delusions and thought disorder. More recently, clozapine and other atypical antipsychotics have shown some promise of greater efficacy in treating negative symptoms and may have benefits for residual functional impairments, as well.

Psychopharmacological Treatment for Other Psychotic Disorders

The pharmacological treatment of many of the other psychotic disorders, particularly brief psychotic episode and schizophreniform disorder, is similar to that described above for acute exacerbations of schizophrenia. For patients with schizoaffective disorder or a mood disorder with psychotic symptoms, a **mood stabilizer** is an important component of the treatment (see Chapter 3, Mood Disorders, and Chapter 16, Psychopharmacology). Antipsychotics are effective for patients suffering from a psychotic disorder due to a general medical condition, although careful consideration must be given to potentially dangerous side effects and medication interactions (e.g., a low-potency antipsychotic, which lowers the seizure threshold, would not be a good choice for a patient with a brain tumor and seizures). Similar caution must be observed in prescribing antipsychotics for substance-induced psychotic symptoms. Low-potency antipsychotics should be avoided in any patient who is at risk of developing alcohol withdrawal (again, to avoid seizures). The one situation in which a psychotic symptom should not be treated with antipsychotics is when a patient has hallucinations associated with alcohol or benzodiazepine withdrawal. A benzodiazepine given in a tapering dosage is effective treatment for all of the autonomic and psychiatric symptoms that accompany sedative withdrawal (see Chapter 7, Alcohol and Substance Abuse Disorders).

Psychosocial Treatment

Medication alone is rarely sufficient for the treatment of patients with schizophrenia. The reasons for this include (1) the relapse rates for patients taking medications average 40% during the first year after hospital discharge and 15% each year for the next several years; (2) the improvement in symptoms is only minimal to modest even in patients who take adequate dosages of medication; (3) patients' social and occupational impairments often persist despite an excellent response to medication; and (4) there are high rates of noncompliance in taking medications because of side effects, patients' denial of illness, and other rational and irrational reasons for refusing to comply with treatment recommendations. Thus, psychosocial treatments for schizophrenia are used to augment medication and improve outcome.

Every nonpharmacological treatment in psychiatry has been used to help patients with schizophrenia accept and recognize their illness, improve their social and occupational functioning, prevent relapse, minimize dangerous behavior, and improve their quality of life. Attaining these goals is especially important for patients with schizophrenia because of the disease's early age of onset and its lifelong duration.

In applying psychosocial approaches to a patient with schizophrenia, the psychiatrist must be careful to provide the appropriate type and level of therapy. Treatment that is too intensive may place demands on the patient that can worsen psychotic symptoms and lead to relapse. On the other hand, lack of sufficient stimulation and expectations can lead to the patient's withdrawal and poor functioning, a situation that occurred, in the past, in large custodial state hospitals, in which patients who were left idle became increasingly socially dysfunctional. The optimal level of intervention varies with each individual and is usually discovered only by trial and error in the context of good working relationships between the patient and the treating staff.

Individual Psychotherapy

Most physicians believe that supportive, structured psychotherapies are more successful than analytically oriented, exploratory psychotherapies for psychotic patients. Exploratory therapy's examination of internal wishes and fears can lead to deterioration in some patients who have schizophrenia because they may confuse their fantasies with reality in ways that make them more anxious and symptomatic. However, therapists can use their own psychodynamic understanding of their patients to help them differentiate between frightening internal ideas and ordinary external reality. Supportive therapy is aimed at helping patients manage their illness by learning about their symptoms and medications and their side effects and how to improve their social and occupational functioning.

Group Therapy

Group therapy for patients with schizophrenia is most effective when it focuses on specific tasks rather than inner fears and feelings. Successful groups teach self-care and social and occupational skills. Through group therapy, the psychiatrist may be able to evaluate effectively patients' abilities to concentrate and get along with others. It can also be an efficient way of educating patients about physical and mental health issues.

Family Therapy

One of the most critical strategies in the treatment of schizophrenia is to preserve patients' existing support network, which is most often the family. Although at one time psychiatrists incorrectly blamed families for the disturbed behavior of schizophrenic patients, today family therapists concentrate on helping family members develop more effective ways of relating to a relative with schizophrenia. Studies suggest that patients do best when families have realistic expectations of patients and can provide emotional support while minimizing criticism and hostility. The term "expressed emotion" has been coined to refer to hostile or overly demanding environments that can increase the chances of relapse in patients with schizophrenia. Family therapy is often essential to reduce expressed emotion and provide support for family members who are coping with ill relatives.

Psychoeducation

Psychoeducation was initially developed to help family members learn more about schizophrenia and its management. It is now a component of most treatments for schizophrenia. Patients and family members are educated about the signs and symptoms of the illness; the medical nature of the unusual phenomena that patients experience; the course and outcome of the illness; the somatic and psychosocial treatments; the strategies for reducing the chances of relapse; and the techniques for handling residual symptoms.

Peer Support and Self-Help Groups

Peer support and self-help groups have grown increasingly popular for both medical and psychiatric disorders. In these forums, people talk about common experiences, exchange advice about illnesses and their management, and offer each other support. In recent years, the self-help movement has undergone a significant expansion among patients with schizophrenia, influencing not only the development of support groups but also of patient-operated vocational programs and counseling activities. It is hoped that these programs will increase the self-esteem and improve the level of functioning of these patients.

Therapeutic Settings
Hospital Treatment

Today, most patients with schizophrenia who need hospitalization stay in the hospital for only brief periods of time. Hospitalization is usually reserved for diagnostic or medical assessments and treatments that would be difficult to perform on an outpatient basis; severe psychiatric symptoms that endanger patients or others; and the management of crises, such as the loss of housing or social supports, that interfere with living in the community. An attempt is made by the staff to resolve the immediate problems and discharge patients as soon as possible.

Although it was common at one time, long-term hospitalization is now reserved for patients with severe unremitting symptoms that are incompatible with living outside of a hospital setting. For a small minority of patients with schizophrenia, this approach is often optimal. The contraction of the once large state hospital system in the United States (deinstitutionalization) is discussed in Box 4–2.

Community Settings

Supervised community settings for mentally ill persons provide housing with varying amounts of supervision and have largely replaced long-term hospital care. Supervised living programs help patients who live apart from their families but cannot live completely independently. These programs may provide help with taking medication; keeping medical appointments; arriving on time for school, work, or day programs; structuring time; grooming; preparing meals; using leisure time; and relating to other residents.

Some community settings, such as nursing homes, may be almost as restrictive as hospitals.

BOX 4–2.   Chronic Mental Illness and the Public Mental Health System

Most people associate the label "chronic mental illness" with schizophrenia. This is valid up to a point. However, the term "chronic mental illness" refers primarily to any severe, persistent mental illness, with continuous or intermittent psychotic symptoms and associated functional disability. This may be true of a number of other serious mental disorders, including bipolar disorder, major depression with psychotic features, and psychosis not otherwise specified. On more careful inspection (e.g., during a research interview), a significant minority of patients with psychosis not otherwise specified who receive the clinical diagnosis of schizophrenia do not actually meet all of the criteria for this disorder. Therefore, they cannot be categorized as having schizophrenia. Patients with chronic mental illness often have more than one disorder. The most frequent coexisting condition is substance use, but mental retardation and neurological impairment are also common.

The controversial public mental health system is largely responsible for the care of patients with chronic mental illness. The number of state hospital beds for such patients was dramatically reduced during the 1960s and 1970s, a phenomenon known as **deinstitutionalization.** Homelessness became a significant problem in the 1980s primarily for social and political reasons, such as family fragmentation, poverty, diminished public funds for housing, reduced entitlement benefits for the poor and disabled, and economic downturns. Deinstitutionalization is actually a misnomer, because the reduction in state hospital beds was offset by the creation of homes for the aged and dependent in the community. Nonetheless, some mentally ill persons have become homeless, and they require extensive outreach efforts by the mental health system.

For most patients, the shift from long-term hospitalization to a community-based system of care has been beneficial. At peak occupancy, typical state hospitals were usually overcrowded and poorly staffed and had little to offer in the way of treatment. Antipsychotic medications, residential programs in the community, and psychoeducational and rehabilitation approaches have improved the outcome of patients with schizophrenia. The patients themselves report that the quality of life outside of a hospital is better.

Others, such as adult homes and board-and-care homes, have limited supervision. Residences are sometimes called halfway houses, community residences, or supervised apartments. At one time, many formerly hospitalized schizophrenic patients lived in inexpensive, single-room-occupancy (SRO) hotels and apartment buildings, usually with no supervision at all. Because of changes in the housing market, little SRO housing exists today. In recent years, the connections between supervised housing and mental health treatment have been strengthened, so that patients living in these settings now receive more effective mental health services.

Day Programs and Rehabilitative Programs

Day programs are group programs that focus on improving self-care, social functioning, occupational skills, and use of leisure time. Program models, which often overlap, are partial hospitalization, day treatment, sheltered employment, vocational rehabilitation, and social skills training. Surveys show that many patients experience the lack of productive activity as their greatest source of dissatisfaction. In recent years, day programs have focused increasingly on rehabilitation, in the hope of helping patients work in volunteer positions or in paid parttime or fulltime jobs. Some rehabilitation programs now take place outside of clinical settings (e.g., in schools or places of employment) and may refer to participants as clients, students, employees, or consumers in order to enhance patients' "nonpatient" identity.

Crisis Intervention, Emergency Services, Outreach Services, and Case Management

Relying less on long-term hospital care and more on a system of community-based services has certain consequences. Some patients avoid the treatment system altogether. Others remain in treatment but continue to suffer episodes of relapse that require urgent intervention. Most patients face the problem of coordinating their own care and entitlement benefits in an increasingly fragmented service delivery system; this has led to an expansion of certain services to help rectify these problems.

Crisis intervention and emergency services are useful during periods of acute psychosis, when the possibility of hospitalization is imminent. Outreach services are most often targeted toward patients who resist needed treatment or are homebound. Case management provides a linkage function, assisting patients with access to mental health services, health care, and entitlement benefits.

References Cited

Gottesman II, S. J. Schizophrenia: The Epigenetic Puzzle. Cambridge, Cambridge University Press, 1982.

Stevens, J. R. Abnormal reinnervation as a basis for schizophrenia: a hypothesis. Archives of General Psychiatry 49:238–243, 1992.

Weinberger, D. R. Implications of normal brain development for the pathogenesis of schizophrenia. Archives of General Psychiatry 44:660–669, 1987.

Selected Readings

Bleuler, E. Dementia Praecox or the Group of Schizophrenias. New York, International Universities Press, 1950.

Hirsch, S. R., and D. R. Weinberger, eds. Schizophrenia. Oxford, Blackwell Science Ltd, 1995.

Johnstone, E. C. Searching for the Causes of Schizophrenia. Oxford, Oxford University Press, 1994.

Kaufmann, C. A. and J. M. Gorman, eds. Schizophrenia, New Directions for Clinical Research and Treatment. Larchmont, N.Y., Mary Ann Liebert, 1996.

McKenna, P. J. Schizophrenia and Related Syndromes. Oxford, Oxford University Press, 1994.

Shriqui, C. L. and H. A. Nasrallah, eds. Contemporary Issues in the Treatment of Schizophrenia. Washington, D. C., American Psychiatric Press, Inc., 1995.

Strauss, J. S., and W. T. Carpenter. Schizophrenia. New York, Plenum Publishing Corporation, 1981.

Torrey, E. F., et al. Schizophrenia and Manic-Depressive Disorder. The Biological Roots of Mental Illness as Revealed by the Landmark Study of Identical Twins. New York, Basic Books, 1994.

CHAPTER FIVE

COGNITIVE AND MENTAL DISORDERS DUE TO GENERAL MEDICAL CONDITIONS

ROBERT E. FEINSTEIN, MD

Psychiatric disorders can be caused by general medical conditions. Cognitive and mental disorders due to general medical conditions present with psychiatric symptoms or behavioral disturbances that result from neurological dysfunction caused by abnormal neuroanatomical structures or neurophysiological processes. (Patients with a "syndrome" such as dementia can have a pattern of similar symptoms that represent different illnesses and etiologies. Patients suffering with a cognitive "disorder," such as vascular dementia, have a similar pattern of symptoms that is presumed to have the same cause. Many of the disorders in the DSM-IV have assumed the label of "disorder," although it would probably be more accurate in some diagnostic categories to have retained the more nonspecific label of "syndrome.") According to the DSM-IV, a cognitive or mental disorder due to a general medical condition can be diagnosed in patients only when their psychiatric symptoms are the direct physiological consequence of a general medical condition, an etiological difference that distinguishes such disorders from primary psychiatric disorders. For patients with general medical conditions that affect the brain, a balanced biopsychosocial approach to the evaluation, differential diagnosis, and treatment of their symptoms is complex but of critical importance.

DIAGNOSTIC AND CLINICAL FEATURES

In the DSM-III-R, mental disorders due to a general medical condition and substance-induced disorders were grouped together with delirium, dementia, and amnestic disorder under the heading "organic mental disorders." In the DSM-IV, this heading has been eliminated and the classification system has been changed. The proponents of the new DSM-IV

system wanted to eliminate the term *organic* because it implied that the primary psychiatric disorders, such as schizophrenia, do not have an organic basis, and, of course, this is not true. Some psychiatrists opposed the new nomenclature because they thought that the change in terminology would create confusion in the literature. They were concerned not only about the departure from the traditional terminology used in the DSM-III-R but also about the departure from the terminology used in the International Disease Classification 10 (IDC-10), which has retained the term *organic*. The proponents of revision prevailed, however, and the category of "organic disorders" does not appear in the DSM-IV. Table 5–1 provides a comparison of the DSM-III-R and DSM-IV systems.

Delirium, dementia, amnestic disorder, and other cognitive disorders are included together in one chapter in the DSM-IV. Many of the mental disorders due to a general medical condition appear in other sections of the manual in order to facilitate their inclusion in the differential diagnosis for the primary psychiatric disorders from which they need to be distinguished. The basic criteria for all of these disorders are as follows: (1) evidence from the history, physical examination, or laboratory findings indicate that the disturbance is the direct physiological consequence of a general medical condition; and (2) the disturbance is not better accounted for by another mental disorder.

The change in classification systems and the use of different instruments for diagnosing cognitive and mental disorders due to general medical conditions have made it virtually impossible to accurately determine the incidence and prevalence of these heterogeneous disorders as a group. However, it is known that 46% of acute hospitalized psychiatric patients have a medical illness. In addition, some im-

TABLE 5–1. Comparison of DSM-III-R and DSM-IV Terminology

DSM-III-R	DSM-IV
Organic mental disorders	**Cognitive disorders**
Delirium	Delirium
Dementia arising in senium and presenium	Dementia
Amnestic disorder	Amnestic disorder
Organic mental disorder not otherwise specified	Cognitive disorder not otherwise specified
	Mental disorders due to a general medical condition
No equivalent	
Organic delusional disorder	Psychotic disorder due to a general medical condition
Organic mood disorder	Mood disorder due to a general medical condition
Organic anxiety disorder	Anxiety disorder due to a general medical condition
Organic personality disorder	Personality change due to a general medical condition
No equivalent	**Substance-related disorders**
Psychoactive substance-induced organic mental disorders	Psychoactive substance-induced disorder
Psychoactive substance use disorders	Psychoactive substance use disorders
Mental retardation	Mental retardation

portant generalizations can be made about these disorders. As a group, the disorders tend to increase in prevalence with age. Primary psychiatric illnesses usually present before age 40 years, whereas most psychiatric syndromes due to general medical conditions occur after this age. In patients who develop new psychiatric symptoms after they have reached 40 years of age, a primary neurological or medical condition that is affecting brain function should be suspected. In other words, if a patient is over 40 years of age and has a new onset of psychiatric symptoms, it is clinically very important to do a complete medical evaluation of the patient.

Cognitive Disorders

Epidemiological information on delirium and dementia is presented in Table 5–2.

Delirium

Patients suffering from delirium experience an acute change in mental status that often leaves them feeling bewildered. The typical signs include confusion, periods of sleepiness alternating with periods of agitation, **deficits in attention and memory,** and changes in the patient's abilities to perceive the outside world and to use and understand language. ➡ For example, a 26-year-old athletic executive, who regularly ran six miles on the beach every day, did not return home from his run one evening. The next day, he was brought to the emergency room by the police, who had found him wandering on a nearby highway in a confused state. He could not remember what had happened to him, and he did not know where he was or where he had been. He had a fluctuating level of consciousness and attention. He was paranoid, illogical, and seemed to be listening to voices. He felt that others wanted to kill him. This patient had some of the cardinal symptoms of delirium. After he was admitted to the hospital, he had a seizure and brain herniation, and he later died. The postmortem diagnosis was delirium due to a ruptured berry aneurysm. ⬅

The cardinal derangement of this disorder has been variously described as a clouding of consciousness, global cognitive impairment, disorientation with memory disturbances, or a deficit in attentional focus that impairs one's ability to acquire new information.

Delirium results from dysfunction of the reticular activating system at the level of the brain stem. When the reticular activating system is functioning normally, a person is awake and alert and has good memory and a normal attention span. When the system is impaired by a disease process, however, the person becomes delirious. Table 5–3 shows the diagnostic criteria for delirium.

Most forms of delirium are clinically indistinguishable from each other, but their etiologies are diverse. Engel and Romano, in their classic paper entitled "Delirium: A Syndrome of Cerebral Insufficiency" (1959), reported the confirmation of suspected deliriums by electroencephalogram (EEG). This clinical observation continues to be valid more than 30 years later. They were the first researchers to describe the neurophysiological changes of delirium as a diffuse cortical slowing of the alpha wave. This pattern directly correlates with fluctuations in attention and the incapacity to acquire new information. Patients with diffuse alpha wave slowing usually have a somnolent, anergic, retarded clinical presentation. Pro and Wells (1977) confirmed that EEG changes always accompany delirious states. They reported that delirious patients can also have a hyperactive, hyperaroused, or agitated clinical presentation, with an EEG pattern of low-voltage, rapid-activity theta waves. As a patient passes from delirium into coma, the EEG may progress to high-voltage delta activity in a bilaterally synchronous or random pattern. When using EEGs to diagnose delirium, the physician must obtain two or more EEGs to improve the chances that the EEG will be recorded during a period of confusion. Alternatively, a computerized EEG, which has a database of EEG recordings that can be used for comparison, can determine whether or not a single EEG recording is abnormal.

Dementia

Patients with dementia may not wish to acknowledge or may not be able to recognize their mental deficits, declining intellectual abilities, or emotional and behavioral changes. ➡ In one case, a 65-year-old

TABLE 5–2. Epidemiology of Delirium and Dementia

Disorder	Prevalence	Age of Onset	Course	Risk Factors
Delirium	10–30% in hospitalized patients	Any age; most common after age 40 years	Variable, depending on etiology	Increases with age
Dementia	Age 60–69, 1.4-1000; age 70–79, 6.4/1000; age 80+, 20.5/1000	Most common after age 40 years	65% chronic, 25% partially treatable, 10% reversible	Increases with age and positive family history
Alzheimer's disease	Represents 50% of all dementias 1.5–2 million people in U.S. From age 70, prevalence doubles every 5 years; from age 90, almost 50%.	Typically after 50s	Progressive downward deterioration	Increases with age; female gender; positive family history of first-degree relative with disorder; head trauma increases risk 3–4 times; Down's syndrome; defects in apolipoprotein E4 allele
Vascular dementia	In 12–20% of patients with dementias	Earlier age than Alzheimer's	Stuttering course: deterioration and destabilization	Cardiovascular (hypertension, abnormal lipid profiles, smoking, history of arrhythmia); diabetes; more common in men; no family correlation known
Dementia due to HIV disease	33% of hospitalized HIV patients	Typically 20s or 30s	Chronic course: deterioration over time	Unknown for HIV dementia. Sexual contact, transfusions, sharing needles for HIV disease
Dementia due to Parkinson's disease	25% of Parkinson patients, usually in end stages	Usually begins between ages 50 and 65 years	Mild dementia for years; later, severe dementia possible in some cases	Males and females equally affected; in U.S. greater risk for African-Americans than whites, for northern inhabitants than southern, for rural areas than urban; family history

landscaper became completely lost while driving his car and was unable to find his way home. He called his wife, who had to go and pick him up because he was so afraid. His wife took him to his physician. She said that her husband had recently been irritable and harshly critical of her for mistakes that he had made (e.g., forgetting to turn off the gas burner on the stove at night, bouncing several checks). The patient said, "I feel like someone is slowly draining my mind . . . of my personality, my thinking, changing my feelings . . . reducing me to rubble." He could not remember the exact date or the day of the week. He could remember only four numbers in sequence and only one out of three objects after five minutes. He was unable to solve simple mathematical problems, even though he had had a high school education. The medical history and physical examination were normal, except for frontal release signs (i.e., release of pathological reflexes, such as the Babinski reflex, rooting reflex, or snout reflex) and soft neurological symptoms, such as left-right confusion, mixed dominance, and drift. The clinical findings suggested dementia of the Alzheimer's type. CT scanning revealed a bilateral frontal brain tumor. The diagnosis was not Alzheimer's dementia but rather dementia due to benign meningioma. ◀▥

The mental, emotional, and behavioral changes caused by dementia usually have a slow or insidious onset and, therefore, are often first recognized by the patient's family, friends, or coworkers. The cardinal feature is a **slow, progressive decline in intellectual abilities** that does not fluctuate over a period of hours or days. The DSM-IV criteria for the diagnosis of dementia are memory impairment, aphasia, apraxia, agnosia, and executive dysfunction (see Table 5–4 for the DSM-IV criteria).

TABLE 5–3.   DSM-IV Diagnostic Criteria for Delirium

A. Disturbance of consciousness (i.e., reduced clarity of awareness of the environment) with reduced ability to focus, sustain, or shift attention.
B. A change in cognition (such as memory deficit, disorientation, language disturbance) or the development of a perceptual disturbance that is not better accounted for by a preexisting, established, or evolving dementia.
C. The disturbance develops over a short period of time (usually hours to days) and tends to fluctuate during the course of the day.
D. There is evidence from the history, physical examination, or laboratory findings that the disturbance is caused by the direct physiologic consequences of a general medical condition.

The steady intellectual decline or cognitive loss and the absence of acute or variable confusion may help to differentiate dementia from delirium. A common initial symptom of dementia is a simple lapse in memory, such as forgetting names, forgetting to turn off lights, or becoming confused about directions. Some patients cannot remember whether they have locked the door at night and repeatedly get out of bed to double-check the lock. Patients may have a gradual decline in cognitive abilities (e.g., they cannot calculate the correct change when shopping, they cannot balance a checkbook, or they get lost when driving). One such patient left home to go to the store and, two hours later, was in a different state. Patients with dementia may become accusatory or paranoid and blame others for their own mistakes. As the dementia progresses, patients may lose track of the time of day, the season of the year, or the geographic location in which they live. Coworkers may notice a slow but dramatic effect on the patient's work. For example, a lawyer who was an expert in contracts began to make uncharacteristic basic mistakes on simple contracts. He also kept asking his secretary to call a client, forgetting that he had previously called the client twice about the same issue. Other changes associated with dementia may include perseveration of speech (i.e., repeating an idea, question, phrase, or word over and over again). In some patients, preexisting personality traits may become altered or increasingly rigid. One woman, for example, who had always been neat and orderly, began to keep her house rigidly neat and to make increasing demands on her spouse to do the same. As the cognitive decline progresses, patients with dementia may appear apathetic, dull, or depressed. Patients with severe lesions of the frontal lobe may present with fluctuating or labile moods; disinhibition; and deteriorating social graces, which may include inappropriate lewdness. For instance, a man who had always acted with sexual propriety propositioned his housekeeper and told his wife's best friend that she had "beautiful breasts."

The dementias due to a general medical condition include dementia of the Alzheimer's type, vascular dementia, and dementias due to HIV disease, Parkinson's disease, head trauma, Huntington's disease, Pick's disease, and Creutzfeldt-Jakob disease. (See Table 5–2 for epidemiological information about the more common dementias.)

Amnestic Disorder

Patients suffering from amnestic disorder have **isolated memory deficits.** Their other cognitive abilities are relatively well preserved, unless they also have delirium or dementia (see Table 5–5 for the DSM-IV diagnostic criteria). ➡ For example, a 20-year-old college student suffered a severe concussion in a motorcycle accident. He came for help because he was failing in his schoolwork. In the three months since his accident, he had been unable to learn or remember new information. He had clear retrograde memories but could not remember the accident, and his intellectual capacities were, for the most part, unimpaired. CT scanning revealed bilateral damage of the mamillary bodies. The diagnosis was amnestic disorder due to head trauma. ⬅ Patients with amnestic disorder often have structural brain damage that affects immediate recall or short-term memory, which makes it difficult to learn new facts. The ability to remember information learned in the more distant past is preserved, as are general cognitive abilities. The sensorium is usually clear; the memory deficits do not fluctuate at different times as they do in delirium; and the intellectual abilities do not progressively decline as they do in dementia.

Mental Disorders Due to a General Medical Condition

The DSM-IV diagnostic criteria for mental disorders due to a general medical condition are listed in Table 5–6.

TABLE 5–4.   DSM-IV Diagnostic Criteria for Dementia

A. The development of multiple cognitive deficits manifested by both
  (1) memory impairment (impaired ability to learn new information or to recall previously learned information)
  (2) one (or more) of the following cognitive disturbances:
    (a) aphasia (language disturbance)
    (b) apraxia (impaired ability to carry out motor activities despite intact motor function)
    (c) agnosia (failure to recognize or identify objects despite intact sensory function)
    (d) disturbance in executive functioning (i.e., planning, organizing, sequencing, abstracting)
B. The cognitive deficits in criteria A1 and A2 each cause significant impairment in social or occupational functioning and represent a significant decline from a previous level of functioning.
C. The deficits do not occur exclusively during the course of a delirium.
D. Additional features may be present, depending on the type of dementia.

**TABLE 5–5.   DSM-IV Diagnostic Criteria
for Amnestic Disorder**

A. The development of memory impairment as manifested by impairment in the ability to learn new information or the inability to recall previously learned information.
B. The memory disturbance causes significant impairment in social or occupational functioning and represents a significant decline from a previous level of functioning.
C. The memory disturbance does not occur exclusively during the course of a delirium or a dementia.
D. There is evidence from the history, physical examination, or laboratory findings that the disturbance is the direct physiological consequence of a general medical condition (including physical trauma)

Specify if:
Transient: if memory impairment lasts for 1 month or less.
Chronic: if memory impairment lasts for more than 1 month.

Psychotic Disorders Due to a General Medical Condition

Patients with psychotic disorder due to a general medical condition develop delusions, hallucinations, or other psychotic symptoms, such as disorganized thinking (e.g., loosening of associations) or bizarre affect, which are caused by a clearly identified medical illness. Patients may present either with delusions or with isolated hallucinations, but only rarely will they have both. ➡ In one case, a 47-year-old man was admitted to the hospital with complaints of fever, weakness, butterfly rash, diffuse joint pain, anemia, and renal failure. The diagnosis was systemic lupus erythematosus. One week later, he became psychotic, with loosening of associations and delusions that the nursing staff wanted to kill him. The psychiatric diagnosis was psychotic disorder with delusions due to systemic lupus erythematosus. ⬅ Other typical paranoid delusions that patients have are that the CIA is "after" them or that they are Jesus Christ. Typical hallucinations are manifested as voices that command patients to take action or that give them directions. Some patients have frightening visual hallucinations and, occasionally, tactile hallucinations (e.g., bugs crawling under the skin). The DSM-IV subclassifies these disorders as psychotic disorders due to a general medical condition with delusions, hallucinations, or mixed features.

Mood Disorders Due to a General Medical Condition

Patients with mood disorder due to a general medical condition develop depression, mania, or mixed features of both. ➡ For example, a 50-year-old former alcoholic began awakening early every morning over the course of three weeks. She inexplicably felt depressed and tearful and had intermittent thoughts of killing herself. She was hospitalized with additional complaints of anorexia, abdominal pain, constipation, and weight loss. Her medical workup revealed jaundice, and ultrasound studies showed an abdominal mass. At surgery, she was found to have pancreatic cancer. Her psychiatric diagnosis was mood disorder with depressed features due to pancreatic carcinoma. ⬅

Mood disturbances can be caused by many medical illnesses. Depressive symptoms, such as a sad mood associated with feelings of hopelessness and helplessness, crying, sleep disturbances, and suicidal thoughts, are commonly reported. Manic symptoms, such as euphoria, talkativeness, irritability, increased energy, and grandiose plans, are also commonly reported, as are mixed depressive and manic symptoms. The DSM-IV subclassifies these disorders as mood disorders due to a general medical condition with depressive, manic, or mixed features, or with major depressivelike episode. Physicians often fail to recognize symptoms of medically induced mood disorders because the symptoms are mild or are incorrectly attributed to the medical condition.

Depression may be the first sign of Parkinson's disease. A parkinsonian-induced depression is usually mild, and suicidal ideation is rare. It is often extremely difficult to discriminate the symptoms of a depressive disorder (i.e., psychomotor retardation, slowed mentation, and decreased concentration) from the symptoms of Parkinson's disease (i.e., rigidity and bradykinesia). The depression is thought to be caused by the disease itself rather than a reaction to having the disease.

Anxiety Disorders Due to a General Medical Condition

Anxiety disorder due to a general medical condition may produce generalized anxiety, panic attacks, obsessive-compulsive symptoms, or social, agoraphobic, or simple phobic symptoms. ➡ In one case, a 35-year-old woman complained of severe anxiety and fears of impending doom that made her unable to leave the house without help from a friend. She also had headaches, excessive sweating, palpitations, and occasional chest discomfort, which she associated with severe work stress. Her physician discovered that she had diastolic hypertension of 140 mm Hg and abnormally high levels of urinary catecholamines. Ultrasound studies and an intravenous pyelogram suggested a right adrenal gland tumor. Surgery confirmed this, and the diagnosis was anxiety disorder with panic attacks due to pheochromocytoma. ⬅

Generalized anxiety symptoms include tremulousness, "butterflies" in the stomach, and uneasiness. Symptoms of panic or agoraphobia, such as

**TABLE 5–6.   DSM-IV Diagnostic Criteria
for Mental Disorders Due
to a General Medical Condition**

A. Psychiatric signs and symptoms are present.
B. There is evidence from the history, physical examination, or laboratory findings that the disturbance is the direct physiological consequence of a general medical condition.
C. The disturbance is not better accounted for by another mental disorder.
D. The disturbance does not occur exclusively during the course of a delirium.
E. The disturbance causes significant distress or impairment in social, occupational, or other important areas of functioning.

those of the patient above, include palpitations, shortness of breath, or feelings of doom. Obsessive-compulsive symptoms may include repetitive worrying or fears or compulsive behaviors, such as excessive hand-washing. Social phobia, agoraphobia, or other specific phobias may include a fear of being seen in public places, a fear of open spaces, or a phobia about dirt or germs. The DSM-IV categorizes anxiety disorders due to a general medical condition with generalized anxiety, panic attacks, or obsessive-compulsive symptoms (see Chapter 6, Anxiety Disorders).

Anxiety syndromes may also be related to caffeinism, nicotine withdrawal, or intoxication with or withdrawal from a wide range of substances (see Differential Diagnosis, below, and Chapter 7, Alcohol and Substance Abuse Disorders).

Personality Change Due to a General Medical Condition

Patients with personality change due to a general medical condition may develop exaggerated forms of preexisting personality traits or new personality styles. Among the subtypes are labile, disinhibited, aggressive, apathetic, and paranoid personalities.

➠ For example, the wife of a 45-year-old accountant who had a past history of alcoholic seizures and an obsessional personality style reported that, throughout the past year, her husband had become more emotional and irritable, less obsessive, and less interested in having sexual relations. He had also developed stringent religious beliefs that did not correspond to his religious upbringing, and he had a new compulsion to record everything in his diary. An EEG revealed new bitemporal abnormalities. The diagnosis was personality change due to partial complex seizures. ◀▥ In other patients with personality changes due to a general medical condition, preexisting personality traits may become more intense and more rigid (e.g., a sloppy person may become sloppier, or a shy person may become reclusive).

Additional changes may be noted in the affective, social, or behavioral spheres. *A diagnosis of personality change cannot be made if delirium or dementia is present.* Disinhibited, apathetic, and akinetic personality changes are all associated with pathological changes in the frontal lobe. Disinhibited patients have the appearance of someone with an antisocial personality disorder. Their personality change is marked by newly impulsive or unpredictable behaviors, distractibility, and poor judgment, although their intellectual capacities remain intact. Some patients exhibit euphoria and express their emotions inappropriately. Apathetic patients appear to have depression with psychomotor retardation and may have problems initiating, organizing, planning, and executing tasks. Akinetic patients may also appear to have depression with psychomotor retardation; speaking very little or not at all; lacking muscular movement (akinesia); and experiencing weakness of the lower extremities, loss of sensation, and, often, incontinence.

Patients with labile personality changes have changeable affects and irritability in association with manic, depressive, or rapidly cycling moods. The aggressive type of personality change is characterized by irritability, anger, or aggression. Minor stress may precipitate impulsive and violent verbal or physical outbursts. Patients with paranoid personality changes are suspicious, mistrustful, and secretive but do not have frank loss of reality testing. Patients with delusions, hallucinations, or loosening of associations should be classified as having a psychotic disorder due to a general medical condition rather than a personality change.

Course of Illness
Cognitive Disorders

Delirium
Urgently **life-threatening delirium** is a medical condition that can result in irreversible brain damage within seconds or minutes. Rapid diagnosis with emergency intervention is essential to prevent permanent brain damage. The man with the ruptured berry aneurysm described earlier probably died because the delirium was not recognized and treated as an emergency.

Immediate-attention delirium requires recognition and treatment within hours to days. ➠ In one case, a 35-year-old research scientist, who had recently returned to the United States from a trip to the Amazon River, felt weak and slightly confused. She developed a high fever, chills, a severe headache, and a stiff neck. The emergency room staff recognized that her delirium required immediate attention. Lumbar puncture revealed pneumococcal meningitis. Within hours, the patient was treated with intravenous antibiotics, and she recovered completely within days. ◀▥

Dementia
Behavioral, affective, and personality changes often herald the increasing intellectual decline found in patients with dementia. The memory gradually erodes from patchy loss of immediate recall to deficits in short-term memory. In general, intermediate-term and long-term memory remain intact until late in the illness. Frequently, patients cannot acknowledge their deficits and may go out of their way to conceal them from others. When one patient with dementia was asked, "Who is the governor of your state?" she tried to conceal a memory lapse with the retort, "Who cares? He's just another idiot politician, anyway." Severely demented patients are generally calm but may be easily startled if they are suddenly disturbed. This vulnerability can result in exaggerated emotional expressions or occasional episodes of unpredictable behavior. At the end stages of dementia, the memory, intellect, and cognitive capacities may decline to the point of complete disorientation. Patients may not recognize immediate family members and may not even know their own names. Patients with severe dementia may be completely unable to care for themselves or carry out the normal activities of daily liv-

ing, such as cooking, shopping, dressing, eating, and toileting. Many patients eventually become bedridden. The mean survival time from diagnosis of dementia to death is approximately seven years.

Dementia of the Alzheimer's type is typical of many dementias in that it has an insidious onset; a slow, steady course; and a downward progression in functioning. The mean life span after diagnosis is 7–10 years. **Vascular dementia** has the usual signs and symptoms of the other dementias but follows a stuttering course. Patients who have stable deficits for years, without the downward deterioration of Alzheimer's disease, may suddenly deteriorate rapidly as new lacunar brain infarcts develop. Some patients may regain stability and retain it again for years.

Amnestic Disorder. The course of amnestic disorder varies with the specific etiology of the disorder, from brief and nonrecurrent (e.g., secondary to a toxic exposure) to brief and intermittent (e.g., with a cerebrovascular etiology) to persistent. Head trauma tends to result in maximal impairment immediately following the injury, with most improvement occurring within two years.

Mental Disorders Due to a General Medical Condition

The course of mental disorders due to a general medical condition varies a great deal depending on the specific medical condition that is responsible for the psychiatric symptoms. As a general rule, the psychiatric symptoms will not remit until the underlying medical condition is treated or otherwise resolves.

THE INTERVIEW

The brain deficits in patients with cognitive or mental disorders due to a general medical condition may be expressed in subtle ways (e.g., inattention, poor concentration, poor comprehension, and minor memory loss) or with obvious behavior (e.g., fluctuating levels of consciousness or an impairment in speech, hearing, or vision). When evaluating these patients, the physician must be especially sensitive to their conditions and must modify his or her usual interviewing style to accommodate their needs. In order to communicate effectively, the physician may have to speak louder than usual, use more hand gestures, express a stronger affect, or write, using a pen and paper. It may be necessary for the physician to get close enough so patients can see his or her lips moving or to speak directly into patients' "good" ear. To focus attention, the physician may hold their hands or repeatedly touch their arms or shoulders. These techniques should be used only if the physician believes that they will improve the therapeutic relationship or help to elicit relevant information. (See also Interviewing Guidelines box.)

The pattern of patient responses depends to a large extent on the characteristics of the disorder. Confusion, befuddlement, or an appearance of being "lost" may occur in patients with delirium or late-

---

Interviewing Guidelines

- Adjust your interview style so the patient can see, hear, touch, and learn from you.
- Maintain a calm environment, privacy, and confidentiality.
- Begin the interview with open-ended questions, which will help you establish rapport and observe the patient and his or her deficits.
- Move to closed-ended questions to assist the patient with difficult answers or to gather vital information quickly.
- Help modulate the patient's anxiety level by avoiding long silences and by explaining the need for all your questions.
- Bolster the patient's self-esteem with realistic reassurance. Be sensitive to the patient's shame about his or her deficits.
- Try to avoid catastrophic reactions by minimizing the test atmosphere, for example, by telling the patient he or she cannot fail a mental status examination.
- Interview the patient's family for information as well as to assess their emotional state and ability to assist in the treatment.

---

stage dementias; somnolence or agitation may also be present in patients with delirium or dementia. Other common characteristics are intellectual slowness in dementia, pseudodementia, and, occasionally, delirium; emotional apathy or lack of concern in dementia or personality change; and rigidity or intensification of preexisting personality characteristics in personality change and, sometimes, dementia. Patients with a psychotic disorder may develop delusions about the physician; patients with a mood disorder may have depressive or manic reactions; and patients with an anxiety disorder may appear anxious, phobic, needy, and clinging.

Patients with severe brain deficits may elicit feelings in the physician of pity, hopelessness, helplessness, disgust, or fear, and the physician may want to keep them at an emotional distance or talk down to them as if they were children. Physicians who are unaware of these possible reactions risk making errors in their approach to these patients. When patients express feelings of hopelessness and helplessness, for example, it is common for the physician to feel unduly pessimistic about their capacity to benefit from psychiatric treatment. By keeping in mind the complex factors involved in their condition that may be producing certain behaviors, the physician can minimize emotional reactions to them and focus instead on gathering information that will lead to accurate diagnosis and appropriate treatment.

Interview Setting

During the interview, the physician should try to be as calm as possible and respect patients' dignity. The setting in which the interview takes place should be as confidential and private as possible, no matter where it is (e.g., in a noisy emergency room area, a relatively quiet intensive care unit, or a general medical or psychiatric unit). If possible, the interview should be held in a separate room or curtained-off area. When privacy is not possible, the physician should ensure confidentiality by not asking sensitive questions or raising personal topics (e.g., patients may not want to reveal their fear of having cancer or AIDS in a setting where others might overhear what is said). To ease the distress of the interview situation and to facilitate communication, patients' physical comfort should be considered. Frequently, a physician will begin the interview by changing the immediate physical environment (e.g., by rearranging the furniture, seating the patient in a chair, or suggesting that the patient lie down), so that it is easier for patients to speak and for the physician to interpret their responses. The physician should also be comfortably situated.

Environmental distractions should be kept to a minimum. When the environment does not have enough normal sensory stimulation, however, normal sounds may need to be introduced. For example, patients in the intensive care unit may be deprived of the sound of human voices but may become overstimulated by a barrage of beeps and buzzers. Turning on the radio in such an environment can mediate the sensory milieu and improve the quality of the interview. It also helps to interview patients when they are fully dressed, are not eating, and are sitting in a comfortable chair. If patients must be interviewed while they are lying in a bed or on a stretcher, they should be wearing hospital gowns and covered by sheets.

Interview Questions

Open-ended questions such as "What brings you here today?" and "How are you feeling?" are useful at the beginning of the interview. Such questions allow patients to feel that they are being understood and are free to express their concerns. They also give patients enough "emotional space" to appreciate the physician's interest in them and thus help to rapidly establish a good rapport between the physician and patient. While listening carefully to their responses, the physician should observe patients, making note of any deficits, such as slurred, dysarthric, or aphasic speech; labile, constricted, or angry emotions; illogical, tangential, circumstantial, or derailed thoughts; or abnormal movements, gestures, or grimaces. By carefully listening and observing, the physician can begin to differentiate brain deficits from primary psychiatric disturbances. The deficits may suggest which underlying disorder is present (e.g., tics and cursing suggest the neurological disorder Tourette's syndrome rather than a primary psychiatric condition).

Long silences or pauses during the interview are stressful to most patients and should be used cautiously. If patients' level of consciousness, attention, concentration, and intellectual ability appear to be normal, the physician can follow the guidelines of a basic psychiatric interview (see Chapter 2, The Psychiatric Interview).

When patients appear to be confused or bewildered or are suffering from intellectual decline, it may be necessary to switch from open-ended to closed-ended questions. Closed-ended questions give the patient several possible answers from which to choose. They may be simple either-or questions or questions that require only yes-or-no answers. Closed-ended questions may be helpful if patients have a restricted capacity because of focal brain deficits or if the physician is trying to obtain specific information quickly (e.g., from a patient who is delirious). The physician might ask, "Did you take drugs? Answer yes or no." "Did you fall down or lose consciousness?" Focal questions such as "Do you know today's date or time?" "Do you recall my name?" "Do you know where you are?" help the physician to quickly establish patients' cognitive orientation and capacity for immediate recall.

If possible, the physician can next gather additional information, such as when, how, and in what sequence the symptoms and illness began and developed.

Therapeutic Interventions

During the course of the interview, it may be important for physicians to help patients modulate their level of anxiety. A friendly atmosphere and frequent reassurance help most patients feel comfortable. Before beginning formal mental status testing, the physician can offer reassurance by saying something like the following: "This is not a test to see how smart you are, but, rather, your answers to these questions will help me learn how you think and what you can remember." The physician should avoid making patients feel as though they are taking a "brain test" that can be passed or failed. This reassurance is especially important in tests involving mathematical problems. One way to build confidence is to start with easy problems so patients can get several answers correct (e.g., "Can you add 1 plus 1?" "2 plus 2?" and so on). Patients with a neurological condition can tolerate only small amounts of anxiety and several brief periods of testing before they become agitated and confused. Excessive anxiety may make some patients seem more neurologically impaired than they really are. When the mental status deficits are subtle, however, they are easier to detect if patients' anxiety level is increased. Longer silences and increasingly difficult cognitive tests, such as complicated mathematical problems or difficult spelling words, may be necessary to discover some deficits. Once the deficits have been recognized and diagnosed, they should not be repeatedly elicited, unless there is a specific medical reason to do so. This guideline is followed to protect patients' often vulnerable sense of self-esteem.

The self-esteem of patients with delirium, dementia, or other cognitive syndromes can be particularly fragile. Patients with dementia often try to conceal their deficits because they are ashamed of appearing stupid. They may deny even to themselves that they have a serious brain disease or may try to protect their families from the deficits. Physicians need to find a balance between respecting patients' needed defenses and obtaining the information necessary for diagnosis and treatment. Reassuring patients that they cannot "fail" the interview and acknowledging their efforts to respond to questions is usually all that is required to avoid defensive responses.

Patients who realize that they cannot remember things or suddenly become fearful that they are losing their intellectual capacity may develop a **catastrophic reaction.** This reaction is a sudden outburst of extreme, intense emotion (e.g., anger, rage, or tears) or violence that may occur when patients first realize, on an emotional level, that their mental capacities are deteriorating rapidly. Patients will later describe a mixture of fear and intense shame. Although novice physicians are more likely to expose patients' mental deficits without tact, even skilled physicians can inadvertently elicit a catastrophic reaction. ➠ One experienced physician did so when he asked a patient who had been a physicist about quark theory. The physician was unaware that the patient had discovered several new subatomic particles that had been predicted by quark theory. A fury of tears and rage erupted in the patient when he realized that his dementia was robbing him of his intellectual abilities and the possibility of doing research in the future. ⬅ Such reactions are more likely when the patients' self-esteem is grounded in intellectual abilities and prowess (e.g., a research physicist is more likely to develop a catastrophic reaction than a construction worker, whose self-esteem is vested in physical abilities). Most catastrophic reactions can be managed and treated psychotherapeutically with empathy and support. In some cases, benzodiazepines can help calm patients.

Once the symptoms have been identified and the entire medical history has been established, the physician should try to develop a differential diagnosis. When patients are feeling less anxious and their medical status has improved or stabilized, it may be desirable to ask more open-ended questions in order to formulate the treatment plan. These questions should focus on the psychological, familial, and social factors influencing the patient's condition.

Family Interview

Family members should be consulted early in the evaluation process. Families are invaluable sources of information because they are usually the best observers of patients' deficits and problems. Some physicians prefer not to interview families because they believe that the evaluation can be done more quickly and in a less complicated fashion by interviewing only the patient. Interviewing the family as a unit, however, allows the physician to hear many different views of patients' problems and can yield important information that distressed or sick patients may not be able to remember or communicate. In addition, families are often the best resources for implementing a treatment plan and follow-up care. They may be able to provide most of the physical care for patients, assist in educating about the illness, and help with specific rehabilitative tasks, such as relearning how to drive or read. A family can be a wonderful source of emotional support and hope, as well, and can give the patient a sense of normalcy.

Family interviews should follow the same basic pattern as individual patient interviews. The family interview can progress from open-ended to closed-ended questions as required. During the interview, the physician should observe the interactions between patients and the various family members, keeping the following questions in mind: Does the family understand the illness? Are patients' deficits highlighted or concealed in the presence of family members? Can the husband, wife, or children help? Are some members frightened of the illness? Are some members good observers and capable of helping? Does the family fight in nonhelpful ways?

The physician can incorporate the family into patients' medical care if the family is interested in, available for, and capable of helping. If the family is too overwhelmed by the illness to be helpful, they may need the support of a professional caregiver or an agency, a hospital, or another social institution.

DIFFERENTIAL DIAGNOSIS

There are three steps in the differential diagnosis of cognitive and psychiatric disorders due to general medical conditions (see Fig. 5–1): (1) differentiate these disorders, as well as the closely related substance-induced disorders, from the category of primary psychiatric disorders; (2) differentiate the specific substance-induced or cognitive disorder or mental disorder due to a general medical condition; and (3) identify the specific medical condition that has produced the psychiatric symptoms.

The medical history taking should determine whether or not patients have a medical or neurological illness or a primary psychiatric disorder, which is the first step in the differential diagnosis. Three factors are especially indicative of a secondary psychiatric disorder: (1) an **acute onset** of symptoms; (2) the development of new psychiatric symptoms in a patient **over 40 years of age** with **no prior psychiatric history;** and (3) use of **drugs** that may have caused the symptoms. Illnesses that have behavioral manifestations and present with an acute or sudden onset (i.e., within hours or days) are usually caused by an anatomical or physiological disruption in the

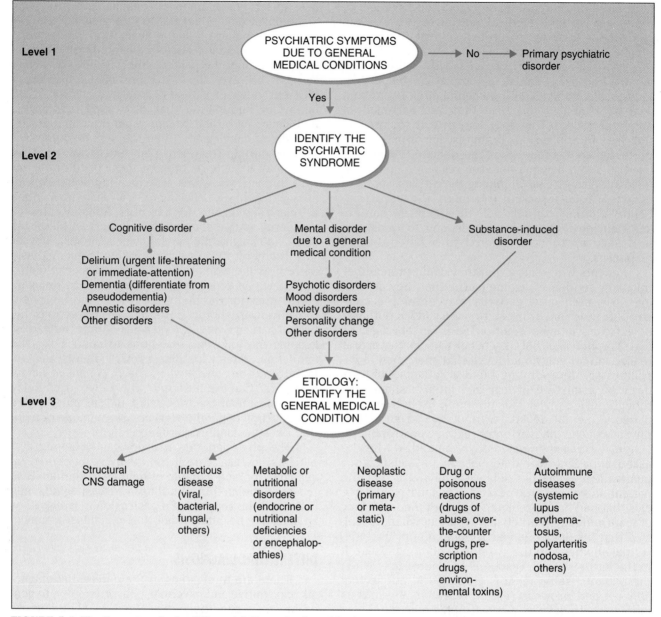

FIGURE 5–1. The three steps in the differential diagnosis of psychiatric symptoms that may be due to a general medical condition. At level 1, the syndrome is distinguished from that of a primary psychiatric disorder. At level 2, the symptoms are classified as one of the disorders due to a general medical condition. At level 3, the cause of the medical condition is determined.

central nervous system (i.e., a general medical condition). Almost all of the major psychiatric illnesses (e.g., schizophrenia, mood disorders, panic disorder) have a slow, insidious onset over a period of weeks, months, or even years. Some exceptions to this general principle exist (e.g., Alzheimer's disease has a slow, insidious onset; brief reactive psychoses and some dissociative states may occur immediately after a catastrophic psychological trauma).

Patients with new psychiatric or neurological symptoms and no history of psychiatric symptoms should also be suspected of having a general medical condition or a substance-related disorder. New symptoms might include disturbances in thinking, affect, or behavior or subtle neurological symptoms,

such as tremors, tics, or other abnormal movements. New psychiatric symptoms can be caused by many medical and neurological illnesses. Physicians who assume that new psychiatric symptoms are medically or neurologically caused until proved otherwise may perform some unnecessary medical workups in patients who are ultimately found to have a primary psychiatric condition. This situation is far more desirable, however, than the dire consequences that may result from incorrectly diagnosing a primary psychiatric disorder and missing a medical or neurological illness. The evaluation should include thorough questioning about the use of prescription and nonprescription drugs, a review of all biological systems, a detailed neurological and physical examination, assessment of the patient's mental and neurobehavioral status, and laboratory testing (see Fig. 5–1, level 1).

Once the physician has determined that the psychiatric syndrome is, in fact, due to a general medical condition, the exact psychiatric disorder due to the medical condition must be identified. The clinical features of the disorder must be distinguished, and they must fit one of the disorders that may be due to a general medical condition. In some cases, the cognitive disorder can be identified (e.g., delirium or dementia) but the medical condition cannot be determined. In other cases, it is impossible to establish the relationship between the medical condition and the psychiatric symptoms. The dilemma may be of the "chicken-versus-egg" variety (e.g., whether a brain tumor is causing depression or whether the depression is the patient's psychological reaction to having a brain tumor). When suspicion is high that the psychiatric disorder is caused by a general medical condition but a causal relationship cannot be proved, the diagnosis of a mental disorder due to a general medical condition can be made anyway. Patients' drug use history, signs and symptoms of drug intoxication or withdrawal, and urine testing can help differentiate substance-related disorders (see Fig. 5–1, level 2, and Chapter 7, Alcohol and Substance Abuse Disorders).

Once the mental disorder and the medical condition have been identified, the specific etiology of the medical condition should be determined, so that a specific medical treatment can be chosen (see Fig. 5–1, level 3, and Etiology, below).

As the following case demonstrates, differentiating between primary psychiatric conditions and psychiatric syndromes due to medical conditions is not always easy. Physicians should make every effort to do so, however, so that tragic results can be avoided.

➡ An 18-year-old college freshman presented to the student health service with sadness, irritability, and inability to concentrate on her schoolwork. She was diagnosed with an adjustment disorder related to conflicts about leaving home. Her symptoms resolved after a brief period of psychotherapy. In her junior year, she complained again of irritability and a depressed mood, and she had intermittent crying spells after she learned that her sister was suffering with a chronic liver disease. The patient's depression resolved quickly after another brief period of psychotherapy and several visits with her sister. At age 25 years, she missed several menstrual cycles and began to "feel different." Her gynecologist made a diagnosis of amenorrhea, etiology unknown. Two years later, the patient developed labile depressed moods, rage without precipitants, and anxiety; she became alcoholic and gained 60 pounds. A neurologist, an internist, and a psychiatrist all felt that her problems were caused by depression, alcoholism, and a mixed personality disorder. She returned to psychiatric treatment for several years. At age 30 years, the patient had an episode of slurred speech when she was clearly sober. She was hospitalized, and her internist

made a diagnosis of mood disorder and dementia due to Wilson's disease. Wilson's disease is a rare genetic defect in copper metabolism that causes copper poisoning of the liver or brain. The patient recovered partially with treatment but sustained brain damage. This patient's psychological symptoms, which had been present for 12 years, were caused mainly by an undiagnosed medical illness. The initial symptoms were not evaluated for medical causes, and none of the physicians made a connection between the sister's liver disease and the patient's symptoms. The sister had the chronic form of liver disease associated with Wilson's disease, while the patient had the psychiatric and central nervous system symptoms of the same illness. Once this unfortunate woman had been given a diagnosis of a psychiatric disorder, consideration was no longer given to the possibility that a medical illness might have been causing her psychological symptoms. Her psychiatric symptoms were approached with a psychological bias that attributed them to conflict, loss, displaced anger, and problems in social adjustment. The tragic result of permanent brain damage could have been entirely prevented if Wilson's disease had been diagnosed earlier and treated. ◄ɪɪɪ

It is vital to obtain a detailed medical history from both the patient and the family (see also Medical Evaluation, below). The physician should ask about risk factors, the mode of onset, and the duration and progression of signs and symptoms and should assess the patient's baseline level of functioning. A detailed psychological and social history should also be obtained (see below), with special emphasis on the patient's current living and family situation and other social supports, including shelter, food, work, finances, and relevant cultural or religious factors.

Special Areas of Concern in Differential Diagnosis

The disorders discussed below are singled out for emphasis because of their frequency or importance in making the differential diagnosis.

Substance-Induced Disorders

Substance-induced disorders are the great imitators of psychiatric illnesses. The wide array of symptoms and syndromes due to drug reactions are frequently indistinguishable from those of primary psychiatric disorders and psychiatric disorders due to a general medical condition. Substance-induced psychiatric symptoms are extremely common. Any type of drug (i.e., prescription, over-the-counter, or illegal) may induce psychiatric symptoms. It is, therefore, extremely important to take a detailed drug history of all patients. This review should cover all medications that are currently being used, how often they are taken, the typical daily dosage, and the time of last ingestion.

Illegal drug use is often the most difficult to uncover. The family may be the best source of information about this problem. **Cocaine-induced panic attacks or mania** may be clinically indistinguishable from panic disorder or bipolar disorder; **chronic phencyclidine (PCP) abuse** produces a syndrome that cannot easily be differentiated from schizophrenia; **glue sniffing** can present as dementia; and **chronic marijuana abuse** can present with an amotivational syndrome that is easily confused with depression. Urine screening is helpful in uncovering drug abuse, but it can be misleading (e.g., a negative drug screening test does not rule out drug withdrawal syndromes or past abuse of drugs).

Caffeine is widely used and abused in the United States. The consumption of two to three cups of coffee per day is enough to produce the signs and symptoms of caffeine intoxication and the symptoms of an anxiety disorder due to **caffeinism.** Associated psychiatric symptoms may include panic and, occasionally, depression. The physical symptoms may include insomnia, tremor, restlessness, abdominal pain, increased heart rate, heart palpitations, or a flushed face. Caffeinism is easily treated by gradually reducing the amount of caffeine that is consumed. Abrupt cessation is not recommended, because it can lead to fatigue, decreased attention span, irritability, and headaches.

A person who is attempting to stop smoking will crave nicotine. Psychiatric symptoms of **nicotine withdrawal** may resemble a generalized anxiety disorder, with nervousness, irritability, restlessness, frustration, poor concentration, and poor cognitive performance. Physical symptoms of nicotine withdrawal may include headaches, sleep disturbances, increased appetite, or weight gain. These symptoms can be prevented by gradually tapering cigarette consumption or by using nicotine replacement medications.

Hallucinosis is commonly associated with acute **alcohol withdrawal,** which may begin 6–24 hours after the cessation of heavy drinking. Hallucinosis is most commonly encountered in patients who have been drinking continuously for more than five years. Patients have a clear sensorium with persecutory, auditory, and, sometimes, visual hallucinations, which usually remit within a matter of days. Some chronic alcoholics have persistent auditory hallucinations that may be readily confused with schizophrenia.

Withdrawal from barbiturates or benzodiazepines may produce syndromes identical to those of acute alcoholic hallucinosis. **Hallucinogens,** such as lysergic acid diethylamide (LSD) or mescaline, can produce visual hallucinations with a clear sensorium during intoxication. Flashbacks, or repeated visual hallucinations, are a frequent sequela.

If a substance-related disorder is misdiagnosed as a primary psychiatric condition, the physician may prescribe the wrong treatment for the patient. Chapter 7, Alcohol and Substance Abuse Disorders, discusses drug reactions in much more detail.

Dementia and Pseudodementia

The possible presence of pseudodementia in elderly patients should not be overlooked. In the elderly, pseudodementia is a variant of depression that has the clinical appearance of a dementia. ➡ For example, a 62-year-old woman told her physician that she was extremely distressed about a "severe memory loss." She said that her memory had changed three weeks earlier, after she had lost her job. She was afraid that she had Alzheimer's disease. Her second husband had had this disease. She seemed to be distressed but was also irritated by the physician's questions and made little effort to answer them. Her response to most of the mental status questions was "I don't know." Her demeanor and responses were typical of a patient with pseudodementia. ⬅

The physician's suspicion that pseudodementia may be present is often the first step in differentiating pseudodementia from dementia. The onset of confusion and memory loss is usually more subacute or more rapid in pseudodementia than it is in dementia. Patients with pseudodementia often have "patchy" memory loss, and their intellectual deficits are not consistent. Patients with dementia have more global memory loss, and their intellectual deficits are persistent, unchanging, or declining. Pseudodementia should be considered in a patient if confusion or a memory problem is triggered by a loss. Patients with pseudodementia tend to focus their attention on their deficits by complaining about them and exaggerating their severity, while patients with dementia often try to conceal their deficits. Patients with pseudodementia seek help, behave in a dependent manner, and make many demands on others. They often make little effort to respond to mental status questions, immediately stating "I don't know" in a resigned tone of voice. They may have a lifelong history of personality problems that are manifested by interpersonal conflicts, repeated job losses, or conversion and other psychosomatic symptoms.

Dementia due to Parkinson's disease is a subcortical dementia. Unlike Alzheimer's disease and the vascular dementias, it is often manifested by memory loss and apathy but the intellectual abilities are relatively well preserved. Aphasia, agnosia, or apraxia is infrequently present. The rigidity and bradykinesia of the disease often cause the patient to appear to have a severe dementia, but, in fact, the dementia is usually mild.

Partial Complex Seizures Causing Psychosis

Partial complex seizures consist of focal cerebral seizure activity that results in an altered state of consciousness, flashbacks, and feelings of déjà vu. The sensorium is clear. These seizures may produce a **psychosis** with paranoia or grandiose delusions that are distinguished from schizophrenia only by the presence of seizure activity on an EEG. Psychotic symptoms can appear between seizure episodes (i.e., interictally) or during seizures. Focal seizures may produce olfactory hallucinations or may affect visual perception (e.g., objects may appear to be a different size or shape than they actually are).

Personality changes resulting from seizures are characterized by a deepening of emotions, a preoccupation with moral or religious issues, and a "viscous" communication style (i.e., tedious, didactic, verbose, and circumstantial). Men have decreased libido, but women may have increased libido.

MEDICAL EVALUATION

Most general medical conditions that produce psychiatric symptoms can be diagnosed and, often, the cause of the condition can be determined on the basis of a comprehensive history; focal review of biological systems; vital signs; detailed physical, neurological, and mental status examinations; neurobehavioral evaluation; and laboratory findings. (See also Differential Diagnosis, above.) Patients who present with a first episode of major psychiatric symptoms should receive a complete, detailed medical and neurological evaluation, including a physical examination, blood tests, CT scanning or MRI imaging of the head, and other sophisticated laboratory tests, as necessary.

Physical and Neurological Examination

An exhaustive review of all biological systems is rarely completed for patients presenting with psychiatric symptoms. Although such a review may be helpful, the physician usually does not have enough time to undertake it. Most physicians perform a focal review of systems that is geared toward the patient's specific complaints. A detailed neurological review is commonly done, as well as a focal review of other systems that may be implicated. A complete neurological review should focus on the following medical problems: headaches, including migraine headaches; seizures, syncope, and head trauma; weakness, paresthesia, and paralysis; atrophy, involuntary movements, tremors, gait disturbances, and incoordination; pain or sensory loss; loss of control of urination or defecation; sweating; learning disabilities; and changes in vision, speech, hearing, equilibrium, swallowing, or taste. Other systems should be reviewed as necessary.

The vital signs are often the earliest objective evidence that a medical condition is producing a change in mental status. The heart rate and respiratory rate, blood pressure, and temperature should be routinely evaluated in all patients. An increased heart rate and slightly bulging eyes might suggest hyperthyroidism; an upper respiratory tract infection, fever, and confusion might suggest encephalitis; and an increase in heart rate, respiratory rate, and blood pressure in the absence of fever might suggest pheochromocytoma. The physical examination should also investigate other relevant signs or symptoms.

A detailed focal neurological examination must be performed in all patients suspected of having a general medical condition affecting the brain. Pyramidal tract signs associated with dementia include brisk deep tendon reflexes, increased muscle tone, and bilateral Babinski signs.

An adjunctive neurological examination may uncover frontal release signs, such as the snout, sucking, rooting, and grasping reflexes; Hoffmann's sign (the physician presses on the fingernail of the patient's middle finger to elicit abnormal flexion and adduction of the thumb); palm-chin reflex (Radovici's sign: the physician scratches the thenar eminence to elicit contraction of the muscles of the chin on the same side); or the glabellar tap (the physician taps repeatedly on the patient's forehead to elicit repetitive eye closings that do not extinguish with time). Soft neurological signs, such as left-right confusion, mixed dominance, drift, or overflow, may suggest learning disabilities, minimal brain dysfunction, or dementia.

General laboratory screening tests may help to confirm or uncover a diagnosis of a general medical condition producing psychiatric symptoms. Special laboratory and technological tests should be reserved to confirm unusual presentations of common illnesses or to diagnose rare or unsuspected illnesses.

Mental Status Testing and Neurobehavioral Assessment

A complete, formal mental status examination should be performed in all patients who have changes in behavior, thinking, or mood. The presence of a neurological or medical condition affecting the brain is often first identified by such an examination. Boxes 5–1 and 5–2 present the tests that are most helpful in differentiating a primary psychiatric disorder from a cognitive or a mental disorder due to a general medical condition.

If there are abnormal or ambiguous findings on the clinical mental status examination, the physician can attempt to localize the deficit further by doing a simple neurobehavioral assessment. This procedure is described in Box 5–3.

ETIOLOGY

Psychiatric disorders due to general medical conditions may have one cause or multiple causes (see Fig. 5–1). The causes fall into six categories: (1) structural central nervous system damage; (2) infections; (3) metabolic or nutritional deficiencies; (4) neoplastic illnesses; (5) autoimmune diseases; or (6) drug or poisonous reactions. The most common medical conditions producing psychiatric symptoms and their causes are reviewed below.

Cognitive Disorders
Delirium

Delirium may be caused by a wide array of pathological processes. It is extremely important to define the exact cause. Some of the most common

BOX 5–1. Mental Status Testing

Mental status tests can help to evaluate neurophysiological brain functions: level of consciousness, orientation, memory, and cognitive ability.

Assessment of the Level of Consciousness
1. Observe the patient to see whether the patient is awake and alert or confused and befuddled.
2. If the patient is awake and alert, note whether the level of consciousness remains the same or fluctuates (waxes and wanes). Fluctuations in the level of consciousness suggest that the patient is delirious.
3. If the level of consciousness fluctuates, note the length of the cycles of fluctuation. The cycles may be short (i.e., apparent during the interview) or long (i.e., occurring over the course of hours or days).
4. Note also whether the fluctuations occur at certain times of the day. It is not uncommon for elderly persons to be fully alert during the day but become delirious in the evening. This phenomenon is called **sundowning** and is often seen in geriatric patients in hospitals and nursing homes.

Assessment of Orientation as to Time, Place, and Person
1. Ask the patient a series of questions to see how well oriented the patient is as to time, place, and person (i.e., the patient's own name).
2. Ask the patient, "What time of the day is it?" "Do you know what day of the week it is?" "What is the date today?" "What year is it?" "Do you know what season of the year it is?"
3. Ask the patient, "Do you know exactly where we are right now?" "What is the name of this place?" "In what institution, city, state, and country are we currently located?"
4. Ask the patient, "Do you know who you are?"
5. Correct answers to all of the questions about time, place, and person are summarized as "oriented × 3."
6. Disorientation caused by a general medical condition always occurs in a certain sequence: time is lost first, place is lost second, and person is lost third.
7. If the sequence is different from in step 6, the disorientation is due to a primary psychiatric disorder (e.g., a patient who knows the time and place but does not remember his or her own name may be suffering from a posttraumatic stress reaction or a dissociative state).

Assessment of Memory
In patients with delirium, memory may be affected as the level of consciousness fluctuates or disorientation occurs. This deficit is due to central nervous system dysfunction, which manifests itself as an inability to learn new information. Four spheres of memory should be tested: immediate recall and short-term, intermediate-term, and long-term memory.

Immediate Recall
1. Introduce yourself, and then ask the patient if he or she can remember your name. If the patient cannot, repeat your name several times and ask the patient again if he or she can remember it.
2. Ask the patient to repeat a span of digits: "I would like you to repeat immediately after me some numbers that I want you to recall. For example, if I say 1 and 3, then I want you to repeat 1 and 3. Let's try it."
3. Start with two digits, then three digits, and so on, up to seven digits.
4. When you say the numbers, keep any cadence out of the tone of your voice. Saying the numbers in a rhythmic tone makes them easier to remember, and this may enable some patients to conceal a memory deficit.

5. Most patients can recall a span of at least five digits. If the patient has a great deal of difficulty in recalling the five digits or can only recall four or fewer digits, there may be additional brain deficits. Further mental status testing should be done in these patients.

Short-term Memory
Test One
1. Give the patient three words to remember (usually, the names of two concrete objects and one abstract idea): "Please remember and repeat the following: ball, telephone, and charity." Ask the patient to repeat the three words immediately. This tests immediate recall and also shows whether the patient can attend, concentrate, and understand what you want him or her to do.
2. Go on to other interview questions. After five minutes, ask the patient to repeat the three words again.
3. If the patient can only remember two of the three (2/3), repeat the test.
4. If the patient has a primary psychiatric disorder, the memory should improve. If the patient has a neurological deficit, the memory will remain impaired.
5. If the patient still cannot remember the third word after step 3, you can say to the patient, "You have forgotten one word. Please pick from this new list of three words the one you have forgotten." This uses recognition memory, which is less readily impaired than immediate recall.

Test Two
1. If the patient has poor short-term recall (i.e., 0/3 or 1/3 after five minutes), alternative short-term memory tests can be administered. One strategy is to give the patient three evocative or colorful things to remember. "Please remember these things that I love: Paul Newman, fast red cars, and chocolate ice cream."
2. After five minutes, ask the patient to repeat these things. If the patient can do so, it means that the poor score on Test One was probably due to anxiety, inability to attend (secondary to delirium), poor concentration, or lack of effort.

Test Three
1. An expanded approach to testing short-term memory uses visual and auditory input to further stimulate the memory. Usually, the patient's performance improves with this test.
2. Take three objects out of your pocket, such as a pen, a quarter, and a set of keys, and place them in front of the patient. Ask the patient to look at the objects and name each one. Hide the objects, and after five minutes, ask the patient to recall them.
3. If the patient cannot remember the objects, repeat the test with three different objects, using visual, auditory, and tactile stimuli. Ask the patient to look at the objects, say their names, and touch them. Hide the objects, and ask the patient to recall them in five minutes. The memory should improve even further.
4. Repeat this test several times. If the memory deficit persists even with the increased sensory input, it is probably due to a severe neurophysiological disorder.

Intermediate-term Memory
1. Ask the patient to recall events that have happened over the last day or week.
2. You can ask the patient what he or she had for dinner the day before, if you can learn what the patient actually had from a source other than the patient.
3. Alternatively, you can ask the patient about current events or recent changes in the weather.

Continued

Long-term Memory

1. Ask the patient to recall events that happened years ago.
2. You can ask the patient "Where and when were you born?" or "Where did you live prior to your current residence?" if you know, from a source other than the patient, the answers to these questions.
3. Alternatively, you can ask the patient to name past presidents of the United States. Before doing this, you must determine whether the patient has had enough education to know about the presidents or has had easy access to information about the presidents in daily life.

Interpreting the Results of Memory Testing

1. The pattern of deficits is more important than any one isolated or specific deficit.
2. The sequence in which neurological function is lost is significant. Patients with memory impairment due to a general medical condition usually lose memory functions in sequence: Immediate recall is lost first, short-term memory is lost second, intermediate-term memory is lost third, and long-term memory is lost last. Patients who lose memory in a different sequence usually have a primary psychiatric disorder or a volitional memory deficit that has no basis in a general medical condition.
3. It is also extremely important to remember that most cognitive and mental disorders caused by a general medical condition have a constellation of neurological deficits. These usually include alterations in the level of consciousness, orientation problems, memory deficits, and disturbances in cognitive functioning. A specific, slight memory deficit that improves rapidly with repeated testing is probably caused by anxiety or a primary psychiatric disorder or it may be a volitional deficit. Some rare general medical conditions do cause specific memory deficits (e.g., thiamine deficiency may result in an amnestic disorder).

Assessment of Cognitive Ability

1. Cognitive ability is tested by asking the patient to do a complex operation (e.g., solve a mathematical problem) that can be performed accurately only if the sensorium is clear and the patient is fully conscious and oriented, has an intact memory, and is able to concentrate. (The patient must also be intelligent enough and well enough educated to do the task.) Simple mathematical problems (e.g., adding numbers) or word problems (e.g., spelling the word "world" backward) are examples of cognitive tests.
2. Before testing begins, find out how much education the patient has had and, in addition, try to minimize the patient's anxiety about the test situation. Ask the patient how far he or she went in school. This information is important in choosing the level of difficulty of the first cognitive test. If the patient is a college graduate, you might start with serial 7 subtraction, beginning with 100 and going backward. If the patient completes this task without difficulty, you can steadily increase the complexity of the mathematical problems (e.g., increasingly complicated multiplication and division problems; then, square root problems; and so on, up to differential calculus problems).
3. If the patient performs poorly on the first test, switch immediately to a drastically simpler test at which the patient is likely to succeed with no difficulty. It is important for the physician to make it easy for the patient to get the next few answers correct because this success will minimize the patient's anxiety, increase the patient's confidence, and improve the patient's performance on subsequent tests.
4. Gradually increase the degree of difficulty, until the cognitive deficits again appear. If a patient makes many mistakes in serial 7 subtraction, ask the patient, "Can you count backward from 21 to 10?" Alternatively, you can ask the patient to add 1 plus 1; then, 2 plus 2; and so on. If the patient still has difficulty, switch to an easy calculation with money, such as "How much money is a nickel and a penny?" Money problems are easier for most patients. A more complex money question might be, "If an orange costs 20 cents, and you buy four oranges, and you give the grocer $5.00, how much change would you receive?"
5. Once you are certain that the patient has a cognitive deficit that is inconsistent with the patient's educational or social background, try to locate the level of the deficit (i.e., altered level of consciousness, disorientation, poor concentration, memory deficit, or intelligence problem). The level of the deficit will suggest whether a cognitive disorder, such as delirium or dementia, or a mental disorder due to a general medical condition is present.

causes are seizures due to structural damage of the central nervous system; metabolic disorders, such as thyroid disease or hepatic or renal failure; infectious diseases, such as HIV infection, herpes simplex encephalitis, or pneumococcal or meningococcal meningitis; primary brain tumors; neoplastic disease, such as breast cancer that has metastasized to the brain; or autoimmune disorders, such as systemic lupus erythematosus or polyarteritis nodosa. Deliriums can also be substance related, such as those due to alcohol or cocaine abuse. The classification of deliriums by one of the six etiologies alone can be extremely helpful in making the diagnosis (Table 5–7). It is also helpful to classify delirium as either (1) delirium that is life-threatening within minutes and requires emergency intervention or (2) delirium that must be recognized immediately but can be treated over a period of hours to days. Table 5–7 shows the most common causes of life-threatening deliriums and gives a partial list of symptoms based on the six etiological categories of disease.

Dementia

Dementias can be caused by primary diseases of the central nervous system or by secondary involvement of the central nervous system by systemic diseases. They can be divided into six etiological categories: (1) structural damage to the central nervous system, such as Alzheimer's disease, vascular dementia, or Parkinson's disease; (2) infectious diseases, such as HIV infection, tuberculous meningitis, or chronic cryptococcus meningitis; (3) metabolic or nutritional disorders, such as hypothyroidism, hyperthyroidism, Wilson's disease, or thiamine or niacin deficiency; (4) neoplastic diseases, such as glioma, astrocytoma, or breast or lung cancer that has metastasized to the brain; (5) autoimmune disorders, such as systemic lupus erythematosus; and (6) drug or poisonous reactions, such as alcohol intoxication or reactions to glue sniffing.

The most common etiologies of the dementias and some of their differentiating features are briefly described below.

BOX 5–2.   Adjunctive Mental Status Testing Performed at the Bedside

---

Clock Test

The clock test (Tuokko et al., 1992) can be administered at the bedside with a pencil and paper. There are three parts to this test: clock drawing, clock setting, and clock reading. Clock drawing is primarily a visual spatial skill located in the non-dominant (usually right) cerebral hemisphere. Clock setting and clock reading require comprehension of the concept of time. They are primarily a function of the dominant (usually left) cerebral hemisphere. In other words, the clock test is a good way of evaluating the cognitive function of both cerebral hemispheres.

1. Clock drawing: Ask the patient to draw a circle, indicate a clock face, and place all the numbers in the proper location within the circle.
2. Clock setting: Have the patient add hands to the clock to indicate a specific time. Try several different times.
3. Clock reading: Show the patient several drawings of clocks that you have made. The clocks should have hands, but no numbers, indicating several different times. Ask the patient to read the different times.
4. Normal elderly persons may have some difficulties in clock drawing but can easily do clock setting and clock reading. About 80% of patients with Alzheimer's disease have difficulty in performing all three tasks.

Set Test With Word Intrusion

The set test with word intrusion (Fuld, 1983) is an easily administered bedside examination.

1. Ask the patient to name 10 objects in each of three general categories, or sets (e.g., "Name 10 cities, 10 foods, and 10 animals.")

2. The maximum score is 30 out of 30 (30/30). A score of 25–30/30 is considered normal. A score of 15–25/30 indicates that either a primary psychiatric disorder or a cognitive or mental disorder due to a general medical condition is present. A score of less than 15/30 strongly suggests that the cause is a general medical condition affecting the brain rather than a primary psychiatric condition.
3. A word intrusion occurs when the patient adds an object from one category to a different category (e.g., when the patient is asked to name 10 animals, the patient includes the name of a city or a food). The more word intrusions there are, the greater is the likelihood of Alzheimer's disease, compared with other dementias. Patients who score less than 15/30 with word intrusions are likely to have Alzheimer's disease. Patients who score less than 15/30 without word intrusions are likely to have another form of dementia.
4. This test does not have much validity if it is used alone. It is helpful as an adjunctive test when other mental status deficits have already been detected. A score of less than 15/30 with word intrusions increases the probability of Alzheimer's disease by 10–20%.

Other Tests

Other, more standardized mental status tests that can be scored can also be used to detect mental disorders due to a general medical condition. Folstein's Mini-Mental State Examination Scale (Folstein, et al., 1975) is one commonly used test. Other research scales, which are more complicated and more cumbersome to administer and interpret, include the Brief Cognitive Rating Scale, Alzheimer's Disease Assessment Scale, and Wechsler Adult Intelligence Scale.

Cognitive deficits in **Alzheimer's disease** may be caused by dysfunction of the cholinergic, muscarinic, or nicotinic receptors. The histopathological findings show senile plaques, neurofibrillary tangles, or cerebral atrophy in the association areas, with sparing of the motor, visual, and somatosensory cerebral cortex. Family studies suggest that some genetic vulnerability to Alzheimer's dementia is inherited via the apolipoprotein E4 allele in at least some cases of the disease.

Vascular dementia is produced by the occlusion of small vessels (i.e., secondary blood vessel damage from hypertension or arteriosclerosis), which leads to focal or lacunar brain infarctions. These lesions are sometimes missed in the clinical examination because they are too small or are confined to the silent areas of the brain. CT scanning or MRI, or both, will reveal these infarcts.

In patients with **HIV infection,** dementia may have a number of causes. It may be caused by primary HIV infection of the brain, by the secondary effects of immunosuppressive drugs, or by drugs for treatment of the infection. All of the dementias associated with HIV disease have the clinical findings of general dementia. The cause of HIV-related dementia can best be differentiated by medical and laboratory testing.

The HIV virus directly infects the brain shortly after seroconversion. The virus is probably carried by macrophages that cross the blood-brain barrier

and produce mild or subclinical meningoencephalitis, which may present clinically as mild delirium. The central nervous system infection may later produce subcortical dementia through an autoimmune reaction. This dementia usually presents years after seroconversion and probably coincides with the gradual deterioration of the immune system. The earliest symptoms of HIV dementia include memory loss, depressive symptoms, decreased flexibility in thinking, personality changes, and difficulty in performing complex actions.

The secondary causes of HIV dementia or other related brain deficits are the result of opportunistic illnesses caused by immunosuppression, which may include brain lymphomas, Kaposi's sarcoma, central nervous system opportunistic infections (e.g., toxoplasmosis, cryptococcosis, cytomegalovirus infection, and herpesvirus infection), or chronic hypoxia due to opportunistic lung infections.

Drugs used in treating HIV infection can also produce central nervous system symptoms. Zidovudine (AZT) may produce adverse mental effects, including depression, hallucinations, and drowsiness. Other common adverse mental effects of AZT include delirium, depression, and a loss of mental acuity that is easily confused with dementia.

Dementia due to **Parkinson's disease** is caused by an imbalance between dopaminergic inhibition and cholinergic stimulation in the basal ganglion,

---

BOX 5–3.   The Three-Dimensional Neurobehavioral Assessment

In addition to the mental status examination, a simple neurobehavioral assessment may help to localize a neurobehavioral deficit further. Smith and Craft (1984) described a three-dimensional model of the nervous system that has three neurobehavioral axes (i.e., the vertical, lateral, and horizontal axes).

1. The vertical neurobehavioral axis extends from the subcortical to the cortical structures of the brain. The basic function, arousal, is controlled by the reticular activating system in the brain stem. This system acts like a dimmer on a light switch. It signals the deep brain structures and the cortex to be fully alert; partially alert, which may cause delirium; or barely alert, which may cause semicoma or coma. The vertical neurobehavioral axis is assessed by observation of the patient's level of alertness and attention and testing of immediate and short-term memory.

2. The lateral neurobehavioral axis extends from the right to the left cerebral hemisphere.
   a. The left brain cortex is the dominant hemisphere in 97% of right-handed patients and in 50% of left-handed patients. The dominant hemisphere primarily controls language. If a patient can name an object and repeat a simple phrase, the functioning of the dominant hemisphere is grossly intact.
      (1) Ask the patient to name an object that you take out of your pocket (e.g., hold up a pen and ask, "What is this?"). This tests Broca's area.
      (2) Have the patient repeat a simple phrase, such as "The boy went to the store to buy some milk." This tests Wernicke's area.
      (3) If the patient has difficulty in answering these questions, it indicates that there are deficits in these specific left hemispheric regions of the brain or in the connection between Broca's area and Wernicke's area.

      (4) Additional simple dominant hemispheric testing can be done by asking the patient to read aloud (test for Broca's area), to comprehend what was read (test for Wernicke's area), and to write a simple sentence (test for the dominant parietal region).
   b. The nondominant brain (i.e., the right hemisphere in most patients) is primarily responsible for spatial relations and pattern recognition.
      (1) Deficits in spatial relations can be elicited by having a patient copy squares, triangles, or other geometric shapes. It is also tested by clock drawing (see Box 5–2).
      (2) Pattern recognition can be tested by showing the patient pictures of famous people in a magazine and asking the patient whether he or she can recognize them, or by tapping a patterned drum beat and asking the patient to repeat the complex pattern of sounds.

3. The horizontal neurobehavioral axis runs along the rolandic fissure, arbitrarily dividing the cortex horizontally.
   a. Deficits of structures in front of the fissure (motor, premotor, prefrontal, and frontal cortex) can often be detected by frontal release signs (i.e., release of pathological reflexes) on the neurological examination or by observing the patient having problems in planning or organization. A simple organizational test is to ask the patient to describe in detail how he or she would go about planning a party.
   b. Deficits of structures behind the fissure (temporal, parietal, and occipital cortex) can be elicited by testing visual fields on the neurological examination or will be discovered by lateral axis testing such as repeating phrases or comprehending a newspaper.

---

which may affect other neurotransmitters, such as serotonin and norepinephrine. Patients lose nerve cells, pigmentation, and cellular Lewy bodies in the substantia nigra, dorsal vagal nucleus, and locus coeruleus of the brain stem. Parkinson's disease does not seem to be a genetic disorder and is probably an acquired disease. Drug treatment of the movement disorder in Parkinson's disease does not seem to affect the development, course, or progression of the disease to dementia. Dementia occurs in 30–40% of patients with Parkinson's disease. It is generally mild and presents late in the course of the illness.

Amnestic Disorder

Amnestic disorders may be caused by any illness that damages the deep brain structures that are associated with memory. These disorders are common in certain populations, such as head trauma victims or patients with thiamine deficiency. Other causes of amnestic disorder include structural damage to the central nervous system associated with partial complex seizures or Alzheimer's disease; infections, such as herpes encephalitis; neoplastic conditions; drugs, such as phencyclidine; and autoimmune vasculitis affecting the posterior cerebral artery.

Traumatic brain injuries due to motorcycle or motor vehicle accidents, falls, or violent assault are usually coup-contracoup lesions (e.g., a blow to the back of the head that injures the frontal or temporal cerebral lobes).

Thiamine deficiency (Korsakoff's disease, or substance-induced persisting amnestic disorder) is usually a result of poor nutrition due to alcohol abuse. It produces severe short-term memory deficits.

Mental Disorders due to a General Medical Condition

Psychotic Disorders Due to a General Medical Condition

The most common medical causes of delusions are substance-induced psychotic disorders, seizures, and lesions of the posterior nondominant cerebral hemisphere. The most common medical causes of isolated hallucinations are alcohol abuse and sensory deprivation.

Stimulants, such as cocaine, amphetamines, methylphenidate, and phencyclidine, commonly produce an acute psychosis that may be clinically indistinguishable from acute paranoid schizophrenia.

TABLE 5–7. Symptoms and Causes of Life-Threatening Deliriums

Disease Category or Agent	Clinical Presentation
Structural CNS damage	
Intracranial bleeding	Headache, or focal neurological signs. Bleeding occurs in 25% of strokes. In young persons, berry aneurysm is most common cause. In general, increased risk of bleeding with advancing age and presence of hypertension
Subdural bleeding	Same as for intracranial bleeding. Often due to head trauma. Increased risk for alcoholics. Can occur long after acute head trauma
Infectious disease	
Bacterial meningitis	Headache, stiff neck, meningeal signs, sudden fever, and increased white blood cell count. Epidemics
Encephalitis (due to virus or opportunistic infections)	Initial flulike prodrome of headache, rhinorrhea, sore throat, fever blisters. Then delirium, neurological symptoms, or seizures. Slight increase in white blood cell count. Can be caused by self-infection or epidemics
Metabolic and nutritional disease	
Decreased cerebral perfusion causing hypoxemia; hypovolemia, hypoglycemia	Decreased blood pressure, glucose, pO_2, or hematocrit; signs and symptoms of cardiac failure (myocardial infarction, congestive heart failure, arrhythmia) diabetes, respiratory distress (COPD, asthma, pulmonary embolism)
Hypertensive encephalopathy	Hypertension, papilledema
Wernicke's encephalopathy	Ataxia, dementia. Seen in 3% alcoholics; 17% mortality rate
Neoplastic and autoimmune diseases	No urgent deliriums
Drug reactions	
Drug abuse	Delirium due to alcohol or cocaine intoxication (most common); delirium due to withdrawal of alcohol, sedative-hypnotics. Status seizures secondary to withdrawal are often life-threatening
Over-the-counter or prescription drugs	Delirium due to use of acetaminophen, sleeping pills, cough preparations; delirium due to use of antidepressants, anticholinergics. At risk for arrhythmias
Poisons (environmental)	Delirium and symptoms specific to poison (e.g., household products such as pesticides, solvents, carbon monoxide, lead)

Chronic abuse of large amounts of crack cocaine may also produce a persistent psychosis. It is probably a result of the **brain-kindling phenomenon,** which is intermittent low-level irritation of the cerebral cortex.

Hallucinations may be caused by acute withdrawal from alcohol or drugs (e.g., barbiturates, benzodiazepines, LSD). When a person is in an environment with inadequate sensory stimulation (e.g., an intensive care unit or a solitary confinement cell in a prison), sensory-deprivation hallucinations may develop. These hallucinations may also occur in patients with cataracts or otosclerosis (usually, elderly patients), who have radically reduced visual and auditory sensory input. In medically ill patients, sensory deprivation should be an etiology of exclusion, in order to avoid missing other causes, such as drug reactions.

Mood Disorders Due to a General Medical Condition

Most mood disorders caused by a general medical condition present with major depression or depressive symptoms. The leading medical causes of depression are the endocrinopathies and drugs. The most common medical causes of mania are antidepressant medications and corticosteroids.

Many endocrine disorders present with depressive or manic symptoms mixed with anxiety symptoms. Often, the hyperactive and hypoactive states have similar neuropsychiatric symptoms but can easily be distinguished by their physical signs and symptoms. Thyroid disease is the most common endocrinopathy causing a mood disorder. Less frequent causes of mood disorders include imbalances of cortisol, calcium, and prolactin.

Patients with **hyperthyroidism** often present with fatigue, weight loss, sweating, heat intolerance, scant menstruation, tachycardia, tremor, and bulging eyes (proptosis). Frequent neuropsychiatric manifestations are insomnia, crying episodes that are easily confused with depression, and anxiety. The most common causes of hyperthyroidism are Graves' disease, inflammatory thyroiditis, excessive thyroid hormone replacement therapy, and, rarely, thyroid or ovarian cancers. The diagnosis is made clinically and confirmed by thyroid function tests and TSH levels. Antithyroid hormone treatment is recommended.

Patients with **hypothyroidism** often present with fatigue, weight gain, constipation, cold intolerance, menorrhagia, goiter, reflex delay, and myxedema (i.e., dryness, hair loss, edema, hoarseness, and muscle weakness). When hypothyroidism is mild, it may present with depression, suicidality, or psychosis. When it is severe and long-standing, it commonly presents as dementia. The most common causes of hypothyroidism are overly zealous treatment of hyperthyroidism by surgery or irradiation, autoimmune thyroid disease, or lithium use. Rarely, it may be caused by pituitary or hypothalamic disease. The diagnosis is made clinically and confirmed by low thyroid function tests and high TSH levels. Thyroid replacement treatment with levothyroxine is recommended.

The list of **prescription drugs** that may cause depression as a side effect is long and impressive. The most common offenders are the antihypertensive drugs, which include central nervous system antihypertensives (e.g., methyldopa); beta-blockers (e.g., propranolol); and adrenergic stimulants (e.g., clonidine). Drugs that are less likely to cause depressive symptoms are diuretics (e.g., hydrochlorothiazide, furosemide); peripheral-acting drugs (e.g., prazosin, terazosin); or calcium channel blockers (e.g., verapamil, nifedipine). Other drugs that commonly produce depression are cimetidine and disulfiram. Withdrawal from steroids may also cause depressive symptoms.

Depressive symptoms are common in persons who abuse alcohol, opioids, phencyclidine, sedatives, or hypnotics and also in those who are in withdrawal from stimulants or alcohol.

Prescription drugs that may produce mania as a side effect are the antidepressants, stimulants, such as methylphenidate and amphetamines, and baclofen. Individuals who have a predisposition toward affective illness are most likely to be affected by these drugs.

Manic symptoms are also common in patients who are acutely intoxicated with cocaine or with appetite suppressants, such as phenmetrazine or diethylpropion. Other drugs that may produce manic features during intoxication include phencyclidine, marijuana, hallucinogens, caffeine, inhalants, alcohol, and anabolic steroids and corticosteroids.

Anxiety Disorders Due to a General Medical Condition

Anxiety disorders are most commonly produced by **cardiac conditions, endocrine disorders** (notably, pheochromocytomas, diabetes, or hyperthyroidism), and **drug intoxication** (e.g., with caffeine and stimulants).

Pheochromocytoma is a catecholamine-secreting tumor of the adrenal medulla or other abdominal paraganglionic sites. It may produce anxiety symptoms, such as a fear of dying, panic attacks, and, rarely, agoraphobia. Physical symptoms include malignant hypertensive episodes, headaches, or severe abdominal, back, or pelvic pain. The tumor may be definitively diagnosed by a 24-hour urine sample that shows high levels of catecholamines or derivatives. Surgical treatment for removal of the tumor is usually required.

Excessive caffeine intake and nicotine withdrawal are common medical causes of generalized anxiety disorder and panic disorder.

Cocaine intoxication or withdrawal, marijuana abuse, and alcohol and opiate withdrawal are also common causes of generalized anxiety disorder and panic disorder. Chronic abuse of large amounts of cocaine and abuse of stimulants can produce an obsessive desire for sex and compulsive masturbation.

Personality Changes Due to a General Medical Condition

The different personality changes are related to the **location of brain lesions.** It has been estimated that 90% of patients with frontal lobe lesions have mental changes. Other locations of brain lesions can also cause a personality change. Labile, aggressive, and paranoid personality changes are caused by more diffusely located brain lesions.

Patients with disinhibition frequently have pathological damage to the orbital-frontal part of the brain following trauma or a brain tumor. Apathy tends to be caused by tumors of or trauma to the frontal cortex convexities or dorsal lateral frontal cortex. Akinetic changes are caused by structural damage from strokes, tumors, or trauma to the medial frontal area of the brain (i.e., the premotor or motor cortex). Lability is usually associated with lesions of the nondominant cerebral hemisphere (usually, the right hemisphere). Diffuse brain lesions due to structural diseases and hyperthyroidism can also produce lability and personality change. Aggressive changes are caused by head trauma or other damage to the frontal, prefrontal, or temporal cortex; the hypothalamus; or the limbic or amygdala regions. The most common causes are motor vehicle accidents and other types of head trauma. Tumors are a less common cause. Strokes, tumors, and hypocortisolism (Addison's disease) may present with paranoid personality changes. Diffuse damage to the frontal cortex or other areas of the brain can also cause this disorder. Personality change associated with seizures occurs interictally (i.e., between seizures). This association implies that it is not the seizures that produce the personality change but rather the progression of the brain lesions. There is controversy as to whether personality changes are caused by all types of seizures or only by partial complex seizures.

TREATMENT

The treatment of cognitive and mental disorders due to a general medical condition often begins with the treatment of the medical condition. Medical treatments routinely involve medications and surgery, as well as general measures to promote good health, such as eating nutritious food, getting enough sleep, increasing the amount of exercise, reducing the level of stress, stopping smoking, and losing weight. Psychiatric treatment may also be needed. The physician must be skillful at combining several types of treatments. The biopsychosocial approach to the treatment of these disorders is an effective one.

The biopsychosocial treatment of patients with medically caused brain deficits is sometimes neglected because some physicians believe that patients with brain damage cannot benefit from psychiatric treatment. Although many patients cannot be "cured," psychiatric treatment can often help restore the optimal level of brain function that the illness, the patient's psychological makeup, and the social situation will permit. Most patients can be helped to do some things that will improve the quality of their lives. The main forms of biopsychosocial treatment for these patients are psychotherapy, behavior therapy, family therapy, and psychopharmacological treatment.

Psychotherapy

Supportive Psychotherapy

Supportive psychotherapy helps patients understand their deficits and adapt to the illness. These goals may be accomplished by the physician's offering a caring, emotionally supportive, safe environment in which patients can talk about the deficits, and their feelings, stresses, and attempts at adaptation. Supportive psychotherapy does not focus on intrapsychic life and conflicts but, instead, focuses on the "here and now." Patients can be helped to develop realistic capacities. Psychosocial support from the family or other social groups can be mobilized, as well.

➡ A 45-year-old man had been in a severe automobile accident. He had had right cerebral hemispheric damage, which resulted in paralysis of the left arm and inattention to the left side of his body. His wife had become increasingly angry with him because, each morning, he would insist that he could dress himself but would only partially complete the task. His wife would try to finish dressing him, but he would insist that he was finished, become furious, and shout at his wife until she left the room. He would remain only partially dressed, and his wife would be ashamed to take him out of the house. Three months after the accident, the physician began supportive psychotherapy. He first reviewed the medical facts with the patient and his wife. The physician explained that the patient's inability to finish dressing himself was based on a persistent neurological syndrome called hemineglect. The patient did not realize that he was not clothed, and he argued with his wife because he thought that she was babying him unnecessarily. The physician also explained the inattention deficits to the patient, who cried during the session as he began to accept and grieve his neurological losses. Once both spouses understood the situation, they were less angry and could work together toward dressing the patient. ⬅

Physicians may suggest that patients use support services (e.g., a visiting nurse), and may help them recognize marital stresses, financial concerns, or other problems of daily living. Other supportive interventions include abreaction (i.e., remembering a traumatic event), catharsis (as with the patient just described), suggestions, guidance, persuasion, environmental manipulation, reassurance, and reality testing. These efforts will usually improve patients' ability to function and decrease vulnerability to their everyday stresses.

Some brain deficits require specific adaptations in psychiatric techniques (e.g., for a patient with attention deficits, the physician may want to eliminate all sensory distractions from the office and use simple sentences with clear, evocative language). Physicians may "lend" patients their capacities (i.e., ego functions) to compensate for deficits (e.g., a patient who has a blunted affect may be helped by a physician who emotes strongly and accentuates his or her feelings with hand gestures). Physicians can encourage patients by praising them for their efforts toward recovery and adaptation to the illness.

The physician's ability to differentiate brain and cortical behaviors from psychological defense mechanisms increases the effectiveness of supportive psychotherapy. The patient discussed above had a neurological cortical deficit in representation of the left side of his body. His wife thought that he was stubborn or was denying his illness. Other patients may not have neurological problems but may use psychological defense mechanisms, such as denial or disavowal, to shield themselves from the psychological pain of being aware of their deficits. If the psychological defenses are pathological, they can be modified by encouraging the patient to use different defenses or by using an interpretive approach. Pathological neurocortical behaviors are better treated by education or environmental manipulation.

Behavior Therapy

Three behavioral approaches are being used increasingly to promote recovery from specific brain deficits: operant-behavior treatment, social learning treatment, and cognitive-behavior treatment. (See also Chapter 15, The Psychotherapies.)

Operant-Behavior Treatment

Operant-behavior treatment is a traditional approach that evaluates the sequence of events that lead up to a specific maladaptive behavior and the consequences that result from the behavior. Altering the preceding events and the consequences of an event can alter the behavior. ➡ Such an approach was used for a patient with Alzheimer's disease who had developed violent outbursts. The outbursts occurred after the patient's spouse attempted to groom him. The consequence of the outbursts was that the spouse would leave in disgust and would be replaced by the patient's favorite nurse. The behavior was modified by having the nurse do the regularly scheduled grooming (positively reinforcing the nonviolent behavior) instead of the spouse (removing the negative reinforcement of the violent behavior) and having the spouse bring the patient a favorite food (positively reinforcing the nonviolent behavior). These changes were completely successful at eliminating the violent episodes. ⬅

Social Learning Treatment

Social learning treatment can be used in combination with other treatments. This approach is based on the theory that neurologically impaired patients with behavioral disturbances can learn to correct the maladaptive behaviors by modeling new behaviors after others who are acting in a socially appropriate manner. This treatment can be carried out in a group or individual setting. A social skills group can help patients relearn how to groom themselves, improve their manners, or reestablish their social graces. These groups rely heavily on modeling, role playing, and positive reinforcements.

Cognitive-Behavior Treatment

Cognitive-behavior treatment focuses primarily on distorted thought processes rather than problematic behaviors. It is based on the theory that patients with psychiatric or neurological brain deficits may develop pathological automatic thoughts that are repetitive and rigid and reflect a distorted style of thinking. These cognitive misperceptions lead to maladaptive behaviors or inhibitions. Cognitive therapy encourages the patient to recognize the distorted thoughts, test their veracity against reality, and change the illogical interpretations of events. Many patients gain a broader perspective about their illness, which gives them more freedom to choose different behavioral responses.

➡ A stroke victim stayed in bed all day, even though he was neurologically capable of mild physical activity. He did this because he felt that he was useless and a burden to his family and thought that the world expected more of him than he could give in his sick condition. His negative view of himself, defeatist attitude, sense of hopelessness, perception of himself as a burden, and experience of the world as demanding were automatic pathological thought processes. The psychotherapist challenged all of these negative views. The patient was asked to observe his negative attitude toward himself and to test reality to see if his family found him a burden. He was also encouraged to use and test his true capacities and abilities. By repeatedly confronting his cognitive distortions, his mood began to improve. Once he was less depressed, he could interpret events more realistically, and this motivated him to change his behavior. He got out of bed and began to move around. ⬅

There are a wide array of **specific cognitive rehabilitative techniques** that may be helpful in the treatment of medical conditions that have caused specific brain deficits. Deficits in memory, orientation, attention, language, or visual and spatial relations can be compensated for by such techniques. Memory can be enhanced by teaching patients to use reminders, cues, or mnemonics. Making lists or using a memory book or a pocket computer may also be helpful. Problems of orientation may be ameliorated by having caregivers repeat the day, date, time, and place. Patients can also be taught to orient themselves through frequent use of a calendar, daily newspaper, or watch. Specific language deficits can be improved by speech therapy, cognitive retraining, and comprehension exercises. Some intellectual deficits can be compensated for by a reeducation process that breaks down an intellectual task into small, manageable steps. Each step can be relearned by using alternative brain capacities. These techniques may be used to teach patients how to drive, do mathematical problems, or read.

Family Therapy

Family therapy is an extremely powerful, effective form of treatment for patients with psychiatric symptoms due to a general medical condition and their families. Family therapy focuses on interactions between patients and their family members, who are trying to cope with the illness and take care of each other. The illness may precipitate changes in the family structure or communication patterns.

The roles of family members often change dramatically in response to patients' deficits. Most patients lose prestige and power and function much differently within the family, which often means that some family members must assume leadership positions and others have to define or assume new roles.

Patterns of communication may also be radically altered when one member of a family becomes mentally disabled. If the patient has specific deficits in communication, this change can create problems. The general patterns of communication within the entire family or between specific dyads within the family may also be altered. ➡ In one family, for example, the mother usually communicated the children's needs to the father. When she developed a dementia, someone else had to fill this role. At first, the father tried to communicate with all of the children, but he quickly became overwhelmed with his roles as primary caretaker of his wife and as breadwinner. The oldest daughter then assumed the mother's role, which altered the communication patterns within the entire family because she communicated differently from her mother. ⬅ If changes such as these are not successfully negotiated, communication problems can readily develop that will decrease a family's cohesiveness and capacity to solve problems together.

Family therapy for patients with a psychiatric disorder secondary to a medical illness is still in the early phases of development. The approach, which uses psychoeducational, structural, and strategic techniques, can be tailored to each family.

Psychoeducational Family Therapy

Most families with patients suffering from a medically caused psychiatric disorder need to be educated about the illness. Families need help in understanding the signs and symptoms of the illness, the stages of deterioration, and the probable course or progression. They should be told which treatments are available, how they can be involved in the treatment, and how they can get help with the daily, routine care of the patient. They should also know about the likelihood of remission or cure and the long-term prognosis. When necessary, they need help in preparing for patients' deaths. In the opening sessions, it is especially helpful to teach families about patients' specific deficits and behaviors and help them to differentiate the true neuropsychiatric deficits from the psychological conflicts or reactions to the illness. This information frequently ameliorates anger toward the patients and fosters a more supportive attitude. It is important to focus on things that can realistically be changed; this will increase hope and promote new family coping strategies. After the educational information has been shared, it is usually imperative to help all of the family members deal with their grief over patients' losses. The stages of grief usually include denial, anger, bargaining, and, eventually, mourning and resolution.

Family Structure Therapy

Family structure is a term used to describe the formal organization of a family. The structure that existed prior to the illness should be compared with the one that has developed since patients became impaired. The physician should ask the following questions: Who was the head of the household before, and who is now the head of the household? Who made and enforced the family rules, and how has this changed since the illness? How did and does the family negotiate with the outside world? How were family disputes settled, and how are they now negotiated? What were and are the roles of the parents and children? How did the parents get along as a couple before, and how are they getting along now? What were and are the different roles of each parent? How do the children interact as siblings? What were and are the different roles of each child?

As the picture of the family structure emerges, specific interventions can be designed to help the family members reorganize and adapt to new roles and positions of power. After several sessions, the entire family may be mobilized to be the major caregivers for patients.

Strategic Family Therapy

Certain issues may arise daily in families that are coping with patients who have a psychiatric disorder secondary to a medical condition. These problems can be treated with strategic family therapy, which focuses on a specific behavioral problem that is troubling to the family. The first step is to establish open, honest, direct lines of communication within the family. Interventions and homework assignments are usually used to improve communication skills and break vicious circles of poor communication. Once good communication is established, families can be helped to develop unique solutions to a specific problem with impaired family members. In addition, families can be assisted in developing a general coping strategy for managing other family problems. Individual strategies and solutions to particular problems of everyday life are emphasized.

Psychopharmacological Treatment

There are many different drug treatments available for cognitive and mental disorders due to a general medical condition. Psychoactive drugs may be used to target specific psychiatric symptoms or a constellation of symptoms associated with neurological or brain syndromes.

When prescribing drugs for elderly or debilitated patients, it is important to remember the following principles: (1) Lower dosages of all medications should be used because elderly or debilitated patients may have slower liver or renal clearance or increased sensitivity to medications, or both. (2) Medications should be chosen either because they have a specific desired effect or because they do not have side effects that would be damaging to the patient. (3) Interactions with other medications must be carefully considered. (4) Prescribing multiple drugs should be avoided whenever possible. Patients who need more than three psychoactive medications are probably not being managed as well as they could be, and their medications should be reevaluated with the goal of simplifying the drug regimen.

A brief review of the main classes and uses of drugs is given below. (See also Chapter 16, Psychopharmacology.)

Antidepressants

Antidepressants can be used to treat a wide array of symptoms seen frequently in patients with psychiatric syndromes due to medical illnesses. In general, they are used for the same symptoms that appear with the primary psychiatric conditions. Antidepressants can be used as one aspect of the treatment of cognitive disorders, mental disorders due to a general medical condition, and substance-related disorders. They are commonly used for depression, panic disorder, generalized anxiety disorder, chronic pain, obsessive-compulsive disorder, and posttraumatic stress disorder. Some of the most common symptoms treated with antidepressants will be highlighted.

Depression is extremely common in patients who have brain damage. It is almost always a sequela of traumatic brain injury. Some authors have noted that 40% of stroke patients have depression. Other brain syndromes that cause depressive affects are central nervous system illness due to HIV infection, chronic fatigue syndrome, and a wide array of dementias. It is common to treat patients empirically with antidepressants when they have dementia with a depressed mood or pseudodementia. The antidepressants most commonly used are those with the fewest side effects, including the selective serotonin reuptake inhibitors (SSRIs) (fluoxetine, sertraline, paroxetine), venlafaxine, trazodone, nefazodone, desipramine, and nortriptyline. Bupropion should be avoided in patients with a neurological disorder because this medication may increase the risk of seizures.

Antipsychotics

Antipsychotic drugs are frequently used to treat delirium or dementia with psychotic symptoms, psychotic disorders due to a general medical condition, or substance-induced psychotic disorders.

It is not uncommon for delirious patients to be agitated. Using restraints or giving appropriate medical treatment directed at the cause of the delirium, or both, should be the first priority. Adjunctive drugs can also be used, if necessary. Mildly agitated deliriums can be managed by giving haloperidol, 1–5 mg orally or intramuscularly at 30-minute intervals, up to approximately 20 mg/d. Extremely agitated patients may be given alternating dosages of haloperidol and lorazepam (an anxiolytic) in order to avoid the high dosages of antipsychotics, which increase the risk of tardive dyskinesia and other side effect syndromes.

Patients with dementia and paranoid delusions or other psychotic symptoms are often helped by low dosages of antipsychotics. The antipsychotics with the least amount of anticholinergic properties are given (e.g., the atypical antipsychotics risperidone and olanzapine or the traditional antipsychotics, such as haloperidol, fluphenazine, or trifluoperazine). Pimozide can be extremely effective in treating pathological jealousy that is related to a dementia. In general, the antipsychotics are not a good choice for managing violence in demented patients, unless the violence is secondary to a psychosis. Nonpsychotic demented patients who become violent can be treated with propranolol, nodolol, carbamazepine, valproate, or lithium.

Atypical antipsychotics or haloperidol and fluphenazine can be used safely in psychotic patients who are at risk for seizures. Drugs that lower the threshold for seizures, such as chlorpromazine, thioridazine, clozapine, and loxapine, are best avoided in patients who are prone to having seizures or who have neurological disorders that are not well defined.

Patients with specific movement disorders and psychotic symptoms are best treated with atypical antipsychotics, such as risperidone, olanzapine, or clozapine, which do not seem to have major extrapyramidal side effects. The more traditional antipsychotics should generally be avoided in these patients.

Antianxiety Drugs

Anxiolytics are usually prescribed as adjunctive treatment for patients with an anxiety disorder due to a general medical condition, substance-induced anxiety disorder, or anxiety due to drug withdrawal. They are usually prescribed for generalized anxiety symptoms, panic attack symptoms, or insomnia.

Patients with an acute generalized anxiety syndrome may be given benzodiazepines for immediate relief. Buspirone is a safe newer drug that is frequently used for chronic anxiety or agitation in patients with dementias. Long-term anxiolytic therapy may be given up to 60 mg/d in divided doses. The effects may not be felt for weeks, so the benzodiazepines are frequently used acutely and are later discontinued.

Drug withdrawal syndromes, including minor alcohol abstinence withdrawal and delirium tremens, are usually treated with the benzodiazepines that have a longer half-life, such as chlordiazepoxide, diazepam, or clonazepam. These drugs may also be used as adjunctive treatment in opiate withdrawal.

Acute drug reactions that may be treated with the benzodiazepines (e.g., lorazepam) include cocaine-induced anxiety, psychedelic "bad trips," or phencyclidine intoxication.

Lithium

Lithium can be used in the treatment of mania or violence caused by mood disorders due to a general medical condition, substance-induced mood disorders, or dementia with marked affective symptoms.

It is extremely important to consider discontinuing other medications that may be producing manic symptoms (e.g., steroids, antidepressants, thyroid hormones, methyldopa, and baclofen). Acute manic symptoms in patients with a mood disorder due to a general medical condition are best treated with lithium. Clonazepam or haloperidol should be given until the effects of lithium can be felt, because it can take several weeks for adequate blood levels to be reached.

Lithium is used to boost the antidepressant response in patients with depression secondary to a general medical condition that has not responded to antidepressant treatment. Lithium has been used with limited success in demented patients who are prone to violence or who have personality changes with hypomanic or manic features.

Anticonvulsants

Anticonvulsants have a wide range of uses in patients with psychiatric disorders secondary to medical conditions. These include seizures, manic symptoms (for which they are used as an alternative treatment after lithium), cocaine-induced psychosis, and violent behavior resulting from severe neurological deficits. While the older standard anticonvulsant drugs, such phenobarbitol, dilantin, or primadone, are still used, the trend in treatment of psychiatric disorders due to general medical conditions is toward carbamezepine and valproate.

New Drugs for the Treatment of Dementia

Many drugs are being developed for the treatment of dementia. Tacrine and donzepil have been released for the treatment of Alzheimer's disease. While they delay the progression of the disease by approximately six months, they have limited effectiveness in reversing memory deficits and have a mild to moderate toxicity profile.

References Cited

Engel, G. L., and J. Romano. Delirium: a syndrome of cerebral insufficiency. Journal of Chronic Diseases 9(3):260–277, 1959.

Folstein, M. F., S. E. Folstein, and P. R. McHugh. "Mini-Mental State": a practical method for grading the cognitive state of patients. Clinical Journal of Psychiatric Research 12:189–198, 1975.

Fuld, P. A. Word intrusion as a diagnostic sign in Alzheimer's disease. Geriatric Medicine Today 2(41):33–41, 1983.

Pro, J. D., and C. E. Wells. The use of encephalogram in the diagnosis of delirium. Diseases of the Nervous System 38:804–808, 1977.

Smith, D. B., and R. Craft. Sudden behavioral change guide to initial evaluation. Neurologic Clinics 2(1):3–74, 1984.

Tuokko, H., et al. The clock test: a sensitive measure to differentiate normal elderly from those with Alzheimer's disease. Journal of the American Geriatrics Society 40:579–584, 1992.

Selected Readings

DeGowin, R. L. DeGowin and DeGowin's Diagnostic Examination, 6th ed. New York, McGraw-Hill, 1994.

Pajeau, A. K., and G. C. Roman. HIV encephalopathy and dementia. Psychiatric Clinics of North America 15(2):455–466, 1992.

Perry, S. W. Organic mental disorders caused by HIV: update on early diagnosis and treatment. American Journal of Psychiatry 147(6):696–705, 1990.

Treves, T. A. Epidemiology of Alzheimer's Disease. Psychiatric Clinics of North America 14(2):251–266, 1991.

Yudofsky, S. C., and R. E. Hales, eds. The American Psychiatric Press Textbook of Neuropsychiatry, 2nd ed. Washington, D. C., American Psychiatric Press, Incorporated, 1992.

CHAPTER SIX

ANXIETY DISORDERS

LESLIE R. VOGEL, MD AND
PHILIP R. MUSKIN, MD

Anxiety is an emotion that everyone has experienced to a greater or lesser degree at some time. Anxiety is a sense of psychological distress that may or not have a focus. It is a state of apprehension that represents an internal psychological conflict, an environmental stress, a physical disease state, a medication or drug effect, or any combination of these. It can occur as a psychobiological circuit. For example, mental distress can give rise to physical symptoms, such as sweating, palpitations, diarrhea, or shortness of breath, which may then potentiate the psychological sense of agitation. Anxiety can be a purely psychological experience with few somatic manifestations. It can be a purely physical experience, with tachycardia, palpitations, chest pain, indigestion, headaches, and so on, with no psychological distress other than a concern about the physical symptoms.

Why some individuals experience anxiety in one way and some in another is puzzling. To some extent, the particular biological disposition of a person may favor certain psychological defenses over others or may generate higher levels of physical responses to a given stimulus. A psychological state can alter a biological response just as definitively as a biological state can modify a psychological response. For example, when a person driving down a city street hears a siren, the effect is noticeably different from what a person experiences upon hearing a siren while driving 80 miles an hour on a highway. The driver in the city might look around for the source of the sound to see if he or she has to move out of the way for an emergency vehicle and might or might not feel annoyed at having to stop. The same driver speeding on the highway might experience fear, a tightening in the stomach, an increase in heart rate, and might suddenly put pressure on the brake pedal. The difference in response to the same stimulus is merely the psychological state of the person at the moment. The awareness that speeding is illegal changes the "mind set" in the highway driver and may even generate a physiological reaction.

Normal and Abnormal Anxiety

Most people experience some anxiety. (This experience is so common that the complete absence of anxiety in a person can suggest the presence of psychopathology.) Anxiety can be a powerful motivator; low levels of it can produce increased attention and improved performance. In its milder forms, anxiety may be a positive adaptive response because it creates a state of optimal mental alertness and motor tension. Anxiety becomes maladaptive when it is constant, regardless of the situation, or when it leads to episodes of extreme vigilance, excessive motor tension, autonomic hyperactivity, and impaired concentration. The following example illustrates three forms of anxiety: a chronic form, an acute but adaptive form, and an acute but maladaptive form. ➡ A 23-year-old male medical student had experienced chronic anxiety about his school performance since he was a child. The anxiety was tolerable and of a low grade. He experienced a mild conscious feeling of anxiety; he continually worried about his grades and was hyperalert in classroom situations and perfectionistic about his homework. The anxiety increased before his first series of national board examinations, creating more discomfort for him but also enabling him to study for hours in a highly organized, effective way. Breaking only to eat and sleep, he reviewed and organized the major basic science courses that he had taken during his first two years of medical school. However, on the plane ride to a nearby city where the examination was being held, he experienced an extreme panic reaction as soon as the door to the plane had been closed. His heart rate accelerated rapidly and became a pounding in his chest, he had difficulty catching his breath, and he felt a sense of impending doom. He begged the stewardess to let him off the plane and was so obviously distressed that she complied at once. Seeing how short of breath he was, she called the ticket agent to get him a wheelchair. The episode passed in 20 minutes, and he was able to board another flight, but was left feeling shaken and worried for several days. ⬅

Some anxiety is normal and may indicate that danger or potential harm exists. Walking down a dark, deserted alley and hearing footsteps creates an anxious physical readiness that will facilitate escape if it is necessary. In contrast with the diffuse worry that anxious persons experience, fear is associated with a specific and focused concern about a situation that is perceived as dangerous and threatening.

At times, anxiety is clearly a primary disabling symptom. Some patients may present with conditions that appear to be entirely physical; these are confusing for the patients and their physicians and may cause physicians to search for nonexistent medical disorders. Experiences that patients may describe as "anxiety" can be caused by many medical disorders and psychiatric conditions other than anxiety disorders. The physical symptoms of anxiety, which are apprehension, tachycardia, palpitations, chest pain, dyspnea, restlessness, insomnia, headaches, difficulty in swallowing, gastrointestinal complaints, frequent urination, paresthesias, blurred vision, lightheadedness, dizziness, and sexual dysfunction, can indicate an anxiety disorder, another psychiatric disorder, a medical condition, or a combination of these conditions.

Finally, anxiety is part of the symptomatic picture of many psychiatric disorders. Patients with mood disorders (both unipolar and bipolar disorders), dementia, panic disorder, psychosis, adjustment disorders, and toxic and withdrawal states commonly complain of anxiety.

DIAGNOSTIC AND CLINICAL FEATURES

The DSM-IV category of anxiety disorders encompasses a wide range of disorders, from discrete episodic outbursts of anxiety to chronic lower-level distress. The anxiety disorders include panic disorder, agoraphobia, specific phobia, social phobia, obsessive-compulsive disorder, posttraumatic stress disorder, acute stress disorder, generalized anxiety disorder, anxiety disorder due to a general medical condition, and substance-induced anxiety disorder.

Panic Disorder

About 9% of persons have a panic attack at least once during their lives; about 3% have recurrent panic attacks (Table 6–1). The lifetime prevalence of panic disorder with or without agoraphobia is 1.5–3.5%. The prevalence of panic disorder in females is approximately twice that in males. Studies of twins appear to support a strong genetic predisposition, and there is a higher rate of panic disorder in relatives of patients (first-degree relatives of patients are four to seven times more likely to develop it) who have panic disorder than in family members of people without panic disorder. The onset is usually between late adolescence and the mid 30s but may occur at any age. See Table 6–2 for the DSM-IV criteria for panic disorder.

➡ A 34-year-old married woman whose job as a corporate executive involved frequent airplane travel had always been anxious when she traveled by plane. Over the course of one year, during which she had flown in rough weather, her anxiety escalated to panic attacks. She would have an occasional attack while she sat at her desk making plans for the next trip. The attack would start as a mounting feeling of conscious anxiety about the trip and the airplane. She would try to handle the mounting panic by referring to her lists

TABLE 6–1.   DSM-IV Criteria for Panic Attack

Note: A Panic Attack is not a codable disorder. Code the specific diagnosis in which the Panic Attack occurs.

A discrete period of intense fear or discomfort, in which four (or more) of the following symptoms developed abruptly and reach a peak within 10 minutes:
  (1) palpitations, pounding heart, or accelerated heart rate
  (2) sweating
  (3) trembling or shaking
  (4) sensations of shortness of breath or smothering
  (5) feeling of choking
  (6) chest pain or discomfort
  (7) nausea or abdominal distress
  (8) feeling dizzy, unsteady, lightheaded, or faint
  (9) derealization (feelings of unreality) or depersonalization (being detached from oneself)
 (10) fear of losing control or going crazy
 (11) fear of dying
 (12) paresthesias (numbness or tingling sensations)
 (13) chills or hot flushes

of airlines with the best safety records, types of planes with the best safety records, and available routes to her destination. This method of handling her anxiety was never very successful, since she knew that all planes and all airlines have some problems. On one occasion, however, the airline and type of airplane for one particular route were definitely not near the top of the safety lists. When she realized this—and that she had no way of avoiding the trip—her hands began to tremble. Within seconds, her heart rate accelerated so fast that she felt light-headed. She became extremely short of breath, and although she realized that she was hyperventilating, she could not slow down her breathing. The more she hyperventilated, the dizzier she felt. When she could not control the episode, her panic mounted and increased in intensity. After suffering with this for five minutes, which felt like five hours, she made an emergency call to her internist. His reassuring voice and episodic prescriptions for diazepam had always helped her in the past, although she had never taken the medicine. She felt somewhat better after talking to him, and, after 10 minutes, the panic began to subside on its own. Feeling tremulous and terrified that she might have such an episode while on the airplane, she decided to fly to a larger city and take a bus back to the smaller city, because this would give her more options about airlines, although it would triple her travel time. ⬛

A **panic attack** is an abrupt onset of intense apprehension (see Table 6–1). One patient described it this way: "It feels . . . like hot all through me, and shaky. And my heart just feels like it's pounding, and I'm breathing really quick." The terror is experienced as a feeling of impending doom, with a fear of dying, going "crazy," or losing control. Physical symptoms of trembling, sweating, and shortness of breath may also occur. Panic-like syndromes have been called "soldier's heart," "neurocirculatory asthenia," or "neurasthenia." Sigmund Freud differentiated this syndrome as an anxiety neurosis. Later, researchers coined the term "panic disorder."

TABLE 6–2.   DSM-IV Diagnostic Criteria for Panic Disorder Without Agoraphobia

A. Both (1) and (2):
   (1) recurrent unexpected Panic Attacks
   (2) at least one of the attacks has been followed by 1 month (or more) of one (or more) of the following:
      (a) persistent concern about having additional attacks
      (b) worry about the implications of the attack or its consequences (e.g., losing control, having a heart attack, "going crazy")
      (c) a significant change in behavior related to the attacks
B. Absence of Agoraphobia
C. The Panic Attacks are not due to the direct physiological effects of a substance (e.g., a drug of abuse, a medication) or a general medical condition (e.g., hyperthyroidism).
D. The Panic Attacks are not better accounted for by another mental disorder, such as Social Phobia (e.g., occurring on exposure to feared social situations), Specific Phobia (e.g., on exposure to a specific phobia situation), Obsessive-Compulsive Disorder (e.g., on exposure to dirt in someone with an obsession about contamination), Posttraumatic Stress Disorder (e.g., in response to stimuli associated with a severe stressor), or Separation Anxiety Disorder (e.g., in response to being away from home or close relatives).

A key feature of panic is the adrenergic surge, commonly referred to as the **fight or flight response,** which is an exaggerated sympathetic response characterized by tachycardia, sweating, and a sense of distress. An inherent feature of this response is that the individual prepares to confront or escape from a perceived threat or challenge. This response is an exaggerated form of the "adrenaline" response that most people experience in situations characterized by excitement or danger.

Panic attacks may be cued or uncued. **Uncued panic attacks** occur without an apparent precipitating factor. **Cued panic attacks** occur upon exposure to or in anticipation of a specific conscious trigger, such as airplane travel. Many patients report that they are not aware of any specific life stressors preceding the onset of panic disorder, although some recall that an emotional stressor, such as the breakup of a relationship or the use of a mind-altering substance, such as cocaine, LSD, or marijuana, preceded the onset of their symptoms. These are **situational panic attacks.**

Although panic attacks can be isolated events, they may evolve into the **triad of panic:** the **acute panic attack, anticipatory anxiety, and phobic avoidance.** Following the experience of an acute panic attack, individuals often fear a recurrence. The anxiety brought on by the feeling that a panic attack will happen again is anticipatory anxiety. These individuals feel that they are at tremendous risk of another attack, which may be associated with specific cued situations. Their psychophysiological reactions are in keeping with this perception.

Triggering situations such as flying in an airplane produce anxiety because they symbolically represent to the patient something that is traumatically overwhelming. Whether or not such situations are inherently traumatic or stressful is not the issue.

The panic attack that a patient has while flying on an airplane, for instance, is the emotional reaction that most people would have if the plane were about to crash.

Patients with panic disorder can often be calmed by the presence of a **"phobic companion"** (i.e., a soothing person). Such patients often have a history of a relationship to a parent of intense anxious attachment, accompanied by intense anger that they are unable to express for fear of abandonment. Even independence within the relationship is seen by both the patient and parent as the equivalent to rebellion. This basic fear is then carried forward through life development, becomes mixed with later developmental fears, and is triggered by situations that symbolize conflicts about competition, ambition, and achievement, all of which come to represent rebellion and abandonment. The universal aspect of the panic experience is a feeling of being terrorized, out of control, and punished.

Most patients with panic disorder see a nonpsychiatric physician before they consult a psychiatrist. Patients may have had extensive evaluations and received a variety of medical diagnoses related to the panic symptoms or to associated benign disorders (e.g., mitral valve prolapse). These diagnoses may be attempts by physicians to validate or put a label on the unexplained but intense symptoms.

Agoraphobia

Anxious patients who are afraid of certain situations, such as being in a public place, but cannot explain why this is so may or may not give a history of panic attacks. If they do, they have cued panic attacks. Such fears may be part of the symptomatic picture of agoraphobia, which is anxiety about having a panic attack in a place or situation from which escape might be difficult or in which help might not be available (e.g., while shopping in a crowded supermarket, traveling across a bridge, or flying in a plane). For instance, a patient with agoraphobia might panic in a crowded supermarket and feel compelled to leave abruptly, even if it means leaving packages and money at the cash register. If the agoraphobia is severe enough, patients eventually avoid these situations. They may become too anxious to go to the supermarket for fear of having another panic attack there, where escape from the crowded aisles might be difficult. Avoidance of these situations may escalate to the point that patients become housebound and are dependent on others to perform every task and activity that involves going outside the home (Table 6–3).

In the clinical context, almost all patients with agoraphobia also have panic disorder. If agoraphobia is going to develop in a patient with panic disorder, it usually does so within the first year of recurrent panic attacks. Recently, researchers reevaluated patients who had reported agoraphobia without panic disorder and changed the diagnoses to specific phobia.

TABLE 6–3. DSM-IV Criteria for Agoraphobia

Note: Agoraphobia is not a codable disorder. Code the specific disorder in which the Agoraphobia occurs.

A. Anxiety about being in places or situations from which escape might be difficult (or embarrassing) or in which help may not be available in the event of having an unexpected or situationally predisposed Panic Attack or panic-like symptoms. Agoraphobic fears typically involve characteristic clusters of situations that include being outside the home alone; being in a crowd or standing in a line; being on a bridge; and traveling in a bus, train, or automobile.

Note: Consider the diagnosis of Specific Phobia if the avoidance is limited to one or only a few specific situations, or Social Phobia if the avoidance is limited to social situations.

B. The situations are avoided (e.g., travel is restricted) or else are endured with marked distress or with anxiety about having a Panic Attack or panic-like symptoms, or require the presence of a companion.

C. The anxiety of phobic avoidance is not better accounted for by another mental disorder, such as Social Phobia (e.g., avoidance limited to social situations because of fear or embarrassment), Specific Phobia (e.g., avoidance limited to a single situation such as elevators), Obsessive-Compulsive Disorder (e.g., avoidance of dirt in someone with an obsession about contamination), Posttraumatic Stress Disorder (e.g., avoidance of stimuli associated with a severe stressor), or Separation Anxiety Disorder (e.g., avoidance of leaving home or relatives).

Phobias

Phobias are fears of specific objects, situations, or experiences, although patients may be unable to articulate the exact nature of the danger that they presume will occur. The feared object, situation, or experience has taken on a symbolic meaning for the patient; both unconscious wishes and fears have been displaced from the original goal onto this external object. The feared object stands for the unconscious wish and fear and, therefore, is associated with anxiety. ➡ For example, a middle-aged man who wished to kill his father by stabbing developed a phobia of knives. The knife became the symbol of his violent, unacceptable wish. When he saw a knife, he felt intense anxiety, which was stimulated by the unacceptable unconscious wish to kill. By avoiding knives, he was able to avoid this intolerable unconscious desire and escape from the anxious feelings. He also avoided the unpleasant conscious experience of anxiety, even though he knew there was nothing to fear from the knife. ⬅ In some cases, the phobic object was present during a childhood trauma and the patient has made the object "guilty" by association. In other cases, the phobic object was of trivial importance in the traumatic event or is a symbolic representation of the trauma or the feared impulse. Although part of this information may emerge during initial interviews with patients, it will become clarified only after a considerable amount of psychological work in therapy.

Specific Phobia

Specific phobia is an irrational fear of a specific object, activity, or situation that is so intense that the phobic stimulus is avoided (e.g., fear of flying). Although individuals recognize that the fear is irrational, they are unable to overcome it. For example, although they know that the chances of being in a plane accident are very low, they continue to be afraid to the point where they will not fly and will do anything to avoid flying. Specific phobia includes the **anticipatory anxiety** provoked by worrying about or confronting the feared object and the resulting **avoidance behavior.** This avoidance can significantly impair occupational and social functioning (Table 6–4).

The degree of debilitation from the phobia depends largely on how central the phobia is in the patient's life. A hospital worker, for example, who has a fear of needles may be chronically anxious because of constant exposure to them. A patient living in Alaska with a phobia about snakes has little opportunity to encounter one, and, therefore, the phobia should play a marginal role in the patient's life. The lifetime prevalence of specific phobia in the United States is 10–11.3%.

Social Phobia

Social phobia is a potentially disabling disease characterized by the persistent **fear of social situations** in which a person is subject to the scrutiny of others and to possible humiliating consequences of such scrutiny. Social phobia may affect public activities, such as eating, drinking, and public speaking, or social activities, such as going to parties, talking to the boss, or asking someone for a date. During the feared scenario, or in the anticipation of it, symptoms include psychic anxiety, sweating, tachycardia, trembling, and a desire to escape. The ramifications of untreated social phobia include avoidance of school and employment, social isolation, and self-medication with alcohol or illicit drugs (Table 6–5).

➡ For example, a 42-year-old man was promoted to a new job requiring that he give small, informal luncheon lectures. As he began to speak at his first lecture, he suddenly experienced profuse sweating, palpitations, and a feeling of faintness, and he was unable to continue. His boss was taken aback but promptly took over the talk. After that experience, the employee began drinking before giving a lecture, because it "calmed him down." Eventually, he needed more and more alcohol and was fired after giving a lecture while he was visibly intoxicated. ⬅ The prevalence of social phobia in adults in the United States is 3–13%, with a slightly higher female to male distribution.

Obsessive-Compulsive Disorder

The cardinal features of obsessive-compulsive disorder are **obsessions,** which are intrusive, recurrent thoughts and impulses that are **egodystonic** (i.e., symptoms that the patient perceives as alien to him or her), and **compulsions,** which are repetitive rituals that the patient cannot resist performing (Table 6–6). Examples of compulsions include com-

TABLE 6–4.   DSM-IV Diagnostic Criteria for Specific Phobia

A. Marked and persistent fear that is excessive or unreasonable, cued by the presence or anticipation of a specific object or situation (e.g., flying, heights, animals, receiving an injection, seeing blood).

B. Exposure to the phobic stimulus almost invariably provokes an immediate anxiety response, which may take the form of a situationally bound or situationally predisposed Panic Attack. **Note:** In children, the anxiety may be expressed by crying, tantrums, freezing, or clinging.

C. The person recognizes that the fear is excessive or unreasonable. **Note:** In children, this feature may be absent.

D. The phobic situation(s) is avoided or else is endured with intense anxiety or distress.

E. The avoidance, anxious anticipation, or distress in the feared situation(s) interferes significantly with the person's normal routine, occupational (or academic) functioning, or social activities or relationships, or there is marked distress about having the phobia.

F. In individuals under age 18 years, the duration is at least 6 months.

G. The anxiety, Panic Attacks, or phobic avoidance associated with the specific object or situation are not better accounted for by another mental disorder, such as Obsessive-Compulsive Disorder (e.g., fear of dirt in someone with an obsession about contamination), Posttraumatic Stress Disorder (e.g., avoidance of stimuli associated with a severe stressor), Separation Anxiety Disorder (e.g., avoidance of school), Social Phobia (e.g., avoidance of social situations because of fear of embarrassment), Panic Disorder With Agoraphobia, or Agoraphobia Without History of Panic Disorder.

Specify type:
Animal Type
Natural Environment Type (e.g., heights, storms, water)
Blood-Injection-Injury Type
Situational Type (e.g., airplanes, elevators, enclosed places)
Other Type (e.g., phobic avoidance of situations that may lead to choking, vomiting, or contracting an illness; in children, avoidance of loud sounds or costumed characters)

plex cleaning rituals and repeated checking to see if lights in the house have been turned off or if the door has been locked. The compulsion can be resisted for a short period of time, but the delay creates a tremendous, anxious tension, which is relieved only by performing the compulsive act. Because these rituals may become extremely time-consuming, patients have little time for work or family relationships, and, consequently, their functioning and quality of life are impaired.

➠ For example, a 16-year-old high school track star had had various rituals and obsessions since early adolescence. He counted, in his head, over and over again from 1 to 3 and had various touching rituals and phobic avoidances. Because he was worried about illness, he traveled a circuitous route to high school, avoiding hospitals, physicians' offices, dentists' offices, and funeral homes. Although this added about 30 minutes each way to school, he rationalized it to his friends as part of his training for running. Unfortunately, his running began to be involved in his obsessive-compulsive symptoms as well. As he raced down the track, he had to move his feet in a rapid sequence of three beats, slight pause, and three beats again. This gave his gait a loping quality, but, more

importantly, it slowed him down. He had begun to notice, to his horror, that his symptoms increased when he was in the lead. He knew that he could have won the last race if his symptoms had not interfered more and more severely as he pulled ahead, so that the student behind him finally won. His coach was furious and thought of kicking him off the team. This was devastating to the patient because his major source of self-esteem was the feeling of strength he experienced while running. ◀▦

The psychodynamics of obsessive-compulsive disorder differ from other anxiety disorders in that punishment and guilt are usually a conscious part of the experience of the anxiety in obsessive-compulsive disorder. Patients believe that if certain thoughts or rituals are not repeated over and over again, they or a loved one will be punished by a catastrophic event. The content of the thought or ritual is more conscious in its elaborated form than in the other anxiety disorders, although the affect appropriate to the thought is not conscious. The physician must elicit the details of the repetitive thought or behavior and associated thoughts during the history taking. Some of the psychological meaning will be-

TABLE 6–5.   DSM-IV Diagnostic Criteria for Social Phobia

A. A marked and persistent fear of one or more social or performance situations in which the person is exposed to unfamiliar people or to possible scrutiny by others. The individual fears that he or she will act in a way (or show anxiety symptoms) that will be humiliating or embarrassing. **Note:** In children, there must be evidence of the capacity for age-appropriate social relationships with familiar people and the anxiety must occur in peer settings, not just in interactions with adults.

B. Exposure to the feared social situation almost invariably provokes anxiety, which may take the form of a situationally bound or situationally predisposed Panic Attack. **Note:** In children, the anxiety may be expressed by crying, tantrums, freezing, or shrinking from social situations with unfamiliar people.

C. The person recognizes that the fear is excessive or unreasonable. **Note:** In children, this feature may be absent.

D. The feared social or performance situations are avoided or else are endured with intense anxiety or distress.

E. The avoidance, anxious anticipation, or distress in the feared social or performance situation(s) interferes significantly with the person's normal routine, occupational (academic) functioning, or social activities or relationships, or there is marked distress about having the phobia.

F. In individuals under age 18 years, the duration is at least 6 months.

G. The fear or avoidance is not due to the direct physiological effects of a substance (e.g., a drug of abuse, a medication) or a general medical condition and is not better accounted for by another mental disorder (e.g., Panic Disorder With or Without Agoraphobia, Separation Anxiety Disorder, Body Dysmorphic Disorder, a Pervasive Developmental Disorder, or Schizoid Personality Disorder).

H. If a general medical condition or another mental disorder is present, the fear in Criterion A is unrelated to it, (e.g., the fear is not of Stuttering, trembling in Parkinson's disease, or exhibiting abnormal eating behavior in Anorexia Nervosa or Bulimia Nervosa).

Specify if:
Generalized: if the fears include most social situations (also consider the additional diagnosis of Avoidant Personality Disorder).

**TABLE 6–6.   DSM-IV Diagnostic Criteria
for Obsessive-Compulsive Disorder**

A. Either obsessions or compulsions:
Obsessions as defined by (1), (2), (3), and (4);
  (1) recurrent and persistent thoughts, impulses, or images
  that are experienced, at some time during the disturbance,
  as intrusive and inappropriate and that cause marked anxiety or distress
  (2) the thoughts, impulses, or images are not simply excessive worries about real-life problems
  (3) the person attempts to ignore or suppress such thoughts,
  impulses, or images, or to neutralize them with some
  other thought or action
  (4) the person recognizes that the obsessional thoughts, impulses, or images are a product of his or her own mind
  (not imposed from without as in thought insertion)
Compulsions as defined by (1) and (2):
  (1) repetitive behaviors (e.g., hand washing, ordering, checking) or mental acts (e.g., praying, counting, repeating
  words silently) that the person feels driven to perform in
  response to an obsession, or according to rules that must
  be applied rigidly
  (2) the behaviors or mental acts are aimed at preventing or
  reducing distress or preventing some dreaded event or situation; however, these behaviors or mental acts either are
  not connected in a realistic way with what they are designed to neutralize or prevent or are clearly excessive
B. At some point during the course of the disorder, the person
  has recognized that the obsessions or compulsions are excessive or unreasonable. **Note:** This does not apply to children.
C. The obsessions or compulsions cause marked distress, are
  time-consuming (take more than 1 hour a day), or significantly
  interfere with the person's normal routine, occupational (or
  academic) functioning, or usual social activities or relationships.
D. If another Axis I disorder is present, the content of the obsessions or compulsions is not restricted to it (e.g., preoccupation with food in the presence of an Eating Disorder; hair
  pulling in the presence of Trichotillomania; concern with appearance in the presence of Body Dysmorphic Disorder; preoccupation with drugs in the presence of a Substance Use Disorder; preoccupation with having a serious illness in the
  presence of Hypochondriasis; preoccupation with sexual
  urges or fantasies in the presence of a Paraphilia; or guilty ruminations in the presence of Major Depressive Disorder).
E. The disturbance is not due to the direct physiological effects
  of a substance (e.g., a drug of abuse, a medication) or a general medical condition.
Specify if:
With Poor Insight: if for most of the time during the current
episode, the person does not recognize that the obsessions and
compulsions are excessive or unreasonable

come obvious as this is done. The life history may
provide the rest of the story.

➡ In one case, a 30-year-old man who had been
raised in a religious home by his mother experienced
obsessive thoughts that blasphemed God, which
triggered a ritual of touching and bowing that was designed to eliminate the dangerous consequences of
these horrible thoughts. His life history revealed
more about a rebellion against his mother, who had
come to symbolize his religious upbringing, than
against God. He was engaged to be married to a
woman whose religious faith had been historically at
odds with his own. The relationship between his
symptoms and this life historical information, which
was so obvious to the interviewer, was not clearly acknowledged by the patient. ◀

The lifetime prevalence of obsessive-compulsive
disorder is approximately 2.5%. It occurs with equal
frequency in adult males and females. The onset is
usually before age 30 years, but it may occur at any
age. Obsessive-compulsive disorder with an onset
in childhood is more common in males. A genetic
link is suggested by the correlations between obsessive-compulsive disorder and Tourette's syndrome and the greater concordance of obsessive-
compulsive disorder among monozygotic twins
than dizygotic twins.

Posttraumatic Stress Disorder

Posttraumatic stress disorder is a syndrome of
psychophysiological signs and symptoms that follows exposure to a traumatic event outside the usual
range of human experience, such as combat exposure, a holocaust experience, rape, or a civilian disaster such as a hurricane (Table 6–7). It was initially
described by Kardiner as an overwhelming life experience resulting in psychological and physiological
sequelae. Pavlov had previously determined that repeated exposure to trauma could cause permanent
autonomic nervous system changes. Posttraumatic
stress disorder first became an official psychiatric diagnosis in 1980 in the DSM-III, but posttraumatic
symptoms had been noted as early as the Civil War,
and the Vietnam War heightened awareness of this
disorder. The original accounts of posttraumatic
stress disorder were based on experiences of sol-
diers in combat, but, more recently, they have per-
tained to experiences of rape and incest.

The prevalence of posttraumatic stress disorder
in the general population is 1–14%, depending on the
diagnostic methods used and the population sam-
pled. Most men with the disorder have been in combat, and most women have a history of sexual or
physical abuse. There is no specific age of onset; it
can occur in childhood or adulthood. Although
about 38% of the population is exposed to so-called
catastrophic stress, only about 9% of these persons
develop a true posttraumatic stress syndrome,
which raises questions about the potential role of
vulnerability: When two individuals are exposed to a
similar stressor, why does one develop posttraumatic stress disorder and the other not?

The three cardinal features of posttraumatic
stress disorder are hyperarousal; intrusive symptoms, or flashbacks, of the initial trauma; and psychic numbing. **Hyperarousal** is a chronic state of
physiological "alertness" during which individuals
brace themselves for a recurrence of the trauma.
The psychophysiological result is a chronically anxious state marked by sympathetic activation, an exaggerated startle response, sleep difficulties, irritability, and impulsive behavior. **Flashbacks** to the
scene of combat or **recurrent nightmares** that recreate the trauma commonly occur. Flashbacks are often triggered by cues that provide a reminder of the
trauma scene (e.g., a sudden loud noise that recalls
the explosive sound of the battlefield). The flashback

TABLE 6-7. DSM-IV Diagnostic Criteria for Posttraumatic Stress Disorder

A. The person has been exposed to a traumatic event in which both of the following were present:
  (1) the person experienced, witnessed, or was confronted with an event or events that involved actual or threatened death or serious injury, or a threat to the physical integrity of self or others.
  (2) the person's response involved intense fear, helplessness, or horror. **Note:** In children, this may be expressed instead by disorganized or agitated behavior.
B. The traumatic event is persistently reexperienced in one (or more) of the following ways:
  (1) recurrent and intrusive distressing recollections of the event, including images, thoughts, or perceptions. **Note:** In young children, repetitive play may occur in which themes or aspects of the trauma are expressed.
  (2) recurrent distressing dreams of the event. **Note:** In children, there may be frightening dreams without recognizable content.
  (3) acting or feeling as if the traumatic event were recurring (includes a sense of reliving the experience, illusions, hallucinations, and dissociative flashback episodes, including those that occur on awakening or when intoxicated). **Note:** In young children, trauma-specific enactment may occur.
  (4) intense psychological distress at exposure to internal or external cues that symbolize or resemble an aspect of the traumatic event.
  (5) physiological reactivity on exposure to internal or external cues that symbolize or resemble an aspect of the traumatic event.
C. Persistent avoidance of stimuli associated with the trauma and numbing of general responsiveness (not present before the trauma), as indicated by three (or more) of the following:
  (1) efforts to avoid thoughts, feelings, or conversations associated with the trauma
  (2) efforts to avoid activities, places, or people that arouse recollections of the trauma
  (3) inability to recall an important aspect of the trauma
  (4) markedly diminished interest or participation in significant activities
  (5) feeling of detachment or estrangement from others
  (6) restricted range of affect (e.g., unable to have loving feelings)
  (7) sense of a foreshortened future (e.g., does not expect to have a career, marriage, children, or a normal life span)
D. Persistent symptoms of increased arousal (not present before the trauma), as indicated by two (or more) of the following:
  (1) difficulty falling or staying asleep
  (2) irritability or outbursts of anger
  (3) difficulty concentrating
  (4) hypervigilance
  (5) exaggerated startle response
E. Duration of the disturbance (symptoms in Criteria B, C, and D) is more than 1 month.
F. The disturbance causes clinically significant distress or impairment in social, occupational, or other important areas of functioning.
Specify if:
Acute: if duration of symptoms is less than 3 months
Chronic: if duration of symptoms is 3 months or more
Specify if:
With Delayed Onset: if onset of symptoms is at least 6 months after the stressor

symptoms appear to be related to the severity of the stressor rather than to the individual's vulnerability before the trauma occurred. **Psychic numbing** is experienced as detachment from others, a reduced capacity for intimacy, and decreased sexual interest.

For example, one patient was a 75-year-old combat veteran of World War II who had been an infantryman in a section of General MacArthur's army and was part of a landing team that invaded island after island in the Allied march toward Japan. From 1943–1945, he was in fairly continuous fighting. Only 6 of his company of 30 men survived the war. Of the 6, several were permanently injured. Throughout his life, the patient had had flashbacks, terrifying nightmares, chronic anxiety with episodic panic attacks, and a feeling of being numb and unconnected to his family, his friends, and the joys of life that he so looked forward to during military service. He had always refused to get treatment because he believed that to do so would be cowardly, especially when he compared his situation with that of his comrades who died. He rationalized their refusal by saying that he had been successful in business and with his family and that he avoided things that he knew would trigger flashbacks. He avoided, therefore, all movies with violence, television news programs, written reminiscences about war, and discussions of his wartime experiences. However, he could not avoid abrupt noises, such as the occasional car backfire, the explosion of Fourth of July fireworks, or the thump when his wife or children occasionally dropped something. Any such noise would trigger intense autonomic arousal, with hyperventilation, rapid heart rate, tremulous hands, profuse sweating, and flashbacks of one of the many times he and his comrades were trapped on the beach with incoming artillery blasting around them. He was fortunate in that his wife intuitively understood these episodes and knew the correct mixture of gentle reassurance and distance that he required at such times. Interestingly enough, about once a year he was drawn to the local shooting range by an urge to practice target shooting with a captured World War II enemy pistol. His anxiety would reach a peak as he started to fire and then instantly disappear for the time that he was at the shooting range. The anxiety would change to an intense, driven, hyperalert, hyperaroused state with great apprehension but also great feelings of rage and triumph. He would be exhausted and drained after such episodes but found that his anxiety was better for a few days to several weeks.

Acute Stress Disorder

Acute stress disorder is a new DSM-IV category of anxiety disorder. The prevalence of acute stress disorder is variable. Its occurrence depends on the severity of the trauma and the degree of exposure.

A patient with this disorder has been exposed to a traumatic event and has specific signs and symptoms resembling those of posttraumatic stress disorder, although they are shorter in duration and their onset occurs more rapidly after the trauma (Table 6–8). The symptomatic reaction is limited to the time that the stressful situation is occurring and its immediate aftermath.

TABLE 6-8. DSM-IV Diagnostic Criteria for Acute Stress Disorder

A. The person has been exposed to a traumatic event in which both of the following were present:
   (1) the person experienced, witnessed, or was confronted with an event or events that involved actual or threatened death or serious injury, or a threat to the physical integrity of self or others
   (2) the person's response involved intense fear, helplessness, or horror
B. Either while experiencing or after experiencing the distressing event, the individual has three (or more) of the following dissociative symptoms:
   (1) a subjective sense of numbing, detachment, or absence of emotional responsiveness
   (2) a reduction in awareness of his or her surroundings (e.g., "being in a daze")
   (3) derealization
   (4) depersonalization
   (5) dissociative amnesia (i.e., inability to recall an important aspect of the trauma)
C. The traumatic event is persistently reexperienced in at least one of the following ways: recurrent images, thoughts, dreams, illusions, flashback episodes, or a sense of reliving the experience; or distress on exposure to reminders of the traumatic event.
D. Marked avoidance of stimuli that arouse recollections of the trauma (e.g., thoughts, feelings, conversations, activities, places, people).
E. Marked symptoms of anxiety or increased arousal (e.g., difficulty sleeping, irritability, poor concentration, hypervigilance, exaggerated startle response, motor restlessness).
F. The disturbance causes clinically significant distress or impairment in social, occupational, or other important areas of functioning or impairs the individual's ability to pursue some necessary task, such as obtaining necessary assistance or mobilizing personal resources by telling family members about the traumatic experience.
G. The disturbance lasts for a minimum of 2 days and a maximum of 4 weeks and occurs within 4 weeks of the traumatic event.
H. The disturbance is not due to the direct physiological effects of a substance (e.g., a drug of abuse, a medication) or a general medical condition, is not better accounted for by Brief Psychotic Disorder, and is not merely an exacerbation of a preexisting Axis I or Axis II disorder.

Generalized Anxiety Disorder

Generalized anxiety disorder has a lifetime prevalence of approximately 5% and is twice as common in females as males. It frequently makes its initial appearance when patients are in their early 20s, although it can occur at any age. Studies support a familial basis for the disorder.

➡ A 40-year-old married woman with two high school–aged children complained of chronic low-grade anxiety with a mildly rapid pulse, mild tremulousness, easy fatigability, preoccupation with anxious worries, and difficulty in falling asleep at night. She had a history of several episodes of depression: two postpartum episodes and one that had occurred after she was fired from a parttime job because of a dispute with her boss. The last episode never completely faded and left her with her present symptoms. Results from a thyroid screening test were normal. ⬅

A person with generalized anxiety disorder experiences continuous, excessive worry, including autonomic nervous system hyperarousal, which causes

some degree of impairment in functioning (Table 6–9). Generalized anxiety disorder is a chronic state of anxious psychic and somatic discomfort. Persons with this disorder do not have the abrupt outbursts found in panic disorder and often have an associated dysphoric mood that is less severe than the dysphoria in patients with major depression but that represents an early or partial manifestation of agitated depression. Despite the mild dysphoria, patients with generalized anxiety disorder are not anhedonic, although they tend to become discouraged when the anxiety interferes with their ability to enjoy life. Major depression is often, but not always, present. The anxiety usually precedes full-blown depression but may also be the remnant of it. Patients complain of constant anxiety without discrete episodes of panic, agoraphobia or other phobias, or obsessions or compulsions. They often medicate themselves with substances such as alcohol.

Many patients with generalized anxiety disorder who do not associate their somatic symptoms with anxiety consult nonpsychiatric physicians, such as cardiologists, neurologists, and pulmonologists.

Anxiety Disorder Due to a General Medical Condition

Anxiety may have a medical etiology, whether the symptoms are somatic (e.g., sweating and tremulousness) or psychological (e.g., a subjective sense

TABLE 6-9. DSM-IV Diagnostic Criteria for Generalized Anxiety Disorder

A. Excessive anxiety and worry (apprehensive expectation), occurring more days than not for at least 6 months, about a number of events or activities (such as work or school performance).
B. The person finds it difficult to control the worry.
C. The anxiety and worry are associated with three (or more) of the following six symptoms (with at least some symptoms present for more days than not for the past 6 months).
   Note: Only one item is required in children.
   (1) restlessness or feeling keyed up or on edge
   (2) being easily fatigued
   (3) difficulty concentrating or mind going blank
   (4) irritability
   (5) muscle tension
   (6) sleep disturbance (difficulty falling or staying asleep, or restless unsatisfying sleep)
D. The focus of the anxiety and worry is not confined to features of an Axis I disorder, e.g., the anxiety or worry is not about having a Panic Attack (as in Panic Disorder), being embarrassed in public (as in Social Phobia), being contaminated (as in Obsessive-Compulsive Disorder), being away from home or close relatives (as in Separation Anxiety Disorder), gaining weight (as in Anorexia Nervosa), having multiple physical complaints (as in Somatization Disorder), or having a serious illness (as in Hypochondriasis), and the anxiety and worry do not occur exclusively during Posttraumatic Stress Disorder.
E. The anxiety, worry, or physical symptoms cause clinically significant distress or impairment in social, occupational, or other important areas of functioning.
F. The disturbance is not due to the direct physiological effects of a substance (e.g., a drug of abuse, a medication) or a general medical condition (e.g., hyperthyroidism) and does not occur exclusively during a Mood Disorder, a Psychotic Disorder, or a Pervasive Developmental Disorder.

of psychic unease). Organically induced anxiety may mimic a variety of "functional" anxiety syndromes because the manifestations of sympathetic nervous system overactivity include tachycardia, palpitations, hypertension, sweating, tremor, and subjective feelings of nervousness (see Chapter 5, Cognitive and Mental Disorders Due to General Medical Conditions).

It is crucial to establish a full medical differential diagnosis before assuming that a patient has a psychiatric disorder. ➡ For example, a 32-year-old woman presented with anxiety, sweating, and weight loss over a six-month period. She was referred to a psychiatrist, who prescribed a benzodiazepine, which had no effect on her symptoms. Eventually, thyroid function tests were conducted, which led to a diagnosis of hyperthyroidism due to Graves' disease. The patient was given the antithyroid medication methimazole but did not consistently take it. She continued to take the benzodiazepine episodically. Although some of her symptoms were masked by the medication, the hyperthyroidism was left untreated. Gradually, she developed exophthalmos, which became more and more pronounced; ptosis; and severe hair loss. She eventually agreed to take a stable regimen of methimazole; once she did, her thyroid function tests became normal, her symptoms disappeared, and she no longer needed the benzodiazepine. ⬅

Numerous medical, neurological, endocrinological, and toxic conditions can cause anxiety (see Table 6–10). Because of the anxietylike symptoms they produce, myocardial infarction, angina pectoris, hyperthyroidism, pheochromocytoma, carcinoid syndrome, and the adrenergic response (i.e., counterregulation) to hypoglycemia in diabetic patients can be mistaken for anxiety disorder. Paniclike symptoms, such as a sense of dread, dizziness, or shortness of breath, can also accompany pulmonary embolism and transient ischemic attacks of the brain.

Substance-Induced Anxiety Disorder

Substance-induced anxiety disorder is a syndrome in which symptoms of anxiety result from the use of, or withdrawal from, substances such as alcohol, caffeine, marijuana, and tobacco, and medications such as benzodiazepines, amphetamines, diethylpropion, methylphenidate, phendimetrazine, thyroid medications, and illicit drugs. A substance-induced anxiety disorder is diagnosed only if the anxiety symptoms are a consequence of the substance itself and do not represent an underlying anxiety disorder (see also Chapter 7, Alcohol and Substance Abuse Disorders, and Chapter 5, Cognitive and Mental Disorders Due to General Medical Conditions).

The presentation of substance-induced anxiety disorders is as varied as the substances themselves. With some exceptions, the anxiety is likely to result either from intoxication with stimulant drugs or from

TABLE 6–10. Medical Causes of Anxiety

Endocrine Disorders
Pheochromocytoma
Thyroid dysfunction
Pituitary dysfunction
Adrenal disorders

Neurological Disorders
Head trauma
Neurosyphilis
Seizure disorders
CNS neoplasms
Cerebrovascular disease
Encephalitis and meningitis
Huntington's disease
Multiple sclerosis

Toxic and Metabolic Disorders
Alcohol or sedative withdrawal
Stimulant intoxication (cocaine, amphetamines, caffeine)
Sympathomimetic agents
Cannabis
B_{12} deficiency
Hypoxia
Ischemia
Anemia

Autoimmune Disorders
Systemic lupus erythematosus
Temporal arteritis
Polyarteritis nodosa

the withdrawal of depressants and opioids from the central nervous system.

Stimulant Intoxication

Anxiety may be caused by acute intoxication with stimulant drugs, which include cocaine, dextroamphetamine, methamphetamine, phendimetrazine, methylphenidate, and diethylpropion. In some susceptible patients, marijuana, caffeine, or tobacco may also act as stimulants. Aside from causing the euphoria for which they are initially selected, these drugs may cause anxiety, irritability, and anorexia. Strong stimulant drugs, such as cocaine, produce an anxiety syndrome so severe that it sometimes progresses to a condition of paranoia that is indistinguishable from the psychosis of schizophreniform disorder. Withdrawal from stimulants causes lethargy and depression.

The side effects of the stimulant can be affected by their route of administration. For instance, natives of the Andes Mountains who chew coca leaves rarely develop anxiety or suspiciousness, although persons living in the urban areas of Peru who smoke coca paste have a high incidence of irritability, stereotypic behaviors, toxic psychosis, and criminal behavior. Stimulant side effects are also influenced by the amount of stimulant used. For example, as the euphoria induced by cocaine becomes progressively more difficult to achieve, users take increasingly larger amounts, which produce an anxiety syndrome that includes the psychophysiological signs and symptoms of adrenergic stimulation. Panic attacks may also occur in acutely intoxicated cocaine users who have no previous history of panic disorder. They may continue to have panic attacks even when they are not intoxicated. The same is true of marijuana users.

Commonly consumed stimulants such as caffeine and diet pills are also anxiogenic. The spectrum of symptoms they can produce ranges from generalized anxiety or discrete panic attacks to obsessive-compulsive symptoms or phobic symptoms. Autonomic nervous system arousal may be evidenced by tachycardia, hypertension, mydriasis, and diaphoresis. The following example illustrates a case of caffeinism. ➠ A 38-year-old man was referred to a nutritionist for advice regarding weight loss. He was 40 kg overweight and had a history of poor sleep, dysphoric mood, and restlessness. He complained of headache, tachycardia, frequent urination, and an inability to lose weight. His dietary history was significant because he drank 10–12 cans of caffeinated cola daily. He was advised to discontinue the cola intake and make other dietary changes. The day after the consultation, he saw his psychotherapist and complained of fatigue, dysphoria, and an intense headache. The therapist arranged for a psychiatric consultation, in which it was determined that the patient's anxiety symptoms were the result of ingesting too much caffeine. Abruptly discontinuing the habit then produced a transient withdrawal syndrome. ⬛

Alcohol Withdrawal

Alcohol is a central nervous system depressant. An anxiety syndrome may result from two types of alcohol withdrawal. "Classic" alcohol withdrawal, which is seen most often in a hospital setting, occurs in alcoholics who either stop or sharply reduce their alcohol intake for several hours to one day. Its symptoms are jitteriness, nervousness, mild tremor, and a mild increase in the heart rate and blood pressure. Panic attacks may also occur. Even an experienced interviewer may mistake a patient's withdrawal from alcohol as generalized anxiety disorder or another anxiety syndrome, since the clinical presentations are similar. The more severe alcohol withdrawal syndrome progresses to delirium tremens, hyperthermia, seizures, and, in some cases, cardiovascular collapse.

The second type of alcohol withdrawal, nocturnal withdrawal syndrome, is also characterized by anxiety but involves a milder, less prolonged process, occurs in nonalcoholics, and is not a function of addiction. Since a small amount of alcohol (e.g., a few glasses of wine) can produce a sedative effect, it is often used as a sleep aid. Initially, alcohol inhibits rapid eye movement (REM) sleep, but because alcohol is rapidly metabolized, its inhibitory effect soon abates, causing a rebound increase in REM. This rebound effect results in insomnia, anxiety, and a sense of unease, symptoms which the individual may try to relieve by drinking more alcohol, thus reenforcing the habit of drinking alcohol.

Withdrawal from Other Central Nervous System Depressants

The central nervous system depressants other than alcohol are the benzodiazepines, barbiturates, and other sedative-hypnotics, such as meprobamate, and glutethimide. The benzodiazepines and barbiturates are most likely to induce an anxiety withdrawal syndrome. The shorter-acting benzodiazepines, like the opiates, tend to produce a more rapid onset of symptoms and a more intense withdrawal syndrome, characterized by jitteriness, a sense of unease, insomnia, mild tremulousness, and increased pulse and blood pressure. There is a concomitant rebound increase in REM during sleep. "Rebound anxiety" may occur as soon as a few hours after the last dose of a short-acting benzodiazepine such as alprazolam is taken. Up to 50% of people taking lorazepam suffer from withdrawal symptoms. "Rebound insomnia" may occur in the early morning hours with triazolam, a benzodiazepine used as a sleep aid. Even an experienced physician may mistake a patient's benzodiazepine withdrawal for a non–substance-related anxiety disorder such as generalized anxiety disorder, panic disorder, or phobia. The extreme form of benzodiazepine withdrawal is characterized by seizures and delirium.

When a patient withdraws abruptly from the prolonged use of high dosages of short-acting barbiturates, he or she becomes anxious, tremulous, nauseated, and weak within approximately 24 hours of taking the last dose. The syndrome peaks around the second or third day of abstinence. Convulsions are rare and occur two to three days after the last dose. With central nervous system depressants, including both barbiturates and benzodiazepines, signs and symptoms of withdrawal may appear within several days of the last dose, and seizures may occur up to a week after the last dose. There may be a mild withdrawal syndrome consisting of anxiety, or a more severe syndrome consisting of frightening dreams, insomnia, visual hallucinations, delirium, hyperthermia, cardiovascular collapse, exhaustion, and even death. The resolution of the delirium may take several days or more, even when the patient is promptly given large dosages of replacement benzodiazepines or barbiturates.

Withdrawal from Opioids

Anxiety syndromes are also caused by withdrawal from opioids, which include morphine, heroin (which is converted to morphine in vivo), methadone, fentanyl, meperidine, and codeine. "Cold turkey" withdrawal (abrupt opioid withdrawal) derives its name from the "plucked turkey" appearance of the skin, which is caused by piloerection, one of the classic physical signs of withdrawal. Acute heroin withdrawal causes marked anxiety that begins 8–12 hours after the last dose is taken. During this phase, the addict has intense cravings for the drug. The subjective anxiety is accompanied by tachycardia, raised blood pressure, mydriasis, restlessness, and tremor.

The withdrawal syndrome peaks at 48–72 hours after the last dose, with piloerection, yawning, sneezing, nausea, vomiting, and diarrhea.

Abrupt methadone withdrawal also causes anxiety and a psychophysiological cascade similar to that produced by heroin withdrawal, although it is generally milder and more prolonged because the longer half-life of methadone allows blood levels of the drug to fall less rapidly after it has been discontinued. The syndrome begins 24–48 hours after the last dose, and mild symptoms may occur up to 6 weeks later. Withdrawal from meperidine begins approximately three hours after the last dose, peaks in about eight hours, and usually lasts approximately four days. Codeine withdrawal is similar to morphine withdrawal but produces a less intense syndrome. The synthetic and semi-synthetic opioids also cause anxiety syndromes upon withdrawal.

The general rule is, the shorter the duration of action of the substance, the more rapidly it disappears from the body, therefore, the more intense the withdrawal syndrome.

Paradoxic Reactions

Certain pharmacological agents that normally cause calming and sedation occasionally have a paradoxic effect in specific groups of patients, such as elderly persons, children, and patients with dementia. Benzodiazepines and barbiturates may occasionally cause anxiety, disinhibition, confusion, and agitation. Central nervous system depressants should be avoided or, if used, should be given in minimal dosages in these individuals, who should be carefully monitored for agitation and confusion.

The concept that an addictive substance may induce an anxiety disorder is intriguing and controversial. Although it may seem illogical that an "anxiolytic" such as alcohol can, in the long run, actually create a permanent anxiety disorder, prolonged alcohol consumption and repeated alcohol withdrawals may sensitize individuals via a kindling effect, in which each successive withdrawal decreases the threshold for anxiety (see Etiology, below). It has also been suggested that the high cortisol levels in patients with alcohol withdrawal syndrome, and in patients with other types of "stress," are associated with hippocampal neuronal damage resulting in alcoholic dementia and a variety of other central nervous system syndromes.

A question that is frequently asked about substance abuse and anxiety is which came first, the anxiety disorder or the substance abuse. Substance abuse is connected to anxiety in two ways: (1) Use of a substance or withdrawal from a substance may be a primary cause of anxiety, and (2) use of a substance may be a way to "medicate" oneself and temporarily relieve feelings of nervousness and worry caused by an underlying anxiety disorder. Careful history taking can reveal which came first.

Course of Illness

The course of **panic disorder with or without agoraphobia** is chronic, with symptoms waxing and waning over a number of years. The onset is typically between late adolescence and the mid 30s. The course ranges from episodic outbreaks with several years of remission between them to continuous symptoms. Suicide and substance abuse are two common complications.

The onset of **generalized anxiety disorder** may occur in childhood, adolescence, or adulthood. The course is chronic, with waxing and waning of symptoms and exacerbations during times of stress. Many patients develop other syndromes, such as panic disorder or a major depressive illness.

Specific phobia has a peak onset in childhood and a second peak in the mid 20s. Phobias that continue into adulthood have a spontaneous remission rate of about 20%. Phobic symptoms may decline with age because life circumstances may have placed the patient in phobic situations that serve as a natural form of "behavior therapy."

Social phobia is characterized by a chronic, fluctuating course, which may be complicated by self-medication with alcohol or other substances. The onset is usually in the mid teens. The patient often has a history of shyness as a child. The onset may also occur after a particularly stressful or humiliating experience (e.g., loss of job, home, or family). The sequelae of self-medication with drugs or alcohol may prove to be worse than the social phobia itself.

Obsessive-compulsive disorder usually begins in adolescence or early adulthood, although it can begin as early as childhood. Generally, the age of onset for males is 6–15 years and for females 20–29 years. The onset is most often gradual but can be acute, and the course tends to be chronic, with waxing and waning of symptoms. About 15% of patients experience a progressive decline in occupational or social functioning.

The course of **posttraumatic stress disorder** is variable, both in terms of the duration of the disorder and the delay between the initial trauma and the emergence of symptoms. Symptoms usually begin within three months of the trauma, but, in some patients, years may go by before symptoms appear. For example, people who survive an earthquake may experience posttraumatic signs and symptoms for a number of months or an entire lifetime, and women who are sexually assaulted may experience a posttraumatic syndrome immediately after the assault or not until several years later. The course of posttraumatic stress disorder may be divided into three stages: (1) an acute response to the trauma; (2) acute posttraumatic stress disorder, which is marked by autonomic arousal, flashbacks, irritability, and phobic avoidance; and (3) chronic posttraumatic stress disorder, which is characterized by preoccupation with the trauma, isolation, withdrawal, and psychic numbing. Factors predictive of a positive outcome include a solid social support system, good psychiatric and medical health before the trauma occurred, a rapid onset of symptoms, and prompt crisis intervention with abreaction. The course is often complicated if the patient attempts to alleviate symptoms of anxiety, autonomic arousal, and irritability through self-medication with alcohol or drugs.

The symptoms of **acute stress disorder** are experienced during the trauma or immediately following it and resolve within 4 weeks. Symptoms persisting beyond this time are usually classified as posttraumatic stress disorder.

THE INTERVIEW

When interviewing a patient who is complaining of anxiety, it is important that the physician listen for clues to the kind of symptoms the person experiences, the times when they occur, and the pattern of the anxiety (see Interviewing Guidelines box). The interviewer should listen for clues to a medical condition or medical treatment that may be causing anxiety-like symptoms. It is important to elicit historical data about life experiences that may have influenced the onset or exacerbation of the symptoms and the patient's prior history of anxiety. This information may reveal the psychosocial components contributing to the symptoms. The physician should apply his or her knowledge about the psychodynamics of anxiety in formulating the diagnostic importance of the information presented and in discerning the conditions that would benefit from psychotherapy or pharmacotherapy.

Patients with anxiety disorders usually describe their symptoms in great detail, focusing on how the symptoms make them feel. The interviewer must elicit **specific information** about the symptoms, such as the onset, duration, distribution, quality, and intensity of the symptoms; the past history of anxiety symptoms; the family history of anxiety symptoms; and whether any other symptoms are associated with the anxiety symptoms. Patients may be surprisingly vague about the parameters of their symptoms, and some persistent questioning by the interviewer may be needed to obtain the details. Some patients, on the other hand, are quite specific from the beginning. The ability to be specific depends partially on the patient's experience of anxiety and whether the symptoms are focal and isolated in mental functioning or whether they are diffuse. It will be easier for the patient to describe an onset that is sharp and sudden than one that is subtle, insidious, and chronic. If the patient is struggling to describe the onset, the physician should suspect that the onset was of the second type. The usual style of interviewing patients with anxiety disorders is to alternate between asking specific questions and listening carefully to the patient's elaboration on various topics. Because depressive symptoms often coexist with anxiety symptoms, the interviewer should ask specifically about symptoms of depression (see Chapter 3, Mood Disorders). At this time, the interviewer should also ask about other conditions that are sometimes associated with anxiety disorder, such as substance abuse or medical disorders such as thyroid disease.

The **life history** is an important part of the interview because it may suggest psychosocial causes of anxiety. Because they do not consider such information to be relevant to their symptoms, many patients do not spontaneously provide an integrated life history that reveals the juxtaposition between their symptoms and what is going on in their lives. The interviewer should take a parallel history, which is divided into two parts according to time sequence: The first part is the history of the symptoms; the second part is the life history. The interviewer might say to the patient, "Please tell me what was going on in your life at the onset of your symptoms." If the patient responds by saying, "Not much," the interviewer should ask the patient to elaborate and then remain silent while the patient organizes his or her thoughts and begins to speak. The patient's starting point may give the interviewer the first clues about the relevant context in which the symptoms have occurred. As with psychosomatic disease, events that might seem negligible to the patient are often quickly identified by the interviewer as the stressors or precipitating events. When they are pointed out, the patient may dismiss or deny them. Even if the patient has some conscious experience of the contiguity and cause of the symptoms, the mediating emotions are usually not known to the patient. The interviewer must understand the emotional dynamics of patients with anxiety in order to help them.

The psychological features of many of the anxiety disorders include conflicts over dependence and independence, attachment and hostility, and sexual or aggressive wishes and punishment. The link to the depressive disorders again emerges in this overlap of the psychodynamics of guilt, aggression, and abandonment. Even in an interview situation, an anxious patient may convey a need for immediate, unrealistic

---

Interviewing Guidelines

- Ask about the specific symptoms of anxiety, including the onset, duration, distribution, quality, and intensity of the symptoms.
- Inquire about associated symptoms, including depression and suicidal ideation.
- Inquire about the patient's life history, listening for psychosocial triggers of anxiety and the context in which they have occurred.
- Ask whether the patient has any theories about the psychological meaning of the symptoms.
- Obtain a complete medical history.
- Maintain a calm, reassuring demeanor. Avoid expressing irritation with the patient.

attention and may elicit rescue fantasies in the interviewer. The patient may try to place extra demands on the physician that intrude upon his or her time with other patients or personal time. This may cause the physician to become annoyed and scold the patient or to avoid or postpone meeting with the patient in the future. The physician may feel guilty for having these negative emotions. By provoking the physician into showing mild signs of anger (e.g., using a sharp tone of voice or making a sharp reply) or abandonment (e.g., avoiding contact), the patient is expressing the attachment anxiety and abandonment psychology that are present in his or her relationship with the physician. The patient is expressing his or her hostile reaction to dependency, but by doing so, fulfills the most feared expectations of abandonment and anger. Recognizing the frightening nature of the symptoms of an anxiety disorder and understanding the psychodynamics that result enable the physician to structure a therapeutic environment that can help contain the patient's anxiety but not overwhelm the physician.

DIFFERENTIAL DIAGNOSIS

Making the correct diagnosis in patients with signs and symptoms of anxiety is complicated by the many medical syndromes that mimic psychiatric syndromes and vice versa (see Chapter 5, Cognitive and Mental Disorders Due to General Medical Conditions). Diaphoresis, tachycardia, and shortness of breath can appear to be psychiatric signs and symptoms but can be caused by a myocardial infarction. The coexistence of a medical condition with panic disorder may deflect the physician's attention from the psychiatric diagnosis and delay appropriate, complete treatment. Another complication of the differential diagnosis is that the same complex of specific signs and symptoms can occur in a variety of anxiety disorders. The demarcation between the subtypes of anxiety disorders is inexact, and there is considerable overlapping among them. Some patients with panic disorder present with symptoms of social phobia, as do some patients with agoraphobia.

The pattern of anxiety is the differentiating factor in the various anxiety disorders. For example, in **generalized anxiety disorder,** the level of anxiety remains constant and the patient finds no internal or external focus for the anxious feelings. The anxiety may increase in intensity over hours or days and may reach a peak level of extreme intensity, as in substance-induced anxiety, but no actual panic attacks accompany it. The anxiety may have a rapid onset, increase to an extreme level of intensity over only a few minutes, and result in panic attacks. When this happens, the patient clearly has **panic disorder.**

The differential diagnosis of **panic disorder** includes anxiety disorder due to a general medical condition, substance-induced anxiety disorder, and other mental disorders that have panic attacks as an associated feature. Panic attacks can occur not only as part of panic disorder but also as part of a social or specific phobia (see below). Panic attacks occur "out of the blue" in panic disorder but are related to an external situation in social phobia, specific phobia, obsessive-compulsive disorder, and posttraumatic stress disorder. Panic attacks occur most frequently in patients with panic disorder and agoraphobia. Other anxiety disorders occur in approximately 20% of patients with panic disorder. Major depression frequently accompanies panic disorder (40–70% of patients), and about 20–25% of depressed patients have a lifetime history of panic disorder. The comorbidity rate of panic disorder and substance abuse is about 15%.

The differential diagnosis of **specific phobia** includes panic disorder with agoraphobia, social phobia, posttraumatic stress disorder, obsessive-compulsive disorder, separation anxiety disorder (a disorder of childhood), and other disorders involving avoidance of various situations or activities.

Social phobia must be distinguished from other mental disorders involving social anxiety and the avoidance of social situations, including panic disorder with agoraphobia, agoraphobia without a history of panic disorder, generalized anxiety disorder, specific phobia, and avoidant personality disorder. It should also be differentiated from common responses such as performance anxiety, stage fright, and shyness.

Obsessive-compulsive disorder should be distinguished from other mental disorders involving recurrent or intrusive thoughts, images, impulses, or behaviors. Some differential diagnoses include anxiety disorder due to a general medical condition, substance-induced anxiety disorder, body dysmorphic disorder, and a specific phobia or social phobia in which there is a preoccupation with a feared object or situation. Persistent brooding in major depression, excessive worry in generalized anxiety disorder, and other disorders with ruminative aspects should also be differentiated. Obsessive-compulsive disorder should not be confused with superstitious and repetitive checking behaviors that may be within the realm of normal, everyday behavior.

The differential diagnosis of **posttraumatic stress disorder** includes adjustment disorder, acute stress disorder, and obsessive-compulsive disorder that is characterized by recurrent intrusive thoughts that are experienced as inappropriate and are not related to an experienced traumatic event. The flashbacks in posttraumatic stress disorder must be distinguished from perceptual disturbances that occur in other disorders, such as schizophrenic disorders, substance-induced disorders, mood disorder with psychotic features, and psychotic disorder due to a general medical condition. The dissociative symptoms that are typical of posttraumatic stress disorder also occur in the dissociative disorders (Box 6–1).

The differential diagnosis of **acute stress disorder** includes posttraumatic stress disorder, anxiety disorder due to a general medical condition, substance-induced disorder, brief psychotic disorder, and an exacerbation of a preexisting mental disorder.

BOX 6–1.   Dissociative Disorder

Dissociation is a ubiquitous human psychological phenomenon. Its function is to relieve anxiety by separating the mental content of a thought that produces anxiety from the unpleasant feeling of anxiety. It may be a mild phenomenon that is a common response to daily life experiences or a severe, incapacitating psychiatric disorder, with various gradations between these two extremes. Biological factors seem to play a role in severe dissociation.

Depersonalization is a dissociative phenomenon in which a person feels slightly removed from his or her body. A 40-year-old business executive is mildly uncomfortable during airplane travel, but he must fly frequently because of his job. He feels quite relaxed and happy as he walks down the ramp to the airplane, but he then begins to feel mildly anxious, with a sensation of being "slightly out of my body." He describes the sensation as a hyperobjective experience of watching himself. In his mind, he is describing his motions to himself as if he were observing another person. "Now he's walking down the ramp, now he's entering the airplane, now he's showing his ticket to the stewardess." These are merely thoughts. He is aware that they are due to anxiety.

Derealization is a dissociative state in which a person experiences his or her surroundings as strange or unreal. A soldier who is having his first experience of combat is being flown by helicopter into a forward area. As the chopper quickly skirts a line of trees and comes down in the landing zone, he sees flare markers shooting into the sky, artillery rounds landing 200 yards away, and infantry troops that have previously landed running into the trees to form a skirmish line. He feels as if the scene is in a movie and not actually real. He has a dual emotional experience of anxiety and of great interest and excitement. He watches the unfolding battle scene as if he is not about to be plunged into its center.

The DSM-IV describes five specific syndromes of dissociation. **Dissociative amnesia** is the forgetting of past events that are usually of a traumatic nature. The material is actively repressed and not just merely overlooked. When the patient retrieves the information during the course of psychotherapy, the patient is often interested and enlightened but not surprised, because the patient has the feeling that he or she has known the information all along in some way. Traumatic episodes that pass in and out of consciousness over many years are more common than complete repression. Examples of such episodes are combat experiences in young adulthood or sexual, abusive, or abandonment traumas of childhood.

Dissociative fugue is characterized by massive repression of all personal information. The syndrome presents as the patient suddenly travels away from home, often far away, and sheds his or her personal identification. It is sometimes associated with some degree of stupor and mild confusion. The patient may be brought to the emergency room by the local police after being found wandering. Some patients may retain their ability to interact superficially with people and to work and may set up a new life. The differential diagnosis of dissociative amnesia and fugue should include malingering about the symptom of amnesia as well as a mental disorder due to a general medical condition or a substance-induced disorder.

Dissociative identity disorder is the latest term for multiple personality disorder. It is characterized by the presence of two or more subjectively felt, distinct identities that are actually personality states divided according to affect. In such states, the patient and the multiples are almost always aware of the presence of the others. The mechanism does not seem to be repression, as in dissociative amnesia or fugue, but rather an inability to integrate different conscious emotional experiences.

Depersonalization disorder has as its main criterion recurrent episodes of depersonalization that cause distress or impairment.

Dissociative disorder not otherwise specified is diagnosed when dissociative symptoms cause significant impairment or distress, or both, but do not meet the criteria for one of the other dissociative disorders.

Hypnosis and intravenous administration of the short-acting barbiturate amobarbital sodium can be useful in the treatment of patients with dissociative amnesia and fugue because it facilitates the recovery of repressed memories. Long-term psychotherapy is required for patients suffering from dissociative identity disorder. Psychiatrists must be careful not to act as if the multiples are truly separate identities, because this approach will cause the patient's condition to worsen. The goal of treatment should be integration, as the following vignette illustrates. A woman is admitted to a psychiatric hospital. She says that she has an "alter" named Mary, who is always getting her into trouble. Mary is an angry young woman, who is constantly acting out aggressively or sexually, or both. The patient's true name is Susan. She presents herself as a calm, loving, organized, and very controlled person. The admitting psychiatrist tells her that while she is on the psychiatric unit, Susan will be held responsible for whatever Mary does and Mary will be held responsible for whatever Susan does. The patient becomes furious and says, "That's not fair!" The psychiatrist says that this may not be fair, but that's the way it is. The patient says angrily, "I hate you!" The psychiatrist says, "Did you hear what you said? You didn't say 'Mary hates you'; you didn't say 'Susan hates you'; you said 'I hate you!' Good! See you tomorrow." The psychiatrist is pleased with the patient's response because, despite her protest, she has taken a step toward integration in identifying herself as "I" and in tolerating anger without dissociating.

Accurate diagnosis is crucial to treatment, and there is no greater camouflage for illness than **generalized anxiety disorder.** Many patients with depression present with depressive anxiety, which is diagnosed as a chronic anxiety disorder. In order to uncover depressive signs and symptoms, the physician must take the patient's history carefully and systematically review the patient's past medical history, which may include depression. For such patients, antidepressants will be much more effective than anxiolytics. Generalized anxiety may be the most prominent symptom of hypomania. The common medical condition of hyperthyroidism should not be overlooked and is usually easily treatable.

Generalized anxiety disorder must be distinguished from anxiety disorder due to a general medical condition, substance-induced anxiety disorder, and other anxiety disorders involving excessive worry, ruminations, or physical complaints (e.g., panic disorder, social phobia, obsessive-compulsive disorder, or posttraumatic stress disorder), as well as hypochondriasis and adjustment disorder. Nonpathological anxiety differs from generalized anxiety disorder in that it is easier to control and interferes less with functioning, is less pervasive, and has a shorter duration.

Anxiety disorder due to a general medical condition should be differentiated from delirium, substance-induced anxiety disorder, and the primary anxiety disorders.

Substance-induced anxiety disorder should be classified as substance intoxication or substance withdrawal, and should be differentiated from a primary anxiety disorder or anxiety disorder due to a general medical condition.

MEDICAL EVALUATION

The patients most likely to present with symptoms that mimic anxiety and that may initially be misdiagnosed as psychiatric symptoms are patients with endocrine, cardiac, and neurological conditions. For example, a 38-year-old mother and businesswoman complained of sudden, unpredictable, brief attacks of tachycardia, pounding headaches, and dizziness. The symptoms did not correspond to a change in her mood or circumstances. Her family physician advised her to see a psychiatrist for treatment of "anxiety attacks," but she never did. A friend referred her to an endocrinologist, who discovered an epinephrine-secreting pheochromocytoma. After the tumor was removed, the woman had no more attacks.

Focusing only on possible medical etiologies, however, can unnecessarily delay appropriate psychiatric treatment, as the following case demonstrates. In December of 1970, a 43-year-old woman presented to the emergency room with the chief complaint of "palpitations"; an electrocardiogram (ECG) revealed that the sinus rhythm was normal with occasional premature atrial contractions. She was reassured that "nothing was abnormal" and was sent home. In July of 1971, she again presented to the emergency room with the same chief complaint. On that occasion, the ECG showed a normal sinus rhythm with occasional premature ventricular contractions, and an echocardiogram revealed "marked to moderate-late systolic posterior prolapse of the mitral valve." In March of 1972, she presented to the emergency room complaining of palpitations and dizziness. She did not complain of chest pain, syncope, or dyspnea. Twenty-four-hour Holter monitoring revealed a mean heart rate of 97 beats per minute and 326 premature ventricular contractions per hour. She was again diagnosed with mitral valve prolapse and was given propranolol. Over the following 10 years, she presented to the emergency room about once a week complaining of palpitations. In April of 1982, lorazepam was added to the propranolol regimen to treat her anxiety. Cardiovascular evaluation confirmed the diagnosis of mitral valve prolapse. In May of 1982, a psychiatric consultation was requested for treatment of her anxiety. She was then diagnosed with panic disorder. By that time, she had stopped working because the palpitations were so bothersome. She was finally convinced to take the antipanic, antidepressant medication imipramine, 25 mg at bedtime. The dosage was increased slowly by increments. On a follow-up visit in November of 1982 (when she was taking a dosage of 75 mg at bedtime),

24-hour Holter monitoring revealed a normal sinus rhythm with a mean heart rate of 78 beats per minute and no premature ventricular contractions. Her anxiety and panic had disappeared.

Mitral valve prolapse appears to occur more frequently in patients with panic disorder than in people without panic disorder, although there appears to be no greater frequency of panic disorder in patients with mitral valve prolapse than in those who do not have it. Mitral valve prolapse and panic disorder share some characteristics, such as palpitations, light-headedness, and chest pain. When both disorders occur together, it is difficult to determine whether the symptoms arise from mitral valve prolapse, panic disorder, or a mechanism involving both. In patients who have both mitral valve prolapse and panic disorder, the "cardiac symptoms" resolve when they are taking imipramine, even though there are continued findings of mitral valve prolapse (i.e., even though the prolapse has not resolved). The imipramine may be treating a neurochemical defect common to both mitral valve prolapse and panic disorder, and the "cardiac symptoms" may not stem strictly from the mitral valve prolapse. When the panic disorder is treated, the "cardiac symptoms" may improve as well.

Physicians pursuing a medical evaluation of patients complaining of anxiety must strike a balance between avoiding excessive workups that delay the prescription of appropriate psychiatric treatment and investigating possible physiological explanations for the anxiety symptoms.

A crucial first step is to take a careful, thorough medical history; review of systems; and review of medications (including prescription drugs and over-the-counter drugs) and other agents (including recreational drugs, alcohol, nicotine, and caffeine) that have recently been consumed by the patient. Taking the patient's vital signs and doing a physical examination that focuses on the signs of endocrinological, cardiac, pulmonary, and neurological diseases are the next steps. Useful laboratory tests may include a complete blood count and tests of thyroid function, blood glucose levels, and arterial blood gas levels. An assessment of cardiac functioning, which may include an ECG, chest x-ray, 24-hour Holter monitoring test, and echocardiogram, should be considered in patients with a recent onset of anxiety symptoms with physical symptoms suggesting cardiac ischemia (e.g., crushing chest pain), particularly in patients over age 40 years. Repeated extensive testing that consistently produces negative results should be avoided.

ETIOLOGY

The etiology, manifestations, and treatment may differ markedly in each anxiety disorder. There is no single theory that fully explains all anxiety disorders, although some unifying features are shared by several disorders.

Specific etiological theories range from the psychoanalytical to the neurochemical. These theories are not mutually exclusive. The neurochemical theories describe physiological mediators and triggers; the psychoanalytical theories describe psychological mediators and triggers. Anxiety is not strictly a biological phenomenon or a psychological phenomenon. Anxiety due to a biological disorder, such as hyperthyroidism, inevitably has some psychological manifestations that share many features of "functional" anxiety (i.e., anxiety for which no medical cause is known). Similarly, anxiety of psychological origin, such as fear of performing before an audience, has biological manifestations, (e. g., light-headedness, tachycardia, sweating, and voice tremor). Once a circuit has been established between the individual psychological and physiological manifestations, it becomes increasingly difficult to determine whether the initial trigger for the anxiety is psychological, physiological, or an indecipherable combination of both.

Approaches to the etiology of anxiety include seemingly opposite views. Sigmund Freud believed that subjective feelings of psychological distress (anxiety) lead to physical symptoms, such as tachycardia and diaphoresis. William James believed that the physical symptoms lead to the subjective feeling of anxiety. According to the James-Lange theory, emotions represent the awareness of visceral activity. After this theory was proposed, it was demonstrated that emotional experience remained intact even after visceral afferent fibers had been severed. This proved that the experience of emotions does not depend on the experience of peripheral visceral activity. In one study of subjects who were given injections of epinephrine, it was found that their psychological experiences depended on the external situation and not on their internal physiological state. In general, studies of human psychophysiology imply that there is some linkage between emotions and the autonomic nervous system but whether the connection is unidirectional, bidirectional, or circuitous is not yet known.

The diversity of the theories described above underscores the point that there is no single biological or psychological cause of anxiety and that, at this point, all theories are speculative. Instead of trying to categorize anxiety as either a biological or psychological phenomenon, it might be more productive to determine how biological factors translate into and influence psychological factors, and vice versa. In other words, what is the summation of the psychosocial and biological processes that together generate human behavior?

Psychoanalytic Theories

Psychoanalysis and psychoanalytic psychotherapy attempt to disassemble the psychological triggers of anxiety. These therapies attempt to do so by finding the specific situations that evoke specific feelings that trigger anxiety states. The focus in these treatments is on discovering the frightening unconscious emotional meanings that are associated with real-life stressors and the conscious thoughts and feelings that trigger and mediate anxiety states. Many patients with symptomatic anxiety states are consciously aware that certain situations have an exaggerated emotional meaning for them. A patient with panic attacks triggered mainly by airplane travel knows that the likelihood of death and dismemberment is much greater when crossing the street than when flying in an airplane, but, nonetheless, fears the airplane as though a catastrophe is imminent and crosses the street with carefree abandon. Psychoanalytically based treatments work by uncovering the emotional complexes that are symbolically represented in the phobic trigger. Once the patient understands which emotional situation is being displaced to the real-life event, he or she may be better able to work through the emotional conflicts and free the reality stimulus from the anxiety it produces. The noxious effect is mediated by conflicted emotions, and when these change, the reality stimulus loses its power. Treatments involve varying measures of exploration, support, and positive suggestion, depending on the phase of the treatment, the severity of the symptoms, the availability of the underlying emotional themes, and whether or not concurrent medication is needed. The psychodynamic theory of anxiety, therefore, focuses on mechanisms of symbolic representation that attach frightening emotional significance to reality events. These events have the capacity, through unknown mediating biological mechanisms, to trigger a neurobiological tendency toward anxiety. The symptoms vary according to the degree of trauma that is triggered by the situation, the sensitivity of the brain centers that mediate anxiety, and the intensity of the response once it has been triggered. This neurobiological-psychological interaction is most similar to that of the mood disorders, with which the anxiety disorders often coexist and overlap.

It is the impression of many psychoanalysts that patients with panic have some common dynamic conflicts in the area of fears and insecurities regarding dependency. These conflicts may derive from early childhood and may be based on actual deprivation, a heightened sensitivity to normal environmental deprivation experiences, or a combination of the two. These dependency issues of early childhood continue throughout life and may become commingled with later issues of competition and achievement, making patients with anxiety vulnerable to situations that symbolically represent these issues.

Neurobiological Theories

The biological vulnerability to certain anxiety disorders varies from person to person. Patients with panic disorder commonly have a family history of panic attacks, suggesting that a heritable neuronal state generates a lower threshold for spontaneous emergency response episodes. This vulnerability may never be stressed, and the person may have no symptoms. Another person may experience panic attacks from smoking marijuana, drinking alcohol, or having a frightening real-life experience. Also, it is logical to assume that psychological changes may alter biological vulnerability. Changes for better or worse may result from life experiences or from having been treated with psychotherapy.

Panic Disorder

Locus Coeruleus

The locus coeruleus is a brain stem structure that contains the majority of noradrenergic neurons in the central nervous system. It may play a pivotal role in mediating the sympathetic flooding that occurs during some fear and anxiety states. Located in the pons, it projects to several important brain structures that are thought to be involved in human emotion, particularly the limbic system, amygdala, hippocampus, and cerebral cortex (Fig. 6–1). The central noradrenergic neurons in the locus coeruleus appear to alert and alarm an individual to potentially threatening environmental factors; in situations of potential "danger," the locus coeruleus sets off a sympathetic discharge that may facilitate responses, ranging from an alerting and adaptive response to one that is anxiogenic and disabling. It is unclear to what extent animal studies of locus coeruleus activity mirror the human scenario of arousal and anxiety, just as it is difficult to distinguish in nonhumans the experience of anxiety from generalized "stress" or fear. The demonstrable connection lies mostly in behavioral and physiological responses. But pharmacological agents that increase locus coeruleus discharge, such as the α_2-antagonist yohimbine, can mimic both the psychic and physical sensations of anxiety, particularly in persons who are vulnerable

to anxiety. Conversely, agents that decrease central noradrenergic release (e.g., the α_2-agonist clonidine) partially or completely alleviate the physiological components of anxiety.

Central Medullary Chemoreceptor and Serotinergic Midbrain Dorsal Raphe

In addition to the locus coeruleus, two other brain stem structures may be involved in the development of panic disorder. These are the central medullary chemoreceptor and the serotonergic midbrain dorsal raphe, both of which are thought to innervate the locus coeruleus. A hypersensitivity of the medullary chemoreceptors to carbon dioxide may result in excessive stimulation of the locus coeruleus, facilitating a paniclike state (see Fig. 6–1).

The effectiveness of the selective serotonin reuptake inhibitors (SSRIs) for patients with panic disorder suggests that **serotonin** may play a role in the pathophysiology of panic disorder. Serotonin may attenuate the activity of the locus coeruleus. The apparent ability of the SSRI fluoxetine to reduce the firing of the locus coeruleus during withdrawal from opiates supports this hypothesis.

In summary, panic and anxiety may be correlated with the dysregulated firing of the locus coeruleus that is caused by input from multiple sources, including peripheral autonomic afferents, medullary afferents, and serotonergic fibers.

The role of the brain stem in panic disorder will continue to be elucidated as knowledge of the neural connections between the brain stem, cerebellum, limbic system, and cortex expands. Because psychotherapy is effective in the treatment of anxiety disorders, it is reasonable to speculate that such therapy acts via the cortex to affect the locus

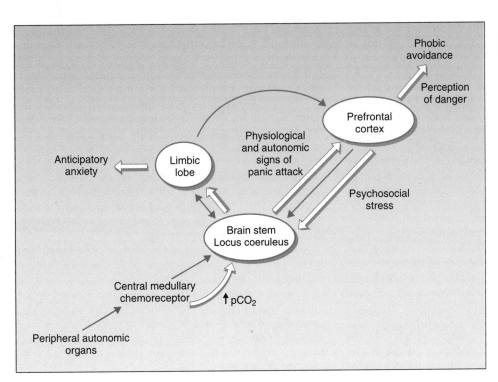

FIGURE 6–1. Theory of the neurobiological basis of panic disorder with agoraphobia.

coeruleus and down-regulate noradrenergic activity. There are known corticoreticular paths that extend from the higher cortex in an inferior direction to the brain stem.

Lactate-Induced Panic

An adrenergic surge and parallel physiological phenomena that characterize a panic attack can be reproduced by chemical agents such as lactate (Pitts and McClure, 1967). An examination of these chemically induced attacks can be used to elucidate which of the neural pathways described above might be involved in the genesis of panic anxiety. It is hypothesized that patients with panic symptoms may have a baseline biochemical vulnerability that makes them susceptible to the effects of lactate infusion. Reiman (1984) has found that patients who develop lactate-induced panic have parahippocampal blood flow asymmetry on positron emission tomography before they receive the lactate infusion.

While discrete physiological events (e.g., tachycardia, hyperventilation, increased blood pressure) during lactate-induced panic have been consistently demonstrated, the biochemical theories of the causes of these events are still speculative. The question that remains is whether lactate induces panic via peripheral metabolic effects, direct effects on the central nervous system, or a circuitry involving both.

One hypothesis is that once lactate is infused peripherally, it is converted to bicarbonate and then to carbon dioxide. When the carbon dioxide crosses into the brain, it theoretically produces a temporary central hypercapnia, which increases the ventilatory rate. In essence, the lactate infusion mimics carbon dioxide inhalation, which (theoretically) stimulates the central medullary chemoreceptors. Klein had initially proposed a suffocation-alarm mechanism in response to central hypercarbia as a possible mechanism of lactate-induced panic. He now posits a somewhat broader deranged suffocation alarm mechanism that, in response to a physiologic misinterpretation, leads to respiratory distress, hyperventilation, and a desire to escape (Klein, 1993).

Recent studies by Coplan and Gorman and by Dager argue against central hypercarbia as the mode of lactate panicogenesis. Instead, they suggest that lactate-induced panic is based on misevaluation or misinterpretation by the individual of peripheral somatic sensations. Lactate infusion causes peripheral somatic sensations resembling those in natural panic attacks. The patient misinterprets these sensations as an impending catastrophic event.

Benzodiazepine Receptors

The effectiveness of the benzodiazepines in relieving anxiety implies some connection between the genesis of anxiety and the action of benzodiazepine receptors. The understanding of the pharmacotherapeutic properties of the benzodiazepines, and, therefore of γ-aminobutyric acid (GABA) has changed markedly since the discovery in 1977 of high-affinity, specific benzodiazepine binding sites, which include certain receptors that are located only in the brain and others in the periphery. The linkage between benzodiazepine and GABA is as follows: The central nervous system benzodiazepine receptor shares a chloride ionophore complex with the GABA receptor. The binding of a benzodiazepine such as diazepam to the benzodiazepine receptor facilitates the action of GABA as an inhibitory neurotransmitter. (The amino acids GABA, glycine, and taurine are the major inhibitory neurotransmitters; glutamate and aspartate are the excitatory neurotransmitters.) On the neuronal surface, the GABA receptor is linked to a chloride channel in the neuronal membrane. When the benzodiazepine binds to its receptor, chloride channels open, sending chloride into the cell. This causes hyperpolarization of the cell membrane and, therefore, inhibition of neuronal firing.

The inhibitory effects of GABA can be blocked by picrotoxin, which binds to the chloride channel and blocks its opening. The β-carbolines, which block binding to the benzodiazepine receptor, are anxiogenic. Therefore, a dysfunction involving the benzodiazepine receptor or its ligands may be responsible for some components of anxiety.

Amygdala

The amygdala is a brain structure that influences fear, vigilance, and rage and may, therefore, play a role in the genesis of anxiety. The fear-potentiated startle reflex is a paradigm of anxiety involving projections between the amygdala and various hypothalamic and brain stem structures.

Synaptic Response

While it is well known that "stress" can induce transient biochemical changes, it is not known whether these changes shape future behavioral patterns by structurally changing the brain. Kandel's work with Aplysia (marine snails) (1979) sheds light on how mental experience might be "converted" into neurobiological symptoms. Conditioning processes in Aplysia lead to microanatomic "hard-wiring" changes. Each change is, in essence, an anatomic "memory" at the neuronal synapse, which then grows new connections and has increased sensitivity for established connections. The finding that memory is linked with microanatomical changes in Aplysia introduces a potential converging point uniting psychodynamics, psychophysiology, neuroanatomy, and cellular biology. It is vastly premature to extrapolate data from marine snails to humans, but the concept of transduction of psychosocial experience into neurocircuitry is a central one. Genes, second messengers, and neurobiological cascades are crucial to the functioning of this circuitry. These correlations offer a hypothesis about how psychotherapy may effect neurobiological changes in the brain.

In the biological process of a "memory," the proto-oncogene c-*fos* is part of a class of "immediate early proteins." These proteins act early in the neuronal process and may function in determining cell plasticity by influencing the subsequent cascade of gene activation that orchestrates cell growth (Kandel, 1989). Thus, c-*fos* may effect longer-term, structural synaptic changes (i.e., "anatomic memory").

It is reasonable to speculate that acute events (stressors) induce the protein c-*fos*, which, through cascades, may induce long-lasting biochemical and neurobiological changes. This is an intriguing but speculative way of understanding how psychosocial stressors might "translate" into permanent neurobiological changes and manifest themselves as future altered behavior patterns and psychiatric disorders.

Rose's group (1991) has studied chicks who learned to avoid a bitter-tasting substance after being allowed to peck at a shiny tube containing the substance. Changes associated with this "learning process" include neurotransmitter changes, glycogen synthesis changes, c-*fos* and other proto-oncogene inductions, as well as alterations in synapse number and density seen under the electron microscope. Others have speculated that these microanatomic changes may remain present, or "anatomically remembered," long after the initial "psychosocial" stressor has been removed from consciousness. This might explain how events that are apparently "forgotten" nevertheless continue to exert permanent psychophysiological effects through their "hidden" presence in the "hard-wiring" of the brain.

Both the magnitude and frequency of the stressor may influence how it is recorded. The age at which the experience occurs and, consequently, the tools of language, perception, and expression available to encode that experience may determine the degree of psychological trauma associated with the event and the brain locations affected. What differentiates a "trauma" from an "adventure" for different adults experiencing the same life event has yet to be determined.

Obsessive-Compulsive Disorder

Obsessive-compulsive disorder can be traced back to medieval days, when afflicted individuals were thought to be possessed by demons and were "treated" with exorcism. By the early 1900s, psychological theories about the disorder had been formulated. Subsequently, the perspective on obsessive-compulsive disorder has broadened, and neurobiological etiologies have been explored.

The neurobiological basis of obsessive-compulsive disorder is now being studied with modern radioimaging techniques. These investigations have focused on the frontal lobes and caudate. Positron emission tomography (PET) has demonstrated increased metabolism in the orbital cortex of the frontal lobes and the head of the caudate nucleus. Increased blood flow in the medial frontal lobes has been demonstrated on single-photon emission computed tomography (SPECT). One theory posits striatal hypofunction as the primary defect, with secondary cortical hyperactivity. The defect may lie somewhere in the **frontal-subcortical circuit** linking the orbitofrontal cortex, caudate nuclei, and globus pallidus. Symptoms of obsessive-compulsive disorder may result from any disturbance within this circuit. Corroboration for this hypothesis is the normalization of glucose metabolic rates in the frontal cortical and caudate regions by pharmacological agents such as fluoxetine and clomipramine, which

affect serotonin transmission, as well as through behavioral treatments (Baxter et al, 1992). This implies that both behavioral and pharmacological treatments for obsessive-compulsive disorder effect long-term changes in the same brain structures.

Another structure that might be involved in obsessive-compulsive disorder is the cingulum. Electrical stimulation of the cingulum causes stereotyped movements, and PET studies have shown increased metabolic activity in the anterior cingulate cortex bilaterally, suggesting that a hyperactive cingulum may cause compulsive behavior. Flor-Henry (1990) has advanced the theory that obsessive-compulsive states are determined by "lateralized dysregulation of the left fronto-caudate network," which causes a defect in the inhibition of frontal systems.

A syndrome that is similar to obsessive-compulsive disorder occurs in neurological disorders, often those which involve the basal ganglia. In addition, obsessive-compulsive disorder occurs with greater frequency in patients with Sydenham's chorea or ischemic injury to the caudate.

Posttraumatic Stress Disorder

The neurobiological bases for posttraumatic stress disorder are also becoming more clear. Kolb and, later, Van der Kolk have hypothesized that excessive, prolonged sensitizing stimulation causes **impaired cortical control** over brain stem structures such as the locus coeruleus and hypothalamus. This impairment leads to a repetitive restimulation of the affective, perceptual, and somatic sense of the original trauma. The theories of Kolb and Van der Kolk share some common ground with Freud's "stimulus barrier" hypothesis, which suggests that the organism possesses a neuroanatomic structure that protects it from excessive stimulation. Posttraumatic stress disorder appears, in some way, to result from stimulation that overwhelms this barrier.

Some of the neurophysiological alterations in patients with posttraumatic stress disorder include increased sympathetic activity, increased hypothalamic-pituitary-adrenal function, and opioid dysregulation. These neurophysiological variables could determine how the initial trauma affects the personality years later.

The etiological relationship between the severity of the stressor and the development of posttraumatic stress disorder is nebulous and certainly does not follow a direct correlation. Clearly, the same magnitude of stressor has different repercussions in one individual than it does in another individual whose psychological vulnerability might be different. Some investigators have found that the likelihood of developing posttraumatic stress disorder after a traumatic event is increased when a history of previous trauma exists. In some individuals without a history of previous trauma, however, a sufficiently severe stressor is enough to cause posttraumatic stress disorder.

Substance-Induced Anxiety Disorder

A process called **kindling** has been proposed to explain why some alcoholics develop an anxiety disorder after years of drinking. (It is possible, of course, that these individuals are suffering from anxiety before they begin to drink.) Some alcoholics who undergo repeated episodes of alcohol withdrawal develop a kindling effect (i.e., the "increase in neural responsivity produced by spaced and repeated epileptogenic stimulation of certain brain structures"; Racine, 1979). Panic and other types of anxiety could conceivably be kindled by repeated, progressively more severe episodes of alcohol withdrawal. The possibility of such a development underscores the importance of adequately treating all episodes of alcohol withdrawal. It has been shown that the blunted responsiveness of the noradrenergic α_2-autoreceptors is correlated with the number of episodes of alcohol withdrawal; this lends support to the kindling hypothesis. Some studies suggest that alprazolam may have significant α_2-autoreceptor agonist effects, thereby reducing noradrenergic overactivity and the signs and symptoms of anxiety.

TREATMENT
Psychotherapy
Panic Disorder and Agoraphobia

The psychological treatments for patients with panic disorder and agoraphobia are psychodynamic psychotherapy and cognitive-behavior treatment. The behavior treatment of panic attacks includes breathing exercises to decrease acute and chronic hyperventilation, as well as cognitive techniques to reduce the patient's overinterpretation of unpleasant peripheral somatic sensations. The objective is for the patient to learn to reinterpret somatic sensations (e.g., dizziness, tremulousness) as benign and conquerable rather than catastrophic and life-threatening. Relaxation training through electromyographic feedback or hypnosis is another technique that produces a general reduction in somatic tension, which in turn reduces the patient's generalized anxiety. Patients with panic disorder are sometimes advised to avoid unnecessary stimulants, such as caffeine, to which they may be unusually sensitive.

For a patient with panic attacks, the therapist uses psychodynamic treatments and psychoanalysis to understand the emotional content of the symbolic representations of reality that trigger the episodes. For a patient without obvious triggers, the therapist attempts to understand the episodes by exploring the patient's conflicted psychological states and connections to ongoing struggles within his or her personality. Reflections of these struggles in interpersonal relationships and life events are carefully explored. Connections to other types of anxiety, such as performance anxiety, achievement anxiety, and depressive anxieties, are most easily seen in these exploratory treatments. Triggers that are often important in patients with panic disorder are separation anxiety and emotional conflicts over dependency needs and feelings of rage that conflict with fears of abandonment.

Because human beings are infinitely complex, one must be wary about making universal dynamic formulations. The content, experience, and secondary elaboration of the psychological factors that produce symptoms vary with each patient. The goal of psychotherapy is to explore with each individual the unique mixture and content of these factors, and it is through interactions with each patient that the experienced physician can develop, over time, an understanding of the psychological causes.

Phobias

The behavior techniques of systematic desensitization and flooding are commonly used in treating a patient with specific phobia. In **systematic desensitization,** as the patient is gradually exposed to the feared scenario, a progressive reduction in anxiety occurs. In **flooding,** the patient is exposed directly to intense anxiety-provoking stimulation until the anxiety dissipates. Supportive psychotherapy may be used as an adjunctive treatment.

The behavior treatments may take place within the context of a psychodynamic psychotherapy that explores the emotionally symbolic meaning of the specifically feared objects or situations. As the patient becomes more aware of what the phobic situation represents emotionally, he or she will be better able to rationally think through the aroused affects instead of only emotionally experiencing the fear they produce. A patient's phobic symptom is often an expression—in the most intensely condensed and obvious form—of one of the many possible emotional conflicts that has infiltrated the functioning of his or her personality. Psychodynamic therapists must be prepared to encounter other emotional conflicts as they follow the trail of psychodynamic causality.

Psychodynamic and cognitive-behavior techniques are also useful for many patients with social phobia. The cognitive-behavior technique attempts to help patients think more rationally about the social phobias that cripple them. The psychodynamic approach attempts to help patients separate the feared situation from the mediating emotions. Social situations have symbolic significance for such patients and understanding these more completely may help them gain better cognitive control over the emotional eruptions that are projected onto the social situation.

Obsessive-Compulsive Disorder

A number of psychotherapeutic approaches have been used to treat patients with obsessive-compulsive disorder, whether it is severe or mild. For severe disorders, medication is used in conjunction with all forms of psychotherapy. Behavior therapy or behavior-cognitive therapy has had some effectiveness in treating symptoms. Psychodynamic treatment may also be used, especially when the dynamic material involved in obsessions and compulsions corresponds with the conflicts that have infiltrated the personality. Patients with obsessive-compulsive disorder and severe personality disorders need a psychodynamic treatment that is geared to all manifestations of their psychological problems. Personality disorders sometimes associated with obsessive-compulsive disorder include obsessive-compulsive and borderline personality disorders.

Posttraumatic Stress Disorder

Abreaction is the process of describing an event and experiencing the emotions that occurred. It is a key therapeutic step in treating trauma victims. Once the individual is over the initial shock of the trauma, abreaction should take place as soon as possible to relieve the immediate distress and prevent chronic signs and symptoms from developing later. Some traumas are disclosed immediately after they occur, so that abreaction can begin soon after the event before the signs and symptoms become entrenched. In other cases, the trauma is buried and "forgotten" for years until it is reactivated by another trauma. Techniques such as hypnosis and the amobarbital interview are sometimes used to facilitate abreaction.

Other nonpharmacological treatments include group therapy with others who have been exposed to similar stressors (e.g., combat veterans) and the behavior techniques of systematic desensitization and flooding. Two other methods, hypnosis and relaxation training, are targeted at the signs and symptoms of chronic autonomic arousal. Psychodynamic treatments explore the emotional meaning and effect of the traumatic episode.

Generalized Anxiety Disorder

Supportive psychotherapies help patients with generalized anxiety disorder to make changes that will decrease the severity of obvious anxiety-causing situations. Cognitive-behavior therapies help patients consciously change patterns of thinking or behavior that keep them in stressful situations or cause stressful states. Biofeedback and relaxation training are used to ease patients' stress; patients are instructed to employ self-directed relaxation techniques at regular intervals during the day. Psychodynamic treatment attempts to understand the basic psychological structures of attitude and character that are integral parts of feedback loops between behavior, attitudes, stressful life events, and emotional meanings and anxiety.

Psychopharmacological Treatment
Panic Disorder and Agoraphobia

The demonstrated success of the tricyclic antidepressants (TCAs), monoamine oxidase inhibitors (MAOIs), selective serotonin reuptake inhibitors (SSRIs), and certain benzodiazepines for the long-term treatment of panic symptoms may hinge on their common mechanism of reducing central noradrenergic activity. However, this does not imply that any agent that reduces central noradrenergic activity or acts on the α_2 receptor is a successful antipanic agent. Clonidine, for example, has very limited clinical effectiveness in panic disorder. The α_2 receptor is only a portion of the neurological substrate.

Of the TCAs, imipramine and clomipramine have been the most successful. Desipramine, nortriptyline, and amitriptyline are also effective. Some antidepressant drugs have not been useful in panic (e.g., maprotiline, amoxapine, trazodone, and bupropion).

In the few weeks before the TCAs and SSRIs begin to be effective, many patients complain of jitteriness, nervousness, and insomnia. These symptoms are usually transient and can be minimized by increasing the dosage slowly. A temporary course of benzodiazepines may be needed in cases of severe anticipatory anxiety or to alleviate the initial jitteriness induced by the antidepressant. Side effects of the TCAs include anticholinergic signs and symptoms, such as dry mouth, blurry vision, and constipation as well as orthostatic hypotension (see Chapter 16, Psychopharmacology). Most patients with panic disorder respond to **TCAs.** Those who do not respond, who have cardiac contraindications to TCAs, or who otherwise find TCAs difficult to tolerate may benefit from an **SSRI,** such as fluoxetine. Other SSRIs, such as sertraline, paroxetine, and fluvoxamine, appear to be effective as well. The side effects of the SSRIs include agitation, gastrointestinal distress, insomnia, headache, and disturbances in sexual function. The MAOIs are effective antipanic agents but are usually difficult to tolerate. The most serious side effects are hypertensive episodes that occur when dietary tyramine is ingested or over-the-counter decongestants or cold preparations are used. These episodes may be fatal. Other side effects include orthostatic hypotension and sexual problems.

There is some question as to whether benzodiazepines given in relatively high dosages might be effective antipanic agents. Sedation is the limiting factor. Some studies suggest that clonazepam, which is a long-acting benzodiazepine used in certain seizure disorders, may be effective in panic disorder.

Patients should be informed of the side effects of their medications, but it is counterproductive to unnecessarily frighten already anxious patients by describing every known side effect. The dosages of antidepressants for the effective treatment of panic disorder are the same as those for major depression.

Once the panic attacks have remitted, treatment should continue for a minimum of six to nine months. It usually takes many months after the panic attacks have ended for patients to effect a change in their behavior.

Social Phobias

Psychopharmacological treatment for social phobia began to be studied in the mid 1980s, with trials of β-blockers and the MAOI phenelzine.

Patients with social phobia often respond to

agents that are conventionally used for panic disorder, such as antidepressants (the SSRIs and MAOIs, in particular) and alprazolam. Some individuals with specific performance phobias (e.g., fear of public speaking and stage fright) respond to treatment with β-blockers (e.g., atenolol) used in conjunction with cognitive-behavioral therapies.

Obsessive-Compulsive Disorder

During the 1980s, it became evident that patients with obsessive-compulsive symptoms improved when they were given an **SSRI** (e.g., fluoxetine) or **clomipramine.** The side effects of clomipramine, which is an analog of the TCA imipramine, include orthostatic hypotension, dry mouth, constipation, sexual dysfunction, and weight gain. The side effects of fluoxetine include agitation, insomnia, gastrointestinal distress, and sexual dysfunction.

Posttraumatic Stress Disorder

There is no one specific pharmacological agent that has been proved to be widely effective in treating posttraumatic stress disorder. Phenelzine has been the most widely studied agent for the disorder. Other antidepressants, such as imipramine, desipramine, amitriptyline, and doxepin, have been studied to a lesser degree. Phenelzine was more effective for intrusive symptoms such as nightmares and flashbacks. Medications other than antidepressants, including propranolol, carbamazepine, clonidine, the benzodiazepines, and lithium, have also been studied. Phenelzine and imipramine significantly relieved posttraumatic stress disorder symptoms in one group of Vietnam War veterans. Further controlled studies with larger patient populations must be done to determine the efficacy of pharmacological agents in this disorder.

Generalized Anxiety Disorder

The mainstay treatment of generalized anxiety disorder is the **benzodiazepines.** A major concern about these agents is their addictive potential. There is no standard dosage of anxiolytic for generalized anxiety disorder. Lorazepam, 0.5 mg two to three times a day, is an average starting dosage for a physically healthy adult. Sedation is a limiting factor for the benzodiazepines. For the benzodiazepines currently used in clinical practice, the anxiolytic and sedative effects generally occur together. Benzodiazepines without active metabolites are preferable for the treatment of generalized anxiety disorder. They can be given several times daily without the risk of drug accumulation. Drugs such as diazepam, with long half-lives, would seem to be ideally suited for once-daily administration. However, because of its wide distribution in the body, diazepam has a relatively short antianxiety effect and must be given in multiple daily doses. Some patients taking the short-acting agent alprazolam develop rebound anxiety between doses and therefore require four to five doses per day. The total daily dosage is not increased but is divided into smaller doses that are given more frequently.

Anxiety Disorder Due to a General Medical Condition

Treatment of secondary anxiety should be guided by the nature of the underlying medical condition. For example, for the tachycardia, diaphoresis, and tremulousness caused by hyperthyroidism, β-blockers may be used temporarily to acutely counteract the sympathetic overstimulation, but the underlying hyperthyroidism needs to be treated promptly with an agent such as propylthiouracil. ➡ In the case of the 32-year-old woman with undiagnosed hyperthyroidism, treatment with the anxiolytic chlordiazepoxide partially masked the anxiety and physical agitation resulting from the hyperthyroidism. This prevented the diagnosis and treatment of the hyperthyroidism, caused irreversible physical changes, and subjected the patient to potentially fatal consequences. ⬅

Substance-Induced Anxiety Disorders

Stimulant intoxication syndromes are treated by discontinuing the stimulant, observing the patient, administering anxiolytics, and treating physical signs and symptoms such as hypertension or tachycardia with β-blockers and other appropriate agents. The anxiety induced by opioid withdrawal is treated with either methadone or clonidine. If clonidine is used, the blood pressure must be carefully monitored.

Alcohol withdrawal is treated with benzodiazepines such as chlordiazepoxide or lorazepam. Lorazepam has the advantage of being effective when given intramuscularly. It also has a shorter half-life and can be used safely by alcoholic patients with liver disease. The major goal of treating alcohol withdrawal is to prevent seizures. Although benzodiazepines are effective in raising the seizure threshold in delirium due to alcohol withdrawal, they do not appear to affect the course of the delirium once it begins. A similar phenomenon is seen in barbiturate withdrawal.

Anxiety syndromes caused by benzodiazepine and barbiturate withdrawal are treated with appropriate doses of benzodiazepines or barbiturates that are then gently tapered. Many clinicians follow the "10% rule" (i.e., the dosage should not be decreased by more than 10% each day). Particularly with short-acting benzodiazepines such as alprazolam, the tapering should be very gradual to reduce rebound anxiety.

References Cited

Baxter, L. R., et al. Caudate glucose metabolic rate changes with both drugs and behavior therapy for obsessive-compulsive disorder. Archives of General Psychiatry 49(9):681–689, 1992.

Coplan, J. D., et al. Effects of sodium lactate infusion on cisternal lactate and carbon dioxide levels in nonhuman primates. American Journal of Psychiatry 149(10):1369–1373, October, 1992.

Dager, S. R., et al. Central nervous system effects of lactate infusion in primates. Biological Psychiatry 27(2):193–204, January 15, 1990.

Flor-Henry, P. The obsessive-compulsive syndrome: reflection of fronto-caudate dysregulation of the left hemisphere? Encephale 16(Special Number):325–329, July-August, 1990.

Gorman J. M., et al. Mitral valve prolapse and panic disorders: effect of imipramine. *In* Klein, D. F., and J. G. Rabkin, eds. Anxiety: New Research and Changing Concepts. New York, Raven Press, 1981.

Kandel, E. R. From metapsychology to molecular biology: explorations into the nature of anxiety. American Journal of Psychiatry 140:1277–1293, l983.

Kandel, E. R. Genes, nerve cells, and the remembrance of things past. Journal of Neuropsychiatry and Clinical Neurosciences 1:103–125, 1989.

Kandel, E. R. Psychotherapy and the single synapse: the impact of psychiatric thought on neurobiologic research. New England Journal of Medicine 301:1028–1037, 1979.

Kardiner, A., and H. Spiegel. The Traumatic Neuroses of War. New York, Paul Hoeber, 1947.

Klein, D. F. False suffocation alarms, spontaneous panics, and related conditions: an integrative hypothesis. Archives of General Psychiatry, vol. 50, April, 1993.

Kolb, C. L., B. C. Burns, and S. Griffiths. Propranolol and clonidine in the treatment of the chronic posttraumatic stress disorders of war. *In* Van Der Volk, B. A., and D. C. Wash, eds. Posttraumatic Stress Disorder: Psychological and Physiological Sequelae. New York, APA Press, 1984.

Muskin, P. R. Panics, prolapse, and PVCs. General Hospital Psychiatry 7:2119–2223, 1985.

Muskin, P. R., and A. J. Fyer. The treatment of panic disorder. Journal of Clinical Psychopharmacology 1:81–90, 1981.

Pitts, F. N., and J. N. McClure. Lactate metabolism in anxiety neurosis. New England Journal of Medicine 277:1329–1339, 1967.

Racine, R. Kindling: the first decade. Neurosurgery 3:234–252, 1979.

Reiman, E. M., et al. A focal brain abnormality in panic disorder: a CBF form of anxiety. Nature 310:683–685, 1984.

Rose, S. P. R. How chicks make memories: the cellular cascade from c-fos to dendritic remodeling. Trends in Neuroscience 14:390–397, 1991.

Van der Kolk, B. A., et al. Endogenous opioids, Stress induced analgesia, and posttraumatic stress disorder. Psychopharmacology Bulletin 25: 417–421, 1989.

Selected Readings

Coplan, J. D., and J. M. Gorman. Treatment of anxiety disorder in patients with mood disorders. Journal of Clinical Psychiatry 51:10 (Supplement), October 1990.

Dubovsky, S. L. Understanding and treating depression in anxious patients. Journal of Clinical Psychiatry 51:10 (Supplement), October 1990.

Freud, S. Inhibitions, symptoms, and anxiety. *In* Strachey, J., ed. The Standard Edition of the Complete Psychological Works of Sigmund Freud. Vol. 20. London, Hogarth Press, 1959.

Gunderson, J. G., and A. N. Sabo. The phenomenological and conceptual interface between borderline personality disorder and PTSD. American Journal of Psychiatry 150:1, January 1993.

Herman, J. L. Trauma and Recovery. New York, Basic Books, 1992.

James, W. The Principles of Psychology. New York, Holt, 1890.

Kessler, R. C., et al. Lifetime and 12-month prevalence of DSM-III-R psychiatric disorders in the United States. Results from the National Comorbidity Survey. Archives of General Psychiatry 51 (1): 8–19, 1994.

Lydiard, B., P. P. Roy-Byrne, and J. C. Ballenger. Recent advances in the psychopharmacological treatment of anxiety disorders. Hospital Community Psychiatry. Vol. 39, No. 11, November 1988.

Shear, M. K., et al. A psychodynamic model of panic disorder. American Journal of Psychiatry 150:859–867, 1993.

CHAPTER SEVEN

ALCOHOL AND SUBSTANCE

ABUSE DISORDERS

FRANCES R. LEVIN, MD, AND
HERBERT D. KLEBER, MD

Alcohol abuse and other substance abuse disorders are among the most common problems encountered in general medical settings (Box 7–1). The Epidemiologic Catchment Area survey conducted by the National Institute of Mental Health to determine the prevalence rates of various DSM-III disorders found that alcohol abuse or dependence had a lifetime prevalence of 5–6%, the highest prevalence of all psychiatric disorders evaluated (Robins et al., 1984). This survey was unusual in that it conducted door-to-door interviews in several communities and determined whether individuals met the DSM criteria for alcohol abuse or dependence, unlike other community surveys that assess individuals for frequency of use. The detection of these disorders is often confused by patients' inability or unwillingness to acknowledge their detrimental use of substances. Although these disorders can include significant physical and emotional complications, patients tend to have limited insight about the impact that the substance abuse has upon their lives and may deny or underreport the extent of their substance use. Detecting alcohol and substance abuse disorders is made even more difficult by the insidious nature of addictive illness. Many people can drink alcohol or use other psychoactive drugs occasionally without any negative effects on their physical or emotional well-being. Only a minority of individuals will develop problematic use. However, it is often difficult to predict who these individuals will be. Another factor that complicates the diagnosis and treatment of substance abuse disorders is that many physicians believe, for a variety of reasons, that attempts to treat these problems are futile. In fact, once substance abuse has been recognized, it can be successfully treated.

DIAGNOSTIC AND CLINICAL FEATURES

The DSM-IV conceptual approach to psychiatric disorders associated with substance use (referred to as substance-related disorders) distinguishes substance use disorders (i.e., substance abuse and substance dependence) from substance-induced disorders (i.e., intoxication, withdrawal, delirium, and dementia, as well as mood, anxiety, and psychotic disorders). These two types of disorders frequently coexist in the same patient (see Differential Diagnosis, below).

Substance Use Disorders

Substance abuse refers to a patient's pattern of use that results in repeated negative consequences (e.g., legal difficulties, psychological distress, and poor functioning at work or school) without loss of control over his or her use, or physical dependence on or tolerance to the substance. The DSM-IV criteria for psychoactive substance abuse stipulate that the patient must be using the substance in a maladaptive manner. What constitutes maladaptive behavior, however, is not always clear. To make a judgment about the patient's behavior, the physician must view it within the context of the patient's individual circumstances and societal strictures (e.g., while it may be socially appropriate for a healthy young adult to drink two glasses of wine at dinner, it is generally not acceptable for a six-year-old or an elderly individual with diabetes to drink in a similar manner). The DSM-IV criteria for substance abuse are listed in Table 7–1. Substance abuse frequently precedes substance dependence.

Substance dependence occurs when a patient has lost control over the use of the psychoactive substance, which has become so dominant in the patient's life that his or her occupational, psychological, or social functioning has deteriorated as a result. Both psychological and physiological features are crucial in making the diagnosis of dependence. Physical dependence and tolerance are two of the possible criteria for substance dependence. Patients have **physical dependence** if they suffer from, or must use a drug to avoid, symptoms of withdrawal. **Withdrawal symptoms** are defined as symptoms that are

BOX 7–1.   Epidemiological Drug Abuse Profile of the United States

General Trends in Illicit Drug Use

In the United States, approximately 12.8 million persons, or 6% of the household population age 12 years or older, use illegal drugs on a current basis (within the past 30 days). This is a decrease of almost 50% from the 1979 high of 25 million persons. Even so, more than one-third of persons age 12 years or older have tried an illicit drug. Ninety percent have used marijuana or hashish; approximately one-third have used cocaine or a prescription-type drug for nonmedical reasons; and approximately one-fifth have used LSD. Fortunately, nearly 60 million persons who used illicit drugs when young have rejected them as adults.

Drug use and its consequences affect persons of every socioeconomic background, geographic region, educational level, and ethnic and racial identity. Some persons are affected more directly than others (e.g., those who live in neighborhoods where illegal drug markets flourish, leading to crime and violence, and those who lack health insurance or have low incomes and cannot afford drug treatment).

In 1995, 1.5 million persons were current **cocaine** users. This is a 74% decline from 5.7 million persons in 1985. In addition, fewer people are trying cocaine. The estimated 533,000 first-time users in 1994 represented a 60% decline from the approximately 1.3 million first-time users per year between 1980 and 1984. While these figures indicate significant progress, the number of frequent users in 1995, which is estimated to be 582,000 (255,000 of whom use crack), has not changed markedly since 1985. One study estimates that chronic users account for two-thirds of the demand for cocaine in the United States. Thus, while the number of cocaine *users* has dropped, the *amount* of cocaine consumed has not declined commensurately.

About 600,000 persons in the United States are addicted to **heroin,** an increase over the estimated number of addicts during the 1970s and 1980s. More chronic users have turned to snorting heroin because of the availability of high-purity forms of the drug. This has caused consumption to increase dramatically compared with a decade ago, when injection of lower-purity forms was the only option available. A 1996 survey found that although most heroin users are older long-term drug abusers, growing numbers of teenagers and young adults are also using the drug.

In 1995, an estimated 9.8 million persons (77% of all current illicit drug users) were smokers of **marijuana,** making it the most commonly used illicit drug. Approximately 57% of current illicit drug users limit their consumption exclusively to marijuana. In 1995, five million persons used marijuana frequently (defined as at least 51 days a year), as compared with an estimated 8.4 million in 1985. However, the annual number of first-time users has risen since 1991, reaching 2.3 million in 1994.

Methamphetamine use is increasing. An estimated 4.7 million persons have tried this drug. In 1995, approximately 6% of adult and juvenile arrestees from all sites tested positive for methamphetamine.

In 1995, the prevalence of current use of **other illicit drugs,** including hallucinogens, inhalants, and prescription drugs, was less than 1%. Only hallucinogen use showed any significant change between 1994 and 1995, rising from 0.4% to 0.7%. "Club drugs," such as Rohypnol, Ketamine, Quaaludes, Xanax, MDMA, and LSD, continue to gain popularity among young adults.

Trends in Illicit Drug Use in Young People

Adolescent drug use rose rapidly in the 1970s, peaking around 1980. There was then a sharp decline of over two-thirds until 1992, when it turned sharply upward again. It is still, however, below the 1980 peak based on the annual high school senior survey in 1996.

Children who use illegal drugs, tobacco, or alcohol have an increased chance of acquiring lifelong dependency problems and greater health risks. Every day, 3000 children begin smoking cigarettes regularly; this will result in a shortened life span for one-third of these youngsters. According to one study, children who smoke marijuana are 85 times more likely to use cocaine than their peers who have never tried marijuana. The use of illicit drugs among eighth graders has risen 150% over the past five years. While this is an alarmingly high rate, the prevalence of drug use among young people has not returned to the nearly epidemic levels of the late 1970s.

In 1995, 10.9% of young persons 12–17 years of age used illicit drugs on a past-month basis. In 1992, the rate was 5.3% (which was the historic low since the 1979 high of 16.3%). One study found that more than half of high school students have used illicit drugs by the time they graduate.

Cocaine use is not prevalent among young people. In 1996, approximately 2% of twelfth graders were current cocaine users (an increase from 1.4% in 1992 but a 70% decrease from 6.7% in 1985), and 7.1% had tried cocaine (an increase from 6.1% in 1992 but a significant decrease from 17.3% in 1985). However, during the last five years, the lifetime use of cocaine has nearly doubled among eighth graders, reaching 4.5% in 1996. The mean age for first-time use of cocaine dropped from 23.3 years in 1990 to 19 years in 1994.

Heroin use is also not prevalent among young people. In 1996, 1% of twelfth graders had used heroin in the past year, and half of 1% had done so within the last 30 days (both figures were lower than the 1995 figures). However, the number of eighth and twelfth graders who had used heroin at some time doubled between 1991 and 1996 to 2.4% and 1.8%, respectively.

Marijuana use continues to be a major problem among young people. Almost one in four high school seniors used marijuana on a past-month basis in 1996. Less than 10% used any other illicit drug with the same frequency. Within the past year, nearly twice as many seniors used marijuana as any other illicit drug. Marijuana also accounts for most of the increase in illicit drug use in 12- to 17-year-olds. Between 1994 and 1995, the rate of marijuana use in this age-group increased from 6% to 8.2% (a 37% increase). Adolescents are beginning to smoke marijuana at a younger age (the mean age of first-time use dropped from 17.8 years in 1987 to 16.3 years in 1994).

Alcohol is the drug most often used by young people. Approximately one in four tenth graders and one-third of twelfth graders had five or more drinks on at least one occasion within two weeks of one survey. The average age of first-time drinking has declined to 15.9 years from 17.4 years in 1987.

Tobacco use is rising among youths. In 1996, more than one-third of high school seniors smoked cigarettes, and more than one in five did so daily. These percentages are greater than at any time since the 1970s.

After marijuana, the second most commonly used class of illicit drugs in young people is **stimulants** (a category that includes methamphetamines). About 5% of high school students use stimulants on a monthly basis, and 10% have done so within the past year. The third most commonly used class of illicit substances is **inhalants.** Use of these drugs declined among eighth, tenth, and twelfth graders in 1996. **LSD,** however, was used by 8.8% of twelfth graders during the past year.

Consequences of Illicit Drug Use

The social and health costs to society of illicit drug use are staggering. Drug-related illness, death, and crime cost the nation approximately $66.9 billion. Every man, woman, and child in the United States pays nearly $1000 annually to cover the expense of unnecessary health care, extra law enforcement, automobile accidents, crime, and lost productivity resulting from substance abuse. Illicit drug use hurts families, businesses, *Continued* and neighborhoods; impedes education; and chokes the criminal justice, health, and social service systems.

Currently, some of the major problems associated with drug abuse are drug-related medical emergencies, which are at a historic high; maternal drug abuse, which is contributing to birth defects and infant deaths; and chronic drug use, which makes users susceptible to diseases such as hepatitis, tuberculosis, HIV infection, and sexually transmitted diseases. The use of alcohol and tobacco by young people can lead to premature death due to automobile accidents or smoking-related diseases. Drug abuse also burdens the workplace because of lost productivity and increased use of health care benefits.

Source: US Office of National Drug Control Policy. America's drug abuse profile. In The National Drug Control Strategy: 1997. Washington, D. C., Office of National Drug Control Policy, Executive Office of the President, 1997.

judged by the physician to occur because the patient has stopped using, or is using less of, a particular drug. In addition, these symptoms must cause distress or functional impairment, according to the DSM-IV (Table 7–2). **Tolerance** means that increasing amounts of a drug are needed to produce the same degree of intoxication, or, to put it another way, that the same amount of the drug produces less of the desired effect.

Although the term **addiction** is not mentioned in the DSM-IV, physicians frequently use it to describe a disease process that is most similar to substance abuse, in which a patient continues to use a psychoactive substance regardless of any physical, psychological, or social harm caused by doing so. The following case describes the sequential development of one patient's substance abuse into substance dependence.

⇒ A 29-year-old female associate attorney at a "high-powered" law firm consulted her gynecologist about an unplanned, unwanted pregnancy. The physical examination showed that the patient had lost 30 pounds since her last visit, which had been two years earlier. At that time, her weight had been normal for her height. Although she initially denied any substance use other than "a glass or two of wine occasionally," she finally reluctantly confided that she had been using cocaine for the past year. She had begun by occasionally "snorting" cocaine at parties, but for the past few months, she had been "freebasing" (smoking), a process that rapidly leads to extremely high levels of cocaine in the blood. She frequently did this when alone, and she had also been using more and more alcohol. The quality of her work at the law firm had been deteriorating.

In the past couple of months, she had broken up with her boyfriend in order to have more time to get high by herself. People at work were suspicious because she was coming in later and later in the morning. She had not shown up for three days during the previous month, when she had been on a cocaine binge. After the binge, she had become concerned that her use was getting out of control and decided to stop using the drug. Despite repeated attempts, she had been able to remain abstinent only for two to three days at a time. She had become pregnant when she had had unprotected intercourse with a man she met at a party while she was high. She was also $50,000 in debt as a result of her drug purchases. ⇐

This case illustrates the distinction between the maladaptive behavior typical of abuse and the loss of control that is central to dependence. As this woman's cocaine use became the all-consuming focus of her existence, she crossed the line from abuse to dependence. Her unsuccessful attempts to abstain were a clear indication of her dependence. Two other aspects of this case are seen quite commonly. First, patients often do not present to physicians complaining of a substance abuse problem; instead, they present with psychiatric or other medical sequelae of the abuse. Second, patients frequently abuse more than one substance. By the time they come to medical attention, these disorders have usually advanced to the stage at which a pattern of multiple substance abuse has developed.

Substance-Induced Disorders

Intoxication occurs when a drug's effect on the central nervous system produces maladaptive behavioral or psychological changes. Intoxication can be either acute or chronic and can occur in the absence of substance abuse or dependence. **Withdrawal** is frequently associated with substance dependence. Other substance-induced disorders tend to occur in the context of either abuse or dependence. Although substance use and substance-in-

---

TABLE 7–1. DSM-IV Diagnostic Criteria for Substance Abuse

A. A maladaptive pattern of substance use leading to clinically significant impairment or distress, as manifested by one (or more) of the following, occurring within a 12-month period:
   (1) recurrent substance use resulting in a failure to fulfill major role obligations at work, school, or home (e.g., repeated absences or poor work performance related to substance use; substance-related absences, suspensions, or expulsion from school; neglect of children or household)
   (2) recurrent substance use in situations in which it is physically hazardous (e.g., driving an automobile or operating a machine when impaired by substance use)
   (3) recurrent substance-related legal problems (e.g., arrests for substance-related disorderly conduct)
   (4) continued substance use despite having persistent or recurrent social or interpersonal problems caused or exacerbated by the effects of the substance (e.g., arguments with spouse about consequences of intoxication, physical fights)
B. The symptoms have never met the criteria for Substance Dependence for this class of substance.

TABLE 7–2.   DSM-IV Diagnostic Criteria for Substance Dependence

A maladaptive pattern of substance use, leading to clinically significant impairment or distress, as manifested by three (or more) of the following, occurring at any time in the same 12-month period:

1. tolerance, as defined by either of the following:
   (a) a need for markedly increased amounts of the substance to achieve intoxication or desired effect
   (b) markedly diminished effect with continued use of the same amount of the substance
2. withdrawal, as manifested by either of the following:
   (a) the characteristic withdrawal syndrome for the substance
   (b) the same (or closely related) substance is taken to relieve or avoid withdrawal symptoms
3. the substance is often taken in larger amounts or over a longer period than was intended
4. there is a persistent desire or unsuccessful efforts to cut down or control substance use
5. a great deal of time is spent in activities necessary to obtain the substance (e.g., visiting multiple doctors or driving long distances), use the substance (e.g., chain smoking), or recover from its effects
6. important social, occupational, or recreational activities are given up or reduced because of substance use
7. the substance use is continued despite knowledge of having a persistent or recurrent physical or psychological problem that is likely to have been caused or exacerbated by the substance (e.g., current cocaine use despite recognition of cocaine-induced depression, or continued drinking despite recognition that an ulcer was made worse by alcohol consumption)

Specify if:
With Physiological Dependence: evidence of tolerance or withdrawal (i.e., either item 1 or 2 is present)
Without Physiological Dependence: no evidence of tolerance or withdrawal (i.e., neither item 1 nor 2 is present)

---

duced disorders are separate entities in the DSM-IV, the two types of disorders frequently coexist in the same patient, making the physician's index of suspicion and detection of substance-induced disorders doubly important.

Psychiatric symptoms that are caused by the substance-induced states of intoxication or withdrawal can mimic symptoms of primary psychiatric disorders. Thus, many substance-induced disorders are actually subtypes of primary psychiatric disorders: anxiety disorder, mood disorder, psychotic disorder, and cognitive and mental disorders, including delirium and dementia. They are distinguished from the primary disorders in these categories on the basis of their etiology, which is substance use. For more information on specific substance-induced disorders, see Chapter 3, Mood Disorders; Chapter 4, Schizophrenia and Other Psychotic Disorders; Chapter 5, Cognitive and Mental Disorders Due to General Medical Conditions; and Chapter 6, Anxiety Disorders.

In order to make an adequate diagnosis and distinguish substance-induced disorders from preexisting psychiatric conditions, it is critically important for all physicians to know which psychiatric symptoms are produced by which classes of drugs at different stages of use. (This is particularly true of symptoms of acute and chronic intoxication and withdrawal.) The most common psychological signs and symptoms of the substance-induced disorders are presented according to the major classes of abused substances.

Alcohol and Other Sedatives

Alcohol and other sedatives (e.g., barbiturates, benzodiazepines, and many other drugs known as "downers" or by a plethora of other street names) are commonly abused. For all of these substances, the symptoms of acute intoxication are the same: **slurred speech, staggering gait,** and **horizontal nystagmus.** When intoxicated, individuals may behave violently with little or no provocation. An individual's age, weight, sex, and level of tolerance and the setting in which the substance is used influence the effect that alcohol has upon the individual's behavior.

When chronic users of large amounts of alcohol or other sedatives abruptly discontinue their use, they can experience dramatic psychiatric symptoms of withdrawal, which include **anxiety, insomnia, tremors, hallucinations** (usually visual), extreme **agitation,** and **paranoia.** They may also have seizures, and, less commonly, delirium (referred to as delirium tremens when withdrawal is from alcohol). Because substance withdrawal delirium can be a life-threatening condition, it is imperative that physicians consider this diagnosis when evaluating delirious patients (see Chapter 5, Cognitive and Mental Disorders Due to General Medical Conditions). Because **delirium tremens** usually occurs in patients who have other medical problems, such as pneumonia or heart failure, physicians must be especially diligent in evaluating alcohol use in patients whom they admit for surgery. The failure to obtain a history of heavy drinking from a patient prior to surgery may result in the development of seizures or delirium due to withdrawal a few days after the operation.

Depression is a less dramatic but nonetheless life-threatening complication that occurs in patients with chronic sedative use and withdrawal. ➡ In one case, a female nurse sought psychiatric help for depression, which she felt was caused by a recent work-related back injury. However, as the physician elicited her history, it became clear that the patient was heavily dependent on alcohol. During periods of heavy alcohol use, she experienced depressive symptoms; when she stopped using alcohol, her depressive symptoms would lift. ⬅ Depressive symptoms associated with sedative withdrawal usually diminish within a few weeks. Persistent depression may require pharmacological intervention or inpatient hospitalization, or both. While inebriated or distressed by withdrawal symptoms, patients may act on suicidal impulses.

Primary psychiatric disorders often coexist in patients with substance-related disorders. In most cases, patients' alcohol or drug use must be treated simultaneously with any coexisting psychiatric disorder, such as a primary mood disorder. Often, the coexisting psychiatric condition may require medication.

Heavy chronic alcohol use is associated with hallucinations and delusions. **Alcohol-induced psychotic disorder with hallucinations or delusions** usually occurs in the context of a clear sensorium and does not represent a medical emergency. These symptoms can also occur during a period of withdrawal or diminished alcohol use. Unlike the hallucinations associated with delirium tremens, alcoholic hallucinations are primarily, but not exclusively, auditory. Also in contrast to delirium tremens, alcoholic hallucinosis and paranoia can persist for several weeks, rather than several days, after alcohol cessation. They can also occur when a person's alcohol intake has decreased and seem to be most closely associated with heavy, prolonged alcohol use (i.e., over a period of years). Fortunately, alcohol-induced psychotic disorder usually remits after a period of abstinence. Chronic heavy alcohol abuse has also been associated with a number of **cognitive deficits,** including dementia and encephalopathy.

Opiates

Persons addicted to opiates are more likely to appear "normal" while intoxicated than are sedative abusers. ➡ For example, an anesthesiology resident began taking fentanyl, a potent opiate that was available to him at work, in order to "deal with" the stress, anxiety, and marital difficulties that he was experiencing. As his use increased, the resident began to miss days at work and became argumentative with colleagues. Despite this behavior, opiate dependence was not suspected. Unfortunately, his abuse was not detected until an overdose brought him to the emergency room. ⬅

When patients are brought to the emergency room with an opiate overdose, the first goal is to ensure adequate respiratory function, which may require ventilatory support and opiate antagonists, such as naloxone. After patients have been medically stabilized, they should be assessed for suicidality. Depression is common among chronic opiate users, and suicide attempts are not uncommon.

In contrast to sedative withdrawal, the withdrawal from opiates is an unpleasant but not life-threatening experience. **Gastrointestinal upset, muscle cramps, rhinorrhea,** and **irritability** are the prominent physical symptoms.

With the recent rapid rise in the rate of HIV infection among intravenous drug users, physicians have become increasingly aware of the secondary cognitive syndromes associated with the infection. Opiate users who describe having memory impairments or have evidence of cognitive dysfunction should be assessed for HIV risk factors. After appropriate counseling, patients may agree to have an HIV blood test.

Stimulants

Acute intoxication from **cocaine, amphetamines** ("speed"), and similar stimulants can produce symptoms that mimic those of several psychiatric disorders. It may induce **maniclike symptoms,** such as a decreased need for sleep, rapid flow of speech and ideas, inflated self-esteem, and distractibility. Acute stimulant intoxication can also induce **paranoid ideation** and **delusions,** as well as auditory and visual **hallucinations.** These symptoms usually subside within a few days. Upon the initial presentation of the patient, it may be extremely difficult to differentiate stimulant-induced psychosis from schizophrenia. Anxiety disorders are also common, particularly **panic disorder** (see Chapter 6). Drug screening, which includes a test for the cocaine metabolite benzoylecognine, can be quite useful, particularly in patients for whom adequate histories cannot be obtained. Upon physical examination, acutely intoxicated individuals have dilated pupils (except in cases of multiple substance use that includes a narcotic, which causes pupillary constriction) or physical manifestations of intranasal use (e.g., nasal septum erosions) or intravenous use (e.g., needle track marks). It is important to repeat assessments over time. Stimulant-induced psychosis usually improves without pharmacological intervention, whereas an acute exacerbation of schizophrenia or mania does not.

Like opiate overdoses, cocaine overdoses can be life-threatening. "Crack" cocaine, which is inhaled via "freebasing" or smoking, results in much higher levels of cocaine in the blood than does intranasal "snorting" of the drug. Myocardial infarctions, arrhythmias, strokes, and symptoms consistent with a neuroleptic malignant syndrome have been related to cocaine use. Medical interventions are usually the first line of treatment. However, because **depression** is common in cocaine addicts, particularly during periods of withdrawal, the possibility that the patient has used the drug to attempt suicide must be considered and aggressively investigated. The depressed mood and suicidal ideation usually abate within a few days, but some individuals continue to experience these psychiatric symptoms and may require appropriate intervention. It is not uncommon for individuals to complain of anhedonia and lack of energy for weeks after their last use of cocaine.

Hallucinogens

Two of the most commonly abused hallucinogens are **lysergic acid diethylamide** (LSD) and **phencyclidine** (PCP). Less commonly abused hallucinogens include psilocybin, mescaline, dimethyltryptamine (DMT), and stimulant hallucinogens, such as 3,4-methylenedioxymethamphetamine ("ecstasy," MDMA, MDA).

Acute intoxication from hallucinogens may cause **anxiety, panic reactions,** and feelings of **depersonalization.** Drug-induced changes in mental status usually resolve within eight hours. Some individuals experience flashbacks of prior drug-induced experiences, which may cause severe anxiety and require psychiatric intervention. As the name suggests, hallucinogens can induce visual, tactile, and auditory **hallucinations.** LSD can also induce **synesthesia** (e.g., hearing a sound produces a sensation of color; seeing an object produces a sensation of sound) and odd sensations of time slowing down and physical boundaries being lost.

Although there are no life-threatening medical complications associated with hallucinogen intoxication, deaths have resulted from psychiatric or physical stress. In a confused, psychotic state, individuals may run out into traffic or jump from a high building because they think they can fly. Psychosis, depression, and confusion may require individuals to be hospitalized in order to protect them from harming themselves or others. **MDMA** is becoming increasingly popular on campuses. Both teens and young adults take part in "rave" dances, which may go on all night, fueled in part by the stimulant effects of MDMA. In England, a number of deaths that were apparently related to dehydration and cardiac effects have occurred following these dances.

No clear-cut withdrawal symptoms are associated with chronic hallucinogen use, except for the **flashbacks,** mentioned above, that some individuals experience after they have ceased using hallucinogens. These are usually of a limited duration and occur in patients who are under stress or are physically ill. Most patients respond positively to verbal reassurance, although some may require pharmacological intervention.

Unless physicians consider the possibility of hallucinogen use, patients may be diagnosed as schizophrenic. There are few physical manifestations that suggest hallucinogen use. One may observe dilated pupils with LSD use or pupillary constriction with PCP use. Many diagnostic laboratories do not screen for hallucinogens. Therefore, observing patients, approaching them calmly, and eliciting their histories from all available reliable sources are crucial steps in making an appropriate diagnosis.

Cannabis

The active component of cannabis, tetrahydrocannabinol (THC), can be found in several different preparations of the hemp plant (marijuana). These preparations (e.g., bhang, charas, ganja, or hashish) vary in potency and quality. Acute intoxication may result in **anxiety** and **paranoid ideation** or frank delusions. It can destabilize patients whose schizophrenia is in remission. Commonly, users describe an altered sense of time and distance perception. Occasionally, auditory or visual hallucinations may be experienced. Large dosages have been associated with delirium. Impairment of short-term memory is common. Evidence is mixed as to whether chronic marijuana use results in an "amotivational syndrome." Considering the effects of marijuana on energy levels and memory, however, it is not surprising that heavy users often do poorly academically. Chronic use can lead to pulmonary problems, as well. One "joint" has the deleterious effect on the lungs of four or five cigarettes. A withdrawal syndrome has been demonstrated in animals but is less commonly noted in humans because of the dosages ordinarily used. There are few physical manifestations associated with marijuana use. The most common ones are an elevated heart rate and conjunctival injection.

Nicotine

Nicotine is highly addictive. However, because it is not an intoxicant, nicotine is usually associated with dependence rather than abuse. The withdrawal symptoms associated with dependence may be intense and result in a craving for the drug. **Depression** is common during withdrawal and is associated with a high rate of relapse.

Other Abused Substances

A wide range of other abusable substances can result in an altered mental status. Steroids and inhalants are two classes of drugs that have become increasingly recognized as substances of abuse. **Steroids** are usually taken by body builders, athletes, and others who wish to improve their physical appearance and increase their muscle mass. A strong inducement for the continued use of steroids is the feeling of euphoria they cause. The wide range of psychiatric symptoms associated with anabolic steroids includes aggressiveness, anxiety, impulsiveness, irritability, impaired judgment, and paranoid delusions. Unless physicians are aware that patients are abusing steroids, these symptoms can lead to a misdiagnosis of bipolar disorder. Withdrawal from steroids has been associated with many physical and psychiatric symptoms, such as irritability, anxiety, and depression.

Inhalants are volatile substances that can produce a state of intoxication. They include paint, correction fluid, glue, gasoline, and many other household substances. Abusers of inhalants are usually young adolescents, who progress later to alcohol and marijuana abuse. If the latter substances are difficult to obtain or too expensive, the solvent abuse may continue as the person grows older. Some severely dysfunctional adults may choose to abuse these substances, as well. Acute intoxication can result in neurological and psychiatric symptoms of disinhibition, disorientation, and ataxia; high dosages can cause dysarthria, aggression, hallucinations, and delirium. Chronic use of some inhalants produces dementia or irreversible neurological damage. Inhalants can cause renal, hepatic, hematological, or pulmonary damage or death from cardiac arrhythmias or other organ system dysfunctions. A thorough physical examination and appropriate laboratory tests are, therefore, crucial for patients in whom solvent use is suspected. Presently, no definitive psychiatric or medical symptoms are associated with discontinuation of chronic inhalant use.

Course of Illness

Patients with a long-standing pattern of heavy drug use are at high risk for developing substance dependence, which tends to have a chronic course characterized by waxing and waning of use, with periods of particularly heavy use alternating with periods of lesser use or even complete abstinence. The evolution of a drug use pattern into abuse and then dependence seems to be related to the onset of each agent's effects and the rate at which the effects diminish or are lost. Intravenous heroin causes a rapid sense of euphoria that has been compared with sexual orgasm; the response gradually diminishes over several hours. Crack cocaine also causes a rapid, intensely pleasurable "high" followed by a rapid loss of the feeling over a period of minutes. This "roller coaster" effect seems to reinforce the drug-taking behavior. Thus, while users of heroin and cocaine tend to move fairly quickly from recreational use to abuse to dependence, dependence seems to occur particularly quickly with crack cocaine.

Perhaps the most well-known work regarding the usual course of **alcohol use** is that of George Vaillant (1983). He found that most individuals progress from asymptomatic social drinking to abuse or dependence over a span of 3–15 years, although some alcohol users drink for more than 20 years before their use can be defined as abuse. The death rate among alcoholics age 40–70 years was approximately three times that of age-matched controls. Other recent studies suggest that women become "sicker quicker" from alcohol. This tendency may be related to biological factors. Women have decreased amounts of the gastric enzyme that metabolizes alcohol before it enters the bloodstream. Consequently, the same amount of alcohol will produce higher blood levels in women than in men and, ultimately, greater organ damage.

Individuals with alcohol-related problems have various outcomes. Some die early as a result of their heavy drinking; some continue to drink heavily into their senior years; some diminish or discontinue their use spontaneously or through treatment; and some develop alcohol problems later in life (late-onset alcoholics). Individuals who develop alcohol dependence in their later years are often reacting to the losses associated with aging, such as the deaths of family members or friends, retirement, or ill health. Early-onset alcoholics are more likely to be maladjusted, have a family history of alcoholism, commit more crimes, and respond less well to treatment. Late-onset alcoholics are more likely to be separated or divorced and suffer medical problems.

Cocaine and **marijuana abuse** also seems to follow a pattern, which may include experimental, social-recreational, circumstantial-situational, intensified, and compulsive phases. Individuals may skip one or more of these phases. Many users have episodes of decreased use or abstinence, although the periods of abstinence are often due to lack of availability of the drug. Over time, many cocaine users progress from a lower to a higher level of use, but some do not progress at all. Hallucinogens and other abused substances tend to be used more intermittently. A person can continue to use them recreationally for years without developing an abusive pattern.

THE INTERVIEW
Substance Abuse History

Any patient who is suffering from psychiatric symptoms must be evaluated for drug use. As described above, each class of drugs can induce psychiatric symptoms. Depression, psychosis, anxiety, and delirium are all common symptoms associated with drug use. Before assuming, therefore, that such symptoms are the result of an underlying psychiatric disorder, the physician needs to consider the possibility of a substance-induced disorder.

Whenever the possibility of a substance use or substance-induced disorder exists, the patient should be asked detailed, specific questions about drug and alcohol use (Diagnostic Guidelines box). Although it is not uncommon for physicians to ask an opening question such as "How much do you drink or use drugs?", this approach does not usually provide fruitful information. Often, patients who have problems with alcohol or drugs respond in a vague manner or claim that they use substances only occasionally. Their responses frequently suffice for physi-

---

Diagnostic Guidelines

Whenever possible, several approaches should be used in tandem in order to attain the proper diagnosis. These include the following:

- Always ask about alcohol and drug use.
- If possible, do not rely solely on the patient for the substance use history.
- Elicit information from family, significant others, and friends, as well.
- Perform a urine or blood drug screening test. The urine test is more useful for determining whether drugs have been used in the past 48 hours, whereas the blood test is more useful for determining the current status.
- Perform a Breathalyzer test to screen for recent alcohol use.
- Examine the patient for physical signs of drug use, including signs related to the route of administration. Monitor vital signs and the neurological status.
- Obtain a biochemical profile. Abnormal liver, renal, or hematological tests may all indicate chronic use.
- Observe the patient for a period of time. The effects of drugs may diminish within a few hours, days, or weeks.

cians who are not sensitive to drug-related issues or who feel rushed.

Patients notoriously **underestimate** the amount of alcohol or drugs they use when asked about their intake. It is better to use other information from the clinical assessment to determine which patients might have a problem with alcohol or drugs and then ask a question such as, "When you drink, do you generally drink two cases of beer (or two fifths of liquor) a day?" Obviously, this is an extremely large amount. Patients may laugh and say that the question is ridiculous and then proudly exclaim that they drink half a case of beer a day or confirm that they drink at the level suggested by the interviewer. In both cases, denial or minimization of alcohol use may be circumvented.

Occasionally, substance abusers, especially those who are afraid of experiencing withdrawal symptoms, will exaggerate the amounts they use, thinking that by doing so they will receive greater amounts of the medication used in opiate or sedative detoxification. Unfortunately, this distortion can lead to difficulties in determining the appropriate dosage of medication for detoxification.

To obtain a thorough understanding of the patient's use of substances, the physician should always ask the following questions:

When did you first use psychoactive substances, including tobacco and alcohol?

Which factors influenced you to start using substances (e.g., pressure from peers or a boyfriend or girlfriend, reaction to family dysfunction)?

When were your periods of heaviest use? What drugs were used? What was the amount and frequency of use?

What were your longest periods of abstinence? What supported your abstinence? What hindered your abstinence?

Have you ever attended AA or NA or been in alcohol or drug treatment? Was it helpful?

What external or internal factors precipitated relapse for you?

What has been the frequency and amount of your alcohol or drug use in the past month?

Screening Tests

A variety of screening instruments can be used to indicate whether or not a patient has a problem with alcohol or drugs. The **Michigan Alcoholism Screening Test (MAST),** which can be administered by a physician or self-administered, is a 25-item instrument that can be scored to determine whether a patient has problematic alcohol use (Selzer, 1971). Two other instruments are the Short Michigan Alcoholism Screening Test (SMAST) (Selzer, Vinokur, and Van Roijen, 1975) and the Drug Abuse Screening Test (DAST).

Commonly used screening devices for alcohol abuse are the CAGE device (Ewing, 1984) and the T-ACE (Sokol, Martier, and Alger, 1989). **CAGE** is an acronym for four questions that the physician asks the patient: Have you ever felt you should *cut* down on your drinking? Have people *annoyed* you by criticizing your drinking? Have you ever felt bad or *guilty* about your drinking? Have you ever had a drink first thing in the morning to steady your nerves or get rid of a hangover (*eye-opener*)? An affirmative answer to two or more questions suggests problem drinking. More recently, the T-ACE was devised to identify pregnant women who may be placing their fetuses at risk by their drinking behavior. It is similar to the CAGE, except that a question about tolerance has replaced the question about guilt. The woman is asked, "How many drinks does it take to feel high?" If the woman answers, "More than two," she is given a score of 2 points. A score of 2 or more on the T-ACE is indicative of high-risk drinking. The CAGE and the T-ACE are both worded to minimize denial and allow for rapid screening.

These instruments merely indicate problem use and do not provide enough information to accurately diagnose the problem or develop an appropriate treatment plan. They can also produce false-positive and false-negative results. Therefore, complete alcohol and drug assessments should be performed whenever problem substance use is suspected.

Family, Social, and Legal Histories

It is important to obtain thorough family, social, and legal histories during alcohol and drug assessment. Clearly, the patient's perception of what constitutes addictive behavior and whether treatment is necessary is influenced by familial patterns of substance use. In taking the family history, the physician should ask questions about the biological parents' and stepparents' use of alcohol and drugs. Any substance use problems among siblings, grandparents, aunts, or uncles should be noted, as should the participation of any family members in drug treatment programs or AA or NA (Narcotics Anonymous) meetings. The patient should be asked whether participation in these programs or meetings seemed to help the relative.

The social history of the patient can provide a wealth of information for the physician. The patient's physical and social environments can strongly affect his or her ability to achieve sobriety. Significant personal losses or physical or sexual abuse can influence a patient's pattern of use. It has been estimated that more than half of substance-abusing women and more than 40% of adolescent male drug users seeking treatment have been sexually or physically abused. In order to obtain a complete assessment, the physician needs to sensitively explore the patient's experience of any abuse of this nature.

Physicians frequently fail to obtain the patient's legal history. Legal difficulties may not only be strong indicators of problem use but also may reveal the circumstances under which the patient is currently seeking treatment. Patients who have been arrested for driving while intoxicated, selling or carrying drugs, or disorderly conduct should be evaluated for problematic alcohol or drug use.

History Timeline

A timeline can be particularly helpful for integrating data about the patient's history. Marks are made on the timeline to show when the patient first used psychoactive substances, the periods of heaviest use for each substance, the periods of abstinence, and significant losses or crises experienced by the patient. If a patient has a significant psychiatric history, another timeline can be drawn that indicates the first manifestations of psychiatric problems, periods of psychiatric symptoms, and hospitalizations. One timeline is then placed above the other, using the same demarcations (Figure 7–1). In complicated cases, the two timelines may reveal relationships between the timing of the psychiatric symptoms and of alcohol or drug use. If a patient has persistent psychiatric symptoms during a period of prolonged abstinence, the physician may prescribe an antidepressant. Conversely, if the patient becomes depressed only during periods of heavy drinking, pharmacological approaches are not indicated. Clearly, this method is limited by the patient's ability to recall past psychiatric episodes and periods of alcohol or drug use.

Assessment of Patient Reliability: Potential Denial of Substance-Related Disorders

Physicians must recognize that patients with addictive behaviors have varying degrees of **denial.** Clues to the presence of a substance use disorder include vague medical complaints, social isolation, or erratic and irresponsible behavior. Substance abusers can use hostility and evasiveness quite effectively to distance themselves from the interviewer, and they tend to avoid self-exploration or outside scrutiny of their alcohol or drug use. Cultural, gender, or socioeconomic differences between clinicians and patients may interfere with the patients' ability to trust the interviewer. Also, if patients feel guilty or ashamed, they may minimize the extent of their abuse and the negative impact it has had on their lives.

When physicians ask questions regarding substance use, they may elicit angry responses from patients. For example, if patients have experienced hostile reactions from friends or family regarding their substance use, they may expect the physician to treat them in the same way. Health professionals may be viewed as adversaries rather than allies. Women may be particularly reluctant to admit to alcohol or drug use because of the increased social stigma associated with female substance abuse. A female patient may have experienced condemnation because of her substance use and carry a heavy burden of guilt. She may assume that if she admits to alcohol or drug use, the physician will judge her harshly. Thus, female patients may be more likely to minimize alcohol or drug use and evade questions regarding addictive behavior during the clinical interview.

The physician must assess the **validity** of the information provided by the patient in the interview. The patient's level of denial and ability to trust the physician can influence the accuracy of the data. On a more basic level, the patient's ability to remember past and present details of his or her life may be impaired by substance use or other psychiatric or medical conditions and must be evaluated in order to assess the reliability of the data obtained. If the patient is a poor historian, other persons, such as family members, health care workers, or friends, should be contacted. When patients resist having the physician contact a spouse or other significant persons, the physician's suspicions of a substance use problem should be heightened.

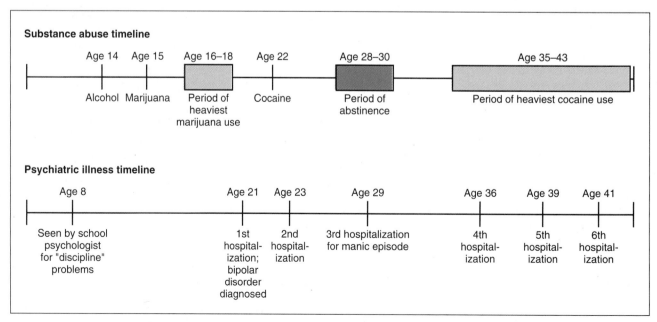

FIGURE 7–1. Timelines showing substance abuse history and psychiatric history.

When patients choose to openly discuss their alcohol or drug use, they make several assumptions and take several risks. First, they assume that the information given will be kept confidential. Second, they assume that physicians will be supportive and nonjudgmental. Third, they assume that physicians are obtaining relevant clinical data in order to help them. All of these assumptions require a significant amount of **trust.** During the initial part of the interview, it is essential that physicians show their sincerity and empathy. Once the patient's trust is elicited, the information the patient provides will be more reliable. It is often useful for the physician to state specifically which aspects of the interview will remain confidential. In a substance-abuse treatment setting, the physician may say something such as the following: "Information obtained during the interview regarding your substance abuse may be shared with the staff, but no information will be released to anyone else without your consent." The physician should also tell the patient, however, that medical records can be subpoenaed by a court of law.

In medical and substance abuse treatment settings, patients may be willing to tell their physicians about the extent of their alcohol or drug use but may stipulate that they do not want family members or employers to be informed about it. Often, once rapport is established, the physician may ask the patient's permission to contact non–drug-using family members and engage them in the treatment. In most cases, family involvement is beneficial. Contacting an employer is not commonly done, since this might result in loss of employment. However, if there is any possibility that the patient might be endangering his or her life or the lives of others because of continued alcohol or drug use (e.g., the patient is an anesthesiologist who is continuing to take opiates), the patient's employee assistance program or an appropriate professional organization must be contacted.

The patient's hostility and minimization of substance use can engender powerful feelings in the physician. When interviewers seek to help patients and are met with belligerence and evasiveness, they may become angry and adopt a more punitive stance. Before they interview substance abusers, physicians must become aware of and understand their own attitudes toward such patients. Their personal experiences with alcohol and drugs can significantly influence their approach. A physician who grew up in an alcoholic household and avoids all psychoactive substances may have little tolerance for substance users. Conversely, physicians who frequently binged on alcohol while in college may minimize the negative consequences of bingeing behavior in their patients.

Patient Engagement: Development of a Therapeutic Alliance

Physicians are frequently unaware of the effect that relatively simple interventions can have on patients with substance-related disorders. If a substance problem is suspected by the physician but denied by the patient, the physician should attempt to bridge this gap and engage the patient rather than turn away and self-righteously regard the patient as a liar or deviant. The physician could suggest that the patient abstain from alcohol or drugs for two weeks and return to see the physician after that time. ➡ In one case, a young mother who was abusing alcohol agreed that she needed to "cut down" the amount she was drinking but did not think that she needed to attend AA meetings or receive other help. After two weeks, she was able to stop drinking but found that it was much harder than she thought it would be. Because she was able to abstain until the next outpatient visit, the benefits of abstinence were reinforced, and she was encouraged to continue to abstain. She agreed to let the physician assess her ability to abstain on an ongoing basis. ⬅ This approach works best for patients whose families do not abuse substances and with whom they have close relationships; the physician can ask families to confirm the agreement that was made and to provide feedback about patients' progress.

When a patient's alcohol or drug use continues despite an agreement to stop, the patient may accept a referral for substance abuse treatment. ➡ One patient, who was an established musician, told his physician that his use of heroin was not a "big deal," despite his heavy weekend use. He agreed to discontinue use for two weeks. After that time, he returned for his appointment and admitted that he had been unable to stop and that he needed "extra help." He agreed to start attending NA meetings regularly. The physician determined that detoxification was not necessary for him. ⬅

Identifying the medical sequelae associated with alcohol or drug dependence can be extremely effective. Even a brief (e.g., 5- to 10-minute) intervention, in which the physician diagnoses a patient with substance abuse, presents the diagnosis to the patient, and offers a treatment referral, can be quite effective in reducing or eliminating substance use.

If substance abuse is suspected and the patient actively denies it, a psychiatrist or substance abuse specialist may be consulted. ➡ For example, a middle-aged man who had been "treating" his excruciating back pain with alcohol developed severe gastritis. When the internist asked whether the patient was having any problems with alcohol, he denied it. After meeting with an addiction specialist at the internist's request, the patient recognized that the gastritis might be alcohol-related. He agreed to take the analgesic prescribed by the physician instead of continuing to use alcohol to numb the pain. The patient still denied having a problem with alcohol, however, even though information obtained by the consultant revealed that he had had extensive problems with alcohol in the past. ⬅

A consultation from an addiction specialist, which is often requested in an inpatient setting by the treating physician, may not be welcomed by the patient, who may regard the interview as an intrusion. The patient may wish to focus only on the medical sequelae of the addiction rather than the underlying addictive behavior. In these situations, physicians should inform patients that a specialist will be meeting with them. By initially focusing on, and demonstrating their concern for, the patient's medical problems, the specialist may be able to facilitate rapport.

In a psychiatric setting, patients are more accustomed to being asked about personal issues. However, it is not uncommon for these patients to view their psychiatric problems as of primary importance and their substance use as a secondary issue. Again, the physician should empathize with the patient's psychiatric problems but also make it clear that an understanding of the alcohol or drug use is necessary to provide effective treatment. ➡ In one case, a patient with bipolar disorder was actively using cocaine. Her physician pointed out that her relapses always occurred after she stopped taking her psychiatric medication. The physician further explained that the use of cocaine exacerbated her manic-depressive symptoms. As her drug abuse was brought into focus as a central problem in her treatment, the patient stopped using cocaine and became more compliant in taking her medications. ⬅

Special Considerations in Children, Adolescents, and Elderly Patients

Physicians should give special consideration to the substance abuse evaluation of children, adolescents, and elderly patients. Generally, the best way to diagnose psychoactive substance abuse in children and adolescents is to look for changes in their lives. Has the child's **academic performance** deteriorated? Has the child broken off contact with old **friends** and acquired new ones? Have there been **personality or behavioral changes?** Have there been changes in the patterns of **sleep or appetite?** Any of these changes may indicate that a child is abusing alcohol or drugs and, therefore, should receive close scrutiny. It is important, however, to remember that such changes could be related to other factors (e.g., depression, parental conflict). Some potential risk factors for adolescents are listed in Table 7–3. The greater the number of risk factors, the more likely it is that an adolescent will use drugs. Substance-abusing adolescents are at a much higher risk for suicide attempts than are their non–substance-using peers. A depressed adolescent who is a substance abuser should be thoroughly evaluated and, if necessary, hospitalized.

Because elderly persons often suffer neurological impairment from other causes, the physician may overlook substance-induced **cognitive changes** in these patients. Social problems related to substance use are not as obvious in senior adults. Because their responsibilities have decreased (e.g., they no longer have to care for children or are retired), a substance use problem may go unrecognized for a longer period of time. A psychiatric and substance use assessment is indicated when an elderly individual shows

TABLE 7–3.   Risk Factors for Adolescent Alcohol and Drug Use

Early alcohol intoxication
Observed adult drug use
Perceived peer approval of drug use
Perceived parental approval of drug use
Frequent absences from school ("ditching")
Poor academic achievement (low grade-point average)
Distrust of teachers
Distrust of parents
Low educational aspirations
Little religious commitment
Emotional distress
Dissatisfaction with life

diminished interest in social activities or becomes more **isolated.**

DIFFERENTIAL DIAGNOSIS

The differential diagnosis of substance-related disorders is extremely complicated. Patients often deny substance use, and more than one substance-related disorder frequently coexists in the same patient, making the physician's detection of substance-induced disorders doubly important. Substance-induced disorders not only require treatment themselves but also serve as clues to a maladaptive pattern of substance use that could benefit from medical attention once the patient acknowledges the self-destructive process.

Other psychiatric syndromes are frequently present in patients with substance-related disorders. **Comorbidity,** or **"dual diagnosis,"** refers to the simultaneous presence of two relatively distinct disorders, one of which is substance related and one of which is not. The term "relatively distinct" indicates that it can be difficult to determine with any certainty whether the two disorders are completely unrelated. For instance, a 30-year-old man with a 10-year history of schizophrenia developed marijuana abuse. He might not have begun using marijuana excessively if he had not been lonely and demoralized by his chronic condition. Some cases show more clearly how substance abuse can begin as a misguided attempt by the patient to self-medicate a preexisting psychiatric disorder. In one case, a woman with panic disorder became alcohol dependent as she drank more and more to try to control her mounting anxiety. Self-medication is sometimes iatrogenic (e.g., a physician may prescribe benzodiazepines for prolonged periods of time without performing a psychiatric assessment or exploring social factors that may be contributing to the patient's anxiety).

Physicians must remember that patients often hide their substance use. When the patient is honest about it, he or she can work with the physician to try to sort out the patterns of causality. Their goals might be to find out whether the substance abuse or the psychiatric syndrome developed first and how much one disorder contributed to the development of the other.

When the patient is not honest with the physician about substance use, the differential diagnosis becomes even more complicated.

The physician's approach to the differential diagnosis varies, depending on whether or not drug use is revealed. For example, a patient who presents to the emergency room in a jittery, suspicious state and admits that he has been binging on crack cocaine for the past two days will most likely receive the diagnosis of cocaine intoxication, with the diagnoses of primary anxiety and psychotic disorders much less likely. The same clinical presentation in a patient who adamantly denies recent drug use would prompt the physician to consider a different diagnostic hierarchy, with primary anxiety and psychotic disorders placed at the top of a list of possible causes.

The differential diagnosis of substance-related disorders should be approached from the following perspectives: When a patient with psychiatric signs and symptoms gives a recent history of substance use, the physician should consider how likely it is that all of the psychiatric findings are substance induced. Alternatively, when a patient presents with psychiatric signs and symptoms but denies substance use, the physician must decide whether the clinical picture suggests that a substance-induced disorder be included in the differential diagnosis. For example, a 25-year-old man with a recent onset of psychosis who denies substance abuse may have schizophrenia but may also be suffering from a cocaine- or amphetamine-induced psychosis. The differential diagnosis sections in other chapters of this text should be consulted for more detailed coverage of the primary psychiatric disorders.

While it is essential that substance-related disorders not be overlooked, it is equally important that general medical conditions not be mistaken for substance-related disorders. Many medical conditions cause syndromes that resemble alcohol intoxication. Some of these are quite common (e.g., hyperglycemia; hypoglycemia; postictal syndrome, which occurs after a generalized seizure; and neurological disorders, such as multiple sclerosis). Any medical condition that can cause delirium can mimic alcohol or sedative intoxication (see Chapter 5, Cognitive and Mental Disorders Due to General Medical Conditions). The general medical differential diagnosis of alcohol and sedative withdrawal is essentially the same as that for anxiety disorders (see Chapter 6, Anxiety Disorders).

MEDICAL EVALUATION

A comprehensive medical history and physical examination can also indicate substance abuse. A variety of medical symptoms or physical signs (e.g., repeated injuries, pancreatitis, gastritis, heart failure, or convulsions) may be related to heavy alcohol use. Repeated bouts of cellulitis, abscesses, or endocarditis suggest intravenous drug use. Even vague complaints, such as insomnia, weakness, or headache, might be secondary to drug use. Table 7–4 shows some of the physical complaints and findings that are related to chronic substance use. Older patients have a decreased tolerance for alcohol and may have toxic effects with amounts that caused few difficulties for them when they were younger. Many elderly patients take benzodiazepines, which may induce a prolonged state of sedation because of decreased plasma clearance and an increased volume of distribution. A thorough mental status examination is crucial in assessing substance abuse (for detailed discussions of the mental status examination, see Chapter 2, The Psychiatric Interview, and Chapter 5, Cognitive and Mental Disorders Due to General Medical Conditions). Many substances can temporarily or permanently affect cognitive functioning.

Laboratory Tests for Alcohol-Related Disorders

Chronic alcohol use may lead to organ damage, which can be revealed by various laboratory abnormalities, including elevated levels of gamma-glutamyl transpeptidase (GGT) and an elevated mean corpuscular volume (MCV) (Table 7–5). These test abnormalities suggest problematic alcohol or drug use, but only information obtained in the clinical interview can confirm the diagnosis.

A wide array of other laboratory abnormalities may be present, including elevations in creatinine phosphokinase (CPK), alanine aminotransferase (APT), aspartate aminotransferase (AST), amylase, or high-density lipoprotein (HDL) cholesterol. It must be kept in mind that heavy alcohol use is not the only cause of these abnormalities; a wide range of medical conditions may produce them as well. Recent alcohol use is more accurately detected by a Breathalyzer test or blood test than by a urine test.

Laboratory Tests for Drug-Related Disorders

An array of blood, urine, and hair sample tests can reveal the use of a wide variety of drugs (see Table 7–5). Each test has a different sensitivity, specificity, and cost. Generally, screening tests such as thin-layer chromatography (TLC) or radioimmunoassay (RIA) are used initially because they are simple, rapid, and inexpensive. If the result is positive, drug use can be confirmed by tests such as gas chromatography or high-performance liquid chromatography, which are more expensive and should be used judiciously. When submitting samples to a laboratory, physicians must specify which drugs should be tested. They cannot merely send the sample to a diagnostic laboratory and ask whether any drugs can be detected. Physicians should be aware that the sensitivity of the laboratory test is not the only factor that affects drug detection. Other factors include the half-life of the substance, the patient's ability to metabolize or excrete the substance, the extent of substance use, the method of collecting the sample, intentional or inadvertent tampering with the sample, and the method used to store the sample.

TABLE 7–4.   Chronic Substance Use

Substance	Related Physical Complaints	Possible Physical Findings
Alcohol	Frequent injuries; abdominal pain, nausea, and vomiting (gastritis, pancreatitis); diarrhea; headaches; vague physical complaints; erectile dysfunction; convulsions; palpitations; insomnia	Hypertension; injuries (e.g., bruises, cigarette burns, unexplained burns); enlarged liver; cutaneous stigmas of liver disease (spider angioma, palmar erythema); ecchymoses on legs, arms, or chest; smell of alcohol on breath; myopathy; peripheral neuritis; congestive heart failure
Cocaine	Fatigue, sinusitis, sore throat, hoarseness, persistent fever, chest pain, sexual problems, bronchitis, weight loss, nausea and vomiting, headaches, muscle jerks and spasms, convulsions, arrhythmia	Cocaine: rhinitis, rash around nasal area, perforation of nasal septum, hypertension, tachycardia. Crack cocaine: hoarseness; parched lips, tongue, and throat; singed eyebrows or eyelashes; stigmas of IV use
Stimulants	Insomnia, weight loss	Worn-down teeth (from tooth grinding), scratches, skin ulcers, dyskinesia
Inhalants (hydrocarbons)	Weight loss, breathing difficulties, fatigue, nosebleeds, weakness, stomach upset, intellectual changes	Halitosis, rash around nose or mouth, mental status changes
Cannabis	Chronic dry cough, bronchitis, sinusitis, pharyngitis, laryngitis	Conjunctival suffusion; distinct odor of burnt leaves on breath and clothes; dilated, poorly reactive pupils
Opioids	False complaints of severe pain made to obtain drugs; infections (especially cellulitis, abscess, pneumonia, SBE)	Needle track marks, skin lesions, constricted pupils, swollen nasal mucosa, thrombosis, lymphadenopathy
Other sedatives	Insomnia, restlessness, convulsions, pneumonia	Slurred speech; needle track marks if IV user (especially with barbiturates); pupillary constriction with glutethimide
Hallucinogens	Palpitations, chest pain (especially in older users); convulsions with PCP	Myopathy; renal failure with PCP

Source: Wartenberg, A., Dubé, C.E., Lewis, D.C., Cyr, M.G. Diagnosing chronic substance use problems in the primary care setting: Related physical problems, psychological problems, physical findings and relevant labs. *In* Dubé, C. E., Goldstein, M.G., Lewis, D.C., Myers, E.R., Zwick, W.R., (eds.) Project ADEPT Curriculum for Primary Care Physician Training. Vol. I: Core Modules. Providence, Rhode Island, Brown University Press, 1989. Printed by permission of the publisher.

ETIOLOGY

For individuals with alcohol or drug problems, there is a complex, unique set of variables that influences their addictive behavior.

Biological Factors

The disease concept of alcoholism is central to most treatment approaches used in the United States. Alcoholics Anonymous strongly endorses this model, which, in essence, views alcoholism as a progressive illness that can be fatal if it is not treated. Loss of control is the dominant symptom. A recovering individual must remain completely abstinent in order to avoid a relapse. As with other chronic diseases, there is no "cure" for alcoholism. (*Cure* is defined as the ability to return to controlled drinking.) Therefore, patients who have stopped drinking alcohol are described as being "in recovery" rather than having "recovered."

Most of the literature about the influence of biological factors on addiction has focused on the familial transmission of or possible **genetic markers** for alcoholism (Box 7–2). Little information about other psychoactive substances exists to either support or refute the possibility of a biologically transmitted dependence. This paucity of information is not surprising, because these other drugs of abuse vary in availability and use, whereas alcohol has usually been widely available and its use socially acceptable.

During the past 20 years, many adoption studies have supported the model of genetic transmission of alcoholism. Adopted men with one biological parent who is an alcoholic are four times as likely to become alcoholics themselves—even if their adoptive parents are not alcoholics—than are those whose biological parents are not alcoholics.

Psychological Factors

During evaluation of a patient who has a psychoactive substance abuse disorder and another psychiatric Axis I or II disorder, it is difficult to determine whether the two disorders are separate entities that developed independently or whether one disorder precipitated the other. Although it might seem that it would be relatively easy to determine which disorder occurred first, often it is not. Chemical use can induce depression, panic attacks, and psychosis (see Differ-

TABLE 7–5. Laboratory Testing for Substance Abuse

Substance	Laboratory Studies
Alcohol	Complete blood count ($\uparrow$MCV, $\uparrow$MCH or cytopenias), liver function tests (GGT, SGOT > SGPT), $\uparrow$uric acid, $\uparrow$triglycerides. Rib fractures on chest x-ray
Cocaine	Immunoassays, chromatography/mass spectroscopy, urine toxicology screening (detection time after last use: up to 12–48 hours)
Stimulants	Urine toxicology screening (detection time after last use: up to 24–48 hours)
Inhalants (hydrocarbons)	Complete blood count, liver and kidney function tests
Cannabis	Urine toxicology screening (detection time after last use: occasional user, 1–3 days or longer; chronic heavy users, 1 month or longer)
Opiates	Urine toxicology screening* (detection time after last use: up to 2–4 days)
Other sedatives	Urine toxicology screening** (detection time after last use: up to 1 week; barbiturates, chronic users, up to several weeks; long-acting benzodiazepines, chronic users, weeks to months)
Hallucinogens	Urine toxicology screening (detection time after last use: PCP, several days to several weeks; LSD, up to 12 hours; LSD metabolites, 2 days). Myoglobinuria, elevated CPK and creatinine/BUN with PCP

Source: Wartenberg, A., Dubé, C.E., Lewis, D.C., Cyr, M. G. Diagnosing chronic substance use problems in the primary care setting: Related physical problems, psychological problems, physical findings and relevant labs. *In* Dubé, C. E., Goldstein, M.G., Lewis, D.C., Myers, E.R., Zwick, W.R. (eds.) Project ADEPT Curriculum for Primary Care Physician Training. Vol. I: Core Modules. Providence, Rhode Island, Brown University Press, 1989. Printed by permission of the publisher.

*If a screening assay is positive for opiates, a confirmatory test specific for morphine or codeine is necessary. Illicit versus clinical use of these substances cannot be determined by test results alone. Further, it is impossible to determine whether heroin, codeine, or morphine has been taken when low concentrations of morphine or codeine are found in the urine. Ingestion of a large quantity of poppy seeds will produce a positive immunoassay result up to 60 hours after ingestion. To distinguish between poppy seed ingestion and heroin use, use GC/MS to test for 6-O-acetylmorphine (a heroin metabolite). Methadone must be analyzed separately; fentanyl and its analogs are not detected by routine methods.

**Alprazolam (Xanax) may not be detected in routine assays. If it is suspected, the laboratory technician should be instructed to use GC/MS to test specifically for this drug.

ential Diagnosis, above). Withdrawal symptoms can be manifested by delirium, anxiety, and protracted insomnia. Therefore, physicians must be extremely cautious when they ascribe alcohol or substance abuse to an underlying mental disorder. The hypothesis that psychoactive substances are used by individuals to treat psychic distress has been referred to as the "self-medication" model of addiction.

There is evidence that depression may predate alcohol abuse in women and that alcohol may be used as an ineffective way to self-medicate a depressive mood state (Rounsaville et al., 1987). Although some physicians might find the **self-medication hypothesis** appealing and although studies have found that some psychiatric disorders may precede substance abuse (Christie et al., 1988), other studies have found the opposite to be true (Woodruff et al., 1973; Breier, Charney, and Heninger, 1986). In addition, psychological factors that do not "qualify" as disease entities may elicit problem substance use. In the psychoanalytic literature, alcoholism and drug dependency have been understood within the context of an individual's psychosocial development. Physicians have theorized that because the dependency needs of addicted individuals were not adequately gratified during the oral stage of their development, oral substitutes (e.g., psychoactive drugs) are used to pacify these needs. Often, substance abusers will assume a "pseudoindependent" stance by rejecting help and support from others (Kaufman and Reoux, 1988). Instead, they will attempt to manipulate and control others. This pattern may seem paradoxical because of the strong dependency needs of these patients. However, in order to accept help from others, these patients must expose their vulnerabilities; this can be particularly frightening for those who have experienced early trauma.

Some physicians, instead of focusing on the psychiatric symptoms or personality disorders that may lead patients to substance abuse, have suggested that individuals with poor coping skills resort to using chemical substances as a means of dealing with life's difficulties and that such use may eventually lead to addiction (Donovan, 1988).

Social Factors

The social factors that influence substance abuse are many, including interpersonal, cultural, and societal factors. Heightened marital conflict is reported more often in homes where childhood alcoholism later develops (Zucker and Lisansky-Gomberg, 1986). Marital conflict may cause children to seek out peers who use alcohol or to participate in antisocial behavior leading to alcohol or drug use. Peer associations are a major influence in the initiation and maintenance of adolescent drug use.

Cultural differences have also been suggested as a factor that influences alcohol and drug use. Differences in drinking behaviors among French and American males males have been noted. Americans with Irish backgrounds may be more likely to be alcoholics than are Italian Americans (Vaillant and Milofsky, 1982). Jewish and Chinese populations in the United States have much lower rates of alcohol problems than the general population, perhaps because neither culture tolerates drinking to the point of losing control (Peele, 1988).

At this point, it remains unclear why the rates of alcohol and drug use are lower in women than in men. Is it biologically or culturally determined? One possible explanation is that although alcoholism in

BOX 7–2. Genetic Influences in Alcoholism

There is evidence to suggest that biological factors may contribute to the development of alcoholism. However, since monozygotic twins have only a 54% concordance for alcoholism, rather than 90–100% (Kaij, 1960), there are undoubtedly other variables that influence the expression of alcoholism.

Schuckit (1984) has done the most work in pursuing genetic markers that may predict a vulnerability to alcoholism. He has compared nonalcoholic young men with first-degree relatives who are alcoholic (group A) and nonalcoholic young men whose first-degree relatives are nonalcoholic (group B). The men in group A were less likely to feel intoxicated after drinking than were the men in group B. Because of this response, the men in group A may be more likely to use alcohol heavily and eventually develop a problematic drinking pattern. (Interestingly, the blood alcohol concentrations and expectations of the two groups did not differ significantly, suggesting that the men in group A somehow perceive the same blood alcohol level differently.) Schuckit's studies are too small to prove that the men in group A are "physiologically different" than the men in group B. Because most physiological studies have not focused on female cohorts, it is less clear whether women with familial alcoholism are likely to have a different physiological response to alcohol or other central nervous stimuli than are women with a negative family history.

Some authors have studied physiological factors that may protect an individual from developing alcoholism. Asians may have an increased sensitivity to alcohol, which is manifested by facial flushing (Wolff, 1972). The flushing may prevent overindulgence in alcohol, which may explain the lower alcoholism rates in Asians. Other researchers have contested this premise by noting that Eskimo and American Indian groups, who also have an increased incidence of facial flushing and other cardiovascular effects related to alcohol use, have high rates of alcoholism, as well.

---

demic, or social difficulties and use alcohol or drugs as ways to cope. When parents are permissive regarding their children's use of psychoactive substances or openly use psychoactive substances themselves, the children are at greater risk for developing substance abuse problems. Additionally, having an older sibling who abuses drugs, having parents with affective disorders, or experiencing family disruption heightens the risk of use and abuse.

TREATMENT
Recovery From Substance-Related Disorders

Recovery from substance addiction is the process by which an individual learns effective coping strategies for leading a substance-free life, which means making a commitment to change addictive behaviors and to maintain these changes. Each stage has a major task to be accomplished, takes a certain period of time, and involves the patient being vulnerable to certain causes of relapse. The treatment plan is designed to help individuals recognize the warning signs of relapse in time to prevent it. (In the past, any return to alcohol or drug use was usually viewed as a treatment failure, but, today, distinctions are often made between a lapse and a relapse. A **lapse** is a brief return to substance use. When patients "slip" in this manner, physicians can work with them to cognitively restructure the situation. Instead of perceiving the loss of sobriety as a personal failure, patients can see it as a chance to understand what prompted them to return to substance use and can learn improved methods of coping so that it will not happen in the future. A **relapse** is a return to excessive or uncontrolled use.)

Recovery can occur spontaneously or with treatment. Regardless of the type of chemical abused, recovery must be seen as a long-term process that is measured in years rather than weeks. If an individual has been abusing a psychoactive substance for a limited period of time and has not had many problems related to its use, spontaneous recovery may be possible.

Successful maintenance of recovery is usually associated with the length of prior periods of abstinence and the involvement of supportive significant others in the patient's treatment. Although it is not clear whether demographic variables, such as income, race, gender, or marital status, can predict the outcome of treatment, income and marital status often reflect social supports that are correlated with a higher probability of a good outcome. The amount or frequency of alcohol or drug use do not seem to be predictive of the outcome.

Because legal substances are obtained in ways that are generally sanctioned by society and because they are used more openly, it usually takes longer for the abuser of such substances to seek treatment. Once alcohol-dependent individuals are engaged in treatment, they are more likely to do well than those who are dependent on illicit substances. Although relapse is common with all substances of abuse, indi-

---

women may be influenced by heredity, the expression of addictive behavior is often suppressed by societal and cultural factors. Women face greater condemnation for out-of-control drinking behavior and experience severe censure if they continue to use chemical substances while they are pregnant.

Societal factors can also influence the extent of addictive behavior. If a psychoactive substance is illegal, it is less widely available and more expensive, and, therefore, fewer individuals are likely to start using it. The use of legal psychoactive substances, such as tobacco or alcohol, is curtailed by prohibiting minors from buying them, but, even so, these substances are easily obtained and widely used by adolescents.

Some specific factors that may lead to abuse in midlife are loss or dissatisfaction with one's job, disruption of relationships (e.g., divorce, separation, children leaving home), emotional distress, and medical ailments. Clearly, most people who encounter these changes do not develop substance abuse. Individuals who develop a chemical addiction during the fourth and fifth decades of life either may have never learned how to handle stress effectively or have not used previously learned coping strategies.

It is unclear why some children begin to use substances. They may be experiencing familial, aca-

viduals addicted to alcohol tend to achieve longer periods of stable recovery than those addicted to illicit substances. One reason for this difference may be the chemical properties of the substances (i.e., cocaine is much more addictive than alcohol). Also, individuals are more likely to develop alcohol-related problems at an older age than cocaine-related problems, and, therefore, they may have better social supports and resources to facilitate recovery.

Individuals who have long histories of substance abuse are often difficult to treat. Some chronic chemical abusers, particularly alcoholics, manage to avoid the substance abuse treatment system altogether. Alcohol dependence is often first detected when the patient has work-related difficulties and is forced to enter an employee assistance program. Some alcoholics are initially diagnosed when they require medical treatment for pancreatitis or liver disease. It may be extremely difficult for these individuals to identify themselves as addicts requiring substance abuse treatment.

Other habitual chemical abusers admit they have a problem with their substance use and repeatedly seek help, but despite the efforts of a myriad of treatment programs, they continue to have difficulties related to their chemical use. Because of their long string of perceived failures, they lose faith that they can be helped. It is the physician's role to remain optimistic and refer these patients to addiction specialists who may be able to offer additional treatment strategies.

Treatment for patients who suffer from chemical dependency uses various approaches and takes place in different settings. The patient's requirements should dictate the strategy, but the availability of community resources or the patient's financial means often determines the mode of therapy.

Treatment Programs

Since the 1960s, the number of treatment options for chemically dependent individuals has expanded tremendously. As physicians have gained a better understanding of addicted patients, they have recognized the importance of matching each patient to the appropriate treatment. The needs of the patient and the patient's conceptual understanding of the addictive behavior must be explored before a treatment plan is designed and implemented. It is important for physicians to recognize that treatment is effective only if it is appropriate and if the patient and the physician are working together. Most patients have a variety of problems related to life functioning. Drug-dependent individuals may lack job skills, may have family or marital difficulties, may suffer from a variety of medical ailments caused by neglect or poor nutrition, and may experience significant emotional distress. Although it may be beyond the scope of one treatment program to address all of these areas, it is crucial that the areas of greatest difficulty or of greatest concern to the patient be recognized.

If the treatment program can provide the appropriate service, the patient can usually remain in that program. However, if the program has inadequate resources for that specific patient, a referral to another program may be necessary. Because patients with severe psychiatric problems tend to do poorly in standard substance abuse programs, they need to be identified and given appropriate pharmacological treatment and psychotherapy. If the chemical treatment program does not have an adequate psychiatric staff or consultants for these patients, they should be referred to a more appropriate program.

An essential part of understanding the individual needs of the patient is recognizing the patient's level of motivation and conceptualization of the addictive behavior. Individuals enter treatment for a multitude of reasons. Some are forced to do so by the legal system or their families. These individuals may not accept that they have a problem with psychoactive substances and, therefore, will be resistant to any form of treatment. Often, these patients require substance abuse education and confrontation regarding the destructive nature of their behavior. Individuals who freely choose to enter treatment may recognize their problems with alcohol or drugs but may believe that they can use chemicals in a controlled manner. Most chemically dependent individuals cannot use psychoactive substances without returning to their earlier addictive behavior patterns.

Substance abusers with concomitant psychiatric symptoms may be more likely to seek either psychiatric or substance abuse treatment than are those without psychiatric symptoms. Individuals with severe psychiatric problems tend to do worse than those with fewer problems. Some types of treatment may be more beneficial for patients with certain psychological characteristics. For alcohol abusers, a depressed or anxious mood may be the most common reason for relapse and situational factors may be the least common. Psychiatric illness must be adequately assessed in addictive patients in order to provide the best treatment.

All patients (and most health professionals) have preconceived views of what causes addiction. Chemically dependent individuals often assume that their addictive behavior is due to moral weakness or a lack of will power. These assumptions cause them to feel enormous guilt and to view treatment as punitive. Unless they are coerced into entering treatment, they may avoid it altogether. For these individuals, a dialog with an addiction specialist who takes a different view (i.e., that addictive behavior can be due to a variety of biological, psychological, and environmental factors) may be extremely productive. If such patients can accept the view that they are not morally reprehensible for having an addiction but are responsible for changing their behavior, they may be willing to embrace treatment.

After physicians and patients agree that treatment is necessary, they must decide whether inpatient or outpatient treatment would be best. It is important to understand the benefits and drawbacks of each setting. In all treatment settings, patients are encouraged to attend AA or NA meetings. In inpatient settings, these meetings are often one component of the treatment. In outpatient settings, these meetings may be the only form of treatment or may be used in conjunction with other therapies. AA and NA meetings are run by lay members of the groups. Using a self-help supportive model, individuals are encouraged to admit their powerlessness over alcohol or other drugs and accept their need for help from a higher power. In AA, the **12-step program** helps the individual to begin a process toward recovery (Table 7—6). Meetings may be closed (i.e., only members or potential members of the group can attend) or open (i.e., any interested person can attend). All physicians should attend at least one open meeting so that they can adequately answer patients' questions regarding these groups.

Inpatient and Residential Chemical Dependence Programs

Inpatient programs are often based in psychiatric hospitals or in freestanding treatment units (i.e., other than hospitals). Psychiatric hospitals often treat adolescents, patients with dual diagnoses, and patients who require close monitoring because of suicidal ideation or other psychiatric symptoms. Patients usually stay for two to four weeks. Patients are first observed medically and may then receive pharmacological agents for detoxification. Alcohol and benzodiazepine dependence can be life-threatening and generally requires **detoxification.** Although withdrawal from opiates may be physically uncomfortable and produce anxiety and sleep disturbances, it is not life-threatening. Various pharmacological strategies can be used to alleviate uncomfortable symptoms. Treatment usually includes individual, group, and family therapy; education; exercise; relaxation techniques; and attendance at AA or NA meetings.

Freestanding units usually use the AA 12-step model of treatment. The focus of these intensive programs is to comprehensively evaluate each patient from a psychosocial approach, develop a treatment plan, and implement the 12-step program. In the past, these programs were often the first treatment option, but with the advent of managed care, they now most commonly treat individuals who have repeatedly relapsed in outpatient settings, have required removal from drug-plagued environments to achieve abstinence, or have been referred by their employers because of occupational difficulties related to substance abuse. Patients are usually admitted for 14–28 days and then referred to substance-free outpatient clinics or encouraged to attend AA or NA meetings. Patients often enter freestanding programs after they have been detoxified in a medical facility. Units with full-time physicians may provide pharmacological treatment for uncomplicated detoxification, but in many cases, the physician's only role is to perform physical examinations and provide medical treatment as needed. Therapy consists of education groups, individual and group therapy, and AA or NA meetings. Treatment is often provided by counselors who are recovering substance abusers, which can be beneficial because formerly addicted individuals can provide a unique perspective. Some programs do a better job than others of identifying and treating individuals with coexisting psychiatric disorders, but many of these programs have no such capability.

Outpatient Programs

Outpatient programs are drug-free or methadone treatment programs. **Outpatient drug-free treatment** (OPDF) refers to a wide range of programs that offer services in several kinds of individual situations. Patients may be new to treatment, referred from other treatment settings, relapsed after treatment, or forced to enter treatment (e.g., by the legal system or an employee-assistance program). Most patients can do well in outpatient programs as long as certain important elements are incorporated. First, the program should carry out a **comprehensive psychosocial evaluation** of the patient to detect major complicating psychiatric, social, or medical problems that may require additional psychotherapy, family therapy, psychiatric medication, or referral to an inpatient program. Second, the program should be structured with clear **clinical criteria** for the particular intensity or mode of treatment (or both) to be used for different patients and situations. Third, **urine testing** must be done frequently to ensure that therapists are aware of the patient's extent of use and to document treatment efficacy.

It is important to emphasize that drug treatment can eventually work for individuals who have frequent relapses. With each treatment attempt, pa-

---

TABLE 7–6. The Twelve Steps of Alcoholics Anonymous

1. We admitted we were powerless over alcohol and that our lives had become unmanageable.
2. Came to believe that a Power greater than ourselves could restore us to sanity.
3. Made a decision to turn our will and our lives over to the care of God as we understood Him.
4. Made a searching and fearless moral inventory of ourselves.
5. Admitted to God, to ourselves, and to another human being the exact nature of our wrongs.
6. Were entirely ready to have God remove all these defects of character.
7. Humbly asked Him to remove our shortcomings.
8. Made a list of all persons we had harmed, and became willing to make amends to them all.
9. Made direct amends to such people wherever possible, except when to do so would injure them or others.
10. Continued to take personal inventory and when we were wrong promptly admitted it.
11. Sought through prayer and meditation to improve our conscious contact with God as we understood Him, praying only for knowledge of His will for us and the power to carry that out.
12. Having had a spiritual awakening as the result of these steps, we tried to carry this message to alcoholics, and to practice these principles in all our affairs.

tients gain new insights and learn more strategies for living a drug-free life-style. Treatment can also be effective for individuals who are reluctant to seek treatment or are forced into it. In fact, substance-abusing individuals who are pressured into therapy by their families, their employers, or the criminal justice system often do at least as well as patients who enter treatment voluntarily.

OPDF clinics often provide individual and group therapy and education groups that teach patients about the negative social, psychiatric, and medical consequences of substance use. They also supply nonaddicting prescription medications (e.g., disulfiram, naltrexone) and encourage abstinence. To better meet the needs of their patients, many OPDF clinics also offer a variety of specialty groups for women, HIV-positive individuals, and adolescents. Other groups may teach parenting skills or help patients learn how to find a job or write a resumé.

If the OPDF clinic is in an outpatient psychiatric hospital or has specially trained staff members (e.g., psychiatrists, psychiatric social workers), the clinic may have a specialized program for patients with dual diagnoses or psychiatric disorders. Some nonpsychiatric substance abuse treatment settings have psychiatric consultants who can evaluate and individually treat patients with psychiatric problems.

Residential Therapeutic Community Programs

Residential programs ("therapeutic communities") stress the importance of having fellow addicts and ex-addicts provide nonprofessional treatment to recovering substance abusers within a residential setting. The communities are often staffed by ex-addicts. Rewards and penalties are used to shape the residents' behaviors, and substance abusers are constantly confronted by their peers regarding the consequences of their behaviors. These programs are highly structured, and residents are required to work. The jobs are ranked from "low" to "high" status and are allocated according to the patient's length of stay in the community, competence, and ability to behave responsibly.

Most residential community programs recommend that residents stay for 12–24 months. Synanon, which was the prototype of the therapeutic community, insisted on a lifetime commitment. Newer programs are advocating at least a six-month stay. Many substance abusers are unwilling to make a 12- to 24-month commitment to a highly structured treatment program and may resist the strict regulation of their behavior. Because these programs rely heavily on confrontation, they are not recommended for psychiatric patients or emotionally fragile individuals. Use of psychotropic medication is uncommon and usually discouraged. Residential programs have been criticized because their dropout rate is high. However, even individuals who leave precipitously benefit from the treatment because the longer they remain in the facility, the more likely they are to reduce their drug use or illegal activities after they leave.

Treatment programs in general have a wide range of strategies for engaging and maintaining patients in therapy, including behavioral or psychological techniques, religious beliefs, and pharmacological interventions. These methods are commonly used in combination.

Psychotherapy

Several psychological strategies used with other types of psychiatric patients have been modified to meet the treatment needs of patients with substance abuse disorders. In supportive therapy, which is frequently used in individual, group, and family settings, an empathetic and nonjudgmental therapist helps patients replace their drug-seeking behaviors with new behaviors that are compatible with a healthier, drug-free life-style. In cognitive and behavior psychotherapy, substance abusers learn how to recognize and manage high-risk situations and feelings that might cause them to use drugs, as well as the early warning signs of relapse. They also learn that one strategy for avoiding relapse is to develop new areas of interest and activities as substitutes for their former drug behaviors.

Supportive, behavioral, and cognitive approaches are usually appropriate for patients during the early stages of their recovery. The goal of early recovery is cessation of the substance use. Uncovering core conflicts and confronting maladaptive defenses produce a significant degree of anxiety. Not until the patient has had an extended period of recovery should a more traditional psychodynamic psychotherapy be applied. Only then is a patient more likely to tolerate anxiety without returning to self-destructive drug use.

At times, issues of loss, past physical or sexual abuse, or other traumatic events impede the patient's ability to achieve prolonged abstinence. For such patients, the therapeutic focus on the present situation may require some modification. These patients have often chosen chemical "solutions" to avoid painful feelings associated with disturbing past events. These events may need to be discussed early in treatment, but the purpose of such discussions should be to teach the patient new strategies for coping with distressing memories and help the patient build self-esteem.

Behavior therapy techniques are based on the psychological theories of operant or respondent conditioning. In **operant conditioning,** a behavior is shaped by the environmental consequences of that behavior. If a behavior is rewarded, it is more likely to be repeated, and if it is punished, it will eventually diminish. When operant techniques are applied successfully to substance abusers, salient reinforcers or punishers effectively compete with the rewarding aspects of drug use. **Contingency contracting** is another technique used to encourage abstinence. Patients may contract to let therapists inform their families, colleagues, or bosses if they break their abstinence and resume using drugs or may receive vouchers redeemable for "prosocial" goods or activities as a contingent reward for a negative urine test.

Respondent conditioning uses aversive stimuli to eliminate or reduce the pleasant effects of drugs or drug stimuli. For example, individuals may be given a chemical that induces nausea while they receive an injection of their drug of choice. The difficulty with all aversive behavioral techniques is finding stimuli that are negative enough to suppress drug use, acceptable to the patient, and ethically and medically responsible.

Psychopharmacological Treatment

Depending on the psychoactive substance that has been abused, various pharmacological strategies may be employed. Antagonists are given to block the pleasant effects of a drug. Other medications produce aversive effects if the abused substance is taken concomitantly. Agonists produce the same effects as the abused substance but with less euphoric effect and fewer physical or psychosocial risks. Other drugs may be used to treat withdrawal symptoms or decrease cravings for a drug. Some classes of drugs tend to be used intermittently (e.g., hallucinogens) and, therefore, do not produce withdrawal symptoms. Detoxifying agents are not needed for patients recovering from such drugs. For other classes of drugs (e.g., stimulants), a safe, less abusable substitution drug has yet to be approved for clinical practice.

Pharmacotherapy is most effective when combined with other forms of treatment. In order to assess which pharmacological approach, if any, is appropriate, the patient's psychological and physical status, as well as motivation for treatment, must be assessed. The symbolic aspect of administering drugs to drug addicts should not be overlooked. Some patients may assume that the therapeutic drug, like the abused substance, can solve all their problems. They must be helped to understand that the medication is being given to help reduce drug abuse. Improvement in other areas (e.g., work, interpersonal relationships) may be facilitated by psychotherapy.

Dependence on Alcohol and Other Sedatives

The pharmacological treatment of alcohol dependence is based on the specific requirements of the patient. Some patients are given **disulfiram,** which produces aversive side effects via the inhibition of aldehyde dehydrogenase. If patients drink alcohol or ingest substances containing alcohol after taking disulfiram, their acetaldehyde levels rise, resulting in flushing, decreased blood pressure, nausea and vomiting, and pounding in the chest. More serious consequences include seizures, myocardial infarction, cerebrovascular hemorrhage, and cardiovascular collapse. Despite the use of this medication for 40 years, deaths have rarely occurred. Disulfiram is generally indicated for highly motivated patients or for those who have had success with the medication in the past. Because of the medical and psychiatric contraindications to this drug, it must be used appropriately and with the informed consent of the patient. **Naltrexone,** an opiate antagonist, was approved by the Food and Drug Administration (FDA) in 1994 for the treatment of alcoholism. By diminishing the reinforcing effects of alcohol, it can prevent a lapse from becoming a relapse. It has the advantage over disulfiram of not leading to any dangerous effects if the patient drinks while taking the medication.

If the patient wishes to be detoxified or is experiencing withdrawal symptoms associated with alcohol or other classes of sedatives (e.g., barbiturates and benzodiazepines), a number of pharmacological approaches can be used. The agent for detoxification is chosen based on the medical status of the patient, intended route of administration, desired half-life, and physician's familiarity with the drug. Although some physicians choose to prescribe barbiturates, such as phenobarbital, for detoxification, the **benzodiazepines,** such as diazepam or chlordiazepoxide, are now the usual drugs of choice. A few studies suggest that carbamazepine or valproic acid may be useful detoxifying agents, especially if there is a prior history of withdrawal seizures, but neither is commonly used for alcohol detoxification. The basic principle of pharmacological detoxification is to rapidly substitute a sufficient amount of the detoxifying agent to prevent withdrawal symptoms and then gradually decrease the drug levels over several days. At times, physicians may choose to detoxify patients with the drugs that they are abusing. Adequate substitution can be estimated using the conversion tables in pharmacology and substance abuse texts.

Opiate Dependence

In emergency settings, physicians often administer naloxone to reverse the effects of opiate overdoses. In substance abuse treatment settings, naltrexone, a long-acting, orally effective antagonist, is sometimes used to maintain abstinence. Unlike methadone, which substitutes for the opiates, **naltrexone** competitively antagonizes their effects. Because naltrexone does not produce an opiate effect, many patients are unenthusiastic about taking it. Patient compliance with naltrexone is also poor because withdrawal symptoms do not occur if the patient misses a dose and because cravings for the opiate may persist. Naltrexone has been most successful for patients who have "much to lose" because of their addiction or who are highly motivated (e.g., physician addicts or opiate addicts under the control of the criminal justice system).

Methadone maintenance is the most established form of substitution pharmacotherapy. Methadone therapy, which is designed specifically for patients who are addicted to opiates (usually heroin), has been used successfully in many individuals for over three decades. Patients are usually required to verify their opiate addiction (i.e., they must have observable physical withdrawal symptoms or precipitated withdrawal symptoms when an opiate antagonist, such as naloxone, is given). Historical evidence may be acceptable if certain standards are met. Prospective patients should have used opiates for one to two years before seeking treatment and should have "failed" other treatments. Unfortunately, up to 75% of patients have a relapse once they stop taking methadone.

Several problems are associated with methadone programs. Individuals often continue to use alcohol and illicit substances, especially cocaine, after they begin taking methadone. In addition, problems may develop if patients are allowed to take the drug home, as is the case in most programs for patients who have demonstrated stable improvement in life functioning and documented periods of no illicit drug use (i.e., some patients take advantage of the situation by selling the drug to other addicts). Methadone diversion to the outside community is possible in any program that allows the drug to be taken home. Methadone overdoses in minors or other heroin addicts are uncommon, however.

Despite such problems, methadone treatment has been repeatedly shown to be effective, perhaps more so than any other form of drug treatment. In well-run programs, patients who take methadone are less likely to commit crimes, use opiates, be unemployed, or become infected with HIV, as compared with opiate-dependent individuals not in methadone treatment.

Methadone is used because it is long acting (i.e., it can be given once a day) and is well absorbed orally, unlike heroin, which has a short half-life and is not well absorbed orally. Methadone does not prevent the euphoric or other psychological effects associated with different classes of drugs, and, therefore, it is not necessarily an effective deterrent against alcohol or cocaine abuse. Because of its opiate effect, patients are more willing to comply with methadone treatment than with naltrexone treatment. However, until the patient demonstrates sustained success with methadone, daily attendance at the methadone clinic and frequent urine tests are required. An opiate antagonist or residential therapeutic community may be a better option for patients who continue to have significant drug problems while they are taking methadone for maintenance.

l-Acetyl-alpha-methadol (LAAM), a synthetic opiate agonist that is similar to methadone, has recently been approved by the FDA. Since the duration of action of LAAM is two to three days and take-home doses are not currently permitted, LAAM is not easily diverted into the community. Detoxification from methadone remains difficult and may be easier with LAAM, although the data are not yet clear on this.

Detoxification from opiates is usually accomplished with methadone substitution and withdrawal. The methadone requirements are found in conversion charts. The alpha-adrenergic agonists clonidine and lofexidine are less frequently used but

may be more effective because they are associated with less postwithdrawal rebound, which may lead to relapse. The rapid detoxification approaches that precipitate withdrawal with the narcotic antagonist naltrexone and then block the symptoms with clonidine and the benzodiazepines are even more successful and much quicker but are also more difficult to use.

Cocaine Dependence

Withdrawal from chronic use of cocaine or other stimulants may result in anhedonia, depression, and fatigue. Desipramine may be somewhat efficacious in treating withdrawal and craving because it reduces these symptoms. Lithium seems to benefit cocaine abusers who have bipolar or cyclothymic disorder, but it is not beneficial for most cocaine addicts.

Because craving is a reason commonly given for relapse, researchers have been trying to use preexisting medications or develop new ones to control craving. Some researchers believe that craving is a psychological manifestation of dopamine depletion and have tried dopamine agonists (e.g., bromocriptine, amantadine), either alone or in combination with neurotransmitter precursors, for the early recovery phase of cocaine treatment.

The selective serotonin reuptake inhibitors (e.g., fluoxetine, sertraline) are also being investigated because cocaine has been shown to impede serotonin uptake. Other drugs that are currently being explored include carbamazepine, mazindol, and buprenorphine, as well as new compounds being developed that target the cocaine binding site on the dopamine transporter. Although over 30 medications have been tried for cocaine treatment, at this time there is no generally effective medication.

Nicotine Dependence

Effective pharmacotherapy is now available for nicotine dependence. The medications work via the principle of drug substitution. Nicotine gum, an intradermal nicotine patch, and an oral nicotine inhaler are now all available. Many patients have had difficulty with the gum because it must be chewed slowly; the saliva must be held in the mouth for a certain period of time; and many pieces of gum must be chewed throughout the day. The nicotine patch appears to have greater patient acceptance. Although most patients who use the patch resume their cigarette use, enough succeed in stopping smoking that the use appears justified. Combining the patch with behavioral treatment appears to double the success rate, but many physicians who recommend the patch to their patients do not help them receive additional therapy. At present, the patch is not recommended for patients who have acute cardiovascular disease, are pregnant, or have an allergic reaction. There has been some concern that patients who continue to smoke while using the patch may be more likely to have a myocardial infarction. Because of the extremely detrimental effects of chronic cigarette smoking, pharmacological strategies that are even partially successful or have some limitations are useful. The antidepressant bupropion was recently approved by the FDA as the first aid for smoking cessation that does not involve nicotine replacement.

References Cited

Breier, A., D. S. Charney, and G. R. Heninger. Agoraphobia with panic attacks: development, diagnostic stability, and course of illness. Archives of General Psychiatry 43:1029–1036, 1986.

Christie, K. A., et al. Epidemiologic evidence for early onset of mental disorders and higher risk of drug abuse in young adults. American Journal of Psychiatry 145:971–975, 1988.

Donovan, D. M. Assessment of addictive behaviors: implications of an emerging biopsychosocial model. *In* Assessment of Addictive Behaviors. Donovan, D. M., and G. A. Marlatt (editors). New York, Guilford Press, 1988.

Ewing, J. A. Detecting alcoholism: the CAGE questionnaire. Journal of the American Medical Association 252(14):1905–1907, 1984.

Kaij, L. Alcoholism in Twins: Studies on the Etiology and Sequelaes of Abuse of Alcohol. Stockholm, Almqvist and Wiksell, 1960.

Kaufman, E., and J. Reoux. Guidelines for the successful psychotherapy of substance abusers. American Journal of Drug and Alcohol Abuse 14(2):199–209, 1988.

Peele, S. A moral vision of addiction: how people's values determine whether they become and remain addicts. *In* Peele, S. (editor). Visions of Addiction: Major Contemporary Perspectives on Addiction and Alcoholism. Lexington, Kentucky, Lexington Books, D. C. Heath and Company, 1988.

Rounsaville, B. J., et al. Psychopathology as a predictor of treatment outcome in alcoholics. Archives of General Psychiatry 44:505–513, 1987.

Robins, L. N., et al. Lifetime prevalence of specific psychiatric disorders in three sites. Archives of General Psychiatry 41:949–958, 1984.

Schuckit, M. A. Subjective responses to alcohol in sons of alcoholics and control subjects. Archives of General Psychiatry 41:879–884, 1984.

Selzer, M. L. The Michigan Alcoholism Screening Test: the quest for a new diagnostic instrument. American Journal of Psychiatry 127:1653–1658, 1971.

Selzer, M. L., A. Vinokur, and L. van Rooijen. A self-administered short version of the Michigan Alcoholism Screening Test (SMAST). Journal of Studies of Alcohol 36:1157–1170, 1975.

Sokol, R. J., S. S. Martier, and J. W. Alger. The T-ACE questions: practical prenatal detection of risk-drinking. American Journal of Obstetrics and Gynecology 160:863–870, 1989.

Vaillant, G. E. The Natural History of Alcoholism: Causes, Patterns, and Paths to Recovery. Cambridge, Massachusetts, Harvard University Press, 1983.

Vaillant, G. E., and E. S. Milofsky. The etiology of alcoholism: a prospective viewpoint. American Psychologist 37:216–232, 1982.

Wolff, P. H. Ethnic differences in alcohol sensitivity. Science 175:449–450, 1972.

Woodruff, R. A., et al. Alcoholism and depression. Archives of General Psychiatry 28:97–100, 1973.

Zucker, R. A., and E. S. Lisansky-Gomberg. Etiology of alcoholism reconsidered: the case for a biopsychosocial process. American Psychologist 41(7):783–793, 1986.

Selected Readings

Galanter, M., and H. D. Kleber (editors). Textbook of Substance Abuse Treatment. Washington, D. C., American Psychiatric Press, 1994.

Goodwin, D. W., et al. Alcohol problems in adoptees raised apart from alcoholic biological parents. Archives of General Psychiatry 28:238–243, 1973.

Helzer, J. E., and T. R. Pryzbeck. The co-occurrence of alcoholism with other psychiatric disorders in the general population and its impact on treatment. Journal of Studies of Alcohol 49:219–224, 1988.

Lowinson, J. H., P. Ruiz, and R. B. Millman (editors). Substance Abuse: A Comprehensive Textbook. Philadelphia, Williams & Wilkins, 1992.

Meyer, R. E. How to understand the relationships between psychopathology and addictive disorders: another example of the chicken and the egg. *In* Meyer, R. E. (editor). Psychopathology and Addictive Disorders. New York, Guilford Press, 1986.

CHAPTER EIGHT

PERSONALITY DISORDERS

MICHAEL H. STONE, MD, ERIC R. MARCUS, MD, AND JANIS L. CUTLER, MD

To a much greater extent than is the case for most other psychiatric disorders, the behaviors and emotions that characterize patients with personality disorders can be observed in most people at one time or another. A crucial difference, however, is that people who have personality disorders continue to repeat certain maladaptive behaviors even though they result in unfortunate social and occupational consequences, whereas people who do not have personality disorders learn from negative experiences and change their behavior in order to avoid negative consequences in the future.

The **stereotyped repetition** of maladaptive behaviors is a key feature of personality disorders. Another is the rigidity with which patients develop such maladaptive behaviors in the first place. Instead of using realistic social and environmental clues to form assumptions of other people and their motives, they rely on their own distorted perceptions. These erroneous assumptions then become the bases for their behavior, which frequently elicits from other people the very reactions they dread. This **pattern** thus reinforces their suspicions about others, and continues the vicious circle. In a way, these patients are trapped in a prison of their own making and do not realize that they hold the key to their release.

➠ One young man, for example, was suspicious of other people because he believed they disliked him. These thoughts made his behavior and attitudes so aggressive and obnoxious that people did, in fact, dislike him, thus confirming his predetermined belief. The patient thought his distrust was a reaction to others' negative feelings for him. He did not realize that his attitude and resulting behavior caused others to dislike him. ⬅

Physicians, in particular, must be careful not to affirm such self-fulfilling prophecies in their patients; instead, they should identify and gradually point out to patients how their pathological attitudes have brought about emotional and behavioral difficulties that negatively affect their social and occupational functioning. (See Table 8–1 for the general DSM-IV criteria for personality disorders.)

Personality disorders are some of the most difficult psychiatric disorders for inexperienced medical students or physicians to understand and recognize. There are several reasons for this difficulty. First, the concept of **personality** is abstract, complex, and not readily definable in clear, concrete terms. In fact, personality is mainly observed only in relation to others. This important aspect is reflected in the word *personality,* which derives from the Latin *per* (through) and *sonare* (to make a sound). This word combination referred to a voice projection technique used by actors before modern amplification systems were invented. Small megaphones inside their masks helped actors project their voices to every seat in the amphitheater, thus magnifying and expressing the personalities of the characters that they portrayed.

Personality is expressed in an infinite number of ways, and the line between functional and dysfunctional personalities is often difficult to determine. Also, patients with personality disorders may appear to be quite normal when first seen, having only a few complaints and exhibiting only minimal signs of psychopathology during an interview. Finally, the diagnosis of personality disorders can be made only after patterns of maladaptive behavior have been discerned, which usually cannot be done during a brief interview.

DIAGNOSTIC AND CLINICAL FEATURES

Personality disorders begin in late adolescence and persist throughout adulthood. Because the personality disorders mainly affect **interpersonal relationships,** they may be extremely disruptive and cause the patient an enormous amount of suffering. In order to encourage physicians and researchers not to overlook personality disorders, as well as to take into account the frequent comorbidity of these disorders with other psychiatric disorders, the multiaxial system of the DSM-IV assigns personality disorders to **Axis II.** Mental retardation is the only other disorder on Axis II because it, too, tends to be a lifelong, core aspect of the affected individual's psychological makeup. All other psychiatric disorders are coded on Axis I. This multiaxial system requires that physicians consider the possibility of a personality disorder for every patient with a suspected psychiatric illness. The psychiatrists involved with the de-

TABLE 8–1. DSM-IV General Diagnostic Criteria for a Personality Disorder

A. An enduring pattern of inner experience and behavior that deviates markedly from the expectations of the individual's culture. This pattern is manifested in two (or more) of the following areas:
  (1) cognition (i.e., ways of perceiving and interpreting self, other people, and events)
  (2) affectivity (i.e., the range, intensity, lability, and appropriateness of emotional response)
  (3) interpersonal functioning
  (4) impulse control
B. The enduring pattern is inflexible and pervasive across a broad range of personal and social situations.
C. The enduring pattern leads to clinically significant distress or impairment in social, occupational, or other important areas of functioning.
D. The pattern is stable and of long duration and its onset can be traced back at least to adolescence or early adulthood.
E. The enduring pattern is not better accounted for as a manifestation or consequence of another mental disorder.
F. The enduring pattern is not due to the direct physiological effects of a substance (e.g., a drug of abuse, a medication) or a general medical condition (e.g., head trauma).

velopment of the DSM were concerned that this consideration might not be given if the personality disorders were included with the disorders on Axis I, especially if one of the more obvious Axis I disorders was also present.

Indications of a personality disorder are chronic unhappiness that has lasted for many years, abnormal social behavior that has disrupted the patient's interpersonal relationships, a pattern of dramatic changes in personality, behaviors or attitudes that so disrupt the physician-patient relationship that rendering medical care is difficult or impossible, failures to succeed at work or to relate well to others on the job or in social situations for a period of years, and failure to progress through the normal phases of developmental maturation.

One distinction between the personality disorders and the Axis I disorders is that personality disorders tend to be **egosyntonic,** which means that patients regard their maladaptive patterns of behavior and emotional responses as part of themselves and not the result of a disease process. In contrast, most other psychiatric disorders are **egodystonic,** which means that patients are aware of and complain about symptoms that they regard as foreign and separate from themselves.

The DSM-IV identifies ten personality disorders that have been fully accepted as psychiatric disorders. They are the paranoid, schizoid, schizotypal, antisocial, borderline, histrionic, narcissistic, avoidant, dependent, and obsessive-compulsive personality disorders. These disorders have well-defined characteristics, based on the observations of many psychiatrists; their manifestations are obvious and consistent; and they are common in psychiatric patients. The DSM-IV categories are discrete and do not overlap (insofar as this is possible). Two other personality disorders, depressive personality disorder and

passive-aggressive personality disorder, have been included provisionally (their validity is still being studied). There are probably more personality disorders, but the ten categories in the DSM-IV are the ones about which there is the greatest agreement. The DSM-IV description of each disorder serves as a useful starting point for the physician. Because most patients have more than one personality disorder, the "pure" form of a personality disorder, which is found in patients with only one personality disorder, is less commonly seen.

In deference to the widespread clinical practice of diagnosing personality disorders on the basis of interrelated collections of traits, the DSM-IV diagnostic criteria are organized **polythetically.** Each disorder is defined by four or more behavioral features. About two-thirds of the features must be present before the diagnosis can be justified, which means that different patients with the same personality disorder may not have the same diagnostic features. In the case of borderline personality disorder, for example, a minimum of five features (from the possible nine) must be present. This may be any five (or more) of the nine (there are 256 different combinations). Some combinations are rarely seen, whereas others are common.

Physicians new to the field of psychiatry may be overwhelmed by the number of personality disorders, each with its own set of behavioral criteria. In clinical practice, it is more important to recognize that a personality disorder is present than to pinpoint the exact disorder, because the best treatment approach does not necessarily require a specific diagnosis. Researchers must make specific diagnoses, however, in order to facilitate epidemiological, phenomenological, and treatment studies.

The number of persons with personality disorders in the general population cannot be easily estimated because different criteria have been used in diagnosing these disorders over the years. Aberrations of personality have a wide spectrum, and the point at which an aberration becomes a disorder is somewhat arbitrary. Wherever the cutoff point is set will determine whether a disorder is rare or comparatively common. In Srole's 1962 Midtown Manhattan epidemiological study, 10% of the 1660 interviewees had a "probable personality disorder," according to the Minnesota Multiphasic Personality Interview (MMPI). In 1984, Robins and her colleagues found that the **lifetime prevalence** of personality disorders was about 3%, according to the DSM-III criteria. In 1986, Casey and Tyrer found, in a random population sample in England, that 10% of their subjects had a personality disorder and another 7% had a significant "personality difficulty" that did not meet the criteria for a disorder. Although these data are dependent on the sampling methods and criteria used and on varying cultural factors, they give some clue as to the prevalence of personality disorders. In 1993, Weissman's update estimated a lifetime prevalence of personality disorders of 10–13% and reviewed the methodological difficulties inherent in obtaining more accurate data. The estimated lifetime rates for specific disorders are paranoid personality disorder, 0.4–1.8%; schizoid personality disorder, 0.5–0.8%; schizotypal personality disorder, 0.6–5.6%; antisocial personality disorder, 3%; borderline personality disorder, 1.1–4.6%; histrionic personality disorder, 1.3–3%; narcissistic personality disorder, 0.4%; avoidant personality disorder, 0.4–1.3%; dependent personality disorder, 1.6–6.7%; and obsessive-compulsive personality disorder, 1.7–6.4%.

The patterns of distribution across gender lines are fairly clear. Paranoid, antisocial, narcissistic, and obsessive-compulsive personality disorders are diagnosed more frequently in men. Borderline personality disorder is more prevalent in women. Histrionic and dependent personality disorders appear to occur with equal frequency in men and women.

Personality Disorder Clusters

In the DSM-IV, the disorders are divided into three clusters: cluster A, the eccentric disorders; cluster B, the dramatic disorders; and cluster C, the anxious disorders. The disorders in each cluster share certain prominent features (Table 8–2). The eccentric cluster is made up of the schizoid, schizotypal, and paranoid personality disorders, in which odd social behavior tends to be the common feature. The dramatic cluster consists of the histrionic, narcissistic, antisocial, and borderline personality disorders, in which a tendency to take action, impulsivity, and externalization (i.e., not taking personal responsibility for behavior; blaming the outside world instead) may be characteristic. The anxious cluster contains the obsessive-compulsive, dependent, and avoidant personality disorders, in which anxiety and inhibition are prominent features. A patient in any of the clusters may not have the most prominent characteristics of that cluster (e.g., many patients with narcissistic, histrionic, and antisocial personality disorders are not impulsive or prone to action).

Eccentric Cluster

The eccentric cluster (schizoid, schizotypal, and paranoid personality disorders) includes patients who tend to have odd interpersonal relationships as

TABLE 8–2. Prototypical Traits of Major Personality Disorder Clusters

Cluster A: Eccentric
  Schizoid: Aloof
  Paranoid: Guarded, touchy
  Schizotypal: Eccentric
Cluster B: Dramatic
  Narcissistic: Self-important
  Antisocial: Glib, thrill-seeking
  Histrionic: Dramatic
  Borderline: Unreasonable, unstable
Cluster C: Anxious disorders
  Obsessive-compulsive: Emotionally constricted
  Avoidant: Timorous, unadventurous
  Dependent: Clingy

TABLE 8–3. DSM-IV Diagnostic Criteria for Schizoid Personality Disorder

A. A pervasive pattern of detachment from social relationships and a restricted range of expression of emotions in interpersonal settings, beginning by early adulthood and present in a variety of contexts, as indicated by four (or more) of the following:
  (1) neither desires nor enjoys close relationships, including being part of a family
  (2) almost always chooses solitary activities
  (3) has little, if any, interest in having sexual experiences with another person
  (4) takes pleasure in few, if any, activities
  (5) lacks close friends or confidants other than first-degree relatives
  (6) appears indifferent to the praise or criticism of others
  (7) shows emotional coldness, detachment, or flattened affectivity
B. Does not occur exclusively during the course of Schizophrenia, a Mood Disorder With Psychotic Features, another Psychotic Disorder, or a Pervasive Developmental Disorder and is not due to the direct physiological effects of a general medical condition.
Note: If criteria are met prior to the onset of Schizophrenia, add "Premorbid," e.g., "Schizoid Personality Disorder (Premorbid)."

a prominent feature. The schizoid and schizotypal personality disorders may be attenuated forms of a genetic predisposition to schizophrenia.

Schizoid patients are withdrawn and aloof (Table 8–3). They have little contact with other people, and the contact they do have tends to be rudimentary and work-related. They do not socialize much and seem not to mind the lack of interpersonal relationships. This lack of concern about their **isolation** is in contrast to the other personality disorders, particularly avoidant personality disorder, in which patients are anxious about their interactions and do have a few relationships. The tendency of schizoid patients to isolate themselves from others is egosyntonic behavior. For this reason, these patients rarely consult a psychiatrist, unless a coexisting egodystonic psychiatric disorder requires attention. ⬛➡ For example, a 40-year-old unmarried woman worked 16 hours a day as an actuarial accountant in the "back office" of a large corporation. She had been a steady, reliable employee for many years. She did not socialize with anyone and had only the most perfunctory contact with her coworkers. She had an active fantasy life, however. She had been composing a novel, in her mind, that progressed from day to day over the course of years. She planned to commit the novel to paper someday, but that day never arrived. She was not terribly upset about this, because she was not sure that she wanted to share this most personal aspect of herself. She did not feel unfulfilled in life but, rather, she felt secretly triumphant. This information was revealed only when she became engaged in psychiatric treatment for a major depressive episode, which occurred after severe hypertension was detected during a routine physical examination. ⬛➡

Schizotypal patients appear to others as quite **odd** (Table 8–4). Their magical thinking, idiosyn-

TABLE 8–4. DSM-IV Diagnostic Criteria for Schizotypal Personality Disorder

A. A pervasive pattern of social and interpersonal deficits marked by acute discomfort with, and reduced capacity for, close relationships as well as by cognitive or perceptual distortions and eccentricities of behavior, beginning by early adulthood and present in a variety of contexts, as indicated by five (or more) of the following:
  (1) ideas of reference (excluding delusions of reference)
  (2) odd beliefs or magical thinking that influences behavior and is inconsistent with subcultural norms (e.g., superstitiousness, belief in clairvoyance, telepathy, or "sixth sense"; in children and adolescents, bizarre fantasies or preoccupations)
  (3) unusual perceptual experiences, including bodily illusions
  (4) odd thinking and speech (e.g., vague, circumstantial, metaphorical, overelaborate, or stereotyped)
  (5) suspiciousness or paranoid ideation
  (6) inappropriate or constricted affect
  (7) behavior or appearance that is odd, eccentric, or peculiar
  (8) lack of close friends or confidants other than first-degree relatives
  (9) excessive social anxiety that does not diminish with familiarity and tends to be associated with paranoid fears rather than negative judgments about self
B. Does not occur exclusively during the course of Schizophrenia, a Mood Disorder With Psychotic Features, another Psychotic Disorder, or a Pervasive Developmental Disorder.
Note: If criteria are met prior to the onset of Schizophrenia, add "Premorbid," e.g., "Schizotypal Personality Disorder (Premorbid)."

cratic thought processes, and unusual beliefs are nearly psychotic, but they are able to engage in reality testing. ➡ For example, a single male mathematics professor in his fifties had a circle of acquaintances who tolerated him but found him to be weird. They were amused by his convoluted, difficult-to-follow theories about world politics and philosophy. He seemed to be unable to develop more intimate relationships and became quite suspicious when anyone tried to get close to him. ⬅ Schizotypal patients tend to have closer emotional connections with other people than do other patients in the eccentric cluster. As with many of the personality disorders, the severity of personality dysfunction varies greatly among schizotypal patients, ranging from a relatively fragmented personality in patients who can barely function socially and occupationally to a more integrated personality in patients who function well at work and in relationships where their eccentricity is tolerated.

Paranoid patients have an **angry mistrust** of other people (Table 8–5). These patients see plots against them wherever they go and feel that all actions by other people are motivated by anger, greed, and a wish to betray others. As one paranoid patient remarked, "Doc, I get up in the morning, I smoke a cigarette, and I think, 'Who's gonna try to screw me today?'" Paranoid patients fall into one of two general categories: those who are relatively warm and outgoing with friends and family but have hostile interactions with the rest of humanity, and those who are guarded, aloof, sullen, suspicious, and interact with few people. Some paranoid patients do marry.

The spouse is often a compliant but distant person who leaves the patient alone or is a warm, involved person who tries to take care of the patient, mediating the patient's suspicious interactions with the outside world and putting up with the patient's anger and abuse.

Dramatic Cluster

The dramatic cluster consists of the histrionic, narcissistic, antisocial, and borderline personality disorders. The most common is the **histrionic personality disorder** (formerly called hysterical personality). Histrionic patients are **dramatic** and highly emotional; their emotional storms are not as severe as those seen in patients with borderline personality disorder. Healthier patients experience disruptions in psychosexual functioning but have deep stable friendships and work relationships. Patients with a more severe form of the disorder experience disruption in almost all of their interpersonal relationships (Table 8–6).

➡ For example, a hard-working, highly successful litigation attorney, who had worked her way up the ranks in a large law firm, was well thought of at work but was prone to temper tantrums, particularly when she was under stress. These tantrums would end as abruptly as they began. The patient felt much relief afterward, but those around her felt shaken and emotionally abused. The attorney was particularly upset about her perception that the firm's senior partners were too busy to spend enough time supervising her. Although she worked long hours, she had a circle of warm friendships. Her best friend was her mature, calm, patient boyfriend, with whom she had been living for three years. Whenever he raised the

TABLE 8–5. DSM-IV Diagnostic Criteria for Paranoid Personality Disorder

A. A pervasive distrust and suspiciousness of others such that their motives are interpreted as malevolent, beginning by early adulthood and present in a variety of contexts, as indicated by four (or more) of the following:
  (1) suspects, without sufficient basis, that others are exploiting, harming, or deceiving him or her
  (2) is preoccupied with unjustified doubts about the loyalty or trustworthiness of friends or associates
  (3) is reluctant to confide in others because of unwarranted fear that the information will be used maliciously against him or her
  (4) reads hidden demeaning or threatening meanings into benign remarks or events
  (5) persistently bears grudges, i.e., is unforgiving of insults, injuries, or slights
  (6) perceives attacks on his or her character or reputation that are not apparent to others and is quick to react angrily or to counterattack
  (7) has recurrent suspicions, without justification, regarding fidelity of spouse or sexual partner
B. Does not occur exclusively during the course of Schizophrenia, a Mood Disorder With Psychotic Features, or another Psychotic Disorder and is not due to the direct physiological effects of a general medical condition.
Note: If criteria are met prior to the onset of Schizophrenia, add "Premorbid," e.g., "Paranoid Personality Disorder (Premorbid)."

TABLE 8–6.   DSM-IV Diagnostic Criteria for Histrionic Personality Disorder

A pervasive pattern of excessive emotionality and attention seeking, beginning by early adulthood and present in a variety of contexts, as indicated by five (or more) of the following:
  (1) is uncomfortable in situations in which he or she is not the center of attention
  (2) interaction with others is often characterized by inappropriate sexually seductive or provocative behavior
  (3) displays rapidly shifting and shallow expression of emotions
  (4) consistently uses physical appearance to draw attention to self
  (5) has a style of speech that is excessively impressionistic and lacking in detail
  (6) shows self-dramatization, theatricality, and exaggerated expression of emotion
  (7) is suggestible, i.e., easily influenced by others or circumstances
  (8) considers relationships to be more intimate than they actually are

issue of marriage, she would procrastinate in making a commitment because she was not sexually attracted to him. Her sexual interest was expressed through a long-standing affair she had been having with a coworker, who was two years older than she and whom she found intensely exciting, dramatically vibrant, but highly unreliable.

She was motivated to consult a psychiatrist because of two issues. First, her boss finally lost his temper when she had a particularly heated outburst. Perhaps more crucially, her live-in boyfriend had set a deadline by which she would either have to accept his marriage proposal or the relationship would end. She had become extremely preoccupied with this life decision and had symptoms of intense anxiety, tearfulness, insomnia, anorexia, and intermittent panic. She felt that if she did not marry her boyfriend, she would lose her dearest friend, but, on the other hand, she did not want to have a sexless marriage and did not want to continue having an affair once she was married. In addition, the man with whom she was having the affair was a bachelor who was busily pursuing his career and other women. She was not really sure whether she could live with him, anyway. She described her dilemma as "life problems." She did not think that a psychiatrist could help her except, perhaps, to prescribe "some valium" for her anxiety. ◄

This formulation is typical of the egosyntonicity and externalization of most people with personality disorders. It is also typical for a patient to seek treatment during a crisis that is complicated by egodystonic symptoms. In this case, the symptoms are anxiety and depression consistent with a diagnosis of adjustment disorder with mixed anxiety and depressed mood. Another common presenting diagnosis for such patients is a major depressive episode.

The above case illustrates the DSM-IV diagnostic criteria for histrionic personality disorder, which include emotional lability, self-dramatization, and the need to be the center of attention. Conflict about sex-

uality also tends to be one of the core issues for patients with this personality disorder.

Patients with **narcissistic personality disorder** struggle with massive problems of self-esteem. They have reparative personality features of **superiority, grandiosity,** and **contempt** for other people (Table 8–7). The degree of dysfunction can range from relatively healthy to nearly psychotic. Their fantasies are always grandiose, and their manner of relating to others varies from haughty and controlling to contemptuously ingratiating.

► For example, a 50-year-old biochemistry professor managed a busy laboratory at a university that was staffed by junior faculty members, teaching fellows, graduate students, and technicians. He was known as a brilliant slave driver who pushed people to their limits and beyond. If a staff member "burnt out" and left, the professor would become angry and complain about what that person had done to him. Always planning the next big breakthrough, he idealized new people when they began working but blamed them later on for failing to "make it big." After this, he ignored them and demoted them in the social hierarchy of the laboratory from a "chosen one" to a common worker. His life was filled with such disappointments in people. He felt that he would be much better known if only he could find good help.

He also saw his wife and children as extensions of his self-esteem system. He and his wife were married when they were both in graduate school. His wife had also been a brilliant biochemistry student, as well as a faithful, loyal person. Her brilliant mind and personal character had attracted him to her. After they were married, however, he demanded that she become highly fashionable, socially ambitious, and politically sophisticated, even though she had no interest in these things. He wanted her to stay at home and take care of their children but was also bit-

TABLE 8–7.   DSM-IV Diagnostic Criteria for Narcissistic Personality Disorder

A pervasive pattern of grandiosity (in fantasy or behavior), need for admiration, and lack of empathy, beginning by early adulthood and present in a variety of contexts, as indicated by five (or more) of the following:
  (1) has a grandiose sense of self-importance (e.g., exaggerates achievements and talents, expects to be recognized as superior without commensurate achievements)
  (2) is preoccupied with fantasies of unlimited success, power, brilliance, beauty, or ideal love
  (3) believes that he or she is "special" and unique and can only be understood by, or should associate with, other special or high-status people (or institutions)
  (4) requires excessive admiration
  (5) has a sense of entitlement, i.e., unreasonable expectations of especially favorable treatment or automatic compliance with his or her expectations
  (6) is interpersonally exploitative, i.e., takes advantage of others to achieve his or her own ends
  (7) lacks empathy: is unwilling to recognize or identify with the feelings and needs of others
  (8) is often envious of others or believes that others are envious of him or her
  (9) shows arrogant, haughty behaviors or attitudes

terly disappointed that she had progressively lost touch with the field of biochemistry and therefore could not help him with his intellectual pursuits. He was sorry that he had married her.

This history makes painfully clear that the patient is grandiose, exploitive of others, and lacking in empathy. The circumstances in which he sought psychiatric treatment are characteristic of narcissistic patients. When an application for a grant was turned down, he became unhappy, bitter, and angry. He tried to make himself feel better by having an affair with a vivacious, outgoing young graduate student who worked in his laboratory. His wife found out about the affair several months later. She threatened to leave him and hired a lawyer to draw up separation papers. The patient felt wronged and misunderstood by her and wondered what had happened to her sense of loyalty and family values. ◄█

Patients with **antisocial personality disorder** (who were formerly known as psychopathic or sociopathic patients) tend to attack the trust and caring of other persons (Table 8–8). The level of severity of the illness varies a great deal, as do the number of other personality disorders that may coexist. Antisocial patients would rather do things illegally than legally. They have a desire to manipulate and cheat, which may be a deep-rooted grandiose motive or a defense against feelings of inferiority and incompetence, or both. Either way, their behavior is devastating to interpersonal relationships. They live in an "eat-or-be-eaten" world surrounded by sycophantic people who they do not really trust or by masochistically submissive people over whom they have a domineering power. A striking feature of these patients is their **lack of remorse** for wrongdoing.

Although the interpersonal relationships of antisocial patients are often troubled, some patients are nonetheless able to rise to very high positions. In some ways, their unscrupulousness can be used to

TABLE 8–8. DSM-IV Diagnostic Criteria for Antisocial Personality Disorder

A. There is a pervasive pattern of disregard for and violation of the rights of others occurring since age 15 years, as indicated by three (or more) of the following:
  (1) failure to conform to social norms with respect to lawful behaviors as indicated by repeatedly performing acts that are grounds for arrest
  (2) deceitfulness, as indicated by repeated lying, use of aliases, or conning others for personal profit or pleasure
  (3) impulsivity or failure to plan ahead
  (4) irritability and aggressiveness, as indicated by repeated physical fights or assaults
  (5) reckless disregard for safety of self or others
  (6) consistent irresponsibility, as indicated by repeated failure to sustain consistent work behavior or honor financial obligations
  (7) lack of remorse, as indicated by being indifferent to or rationalizing having hurt, mistreated, or stolen from another
B. The individual is at least age 18 years.
C. There is evidence of Conduct Disorder with onset before age 15 years.
D. The occurrence of antisocial behavior is not exclusively during the course of Schizophrenia or a Manic Episode.

their advantage in the progression of their career. The following example is typical of the circumstances in which the more highly functioning, less severely impaired patients might find themselves. The information provided is not sufficient to meet the DSM-IV diagnostic criteria for antisocial personality disorder, because a long-standing pattern of behavior is not described. However, if a history similar to the following is elicited from a patient, the psychiatrist should look for such a pattern.

█► A 36-year-old accountant at a major Wall Street firm felt that he was being unfairly treated and not given enough recognition and support at work. He wanted to transfer to the trading desk, where the excitement and action were, but because he did not have a graduate business degree, his boss thought that it was not worth the effort required to train him. He was competent at performing routine, mundane tasks, but he wanted more and felt that his ambition had been thwarted. He decided to prove himself by making a few trades on his own, using his boss's name to execute the orders.

At first, he used his own savings and did moderately well. After several months, he began "borrowing" small and then moderate sums from other accounts and entered into riskier trading situations that he thought he understood. Knowing when audits would occur, he moved money from one account to another to avoid the day of reckoning. He might have gotten away with this scheme for longer than he did if he had not been tempted to show his boss how well he was doing after he had had a successful week of trading "on paper." He still hoped to get transferred to the trading desk, where he might rapidly recoup his losses and pay off his debts. His boss, who was nobody's fool, wondered how he had managed to do so well. He also pointed out that the employee did not have permission to dabble in this area. Because the employee responded with anger, the boss began to ask pointed questions about the reasoning and rationale behind the trades. The patient answered glibly, revealing his superficial level of knowledge and increasing the boss's suspicions. A full-scale audit of the trades was conducted, which exposed the entire affair and the actual long-term losses.

In order to spare the firm notoriety, the boss bailed out the patient, covered the losses, and switched the account to an experienced trader to recoup some of the money. He also fired the patient. The patient's wife insisted that he go to a psychiatrist, which totally perplexed him because he did not feel that there was anything wrong with him. In fact, he believed that if his boss had only been more understanding and given him another couple of months, everything would have worked out fine. He saw this incident as just one more example of how the world had always treated him unfairly and how following the rules was useless. He claimed that nobody in his business followed the rules, and he could not see what was so different about what he had done. ◄█

The last disorder in the dramatic cluster is **borderline personality disorder.** The term *borderline* originally referred to the "border" between psychosis and neurosis but is currently used to describe a specific personality disorder, which has been given a new set of descriptors in the DSM-IV. In the past, the descriptor *psychotic* frequently described a patient who was severely disturbed; it is now used in a much more precise manner to indicate an absence of reality testing (see Chapter 1, The Psychiatric Interview). The DSM-IV diagnostic criteria for borderline personality disorder focus on emotional and interpersonal **instability** and **impulsivity.** Abnormal feeling states and **self-destructive behavior** are the main features (Table 8–9).

Many clinicians believe that patients who do not meet all of the DSM-IV criteria for borderline personality disorder should be considered to have a **"borderline character structure,"** according to the original meaning of the term. Otto Kernberg, a psychoanalyst and psychiatrist with a particular interest in these patients, conceived of this character structure as encompassing three key features: **identity diffusion, primitive defense mechanisms,** and **intact reality testing.** The presence of the first two characteristics distinguishes these patients from those who function with a healthier "neurotic character structure," while the presence of the third characteristic distinguishes them from patients who are overtly psychotic. According to this approach, most patients in the eccentric cluster and most with narcissistic and antisocial personality disorders have a borderline character structure. Some patients in the dramatic and anxious clusters may also range between neurotic and borderline. The distinction between these two categories

may be more useful than the DSM-IV categories in predicting the prognosis and suggesting appropriate therapeutic interventions (see Treatment, below).

Identity diffusion is associated with behavior that lacks social and professional direction. Patients have a chameleonlike capacity to fit into any group they are with at any time, e.g., being the life of the party with boisterous college buddies but quietly contemplative with other friends. Although many people show different aspects of themselves in different settings, patients with identity diffusion take this characteristic to an extreme. They genuinely seem to have no coherent sense of themselves and, thus, their entire persona seems to change effortlessly. This fluidity extends to their perceptions of other people as well. These perceptions also shift in response to immediate circumstances and are closely linked with the primitive defense mechanisms of splitting and projection. In **splitting,** ambiguity and shades of gray in interpersonal relationships are eliminated, so that the patient sees the self and others in clearly demarcated categories of black and white. **Projection** attributes thoughts and feelings that are uncomfortable to acknowledge as one's own to other people . ➥ For example, a 23-year-old woman was angry with her sister for not returning her phone call. She described her as "unreliable, self-centered, and cold." That evening, the sister did call, and the next day, the patient spoke lovingly of her as "warm and supportive, the perfect big sister." ◄▪

One primitive defense mechanism particularly characteristic of patients with borderline personality disorder is **acting out.** Patients put their feelings into actions in order to avoid the feelings (which are usually, but not always, unpleasant) and soothe themselves. The emotional state of such patients is labile and intense, and the connections between their feelings and actions are not consciously apparent to them. As with all defense mechanisms, the entire process occurs at an unconscious level. Impulse control tends to be impaired, and the actions may be quite destructive. ➥ For example, a patient with a history of alcohol abuse had been abstinent for six months. While her psychiatrist was away on vacation, she went to a bar and got drunk. She woke up the next morning in bed with a man whom she vaguely remembered meeting in the bar. The patient was not aware of any connection between the feelings of anger and loneliness caused by her psychiatrist's absence and the self-destructive behavior until her psychiatrist pointed it out to her. ◄▪

Drug and alcohol abuse, binge eating, sexual promiscuity, self-mutilation, and suicide attempts are typical of the extreme forms that acting out can take. Obviously, such behaviors can have deleterious consequences, and they must be addressed early in treatment. The self-destructive behavior of the patient described above was actually significantly healthier than it had been several months earlier. On two previous occasions when her psychiatrist was on vacation, she had taken a drug overdose.

TABLE 8–9. DSM-IV Diagnostic Criteria for Borderline Personality Disorder

A pervasive pattern of instability of interpersonal relationships, self-image, and affects, and marked impulsivity beginning by early adulthood and present in a variety of contexts, as indicated by five (or more) of the following:

(1) frantic efforts to avoid real or imagined abandonment. **Note:** Do not include suicidal or self-mutilating behavior covered in Criterion 5.

(2) a pattern of unstable and intense interpersonal relationships characterized by alternating between extremes of idealization and devaluation

(3) identity disturbance: markedly and persistently unstable self-image or sense of self

(4) impulsivity in at least two areas that are potentially self-damaging (e.g., spending, sex, substance abuse, reckless driving, binge eating). **Note:** Do not include suicidal or self-mutilating behavior covered in Criterion 5.

(5) recurrent suicidal behavior, gestures, or threats, or self-mutilating behavior

(6) affective instability due to a marked reactivity of mood (e.g., intense episodic dysphoria, irritability, or anxiety usually lasting a few hours and only rarely more than a few days)

(7) chronic feelings of emptiness

(8) inappropriate, intense anger or difficulty controlling anger (e.g., frequent displays of temper, constant anger, recurrent physical fights)

(9) transient, stress-related paranoid ideation or severe dissociative symptoms

TABLE 8–10.   DSM-IV Diagnostic Criteria for Obsessive-Compulsive Personality Disorder

A pervasive pattern of preoccupation with orderliness, perfectionism, and mental and interpersonal control, at the expense of flexibility, openness, and efficiency, beginning by early adulthood and present in a variety of contexts, as indicated by four (or more) of the following:

(1) is preoccupied with details, rules, lists, order, organization, or schedules to the extent that the major point of the activity is lost

(2) shows perfectionism that interferes with task completion (e.g., is unable to complete a project because his or her own overly strict standards are not met)

(3) is excessively devoted to work and productivity to the exclusion of leisure activities and friendships (not accounted for by obvious economic necessity)

(4) is overconscientious, scrupulous, and inflexible about matters of morality, ethics, or values (not accounted for by cultural or religious identification)

(5) is unable to discard worn-out or worthless objects even when they have no sentimental value

(6) is reluctant to delegate tasks or to work with others unless they submit to exactly his or her way of doing things

(7) adopts a miserly spending style toward both self and others; money is viewed as something to be hoarded for future catastrophes

(8) shows rigidity and stubbornness

Anxious Cluster

The three disorders in the anxious cluster are the obsessive-compulsive, avoidant, and dependent personality disorders.

Patients with **obsessive-compulsive personality disorder** have extremely controlled and controlling personalities and rigidly repress all emotions except anger. Their ability to confide in others and reveal themselves in an intimate setting is severely **constricted** (Table 8–10). The most successful patients are hard working, focused, and quite efficient and are therefore unusually productive. Anxiety, procrastination, and compulsive attention to detail rather than the "big picture" interfere with the productivity of the more severely ill patients. They fail to live up to their own ego ideal of being a "well-oiled machine." ➡ One such patient, a lawyer, was so meticulous about drafting each document assigned to her that she was constantly behind in her work. Her colleagues reviewed each draft once and then moved on to the next and were much more productive. ◄

Patients with **avoidant personality disorder** are chronically **anxious,** timorous, and unadventurous (Table 8–11). They respond to their fear of social situations by avoiding them, which can have serious repercussions in their work and personal lives. These patients are unable to find other ways of dealing with their fears. They worry that social situations will overwhelm them. This worry seems to represent an awareness on some level that their particular psychological conflicts will be stimulated beyond the capacity of their repertoire of defense mechanisms to maintain inner comfort. This personality disorder frequently coexists with narcissistic, histrionic, or paranoid personality disorders. ➡ For example, a 23-year-old aspiring novelist became "paralyzed" with anxiety whenever he thought about writing a story down on paper. He was excited about his ideas for characters and plots and would imagine himself as a famous best-selling author who was the center of attention. But the possibility of writing anything less than a perfect, astonishing first novel made him so anxious that he could never get beyond writing a rough outline. ◄

Patients with **dependent personality disorder** attach themselves to other people in an intense, desperate way, like anxious children clinging to parents. They are extractive and demanding (Table 8–12). Like avoidant patients, they may have a variety of coexisting Axis I or II disorders. Depression is common, as are histrionic, borderline, and narcissistic personality disorders. ➡ For example, a 26-year-old elementary schoolteacher who lived with her parents presented for treatment with major depression, which had developed during a three-month relationship with a fellow teacher. Although this man appeared to be quite interested in her and saw her every weekend, she ruminated during the week about why he did not call more frequently and whether he really cared for her. As they became more involved, she called him twice a day and still felt that it was not enough. ◄

Course of Illness

Many factors affect the course of illness in patients with personality disorders. The course varies from one personality disorder to another, as does the severity of each patient's disorder. The prognosis often depends more on the severity of the disorder than on the particular disorder that is present. The balance between positive and negative traits can also play an important role in the course. For example, the positive trait of "agreeableness" is associated with a good prognosis, regardless of any coexisting negative traits. By the same token, the negative trait of unlikableness (e.g., chronic hostility) predicts a

TABLE 8–11.   DSM-IV Diagnostic Criteria for Avoidant Personality Disorder

A pervasive pattern of social inhibition, feelings of inadequacy, and hypersensitivity to negative evaluation, beginning by early adulthood and present in a variety of contexts, as indicated by four (or more) of the following:

(1) avoids occupational activities that involve significant interpersonal contact, because of fears of criticism, disapproval, or rejection

(2) is unwilling to get involved with people unless certain of being liked

(3) shows restraint within intimate relationships because of the fear of being shamed or ridiculed

(4) is preoccupied with being criticized or rejected in social situations

(5) is inhibited in new interpersonal situations because of feelings of inadequacy

(6) views self as socially inept, personally unappealing, or inferior to others

(7) is unusually reluctant to take personal risks or to engage in any new activities because they may prove embarrassing

TABLE 8–12.   DSM-IV Diagnostic Criteria for Dependent Personality Disorder

A pervasive and excessive need to be taken care of that leads to submissive and clinging behavior and fears of separation, beginning by early adulthood and present in a variety of contexts, as indicated by five (or more) of the following:

(1) has difficulty making everyday decisions without an excessive amount of advice and reassurance from others
(2) needs others to assume responsibility for most major areas of his or her life
(3) has difficulty expressing disagreement with others because of fear of loss of support or approval. **Note:** Do not include realistic fears of retribution.
(4) has difficulty initiating projects or doing things on his or her own (because of a lack of self-confidence in judgment or abilities rather than a lack of motivation or energy)
(5) goes to excessive lengths to obtain nurturance and support from others, to the point of volunteering to do things that are unpleasant
(6) feels uncomfortable or helpless when alone because of exaggerated fears of being unable to care for himself or herself
(7) urgently seeks another relationship as a source of care and support when a close relationship ends
(8) is unrealistically preoccupied with fears of being left to take care of himself or herself

poor outcome, even in disorders that are considered less serious (e.g., a likable paranoid person may do better than an unlikable histrionic person).

By definition, all personality disorders begin in adolescence or early adulthood. The degree to which they are disruptive can vary a great deal, depending on the particular circumstances of the patient's life at any given time. (See the discussion of psychosocial changes across the adult life cycle in Chapter 13, Life Development.) The age at which the patient presents for psychiatric treatment varies from late adolescence through middle age. Two disorders for which there seems to be a particular pattern of presentation are narcissistic personality disorder, which tends to present in middle age, and borderline personality disorder, which tends to present in young adulthood.

Whether or not a patient seeks treatment is an important factor in predicting the course. As with other psychiatric disorders, the reasons patients do or do not seek help can be complex; receiving the treatment is ultimately more important than the underlying reason why it is sought. Some patients with personality disorders seem to be capable of growing and maturing as they deal with life's experiences. This may explain why, for example, in patients with borderline personality disorder, the disorder seems to "burn out" when they reach middle age. Much more research is needed to clarify further the different patterns of course for the personality disorders and the factors affecting those patterns.

Eccentric Cluster

Patients with **schizoid personality disorder** rarely seek help and, when they do, seldom benefit from it, which is unfortunate because such people tend to isolate themselves from others and do poorly at work. Their lives are usually limited in many areas. A few patients, who are highly intelligent and work in a profession that does not involve much interaction with other people, do well. Treatment can help them, should they seek it out, particularly if it is warmly supportive, unintrusive, and focuses on improving interpersonal relationships.

Patients with **schizotypal personality disorder** are more amenable to treatment. Their recovery tends to be marginal to fair because of their persistent problems in grasping the intentions of other people. Some patients engage in long-term treatment. A supportive relationship with the psychiatrist and dynamically based psychoeducational approaches that focus on improving relationships with other people may be augmented by low dosages of antipsychotic medication.

Patients with severe **paranoid personality disorder** have a poor long-term outcome. Their extreme mistrustfulness extends to the treatment process and leads to a wariness of therapists and misunderstandings with all people. Many paranoid patients eventually do undergo treatment. The best approach is sophisticated, long-term psychodynamic psychotherapy that explores their paranoid attitudes and the bases for their massive mistrust of other people.

Dramatic Cluster

Patients with **histrionic personality disorder** who do not engage in treatment have a variable course, depending on the severity of the illness. Inhibitions and chaotic work and interpersonal relationships mark the most severely affected patients. The more mildly affected patients reveal their chaotic emotional disruptions only in intimate relationships. Some of these patients respond well to intensive, long-term psychodynamic psychotherapy. The success of treatment depends on the severity of the disorder and whether there are coexisting illnesses such as depression.

Patients with **narcissistic personality disorder** usually have a fair to good outcome, if they are treated with intensive psychodynamic psychotherapy. Patients who do not receive treatment may do poorly or extremely well in their work but usually have a series of disastrous interpersonal relationships that lead to a general feeling of unhappiness and, often, recurrent depressive episodes.

Patients with **antisocial personality disorder** seldom seek therapy and seldom improve even when they receive therapy. A certain mellowing seems to occur with age, however, and antisocial tendencies tend to abate after age 40 years. Antisocial patients do especially poorly when they act on their destructive tendencies. They may have many career disruptions and failed marriages. Some smoothly functioning patients do extraordinarily well in their work. They may reach positions of power and "cheat" just enough to become notorious but not enough to end up in jail. A strong tendency toward violence suggests a poorer prognosis.

Many patients with **borderline personality disorder** do well if they receive treatment. A follow-up study of a group of patients who had been hospitalized was done 10–25 years after their release (Stone, 1990). Seventy-five percent of the patients were doing surprisingly well. The suicide rate was 8–10%, however, which is similar to the rate for patients suffering from bipolar disorder and schizophrenia. Factors correlated with a successful outcome (i.e., with a dramatic decrease in symptoms and better life functioning) were high intelligence, physical attractiveness, self-discipline (i.e., mildly "compulsive" traits, such as interests in hobbies and reading), and artistic talent in any form. For patients with a history of alcohol abuse, continued involvement with Alcoholics Anonymous was also a positive factor. Factors correlated with a poor outcome were continuing severe symptoms, frequent hospitalizations, life failures, a history of sexual or physical abuse in childhood (especially before age 14 years), antisocial behavior, marked irritability and ragefulness, chaotic impulsivity, and schizotypal traits.

Anxious Cluster

Most patients in the anxious cluster do well eventually because their less primitive, higher level of defenses limits chaotic action. Although their work performance is generally good, their anxious inhibitions may prevent them from fully realizing their capacities. The patient may "latch onto" a long-standing personal relationship, but the happiness of both parties is greatly interfered with by the patient's chronic anxiety, worrying, and intrusive controlling. Intensive, long-term psychodynamic psychotherapy is generally the treatment of choice, accompanied by medication for patients with a coexisting Axis I anxiety or depressive disorder.

THE INTERVIEW

Interviewing in any field of clinical medicine is both a science and an art. It is perhaps the most accurate diagnostic tool there is, and one that takes considerable practice to master. In no area of psychiatry is the need for art and skill in interviewing more apparent than in the area of personality disorders, and in no area is the interview more crucial. The diagnosis of personality disorders is especially challenging because the symptoms may be subtle and easily confused with the symptoms of more obvious psychiatric disorders. Assessing patients with personality disorders is difficult because these patients do not view their problems as egodystonic. Instead of recognizing that the source of their problems lies within themselves, they tend to blame life circumstances for their difficulties. They see their pathological traits, which are long-standing and have been particularly adaptive for them, as normal or as parts of "who they are" and, therefore, unchangeable. Personality disorders may not be detected by a personality assessment scale (Box 8–1), and patients may be skillful at hiding their problems. The interviewer must be able to conduct the interview at a deep enough level and for a sufficient amount of time to find the behavioral clues to these disorders. The following general guidelines may be helpful for inexperienced interviewers.

First, the interviewer must realize that the goal of the interview is to elicit the patient's history as if it were a story with a plot line. This story will reveal how the patient relates to other people, what motivates the patient, and what the patient fears in life. If the interviewer merely tries to gather a series of facts, the information obtained will be superficial. The patient is likely to evade important topics or go off on tangents. If a clear picture of the patient's object relations does not emerge, the personality assessment will be incomplete.

Second, the interviewer must know what kind of questions to ask and when to ask them. The only questions that are appropriate are those that encourage the patient to continue talking. The interviewer should not interrupt the patient repeatedly, because this will prevent the patient from telling a coherent story. The interviewer should not ask irrelevant questions about minor details of the story, such as when or where an event took place, because this may obscure more important information, such as what motivated the patient's behavior or how the patient felt. The interviewer should interrupt only if it is truly necessary to clarify important aspects of the story.

Third, the interviewer must be familiar with the personality disorders and their many diagnostic criteria. These criteria must be kept in mind as the interview progresses. The interviewer must be able to recognize the behavioral patterns that emerge from the patient's story and understand their significance in diagnosing a personality disorder.

Fourth, the interviewer should be aware that a patient with a personality disorder may not be receptive to a diagnostic interview. This negative attitude may be the most difficult aspect of the interview. The patient may be hostile or uncooperative, may feel that there is nothing wrong with his or her personality, and may regard the interview as pointless. Some personality disorder symptoms that have caused other people to feel uncomfortable around the patient may also have the same effect on the interviewer. For example, a paranoid patient may elicit feelings of fear in the interviewer; a narcissistic patient may elicit feelings of inadequacy; and a histrionic patient may elicit feelings of agitation. The physician may become so uncomfortable that he or she conducts the interview at only a superficial level or decides to end it after only 10–15 minutes. When such feelings are evoked, physicians should remind themselves that these feelings reflect how other people are influenced by the patient's behavior and, therefore, are useful clues to the diagnosis.

Interviewing Techniques

The best technique for interviewing a patient with a personality disorder is to listen carefully and attentively as the patient tells his or her life story and emotional history (see also Interviewing Guidelines box). The interviewer should take note of **repeated themes, attitudes,** and **behaviors,** which are often revealed when the patient describes how other people react to him or her. The interviewer should also try to determine what motivates the patient. In general, the more severe the disorder, the more obvious the pathological attitudes and behaviors.

While listening, the interviewer should be weighing his or her observations against the DSM-IV criteria for the various disorders. Inexperienced interviewers may systematically ask the patient about each criterion for the ten disorders. Obviously, this is a tedious process, and, more importantly, it is usually not helpful in distinguishing important behavioral patterns. It is far better to use an open-ended approach and let the patterns emerge spontaneously from the patient's story. The only situation in which the more systematic technique may be helpful is when gathering research data from a large number of patients. Researchers often use the Personality Disorders Examination (see Box 8–1).

It is natural for patients to try to appear more "normal" than they really are during the first interview. They may not want to reveal embarrassing or humiliating information about themselves. The interviewer should pay careful attention to the patient's words, tone of voice, manner of dress, and body language. These details can provide the interviewer with a general picture of the patient's personality. It usually takes at least four weekly sessions before patients reveal all of the relevant facets of their personalities (e.g., how they behave when under stress; how they interact with coworkers and intimate friends). This is especially true for patients with anti-

social personality disorder, who can pull the wool over the eyes of the most astute interviewers for long stretches of time.

The interviewer may be able to draw the patient out by using appropriate questions or a certain tone of voice. If a patient boasts in a quiet way about his advanced degrees, honors, and publications but seems to be leading an unhappy life and talks in a complaining tone, he may be downplaying his grandiosity and envy. The interviewer might comment on the patient's impressive level of accomplishment, which may encourage the patient to complain bitterly that "others in my department don't recognize my worth, don't invite me to their parties, and don't understand that I should have been appointed to the top spot instead of the guy who just got promoted." This dialog clearly reveals the patient's narcissism (and his loneliness). It will help the interviewer to make the diagnosis with greater certainty.

The interviewer should vary the approach for patients in the different personality disorder clusters. Patients in the eccentric cluster tend to be emotionally fragile. The interviewer should respect this vulnerability and should be wary of directly confronting patients' statements until a solid therapeutic alliance has been forged. Attempts at humor or overt expressions of warmth or empathy should be avoided, because these patients tend to look for evidence of mockery and are suspicious of the motives of anyone who tries to get too close to them emotionally. Patients in the dramatic cluster tend to express their emotions but are vague about their histories. Expressions of warmth and empathy are appropriate but should be combined with a firm, unrattled, take-charge manner. This approach will help the interviewer to gain the trust of these patients. Warmth and empathy are also helpful for patients in the anxious cluster. These patients need much more help in identifying their feeling states, however, and also in becoming aware of their unconscious worries and conflicts.

A few sample dialogs and typical patterns of patients with personality disorders may be helpful in learning the art of interviewing. The first dialog is typical of a patient with obsessive-compulsive personality disorder. These patients tend to dress in a "correct," conventional, severe fashion; sit stiffly in a chair; have an immobile expression; and talk in a boring manner about irrelevant details. The patient's speech is often filled with set phrases that keep emotions at a distance, as the following interchange demonstrates:

Patient: "There was a death in the family last week."
Interviewer: "My goodness! What happened?"
Patient: "The mother passed."
Interviewer: "Your mother?"
Patient: "That is correct."
Interviewer: "But it must have been very wrenching and . . ."
Patient: "There was some sadness, of course."

Interviewing Guidelines

- Use an open-ended approach to elicit the patient's history rather than systematically asking the patient about the criteria for each of the personality disorders.
- Obtain a description of the patient's relationships with others, taking note of repeated themes, attitudes, and behaviors.
- Look for and encourage the patient to elaborate on behavioral patterns that suggest the various personality disorders.
- Specifically ask about other people's reactions to the patient.
- Be aware of emotional reactions to the patient (e.g., inadequacy, fear) that may interfere with developing a working alliance.
- Avoid expressions of warmth or empathy with eccentric cluster patients.
- Assume a firm, take-charge approach with dramatic cluster patients.
- Help anxiety cluster patients to identify and tolerate their feelings.

During the initial diagnostic evaluation, the patterns should be noted and the patient's motivation for maintaining them should be respected. Only in a safe, ongoing therapeutic relationship will this patient be able to begin to deal with the grief that is being intensely denied and isolated.

Histrionic patients use emotional words, speak in an animated manner, often dress seductively or flamboyantly, and focus more on feelings than on factual details or time sequences. Paranoid patients demonstrate their guarded, controlling, suspicious attitudes toward people and situations in every aspect of their life stories.

It is important to remember that personality *traits* are not the same as personality *disorders*. In the following dialog, the interviewer makes observations about the patient's personality style and also elicits information about specific behavioral patterns that might indicate a diagnosis of a personality disorder.

Interviewer: "Please tell me why you're here."
Patient: "I don't really know."
Interviewer: "Oh?"
Patient: "Yes."
Interviewer: "Well, how did you decide to come to see a doctor?"
Patient: "My wife told me I had to."
Interviewer: "Why did she say that?"
Patient: "I don't really know why she said it."

BOX 8–1.   Personality Assessment Scales and Profiles

Personality assessment scales attempt to identify traits that are relevant to personality disorders. A broad-based scale is required to comprehensively assess all of the various types of personalities, both normal and abnormal.

Minnesota Multiphasic Personality Index

The Minnesota Multiphasic Personality Index (MMPI) assesses the full spectrum of personalities, ranging from the normal to the severely disturbed. The MMPI is a self-rating test, consisting of 644 true-or-false questions, 535 of which relate to the ten dimensional scales of hypochondriasis, depression, hysteria, psychopathic deviative, masculinity and femininity, paranoia, psychasthenia, schizophrenia, hypomania, and social introversion. These scales do not directly correspond to the DSM-IV personality disorders. The remaining questions pertain to atypicality, validity, and deception. The results of the

test are plotted on a line graph. The line is the profile of the patient's personality; any peaks and valleys would occur at those scales where the patient's scores either greatly exceed or fall significantly below the average scores in the general population. The profile of a patient with a fairly serious personality disorder is usually a jagged line with peaks and valleys. The figure below shows the typical profile for a patient with borderline personality disorder: high scores on the 8, 6, and 2 subscales; a slightly lower score on the 4 subscale. This 8-6-2-4 pattern is common in patients with borderline personality disorder.

Self-rating scales such as the MMPI are not foolproof. As many as 10% of patients who have been diagnosed with antisocial or borderline personality disorder or other serious psychiatric disorders in a hospital setting may produce a "normal" profile.

Continued

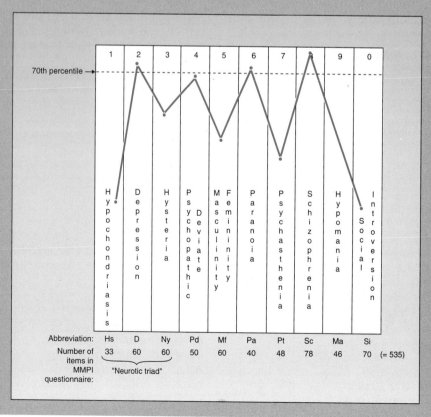

Abbreviation:	Hs	D	Ny	Pd	Mf	Pa	Pt	Sc	Ma	Si	
Number of items in MMPI questionnaire:	33	60	60	50	60	40	48	78	46	70	(= 535)

"Neurotic triad"

Personality Disorders Examination

The Personality Disorders Examination (PDE) is a structured questionnaire, administered by a trained interviewer, that was developed specifically to identify DSM-IV personality disorders. The questions elicit information on the approximately 100 personality traits, such as shyness, suspiciousness, impulsivity, and theatricality, that are listed in the DSM-IV diagnostic categories for personality disorders. Because the PDE can identify all disorders that meet the DSM-IV criteria in any patient, it takes on a dimensional quality as well. In the figure below, each DSM-IV category is set up as a dimension, which allows for gradations in the assessment of personality. The profile shown is typical of a patient with borderline personality disorder whose scores also meet the criteria for narcissistic, histrionic, dependent, and passive-aggressive personality disorders.

Personality Assessment Schedule

The Personality Assessment Schedule (PAS) is a dimensional scale that lies somewhere between the MMPI and the DSM-oriented instruments. Developed in Great Britain by Tyrer and Alexander (1988), this scale relies on 24 dimensions, to each of which the rater must assign a score between 0 and 5.

When the PAS is used to assess patients with DSM-IV personality disorders, a different profile emerges for each disorder. For example, a patient with a histrionic personality disorder would have high scores on the PAS dimensions of dependence, lability, childishness, vulnerability, and irresponsibility, and moderately high scores on the dimensions of anxiousness and sensitivity. A normal person might have high scores on optimism and conscientiousness, modest scores on introspection and sensitivity, and low scores on the remaining dimensions. One advantage of the PAS is the everyday language it uses to label trait dimensions. With the exception of the dependent and avoidant personality disorders, the DSM-IV uses technical words to label the personality disorders (e.g., paranoid personality disorder) rather than ordinary words (e.g., shy, irritable, childish, suspicious).

Personality Profile

The interviewer of a patient with a suspected personality disorder must know which traits and characteristics are ideal and normal for the patient, taking into consideration his or her cultural background, life situation, socioeconomic circumstances, and general goals. The zigzag profile, which is comparable to the MMPI and other dimensional devices, although more detailed, is a basic instrument designed to schematically summarize the extent to which the patient's traits deviate from the ideal. The traits are arranged in five columns. Normal traits are placed in the middle column and deviant traits in the other columns, with the most deviant traits placed in columns 1 and 5. A line is drawn to connect the traits of the patient

In the figure below, the line, which connects 24 traits, provides a zigzag profile of personality traits for a patient with obsessive-compulsive personality traits. The patient is a 54-year-old divorced male engineer who lives with his girlfriend two to three days a week. As the zigzag line reflects, he is remarkably compulsive, stingy, and domineering. He insists that everything has to be done his way and allows no disagreement about this. For example, when traveling long distances in the car with his girlfriend, he refuses to stop at a convenient place along the way when she has to use the restroom. He drives 20 miles to get a "bargain" on a jar of peanut butter, spending two dollars' worth of gas to save one dollar on the peanut butter. Just to save money, he insists on walking in the pouring rain, refusing to take a cab even though his girlfriend offers to pay for it. In the nine years they have been together, he has never given his girlfriend a card or a gift. These abnormalities stand out clearly on the diagram and highlight his obsessive-compulsive traits, which would become the major psychotherapeutic focus for this patient.

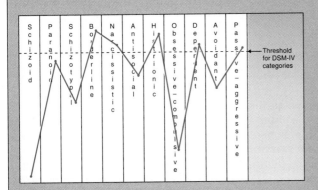

S c h i z o i d	P a r a n o i d	S c h i z o t y p a l	B o r d e r l i n e	N a r c i s s i s t i c	A n t i s o c i a l	H i s t r i o n i c	O b s e s s i v e – c o m p u l s i v e	D e p e n d e n t	A v o i d a n t	P a s s i v e – a g g r e s s i v e

← Threshold for DSM-IV categories

Extreme Traits		Average/Typical Traits		Extreme Traits
Abrasive	Tactless	Polite	Courtly	Obsequious
Stingy	Tight	Thrifty	Generous	Prodigal
Irresponsible	Procrastinating	Punctual	Compulsive	Punctilious
Unfeeling	Cold	Sympathetic	Oversensitive	Maudlin
Vampish	Seductive	Receptive	Coy	Prudish
Randy	Pushy	Assertive	Reserved	Inhibited
Domineering	Bossy	Abrasive	Unassertive	Submissive
Paranoid	Suspicious	Trusting	Naïve	Gullible
Abusive	Irritable	Calm	Phlegmatic	Spineless
Ruthless	Exploitative	Fair	Deferential	Meek
Chaotic	Sloppy	Neat	Meticulous	Fussbudget
Vengeful	Bitter	Forgiving	Philosophic	Altruistic
Brittle	Rigid	Flexible	Yielding	Flabby
Aggressive	Hostile	Agreeable	Friendly	Overfriendly
Defiant	Uncooperative	Cooperative	Superaccommodating	
Bigoted	Dogmatic	Openminded	Easily swayed	"As-if"
Unscrupulous	Devious	Honest	Scrupulous	Abrasive
Garrulous	Talkative	Communicative	Laconic	Taciturn
Extroverted	Outgoing	At ease	Shy	Reclusive
Disloyal	Uncommitted	Faithful	Fawning	Clingy
Pretentious	Affected	Modest	Humble	Self-effacing
Reckless	Impulsive	Spontaneous	Hesitant	Fearful
Obnoxious	Disagreeable	Likable	Charming	Charismatic
Boorish	Philistine	Cultured	Mannered	Precious

Interviewer: "Well, what did she say?"

Patient: "She said I'm impossible to live with, and if I didn't come to see a doctor, she would leave me."

Interviewer: "Why did she say you're impossible to live with?"

Patient: "She thinks that I believe everyone in the whole world is a son of a gun."

Interviewer: "Do you?"

Patient: "Doctor, if you had to deal with the idiots that I have to deal with everyday, you'd think the whole world was full of sons of guns, too!"

Interviewer: "Please tell me about it."

Patient: "My boss is totally unreliable. Sometimes he backs me, and sometimes he doesn't. He blames me for things I didn't do. And he never appreciates what I contribute."

Interviewer: "What seems to be the basic problem?"

Patient: "He doesn't know how to do his job, and I do. Therefore, he doesn't like me and is constantly critical. I know that my way is better, and he might, too, except for my coworkers, who are constantly currying favor with him at my expense. They jockey me for position, put me down, and take credit for what I do. No wonder the boss is confused!"

Interviewer: "Has this happened at other places of employment?"

Patient: "It always happens! That's the way people are, you see. Everybody is out for the buck; everyone's out for the next rung up the ladder; everyone's out to sell their coworkers at the drop of a hat. In addition, most people don't really want to work or even know how to do their job well. They do the minimum, cover up, and blame other people when things go wrong. This is the way people are, and this is the way the world is."

Interviewer: "And your wife, you said she told you to come here."

Patient: "Yes. My wife is part of this story, too. Her in-laws are the same as my boss! Ha! Nosy, controlling, always 'know best,' yet totally incompetent. They basically don't like me, and I don't like them."

Interviewer: "How do you get along with your wife?"

Patient: "Doctor, my wife and I get along fine when she lets me be the head of the house. A ship needs one captain. Anything else just confuses the kids and at times may be downright dangerous."

Interviewer: "What's your wife's point of view about this?"

Patient: "She says I'm bossy, controlling, fly off the handle over small details, that I don't listen to her or to other people, and a lot of the times it doesn't seem as though I really like her."

Interviewer: "Do you like her?"

Patient: "I like her until she does something totally contrary to the way I told her."

Interviewer: "Why does she do that?"

Patient: "I don't know. I think it's just to get me. She knows very well what the rules are. I'm not that unpredictable. It's simple. All she has to do is do it my way. But no, she'll side with the kids against me or with her parents against me, and I tell you, doctor, I can get pretty annoyed. One thing I appreciate at home is a little loyalty. I work hard, I bring home some money, the least I can get is a little respect on the home front. Now she goes and does this to me!"

Interviewer: "What to you?"

Patient: "Sends me to the head shrinker!"

In this interview, the physician asks questions that encourage the patient to continue talking and elaborate on his recent life history as it relates to the chief complaint from his wife. The attitudes of self-centeredness, self-righteousness, and self-inflation and the controlling, denigrating anger at other people are all readily observable. They suggest a diagnosis of coexisting narcissistic and paranoid personality disorders.

Interviewing the Patient's Family and Friends

It is sometimes helpful to interview the patient's family and friends to find out how the patient expresses his or her personality to them. These persons often have the clearest understanding of the patient's personality. Of course, no one human being can possibly know every facet of another human being's personality. A patient may be kind to his children, stingy with his wife, obsequious with his boss, cranky with his coworkers, and a model of sportsmanship with his buddies on the Saturday softball team. The integrated perceptions of all of the people with whom a person interacts would be needed to create a complete picture of the person's personality.

If patients do not want others to be interviewed, or if such interviews would be difficult to arrange, it is useful to ask patients how they think their relatives and friends would respond to questions about their behavior.

Referring Patients

Internists, family practitioners, and other nonpsychiatric physicians and health professionals may find that patients who seem to be suffering from a personality disorder are not receptive to the recommendation of a referral to a psychiatrist. The physician should avoid arguing with patients about their assessment of their problems (i.e., the physician's view that they are internally generated, as opposed to the patient's view that they are external). Instead, the physician should merely reiterate the difficulties as presented by the patient, using the pain and suffering caused by these difficulties as the rationale for the referral to a psychiatrist. If patients are still reluctant, the physician may explain to them that psychiatrists are trained to provide help with all kinds of problems, including life problems, and may suggest that patients try a few sessions and see what they think. Once they enter the psychiatrist's office, it is up to the psychiatrist to help them understand the need for treatment.

DIFFERENTIAL DIAGNOSIS

Three important principles underlie the differential diagnosis for patients who appear to have personality disorders. Patients with Axis I disorders or medical disorders that affect the personality may be misdiagnosed as having personality disorders, and vice versa. Patients with personality disorders often have a coexisting Axis I disorder, which may be overlooked. Also, coexisting personality disorders are common and should not be missed in the differential diagnosis.

Patients with Axis I disorders may be mistakenly diagnosed with a personality disorder because many of the behavioral characteristics are the same (e.g., significant disturbances in affect, interpersonal functioning, and cognition). For example, a patient with a mood disorder may have the same maladaptive behavior in dealing with other persons as a patient with a personality disorder. Manic patients who are overwhelmed by an intensely euphoric affect may behave in a disruptive manner similar to that of a dramatic histrionic patient. In a severely depressed patient, especially one with symptoms of irritability, the depression may overwhelm the patient's personality defenses and permit the acting out of anger and destructive impulses in social interactions. An important rule of thumb is that a personality disorder should not be diagnosed in the initial evaluation of a patient with active Axis I psychopathology.

In rare but devastating cases, central nervous system disease may cause behavior similar to that of a personality disorder. Demyelinating illnesses, such as multiple sclerosis, or brain tumors that are impinging on the frontal lobes are two classic illnesses that may alter the personality. Alzheimer's disease and multi-infarct dementia may also cause disinhibited personality exaggerations and deteriorations.

A search for the signs and symptoms of **mood and cognitive disorders** must be part of the routine differential workup for patients who present with personality disorders, especially those who are middle-aged and older. If a middle-aged or elderly patient appears to have a personality disorder, it may actually be a medical condition or an Axis I disorder.

The second principle of differential diagnosis is that personality disorders may be complicated by a variety of **Axis I illnesses,** especially the mood and anxiety disorders. Therefore, physicians must be careful not to overlook the presence of an Axis I disorder in patients with personality disorders.

The third principle is that personality disorders frequently overlap with one another, and it is therefore important to keep in mind the possibility of **coexisting personality disorders.** This comorbidity may have important therapeutic and prognostic im-

plications. ➡ For example, a 23-year-old male law student presented to a physician in his health service complaining of indecisiveness with regard to his career plans and his relationships with women. He was having second thoughts about whether law was really the best field for him, and he described a pattern of withdrawing from relationships with women just as they became intimate. The physician elicited a number of behavioral patterns that seemed to be consistent with obsessive-compulsive personality disorder. The student was unable to prioritize his material when studying and memorized many unrelated facts without having a sense of the big picture. He also had an intellectual rigidity in class discussions that frequently alienated the faculty. His intrapsychic functioning seemed to be mainly at a neurotic level. An evaluation that had ended at this point might have suggested a good prognosis for this patient, if he were willing to engage in intensive insight-oriented psychotherapy. Further exploration, however, revealed many features of more primitive psychopathology. These features were consistent with a borderline character structure and the presence of comorbid narcissistic and paranoid personality disorders. For example, he felt that all of his classmates disliked him and enjoyed seeing his discomfort when he felt humiliated in class. While intensive psychotherapy might still have been the treatment of choice (see Chapter 15, Psychotherapy), the prognosis was more guarded. The patient's primitive fantasy life and tendency to regress would have to be approached with caution. ◀

The relationship of any Axis I illness to one or several of the personality disorders needs to be investigated in each patient. The effects of mixed disorders are complex and variable. These issues of differential diagnosis are sometimes clarified only during intensive ongoing treatment.

MEDICAL EVALUATION

A careful psychiatric history should confirm that the signs of a personality disorder have been present throughout adult life. A thorough cognitive evaluation via the mental status examination should reveal no positive findings. If the history is equivocal or the cognitive examination is abnormal, a thorough medical evaluation is indicated. Particular attention should be paid to the neurological examination (see Chapter 5, Cognitive and Mental Disorders Due to General Medical Conditions).

ETIOLOGY
Biological Factors

The innate or constitutional qualities of personality, called **temperament,** include genetically programmed tendencies to react to stimuli in certain ways.

The recognition of innate qualities dates back at least to the ancient Greeks, who distinguished four temperaments: sanguine (cheerful, optimistic), choleric (hot-tempered, irascible), melancholic (sad, depressed), and phlegmatic (dull, apathetic). Each temperament represented an excess of one of the four elements—air, fire, earth, and water—of which all things on earth were thought to be composed. Each temperament was associated with a substance found in the body: blood (sanguine), yellow bile (choleric), black bile (melancholic), and lymph (phlegmatic). Although this theory now seems quaint, it is not totally erroneous. Temperaments such as those described above still exist, and the inherited nature of temperament has been scientifically validated. For example, bipolar patients and their close relatives have an increased tendency to be hypomanic (sanguine), irritable (choleric), or depressive (melancholic), or some combination of the three. Patients suffering from schizophrenia and their close relatives are more likely to be innately aloof (schizoid) or mistrustful (paranoid). Modern research has revealed the effects of biochemical factors on mood. The theory of the ancient Greeks can be seen as a primitive prototype for current theories of temperament.

The more the inborn temperament varies from the cultural norm, the greater the need for the personality to adapt to the norm. Temperament predisposes a person to certain personality aberrations and disorders. Recent twin studies have shown that temperament is highly heritable. **Heredity** may account for about half of the variance of personality traits in each person.

The influence of **biochemical factors** on temperament and personality is now being shown. Researchers have drawn attention to compounds that are active in the central nervous system. Male hormones in high concentrations, for example, are associated with heightened aggressiveness and disinhibition. Low basal levels of γ-aminobutyric acid are associated with heightened anxiety and, by extension, increased susceptibility to guilt and highly emotional behavior. Studies of the neurotransmitter serotonin have shown that low levels of the serotonin metabolite 5-hydroxyindoleacetic acid (5-HIAA) in the cerebrospinal fluid are associated with impulsivity. In persons prone to violent acts (e.g., murder; suicide by gunshot or jumping from a height), 5-HIAA levels are particularly low. High levels of serotonin are associated with decreased impulsivity and increased conscientiousness (i.e., self-control).

A person's constitution may be influenced by organic changes in the **central nervous system** during fetal development or at birth (e.g., maternal drug use, malnutrition, perinatal hypoxia, birth trauma, or other noxious factors). **Sex hormones** are also associated with certain personality attributes. When gender differences are pronounced, they may reflect innate features of the temperament. Women tend to emphasize cooperative relationships and express emotions readily. Men tend to be more aggressive and compulsive.

Interesting correlations exist between brain lesions in specific areas and certain abnormalities of personality. Brain tumors and traumatic injuries in the frontal lobes have been associated, depending on their precise location, with paranoid traits, irritability, or lack of customary orderliness. Interestingly, abusers of anabolic steroids have experienced paranoid changes and marked aggressiveness.

Environmental Factors

Life events play an important role in personality formation. The environmentally influenced component of personality is **character.** The crucial environment for human psychological growth is the interpersonal environment—first, the mother, father, and siblings of the nuclear family and, later, peer groups and the culture at large. Positive or negative events in the child's life can also be formative. These include obviously stressful events, such as sexual abuse or the death of a parent, as well as more subtle experiences, such as constant teasing by an older sibling. These events may be especially formative if they occur during certain critical phases of growth. As children grow up and progress through different phases of development, they adapt their personalities to the environment around them. They form complex self and object representations, which, when slowly integrated throughout a lifetime, form the content and organization of personality function.

The aberrations of attitude and behavior in the different personality disorders are characterized by different extreme object relations scenarios and clusters of self and object representations. The story line for each disorder will reflect these characteristic interactions, although it will, of course, also be unique for each individual. Dynamic psychotherapy attempts to analyze these **object relations** and understand how the innate personality has adapted to the environment, so that better ways of adapting can be integrated into the personality.

An example is the following hypothesis regarding the etiology of borderline personality disorder, which has not been proved but is supported by clinical observations. It is a useful example because patients with this disorder suffer from particularly distorted object representations and tend to have a characteristic temperamental orientation. As children, they tend to have intense affective experiences that they have particular difficulty in modulating. Their caregivers may respond to these cranky, difficult children with irritability, which may not only be a reaction to the children but may also reflect the temperament and environmental influences of the caregivers.

Children with an inborn affective lability and sensitivity who grow up in an environment that exacerbates rather than calms their insecurities may become "stuck" with primitive, powerful self and object representations that lack integration. ⇒ Such distorted representations were an underlying factor in the behavior of the patient described earlier who felt angry and lonely when her psychiatrist was on vacation. The anger resulted from her feelings of abandonment and rejection. Because her sense of herself and others was so fragile, she soon forgot that the psychiatrist had not had a vacation in eight months and had always been extremely reliable and understanding. The patient was frightened by her anger and felt guilty about wishing that he would suffer for leaving her. The guilt was transformed into fear that she may have destroyed him with her anger. Getting drunk and "picking up" a man in a bar may have been the only way she could convince herself that she was a good and lovable person and that she could find someone who would take care of her. Unfortunately, the man was not trustworthy. She was lucky to have survived this episode of acting out her anger and hurt on the basis of these unconscious object representations. ◀▥

Several theories and models of personality and personality psychopathology are discussed in Box 8–2.

TREATMENT
Psychotherapy

The mainstay of treatment of the personality disorders is psychotherapy. The goal is for the patient to see maladaptive personality traits as egodystonic instead of egosyntonic and then develop more positive attitudes and behaviors. At first, the therapy proceeds slowly so that it will be tolerable to the patient. The therapist mainly listens to the patient until the pattern of behavior has been drawn out and understood. Only then is the therapist in a position to point out that the behavior is more detrimental than beneficial. Once the patient has assimilated this idea and the recommendations for changing the behavior, he or she may be able to slowly change his or her personality. ▥▶ For example, a crotchety, compulsive man often came home from work in an irritable mood. He would "squawk" at his wife, tell the children to "shut up," and complain about his "hard day" until he had spoiled everyone else's dinner. He had so alienated his wife that she was not interested in his sexual advances, which made him even more crotchety. It was a vicious circle. The patient felt that his complaints were totally justified. At the appropriate time, the psychiatrist asked him, "Well, why exactly should your wife love you, if you treat her like a slave? If you were to stop the stream of complaints, be kinder to the children, be attentive to your wife's needs, and express your appreciation through words or gifts, your wife would be more receptive and the children would no longer cower when Daddy comes home. The circle would begin to spin in the right direction." The psychiatrist made the querulousness an egodystonic trait and also suggested how the patient could go about creating a better environment at home for himself and everyone else in the family. ◀▥

In a slow, careful, and supportive manner, the physician helps the patient to recognize **dysfunctional personality patterns.** As therapy continues, the patient finds it easier to view these aspects of himself or herself as alien and unnecessary although understandable results of temperament and overdetermined life history. After this phase of enlightenment, the middle phase of treatment begins, in which the therapist helps the patient alter the adaptational patterns.

It is not possible to definitively rank the personality disorders in the DSM-IV as to their amenability to psychotherapy. As a rule of thumb, however, disorders that mainly involve traits of inhibition (e.g., self-criticalness, shyness, unassertiveness, overscrupulousness) are the easiest to treat. Obsessive-compulsive, dependent, avoidant, and histrionic patients are the best candidates for one-to-one psychotherapy. In descending order of amenability are the narcissistic, borderline, schizotypal, paranoid, schizoid, and antisocial personality disorders. Mildly paranoid patients with a high motivation for treatment will benefit more from therapy than will severely narcissistic patients who are openly contemptuous of treatment.

Patients in the eccentric cluster tend to defeat psychotherapy through their aloofness or guardedness. Paranoid patients take the therapist's suggestions as criticisms. They need to be handled with great tact and deftness. The therapist should not challenge all of the patient's (often bizarre) assumptions at first but should lead the patient slowly and gently away from them by suggesting other possible, more positive alternatives.

Most research data indicate that both short-term and long-term psychotherapies are effective. If the patient is able to engage cooperatively in treatment, gains are almost certain to be made. More extensive gains require a longer period of treatment. Therefore, the longer the period of treatment that the patient can tolerate, the better the chance will be for making long-term changes. There is much active research on these issues, and in the coming years, there may be further validation of the above statements.

Supportive Short-Term Psychotherapy

One type of short-term treatment is mainly supportive in nature. Its goal is to help the patient cope with a life crisis and the resulting decompensations of personality function to which patients with personality disorders are particularly vulnerable. This work may take only weeks to months. At the conclusion of treatment, the patient will be able to function as well as he or she did before the crisis occurred.

Short-Term Psychodynamic or Cognitive-Behavior Psychotherapy

The other form of short-term treatment is more aggressive. The goal is to help the patient make permanent, long-standing changes in maladaptive personality traits. Either a psychodynamic or a cognitive-behavioral approach is used. Early in treatment, the most obvious and troubling maladaptive personality traits are identified and brought to the patient's attention. In cognitive-behavior psychotherapy, the maladaptive traits are dispassionately and logically sepa-

BOX 8–2. Models of Personality

As recently as the 1890s, psychiatric theories, relying simplistically on the four temperaments–sanguine, choleric, melancholic, or phlegmatic–classified each "personality disorder" as an excess of one or more of these temperaments. For example, a newly hospitalized patient might have been described as follows: "The patient is a 37-year-old mechanic with a sanguineocholeric temperament" (i.e., has a nature that is alternately happy-go-lucky and irritable). The term *personality* would not enter common psychiatric parlance for another 50 years. At the turn of the century, Freud and other pioneering psychoanalysts hypothesized that variations in "character" resulted from traumatic events that occurred during the developmental stages. Trauma during the oral, anal, and genital stages, they believed, gave rise to depressive, compulsive, and hysterical types, respectively. Further subdivisions were made later on (e.g., "phallic-narcissistic" character resulted from trauma during the postulated urethral stage, which occurs just before the genital stage). There were many problems with this system. One major misconception was that the earlier the stage at which trauma occurred, the more serious the resulting disorder (i.e., a compulsive patient was more disturbed than a hysterical patient). This is not true.

Three-Dimensional Models

One of the most influential theoreticians at mid-century was Hans Eysenck in England. He elaborated a three-dimensional system that was built on three superfactors: **e**xtroversion, **n**euroticism, and **p**sychoticism. These abstract terms correspond to broad concepts relating to socialization, emotional stability (the "opposite" of neuroticism), and both eccentricity and (aggressively tinged) impulsivity. The personality could be rated high or low on the three scales. Eysenck's system generates 2^3 or eight different personality types. An avoidant person, for example, might score high on the N scale, low on the E scale, and low on the P scale (neurotic, introverted, not psychotic).

In 1981, Millon advocated a different three-dimensional system, which was based on the polarities that Freud thought governed all mental life (i.e., active versus passive; self versus object; pleasure versus pain). The questions that were addressed by these polarities include: How much initiative does the person take? Is the person self-reliant or dependent on others? Does the person move toward what is pleasurable or simply move away from what is painful? Someone with a hysterical personality, in the Millon system, would, for example, be active/dependent/gregarious (moving toward pleasure).

In 1986, Cloninger proposed a three-dimensional system rooted in neurophysiological phenomena. Three major neurotransmitter systems were correlated with three psychological traits. System A, low basal dopaminergic activity, was correlated with novelty seeking; system B, high serotonergic activity, was correlated with harm avoidance; and system C, low basal noradrenergic activity, was correlated with reward dependence. This scheme situates the personality disorders on a three-dimensional diagram (see figure below). Cloninger's model is especially important because it is based on biological phenomena, which can be tested and objectively validated by biochemical measures instead of subjective psychological factors.

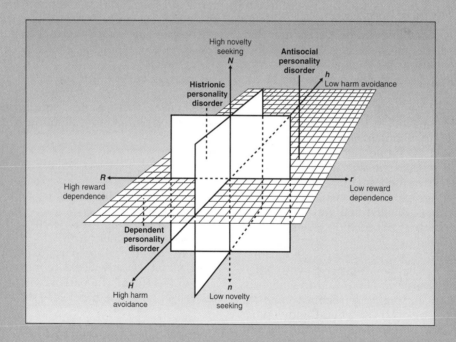

Five-Factor Model

Most recently, the five-factor model has been championed by many of the outstanding contemporary theoreticians of personality. The stimulus for this theory was the lexical approach of the 1920s and 1930s. The dimensions into which the word-lists could be condensed seemed capable of still further distillation—into smaller numbers of large-scale dimensions, or superfactors. These superfactors were similar to some of the major factors that had been suggested by Eysenck, Millon, and Tyrer. It was originally proposed by Tupes and Christal in 1961. The five superfactors cannot be

Continued

condensed further, and there is no need for additional factors. There are precisely five superfactors (or "supertraits") for the same "reason" that the earth has 92 chemical elements: This is all that nature put there. Each of the five superfactors is a pair of opposites:

The Superfactors of the Five-Factor Model

Extroversion (E)	Introversion
Agreeableness (A)	Antagonism
Neuroticism (N)	Emotional stability
Conscientiousness (C)	Unruliness
Openness (O)	Conventionality

The five-factor model is the basis for a comprehensive system of describing personality, and it embraces the disorders in the DSM-IV. Widiger has recently worked out the correlations between the five-factor model and the DSM-IV diagnostic criteria. Most of the DSM-IV disorders are placed in the "minus" column for the five factors. −E (introversion), for example, is notable in both avoidant and schizoid persons; −A (disagreeableness, antagonism) is prominent in passive-aggressive and antisocial persons. The most recently discovered superfactor, openness, describes a person's ability to become absorbed in interests and pursuits and to view the world with an artistic sensitivity (i.e., an openness to new ideas). The only disorder correlated with the O factor is schizotypal disorder, which has the feature of eccentricity or unconventionality.

Each of the three-dimensional systems discussed above and in Box 8–1 embodies several of the five superfactors (e.g., Eysenck uses the E and N factors; Tyrer's personality assessment schedule uses the E, N, A, and C factors). All of the theories and systems converge toward the five-factor model, just as all of the lexical systems can be distilled into the five-factor model. The five-factor model is the final common pathway in all of the attempts to grasp the essence of personality.

rated from other traits involved in regulating self-esteem. The patient and therapist use specific techniques to change specific behaviors. The underlying causes of the personality disorder and the deeper attitudinal problems are not addressed. This approach assumes that treatment will set the stage for deeper psychological growth over the long term, even though it focuses on short-term situational changes. Short-term psychodynamic psychotherapy has the same goal as cognitive-behavior psychotherapy. However, there is more emphasis on uncovering the entrenched, intense affective experiences that underlie the rigid, maladaptive personality defenses. Cognitive behaviorists tend to avoid using transference and countertransference, but in short-term psychodynamic psychotherapy, the identification and interpretation of transferential patterns is the main vehicle of treatment.

Long-Term Psychotherapy

The long-term treatment of patients with personality disorders usually involves formal psychoanalysis or psychodynamic psychotherapy. Both attempt to investigate the affective experiences of self-relations and object-relations scenarios, which are organized in conscious and unconscious fantasies in the emotional lives of patients. Attitudes and behaviors result from these fantasies. Self and object relationships involve memories of actual events, past fantasy experiences, present reality experiences, and present fantasy adaptations. Because the condensations of the past and present and fantasies and reality are complex and multidetermined, the work requires great persistence. Frequent sessions over a period of several years are necessary. These fantasies mediate the motivations of hopes and fears that form the basic psychological structure of the personality disorders.

Kernberg and others have adapted the psychodynamic method for patients with borderline personality disorder. Patients who are acting out express their conflicts through maladaptive actions outside the arena of treatment. They often need a psychodynamic approach that specifically focuses on the consequences of impulsive behavior and that uses cognitive and behavioral techniques, as well. Supportive techniques are sometimes required as the backbone of therapy for such patients. Encouragement, reassurance, and education about life are sometimes necessary, as are active discouragement and confrontation when the patient is about to engage in self-defeating, hostile, or otherwise grossly maladaptive behavior. Whereas analytically oriented therapies with healthier patients try to uncover the early life experiences that may underlie the pathological patterns, therapy with borderline patients will tend to emphasize the patient's distorted assumptions of his or her current interpersonal world (e.g., "Bosses are all power-hungry sadists, and I'm just a failure with nothing to contribute to the company"). The therapist appeals to the patient's reason, or cognition, to help the patient change the crippling distortions. The next step is to help the patient to change his or her behavior to correlate with the newly acquired, more realistic assumptions (e.g., "Some bosses can be okay; I do have something valuable to contribute"). The **limit-setting** on self-destructive behaviors that these patients require may not always be achieved in one-to-one therapy. A team of mental health professionals is sometimes preferable for maintaining rules and allowing the patient to feel supported. Group therapy based on the 12-step program of Alcoholics Anonymous may be necessary.

Group or Couples Therapy

Because of the egosyntonic nature of personality disorders, the patient may not be aware of many of his or her maladaptive traits. Information from the patient's friends and relatives is often needed to shed light on concealed facets of the patient's nature. Group or couples therapy may be helpful in revealing hidden traits that can be addressed in the group as well as later in one-to-one sessions.

Outcome

One should never expect a rapid or wholesale change in personality. The process of shedding old habits and acquiring new ones is necessarily slow. A hermit will never become the life of the party; a histrionic person will not become a certified public accountant. Small, quantitative changes may eventually lead to large, more global, qualitative, desirable effects, however (Fig. 8–1).

➠ A 28-year-old male patient came to treatment because he was unable to work or to get along with his parents, on whom he was emotionally and financially dependent. He was self-centered and intensely preoccupied with his appearance. He was also irritable to the point of occasionally striking his parents if they asked him to do errands or made the slightest criticism of him. He felt pessimistic about his prospects for the future and was known as a worry-wart. He was discouraged about dating women because he was convinced that all women, no matter how pleasant and undemanding they might seem at first, would turn out to be hypercritical and overly demanding. At the beginning of treatment, the patient had significant paranoid, dependent, depressed, passive-aggressive, narcissistic, and irritable traits. At the end of treatment, four years later, the profile was exactly the same (as would be anticipated), but all of the measures were below the maladaptive threshold (e.g., between offending others considerably and becoming more tolerable). He had grown more trusting of women, although he still harbored some suspicions. He was less irritable and no longer lashed out against his parents. He was able to work, although not up to his capacity, and he was less pessimistic and more self-sufficient. He still took excessive pains with his appearance but fretted less over his incipient balding. Family members and coworkers would describe this patient as a "different person." Actually, he is the same person and has the same type of personality, but he has made positive adaptations so he is easier to get along with. ◄▦ This

outcome, which is characterized by a diminution in extreme behaviors, is typical for a patient with a personality disorder who has received treatment. Thus, psychotherapy of one form or another can be *lifesaving* for many patients with personality disorders.

Psychopharmacological Treatment
Personality Disorders

Because maladaptive personality traits tend to be egosyntonic, they may not be "target symptoms" that are amenable to psychoactive drugs (i.e., there are no drugs for stinginess, rudeness, bluntness, or meanness). Several of the personality disorders do have (or are associated with) symptoms that respond favorably to drugs. Anxiety is a common symptom associated with the anxious cluster disorders, especially the avoidant and dependent personality disorders. Anxiolytic drugs of the **benzodiazepine** group are often useful in these disorders. When the anxiety is more focal and of short duration (e.g., before an examination or a speech) and is due to performance anxiety or narcissistic perfectionism, β-blockers such as propranolol or atenolol may be useful if they are taken one hour before the anxiety-laden event. They inhibit the expression of anxiety by the autonomic nervous system, so that the patient is not aware of the anxious state and will not present an anxious demeanor to the audience.

In the eccentric cluster disorders, low dosages of **antipsychotic medications** are sometimes useful, particularly for schizotypal patients and, to a lesser extent, for paranoid patients. The latter tend to feel threatened if they are not constantly "on the alert"; they may feel worse if too much medication makes them feel benumbed to possible dangers. Schizoid traits such as aloofness and reclusiveness do not respond to psychoactive medication.

Patients with borderline personality disorder, as defined in the DSM-IV, are especially challenging to treat. Therefore, most of the literature on drug treat-

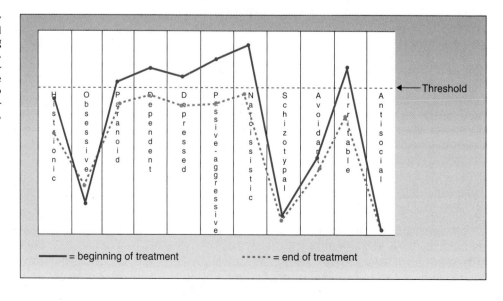

FIGURE 8–1. In the therapy of personality disorders, small quantitative changes can bring about large qualitative changes. The patient's personality is basically the same, but it is more adaptive and less offensive to others. Solid line, profile at beginning of treatment; dotted line, profile at end of treatment.

ment for personality disorders focuses on these patients. The irritability and rage that commonly accompany borderline personality disorder can be treated with low dosages of antipsychotics, lithium, or carbamazepine. (See Chapter 16, Psychopharmacology.)

Coexisting Axis I Disorders

Because Axis I disorders are often present in patients with personality disorders, their symptoms may require drug treatment. The most common disorder is depression, for which **antidepressants** may be given as psychotherapy continues. The identification of Axis I disorders with the prescription of appropriate medication is still the most frequently overlooked aspect of the treatment of personality disorders. In patients without target symptoms but with severe ongoing personality disorders of either the impulsive, action-oriented type or the inhibited, rigid type, the search for coexisting Axis I illnesses is crucial. Affective illness is the most common. It may exacerbate impulsive acting out and intensify rigid character defenses. The key to recognizing affective symptoms is the presence of an intense affect, whether it is acted upon or not. A patient with an action-oriented or rigidly controlled personality may have a bipolar disorder. **Mood stabilizers** have been extremely important in treating this illness. Associated posttraumatic stress disorder may respond to antidepressants.

Now that effective, more easily tolerated antidepressants are available, there seems to be a growing reluctance on the part of patients and therapists to undertake psychotherapy. Perhaps this age of fast food and high-speed communication via computer networks and fax machines has contributed to the understandable wish for immediate gratification. A growing emphasis by managed care companies on the most economically efficient treatment may have contributed to this trend, as well. Unfortunately, any attempt to view personality disorders as being responsive to drug treatment, at least at the present time, risks doing a great disservice to patients. If no target symptoms or Axis I disorders are present, the need for psychotherapy cannot be avoided by a drug-treatment shortcut. ➡ For example, one patient, an aspiring actress, functioned well in her job as a waitress but said she was unable to achieve her personal and professional goals. She did not have a long-term intimate relationship and "spun her wheels" without direction as she drifted from one acting class to another. This lack of initiative was demonstrated in other ways as well (e.g., she constantly bounced checks because she "never got around to" balancing her checkbook). Despite these maladaptive patterns, there was no evidence of an Axis I disorder. The patient was euthymic, got pleasure from acting and music, and had little anxiety. She described her therapy as quite useful in increasing her self-understanding but noted that the insights had not carried over into modifications in behavior.

The therapist referred the patient to a psychiatrist for consultation. The psychiatrist's recommendations were as follows: (1) The woman's difficulties seemed to be fully attributable to an avoidant personality disorder, and, therefore, medication was not indicated. (2) The therapy had been promoting a superficial understanding of the patient's problems but had not reached the level of deeper emotional experience. This is one of the risks of once-a-week sessions, which are often inadequate for insight-oriented work (see Chapter 15, Psychotherapy). (3) A more intensive form of psychotherapy was indicated, with at least two sessions per week. ◀

References Cited

Casey, P., and P. Tyrer. Personality, functioning, and symptomatology. Journal of Psychiatric Research 20:363–374, 1986.

Cloninger, C. R. A unified biosocial theory of personality and its role in the development of anxiety states. *In* Guze, S. B. and M. Roth, eds. Psychiatric Developments. New York, Oxford University Press, 1986.

Eysenck, H. J. The Dimensions of Personality. London, Kegan, Paul, Trench, and Trubner, 1947.

Loranger, A. W. Personality Disorder Examination Manual. Yonkers, New York, DV Communications, 1988.

Millon, T. Disorders of Personality, Axis II. New York, Wiley Interscience, 1981.

Robins, L., et al. Lifetime prevalence of specific psychiatric disorders in three sites. Archives of General Psychiatry 41:949–958, 1984.

Srole, L., et al. Mental Health in the Metropolis: The Midtown Manhattan Study. New York, McGraw-Hill, 1962.

Stone, M. H. The Fate of Borderline Patients. New York, Guilford Press, 1990.

Tupes, E. C., and R. E. Christal. Recurrent personality factors based on trait ratings: U.S. Air Force ASD Technical Reports (#61–97). *Reprinted in* Journal of Personality 60:225–251, 1961–1962.

Tyrer, P., and J. Alexander. Personality assessment schedule. *In* P. Tyrer (editor). Personality Disorders: Diagnosis, Management and Course. London, Wright, 1988.

Weissman, M. M. The epidemiology of personality disorders: a 1990 update. Journal of Personality Disorders 7(Supplement Spring):44–62, 1993.

Widiger, T. A., and J. H. Rogers. Prevalence and comorbidity of personality disorders. Psychiatric Annals 19:132–136, 1989.

Selected Readings

Beck, A. T., and A. Freeman. Cognitive Therapy of Personality Disorders. New York, Guilford Press, 1990.

Clarkin, J. F., and M. F. Lenzenweger (editors). Major Theories of Personality Disorder. New York, Guilford Press, 1996.

Horowitz, N., et al. Personality Styles and Brief Psychotherapy. New York, Basic Books, 1984.

Kernberg, O. F. Severe Personality Disorders: Psychotherapeutic Strategies. New Haven, Yale University Press, 1984.

Stone, M. H. The Borderline Syndromes. New York, McGraw-Hill, 1980.

Zuckerman, M. Physiology of Personality. New York, Cambridge University Press, 1991.

CHAPTER NINE

EATING DISORDERS

MICHAEL J. DEVLIN, MD

The overwhelming majority of patients with eating disorders—anorexia nervosa, bulimia nervosa, and related syndromes—are young women who, as a result of their disorders, face serious psychosocial and health consequences.

An important and difficult question raised by these disorders concerns the boundaries of psychopathology in a cultural context: When does dieting, in a society that idealizes thinness, become pathological? The eating disorders present particularly clear examples of the challenge to physicians to understand their patients' illnesses not only on a psychological level but also on biological, social, and cultural levels. All of these factors must be taken into account as physicians evaluate the onset and maintenance of eating disorders and devise appropriate treatment strategies.

DIAGNOSTIC AND CLINICAL FEATURES
Core Features of Eating Disorders

The eating disorders share a core behavioral feature, which is a disturbance of eating habits, and a core psychological feature, which is a preoccupation with or disturbance in the perception of body image. In anorexia nervosa, the eating disturbance takes the form of undereating, while in bulimia nervosa or anorexia nervosa binge-eating/purging type, it takes the form of severely restrained eating alternating with loss of control and consumption of large amounts of food. Binge-eating disorder is also characterized by episodic uncontrolled eating, frequently in a lifetime context of intermittent attempts at dieting, but without fasting, vigorous exercise, purging, or other attempts to compensate for the binge-eating episodes. Patients with binge-eating disorder consider themselves "compulsive eaters" and often gain large amounts of weight during periods of extreme binge eating.

The second feature shared by the eating disorders is a preoccupation with or disturbance in the perception of body image. Most evident in anorexia nervosa, this excessive concern about body weight and shape is also a major component in bulimia nervosa and binge-eating disorder. This feature was added to the diagnostic criteria for bulimia nervosa in the DSM-III-R and has been retained in the DSM-IV. Some consider it to be the central characteristic of these illnesses and the source of the behavioral disturbances. Many patients with eating disorders consider body weight and shape to be the most important factors in determining how they feel about themselves at a given moment. These factors are more significant to these patients than their performance at work or school; their relationships with friends, spouses, or children; or any other aspect of their lives that might contribute to a sense of well-being. It is not unusual for a patient to feel that the day has been ruined if she finds that she has gained a pound when she steps on the scale in the morning.

Anorexia Nervosa

Anorexia nervosa is characterized by severe restriction of food intake, leading to weight loss and the medical sequelae of starvation. Patients with anorexia nervosa, unlike those who lose weight for other reasons, are unable to acknowledge their emaciated state and are continually afraid of becoming fat.

The first criterion for diagnosing anorexia nervosa is **weight loss** or absence of expected weight gain in a person who refuses to maintain a minimum healthy weight. The minimum healthy weight is usually defined as 85% or more of the recommended weight, often taken from insurance tables, for a person of the same age and height. The diagnosis cannot be based on this criterion alone, however, because it is not unusual for women, especially, to weigh less than the minimum healthy weight. In postmenarcheal women, amenorrhea must also be present for the diagnosis of anorexia nervosa to be made. **Amenorrhea** is a physiological indicator of abnormally low weight and insufficient fat stores, and, in a substantial number of patients with anorexia nervosa, it coincides with, or even precedes, a significant weight loss. After normal weight has been achieved, several months often pass before normal menstrual cycling resumes.

In addition to these behavioral and biological features, the diagnosis of anorexia nervosa requires two psychological features: an **intense fear of gaining weight,** and a **body image disturbance.** The latter is especially difficult to manage because patients with anorexia nervosa usually see themselves or parts of their bodies as fat, even though they appear emaciated to others. Some patients, often older or chronic patients, will admit that they are thin, but are unduly invested in maintaining this degree of emaciation or seem not to appreciate the consequences of maintaining such a low weight. According to the DSM-IV criteria, these patients may also receive the diagnosis.

The DSM-IV recognizes two subtypes of anorexia nervosa. **Anorexia nervosa restricting type** is seen in underweight patients who have engaged in dieting, fasting, or excessive exercise but, during the current episode, have not engaged in binge eating or purging. **Anorexia nervosa binge-eating/purging type** is seen in underweight patients who engage in a cycle of binge eating and purging (Table 9–1). Several studies have shown that anorectic-bulimics have more impulsive behaviors (e.g., stealing, abusing drugs, mutilating themselves, and attempting suicide) and more maladaptive personality traits than anorectic-restrictors. In addition, they more commonly have a personal and family history of obesity and more frequently report psychiatric illness in their parents.

Patients with anorexia nervosa display a number of characteristic behaviors in addition to those described above. Initially, they may be enthusiastic about the discipline involved in dieting, exercising, and continuing to lose weight. As starvation progresses, a depressed mood may develop, which is accompanied by lethargy, irritability, social isolation, and decreased interest in sex.

Patients with anorexia nervosa are **preoccupied with food.** They usually take great interest in preparing food for others and often work in food-related jobs. They may engage in **ritualized behaviors** concerning food, such as eating only specific amounts of specific foods prepared in specific ways, prolonging

the eating of small amounts of food, or hoarding food. They may also engage in rituals concerning weight, such as weighing themselves repeatedly, gazing into mirrors, or measuring parts of their bodies. A patient might make a point of dividing each item on her tray into quarters and eating exactly one-quarter of what is served. These seemingly compulsive behaviors and obsessions about "counting calories" and following weight have led to speculation that there may be a relationship between anorexia nervosa and obsessive-compulsive disorder. Although most patients with anorexia nervosa do not suffer from a clinically defined obsessive-compulsive disorder that can be distinguished from their preoccupations with weight and food, the prevalence of an obsessive-compulsive disorder that appears to be separate and distinct from the eating disorder is higher than would be expected among these patients.

Bulimia Nervosa

Bulimia nervosa, which is usually diagnosed in patients of normal weight, is also characterized by attempts to restrict food intake, but the eating behavior is somewhat different from that found in anorexia nervosa. The attempts at restriction are interspersed with **binge eating,** periods of uncontrollable consumption of large amounts of food followed most frequently by the compensatory behavior of vomiting. The use of syrup of ipecac, which is an emetic that is available without prescription, can result in a potentially lethal cardiomyopathy, and, because patients may not volunteer such information, the physician should specifically ask about the use of syrup of ipecac. Other methods of compensation include laxatives and over-the-counter or prescription diuretics. Stimulant laxatives may be taken in amounts that far exceed the recommended dosage. Some patients use vigorous exercise and fasting to prevent weight gain. The diagnosis of bulimia nervosa has been divided into the purging and nonpurging subtypes in the DSM-IV in the hope that this will facilitate further study of the nonpurging patients, who have been the focus of relatively few systematic studies. **Bulimia nervosa purging type** is seen in patients who have regularly engaged in self-induced vomiting or purging during the current episode. **Bulimia nervosa nonpurging type** is seen in patients who have engaged in fasting or excessive exercising but not in self-induced vomiting or purging during the current episode (Table 9–2).

During eating binges, patients feel a **loss of control** over what or how much is eaten. ➡ One young woman described her eating pattern, which clearly fits the criteria for a binge, as follows: "My worst binges happened at night. I would go down to the basement and grab food out of the refrigerator . . . a pound of roast beef (which I would never usually let myself eat), bagels, a whole cake, and top it off with ice cream. Many mornings, I woke up on the floor in front of the refrigerator, burned out and disgusted

---

TABLE 9–1. DSM-IV Diagnostic Criteria for Anorexia Nervosa

A. Refusal to maintain body weight at or above a minimally normal weight for age and height (e.g., weight loss leading to maintenance of body weight less than 85% of that expected; or failure to make expected weight gain during period of growth, leading to body weight less than 85% of that expected).

B. Intense fear of gaining weight or becoming fat, even though underweight.

C. Disturbance in the way in which one's body weight or shape is experienced, undue influence of body weight or shape on self-evaluation, or denial of the seriousness of the current low body weight.

D. In postmenarcheal females, amenorrhea, i.e., the absence of at least three consecutive menstrual cycles. (A woman is considered to have amenorrhea if her periods occur only following hormone, e.g., estrogen, administration.)

Specify type:

    Restricting Type: during the current episode of Anorexia Nervosa, the person has not regularly engaged in binge-eating or purging behavior (i.e., self-induced vomiting or the misuse of laxatives, diuretics, or enemas)

    Binge-Eating/Purging Type: during the current episode of Anorexia Nervosa, the person has regularly engaged in binge-eating or purging behavior (i.e., self-induced vomiting or the misuse of laxatives, diuretics, or enemas)

TABLE 9–2. DSM-IV Diagnostic Criteria for Bulimia Nervosa

A. Recurrent episodes of binge eating. An episode of binge eating is characterized by both of the following:
   (1) eating, in a discrete period of time (e.g., within any 2-hour period), an amount of food that is definitely larger than most people would eat during a similar period of time and under similar circumstances
   (2) a sense of lack of control over eating during the episode (e.g., a feeling that one cannot stop eating or control what or how much one is eating)
B. Recurrent inappropriate compensatory behavior in order to prevent weight gain, such as self-induced vomiting; misuse of laxatives, diuretics, enemas, or other medications; fasting; or excessive exercise.
C. The binge eating and inappropriate compensatory behaviors both occur, on average, at least twice a week for 3 months.
D. Self-evaluation is unduly influenced by body shape and weight.
E. The disturbance does not occur exclusively during episodes of Anorexia Nervosa.

Specify type:
   Purging Type: during the current episode of Bulimia Nervosa, the person has regularly engaged in self-induced vomiting or the misuse of laxatives, diuretics, or enemas
   Nonpurging Type: during the current episode of Bulimia Nervosa, the person has used other inappropriate compensatory behaviors, such as fasting or excessive exercise, but has not regularly engaged in self-induced vomiting or the misuse of laxatives, diuretics, or enemas

from the night before, but needing to somehow get myself together for another day." ◀▦

Eating binges are usually triggered by unpleasant feelings or circumstances (e.g., a disappointing personal relationship, stress at work or school) or by an experience that affects the patient's perception of her body (e.g., trying on clothes that no longer fit). The bingeing and purging cycle may relieve or neutralize these feelings for a short period of time but later often results in an overall decline in self-esteem.

The structure and context of the binging and purging behavior usually vary little from episode to episode. The preparation and consumption of food often take place in secret, and patients often feel an extreme sense of alienation because of the secrecy. The eating episode is terminated when the patient becomes excessively full, is interrupted by someone or something, or attempts to compensate by purging. One recovered patient remarked on the novelty of being able to concentrate on the dinner conversation when eating out with friends rather than worrying about when and where she would purge. Although physicians who work with bulimic patients usually focus on the binging behavior, they should be aware that other eating behaviors of these patients are also often quite abnormal. Some patients consume little or nothing until the evening hours and then lose control and binge eat. In order to normalize their eating, such patients must not only avoid binging episodes in the evening but must also allow themselves to eat a reasonable amount during the earlier part of the day.

When patients with bulimia nervosa are asked to evaluate their appearance and overall self-worth,

most express undue concern with body shape and weight. These patients are usually of normal weight, although occasionally they may be obese or somewhat underweight. It is normal in the United States for physical appearance to influence a person's overall self-esteem, but patients with bulimia nervosa often consider body weight and shape to be *the* most important factors in determining how they feel about themselves. They derive less satisfaction from other areas of life, such as personal relationships or achievements at work or school.

▦▶ The following patient's story illustrates the way in which this psychological disturbance can lead to the binge eating and purging characteristic of bulimia nervosa: "I had always been overweight as a child, but when I started competitive swimming, I slimmed down and started getting a lot of compliments. I was more popular at school, and guys started showing some interest. Finally, I felt good about myself. The problem came in when I injured my back and had to quit swimming. The weight started coming back on, and I didn't know how to stop it. Vomiting seemed like the perfect solution at first. Only later did I realize that I couldn't control it." ◀▦

Binge-Eating Disorder

Binge-eating disorder is characterized first and foremost by recurrent **uncontrolled eating binges.** The binges are similar to those in bulimia nervosa but cannot be broken down into discrete episodes because they often occur continuously over several hours and are not punctuated by purges. In order to be diagnosed with this disorder, patients must experience a loss of control as well as exhibit the behavioral indicators of **loss of control.** Loss of control differentiates these episodes from "normal" overeating. They must have significant distress related to eating. Patients with binge-eating disorder often feel that their lives are dominated by eating and have significant impairment in their abilities to work and relate to others.

Because binge-eating disorder is a relatively new entity, little is known about its descriptive features and psychopathology. There is an association between binge-eating disorder and obesity, but binge-eating disorder is not synonymous with obesity. Obesity is considered to be a medical rather than a psychiatric disorder, although some obese individuals probably do have an eating disorder, and recent efforts have been made to study, diagnose, and treat such individuals. The DSM-IV category of binge-eating disorder, characterized by uncontrollable binge eating in the absence of purging or other compensatory behaviors, has been proposed for these patients. Criteria for further study are given in Appendix B of the DSM-IV (Table 9–3). It is not yet known what proportion of obese individuals suffer from the disorder or what proportion of individuals with the disorder are obese. Preliminary studies demonstrate that persons of normal weight as well

TABLE 9–3. DSM-IV Diagnostic (Research) Criteria for Binge-Eating Disorder

A. Recurrent episodes of binge eating. An episode of binge eating is characterized by both of the following:
   (1) eating, in a discrete period of time (e.g., within any 2-hour period), an amount of food that is definitely larger than most people would eat in a similar period of time under similar circumstances
   (2) a sense of lack of control over eating during the episode (e.g., a feeling that one cannot stop eating or control what or how much one is eating)
B. The binge-eating episodes are associated with three (or more) of the following:
   (1) eating much more rapidly than normal
   (2) eating until feeling uncomfortably full
   (3) eating large amounts of food when not feeling physically hungry
   (4) eating alone because of being embarrassed by how much one is eating
   (5) feeling disgusted with oneself, depressed, or very guilty after overeating.
C. Marked distress regarding binge eating is present.
D. The binge eating occurs, on average, at least 2 days a week for 6 months.
E. The binge eating is not associated with the regular use of inappropriate compensatory behaviors (e.g., purging, fasting, excessive exercise) and does not occur exclusively during the course of Anorexia Nervosa or Bulimia Nervosa.

as overweight persons may meet the criteria for binge-eating disorder and that most obese patients in weight loss clinics do not fulfill the criteria. There is some evidence that obese patients who engage in binge eating, many of whom probably meet the criteria for binge-eating disorder, have increased psychopathology, particularly depressive symptoms, compared with obese persons who do not engage in binge eating. It is not certain whether binge-eating disorder will become a permanent diagnostic category in the psychiatric classification system. New approaches to the classification and treatment of obese patients are needed, however, as it becomes increasingly clear that long-term weight loss programs are largely ineffective.

Eating Disorder Not Otherwise Specified

The category of eating disorder not otherwise specified is used for patients who have clinically significant eating disorders that do not fulfill the criteria for other diagnoses. Patients with bulimialike syndromes include those who engage in vomiting or laxative abuse in the absence of binge eating (i.e., vomiting after consuming only small amounts of food) or those who chew and spit out large amounts of food. Patients with anorexia-like syndromes include obese individuals who lose a large amount of weight, to the point where their weight is within the statistically normal range, and maintain that weight but develop the psychological and behavioral features of anorexia nervosa. Patients with binge-eating disorder can also be included in the category of eating disorder not otherwise specified.

Associated Physical Symptoms and Signs
Anorexia Nervosa

Anorexia nervosa has a number of physical symptoms and signs, including constipation, abdominal discomfort, and cold intolerance. Typical findings on the physical examination include bradycardia, hypotension, hypothermia, dryness and yellowing of the skin (which is attributed to hypercarotenemia), the presence of lanugo (fine body hair), and peripheral edema. Laboratory findings include leukopenia and elevated blood urea nitrogen levels resulting from dehydration. Results from liver function tests are elevated either at baseline or during refeeding. Electrolyte and trace element disturbances can occur, particularly in anorectic-bulimics. Neuroendocrine abnormalities, which are thought to be hypothalamic in origin, include low estradiol levels, decreased secretion of luteinizing hormone and follicle-stimulating hormone, high cortisol levels, high growth hormone levels, and low triiodothyronine levels with high reverse triiodothyronine levels. The resting metabolic rate is usually low. CT scanning often shows mild atrophy and an increased ventricular-brain ratio. The electrocardiogram (ECG) rarely shows arrhythmias other than sinus bradycardia, but when the QT interval is prolonged, there is an elevated risk of sudden death. Osteoporosis is increasingly recognized as a complication of anorexia nervosa, especially in patients with the more chronic form of illness. All of these abnormalities are characteristic of starvation. Abnormalities arising from purging behavior (see Bulimia Nervosa, below) may be seen in anorectic patients of the binge-eating/purging type. (See also Medical Evaluation, below.)

Bulimia Nervosa

Patients with bulimia nervosa may also have medical complications. They are usually related to purging (e.g., dental sequelae of vomiting, such as erosion of enamel; salivary gland enlargement; electrolyte disturbances, such as hypokalemia, hyponatremia, hypochloremia, and hypomagnesemia; and mildly elevated serum amylase levels). The presence of ulcerations and calluses on the dorsum of the hand secondary to the manual induction of vomiting is known as Russell's sign. Patients occasionally report flecks of blood in the vomitus, which are usually the result of trauma from repeated vomiting. Excessive vomiting may also cause metabolic alkalosis. Prolonged laxative abuse can lead to large bowel abnormalities, laxative dependence, dehydration, and metabolic acidosis. A substantial proportion of patients with bulimia nervosa have menstrual irregularities and, occasionally, amenorrhea, even if their weight is normal. Neuroendocrine abnormalities are not as pronounced as those in patients with anorexia nervosa, although disturbances in gonadotropin secretion and abnormal cortisol responses to dexamethasone occur in a few patients. Rare but catastrophic complications include esophageal tears, gastric rupture, cardiac arrhythmias stemming from electrolyte imbalance, and cardiomyopathy resulting from excessive use of syrup of ipecac. (See also Medical Evaluation, below.)

EPIDEMIOLOGY

One of the practical reasons for studying epidemiology is to better understand the ways in which an illness is contracted and dispersed. Although this model may be more easily applied to infectious diseases, it is nonetheless applicable to psychiatric disorders. Eating disorders may be considered, in some ways, "communicable." Many patients with bulimia nervosa report that they first got the idea of binging and purging from friends or from television programs designed to discourage eating disorders. Although it is overly simplistic to view such influences as being entirely responsible for the development of these disorders, they may be significant contributing causes. Another significant influence may be the pervasive societal promotion of thinness, which may lead to a preoccupation with dieting, a core feature of anorexia nervosa and bulimia nervosa, and to the development of eating disorders at least in some individuals predisposed to the disorders.

Incidence and Prevalence

Anorexia nervosa has an overall incidence of 0.24–7.3 new cases per 100,000 persons per year. The figures increase by an order of magnitude when the population base is restricted to young women. In this group, the prevalence is 0.2–0.8%, with higher rates of subthreshold cases. Studies conducted in Sweden, northeast Scotland, and the United States have suggested that the prevalence of anorexia nervosa is increasing, although there is some disagreement on this point.

Bulimia nervosa is more common than anorexia nervosa. Its prevalence is estimated at 1–5%, with most studies reporting a prevalence of 1–2% among young women. A recent genetic study confirms the general impression that the risk of bulimia nervosa is greater among more recent cohorts, especially women born in or after 1960, but it is not known whether the prevalence is continuing to increase or has reached a plateau.

One of the most striking epidemiological features of the eating disorders is the extreme imbalance between males and females. Most studies report that 90–95% of affected individuals are **female.** Both anorexia nervosa and bulimia nervosa occur in males as well, and homosexual males appear to be at increased risk.

Age of Onset

The mean age of onset for anorexia nervosa is 16–17 years, with a bimodal distribution that peaks at age 14 and 18 years. Bulimia nervosa also usually has its onset in adolescence or early adulthood. Although it is relatively uncommon for preteenage children to present with clinical eating disorders, it is not uncommon for them to begin dieting and, perhaps, unwittingly lay the groundwork for future eating disorders. Dieting seems to be a risk factor for these disorders; in the vast majority of cases, onset occurs during or following a period of dieting. Persons who are under pressure to diet (e.g., ballet dancers, models, and actresses) are at a particularly high risk of developing bulimia nervosa as well as anorexia nervosa. For both disorders, there is a relatively high prevalence of subthreshold or transitory cases in high-risk populations (i.e., women of high school or college age, especially those who are dieting).

The age at which patients first present for treatment is often very different from the age of onset. Patients with anorexia nervosa and bulimia nervosa tend to present within a fairly narrow age range that extends from the early teenage years up through early adulthood. The presentation may be different in the different age-groups. Family issues tend to be more of a concern in younger patients who are living at home, and these patients are more likely to be brought in by family members, sometimes unwillingly. Patients who are older at the time of presentation are more likely to have experienced adverse effects from the disorder and may have a somewhat higher motivation to take part in treatment.

Morbidity and Mortality

Anorexia nervosa is one of the most lethal psychiatric illnesses. Long-term studies have reported alarmingly high mortality rates of 15–18%. Most of these deaths result from starvation and a few from suicide. More recent shorter-term studies have suggested that in patients who receive adequate treatment, these figures may be somewhat lower. Bulimia nervosa is less frequently lethal, but catastrophic complications of vomiting, such as gastric rupture or esophageal tears, cardiac arrhythmia secondary to severe electrolyte imbalance, and cardiomyopathy resulting from abuse of syrup of ipecac can lead to death. Medical and dental complications of anorexia nervosa and bulimia nervosa are noted above. The severely disruptive effects of an eating disorder on personal development (i.e., on the tasks of young adulthood, such as forming intimate relationships, obtaining an education, and setting career goals) should not be underestimated.

There is substantial comorbidity of anorexia nervosa and bulimia nervosa. About 40% of patients with anorexia nervosa develop bulimia nervosa within two years of onset, and about one-half of patients with bulimia nervosa who are of normal weight report a history of anorexia nervosa. Patients with anorexia nervosa and bulimia nervosa are at increased risk for certain other psychiatric disturbances. Studies over the past decade have revealed that roughly one-third to one-half of patients with eating disorders suffer from concurrent **major**

depression, and about one-half to three-quarters have a lifetime history of depression. Patients with bulimia nervosa and with anorexia nervosa binge-eating/purging type have a higher than expected prevalence of **substance abuse disorders,** especially alcohol and stimulant abuse or dependence. Stimulants are often used in an attempt to lose weight. Some physicians view bulimia nervosa as a form of substance abuse, with the substance being food, and point to common features such as craving for a substance; impaired ability to cope with difficult situations or feelings; financial, psychological, and physical complications; and repeated unsuccessful attempts to regain control. However, the analogy is limited in that abstinence from alcohol or drugs leads to better health, whereas abstinence from food leads to another eating disorder, namely, anorexia nervosa.

Researchers have also been interested in the co-morbidity of eating disorders and **personality disorders.** Most studies agree that patients with eating disorders have elevated rates of the DSM-IV personality disorders in Cluster B (antisocial, borderline, histrionic, narcissistic) and Cluster C (avoidant, dependent, obsessive-compulsive). The Cluster B disorders, including borderline personality disorder, are especially common in patients who engage in binge eating and purging. The reported rates of personality disorders vary widely, depending on the methods of assessment used. Sexual abuse has been reported in a substantial proportion of patients with bulimia nervosa, but the rate does not appear to exceed that in other psychiatric patients.

Course of Illness

The following case illustrates the fairly typical downward spiral in functioning that patients with eating disorders experience. ➧ A 21-year-old single college student presented for treatment of binge eating and vomiting that had been occurring since she was age 16 years and that, as she put it, "has taken over my life." When asked about the origin of her eating disorder, she stated, "I have never eaten normal meals . . . I've always been a dieter." She initially got the idea to purge after seeing a television program about eating disorders. Although the program was intended to discourage eating disorders, it seemed at the time to be describing to the patient the ideal method of "eating whatever I wanted and not having to pay the consequences." However, once she started to induce vomiting after normal meals, she soon found herself eating large quantities of food and vomiting on a daily basis. During the current semester, when she had broken up with her boyfriend and was taking a particularly heavy course load, her binge eating and vomiting had gone from once per day to four or five times per day. Much of her day was spent planning her next binge and making sure that she would have the opportunity to vomit without being detected. She was ashamed to relate that, at times, she had taken her roommates' food during a

binge and was not always able to replace it. Although she had always taken pride in being a good student, she was beginning to miss her morning classes after she had stayed up eating and vomiting. She had initially lost weight when she started vomiting, but her weight had now returned to the low normal range. Despite her apparent thinness, she was distressed by what she perceived as her "fat thighs," so much so that she avoided seeing herself in the mirror and had gone from weighing herself several times per day to completely avoiding the scale. In her words, "I hate myself and I hate what my life has become. I can't find my way out of this trap." ⬳

Anorexia Nervosa

Although the number of published longitudinal follow-up studies of patients with anorexia nervosa is relatively small, certain findings have emerged fairly consistently. Patients who have an older age of onset, bulimic symptoms, longer duration of illness before presentation for treatment, lower weight, personality disturbance, social and family difficulties, and failure to respond to previous treatments have a poorer prognosis. Patients who are ill for 5–7 years or longer are likely to have a chronic course and are at increased risk of death. It is possible for patients to recover even after many years of illness, however.

Most patients in inpatient refeeding programs attain a weight within the normal range by the time of discharge. At long-term follow-up (4–12 years), about half of these patients continue to maintain a normal weight and are menstruating and 10–20% are still markedly underweight. About two-thirds of patients continue to be preoccupied with weight and body shape and do not have a regular pattern of eating. As noted above, a substantial proportion of patients with anorexia nervosa develop bulimic behaviors at some point in their illnesses. The longest-term follow-up studies suggest that over the course of time, most patients either recover to a significant degree or die from their illnesses.

Bulimia Nervosa

Relatively little is known about the course of bulimia nervosa because the illness has only been recognized for a little more than a decade. Most of the available information on prognosis is derived from treatment studies that have followed patients for the short term. Certain patterns are beginning to emerge. In the most successful outpatient studies, particularly psychotherapy studies, approximately half of patients are in remission and most of the remaining patients have improved significantly from their baseline status. A small number of patients lose a significant amount of weight during or following treatment. It is also becoming clear that patients who fail to respond to one treatment approach may respond more favorably to a different approach. Therefore, patients who are persistent and motivated to accept treatment are more likely to do well.

Bulimic patients who are treated as inpatients are, for the most part, a more severely ill group. A follow-up study done on the author's inpatient unit found that of patients contacted 2–9 years following hospitalization, about 40% had recovered, 40% still met the full criteria for bulimia nervosa, and 20% had an intermediate outcome.

As more becomes known about the effective treatment of bulimia nervosa and the patient factors that predict success with a particular form of treatment, it makes increasing sense to regard most cases of bulimia nervosa as treatable rather than chronic. A few patients may have a more chronic course and require long-term treatment, however. More chronically ill patients tend to have impaired functioning in maintaining interpersonal relationships and performing occupational activities, in part because of the length of their illness. A small number of patients are able to accommodate the eating disorder and maintain a relatively high level of functioning. Some older patients with bulimia nervosa report that their level of concern with body shape and weight has decreased over the years but that they have become so accustomed to binge eating and purging that it is hard to imagine living any other way.

Binge-Eating Disorder

There is little firm information on the course of binge-eating disorder. Preliminary studies show that these patients, like those with bulimia nervosa, usually begin binge eating in late adolescence or early adulthood. The disorder appears to be relatively chronic, but this view may be revised as more studies are undertaken and more effective treatments are developed.

THE INTERVIEW

Once an eating disorder is suspected, the physician should obtain a thorough history, including the patient's lifetime patterns of weight fluctuation and dieting, the menstrual history, personal and family attitudes toward eating and weight, and the onset and progression of binge eating. The patient should be questioned carefully concerning methods of attempted compensation, including fasting, vigorous exercise, and the use of syrup of ipecac or over-the-counter, prescription, or illicit drugs to control weight. The physician should determine whether symptoms of depression, anxiety, or alcohol and drug abuse or dependence are present, and whether the patient is engaging in behaviors such as impulsivity, self-mutilation, or the stealing of food. It is often useful for family members to be interviewed, especially if the patient is young. Common presenting complaints of patients with eating disorders are given in Table 9–4. Each patient should have a thorough medical evaluation (see below).

During the interview of a patient with an eating disorder, the first priority is for the physician to **establish an alliance** with the patient. The physician

TABLE 9–4. Presenting Complaints of Patients With Eating Disorders

Obsession with dieting or thinness, or both.
Fatigue, inability to exercise, or other sequelae of malnutrition.
Uncontrolled binge eating or purging, or both.
Depressed mood or other symptoms of depression.
Functional impairment (e.g., inability to concentrate at school or work due to one or more of the above factors).
Family or marital discord related to eating disorder.
For patients presenting to dentists: dental erosion or salivary gland enlargement.
For patients presenting to physicians: weakness, light-headedness, amenorrhea, bloating, abdominal discomfort, blood in vomitus, or other symptoms resulting from malnutrition, binge eating, or purging.
For patients presenting to weight loss centers: desire to lose weight despite, in many cases, being of normal or low weight.

must try to understand the patient's view of herself and determine what caused the patient to seek treatment at this time (see Interviewing Guidelines box).

Anorexia Nervosa

Fully developed anorexia nervosa is usually quite obvious, although patients and families sometimes deny the presence of the illness for a surprisingly long time. Patients who are thought to be at risk should be asked about the methods they use to lose weight and should be encouraged to discuss their attitudes toward food, body weight, and body shape. Patients whose weight loss has been entirely voluntary are at the highest risk for anorexia nervosa. Patients who initially lose weight because of an illness or some other external factor but then decide to "keep going" and lose more weight have a somewhat lower risk. Patients who deny their weight loss or are not appropriately concerned about its medical sequelae, such as amenorrhea, should be evaluated carefully for the other symptoms of anorexia nervosa.

Patients with anorexia nervosa are frequently motivated by the physical manifestations of their low weight to ask for professional help. For example, a patient may be so malnourished that she can no longer carry out activities that are important to her, such as exercise or work. Occasionally, a patient will ask for help because she wants to have children and is seeking treatment for amenorrhea. At some level, a patient with anorexia nervosa knows that she needs to gain weight, and the physician must ally himself or herself with this goal. The physician must be aware, however, that the patient is extremely ambivalent and tremendously fearful about giving up what has become the central focus of her life. Although the physician needs to understand the patient's resistance to eating and fear of uncontrolled weight gain, he or she must tell the patient that treatment cannot be successful without weight gain and must not collude with the patient in her attempts to defer it. Once the patient feels that she can trust the physician, she will be able to risk gaining weight and may realize that this is not as unmanageable as she may have

Interviewing Guidelines

- Obtain a thorough history from the patient and the patient's family of eating patterns and fluctuations in weight; important life events and transitions; attitudes toward the body and overall self-esteem; depression, substance abuse, or other psychiatric symptoms; medical disorders; and previous treatments and responses.
- Convey an attitude of understanding and expertise. Avoid statements that evoke shame or guilt.
- Ascertain why the patient is presenting for treatment at this particular time.
- Find out what the patient desires from treatment. Ask how the eating disorder is interfering with her life at the present time or preventing her from attaining her goals. Use this information to form a treatment alliance.
- Inform the patient fully about the structure of, rationale for, and expected outcome of treatment.
- Recognize the patient's anxiety about sudden drastic changes (e.g., rapidly gaining a large amount of weight), and provide reassurance that treatment will take place one step at a time and that the patient will be assisted in maintaining control.
- It may be helpful to interview family members or other informants in order to understand the background and family context of the eating disorder. This is especially important for extremely undernourished patients who are cognitively impaired.

thought. The patient's malnourished state is likely to affect her ability to think. Extremely cachectic patients tend to have concrete, rigid thought patterns. Initially, therefore, much of the focus is on weight gain, and only later is it possible to shift the focus to other important issues in the patient's life that may underlie the eating disorder.

There are some common themes in the responses that patients suffering from anorexia nervosa have to their physicians. The patient often sees the therapist as an authority figure who is acting as a dictator by telling her how much weight she is expected to gain. Depending on the patient's psychological makeup, she usually reacts with covert or open rebellion. The therapist may become frustrated by the rigidity of the patient's thinking and her resistance to efforts to help.

Bulimia Nervosa

Patients with bulimia nervosa tend to have surprisingly few medical sequelae of their behavior. Bulimia nervosa is often more subtle in its presentation than anorexia nervosa because most patients are of normal weight. Patients tend to be extraordinarily ashamed of their behavior, and even if they have reached the point where they want help, they will often not come forward with their concerns unless the physician conveys a sense of understanding and familiarity with the disorder. Occasionally, patients will admit to recurrent vomiting but not to the voluntary induction of vomiting and will be subjected to extensive gastrointestinal workups. In order to diagnose bulimia nervosa as quickly as possible in patients who do not complain of binge eating or purging, the physician should bear in mind the risk factors for this illness. Women of high school or college age, particularly those who have had significant weight fluctuations, who are known to be dieting strictly, who have a rigorous exercise regimen, or who suffer from depression or substance abuse should be considered to be at risk. Unanticipated dental problems or unexplained electrolyte disturbances, particularly hypokalemia, should raise the index of suspicion.

Patients often present for treatment when they have become aware of the destructive effects of binge eating and purging on their lives and their inability to control this behavior. They are often extremely ashamed of their bingeing and purging episodes and associated behavior (e.g., stealing food) and expect others to be repulsed by it. Not uncommonly, the physician is the first person that they have told about the problem. When asked to describe their bingeing behavior in detail, however, some patients describe episodes that do not fit the usual classification of bingeing. A patient may say that she had eaten a large amount of food, particularly if she thinks of the food as fattening or forbidden, and felt that purging was necessary, even though she had eaten only a small amount, such as three cookies or a candy bar. The physician must ask for specific details about the amount and type of food consumed. Patients often find this difficult to discuss because they are afraid that the physician will be shocked by the details of their eating. Therefore, it is important for the physician to assume an empathic but matter-of-fact attitude when questioning patients and to let them know that he or she is familiar with and not disgusted by the amount of food that may be consumed during a bingeing episode, is experienced in working with the disorder, and wants to find out more about the particular difficulties.

Like patients with anorexia nervosa, patients with bulimia nervosa are usually terrified of gaining weight. A surprisingly large number of patients state, at least initially, that even though they are truly distressed about their bulimic behaviors, they would not be willing to accept a 10-pound weight gain in exchange for remission of the disorder. The physician must create a bond of trust with patients so that they are willing to change their eating habits and take the risk of gaining weight (although most patients do not gain a significant amount of weight as they recover from bulimia nervosa).

Patients with eating disorders often provoke intense reactions in the physician. These patients are often young adults who are functioning at a reasonably high level in other areas of their lives. Younger physicians tend to identify strongly with them. Bulimic patients of normal weight may have an appearance and style of interaction that is quite appropriate, which may cause the physician to underrate the severity of the illness. This may be a serious problem if the physician discharges a patient from an inpatient unit on the assumption that she will continue to do well but has not given the patient enough education on how to prevent relapse and how important it is to do so. Physicians sometimes view the illness as self-inflicted and may become angry and frustrated when patients refuse to give up their self-destructive behavior. (Patients are likely to provoke these feelings in their family and friends as well.) When the physician becomes aware of these feelings, he or she should remember that patients' perceptions of their bodies are seriously impaired; that their behavior is deeply entrenched; and that this behavior makes a certain amount of sense when seen from their point of view.

DIFFERENTIAL DIAGNOSIS

The differential diagnosis for anorexia nervosa includes medical causes of wasting, such as occult **malignant tumors** or, rarely, lateral hypothalamic tumors or trauma. Psychiatric syndromes, such as major depression, may also be associated with weight loss. Patients with these diagnoses may feel unable to eat enough to maintain their weight but rarely display the psychological features of anorexia nervosa. The differential diagnosis between anorexia nervosa and **depression** can at times be difficult because patients with anorexia nervosa not uncommonly suffer from major depression. Patients who are depressed may say that they realize they are thin and need to gain weight, but if they are also suffering from anorexia nervosa, their unexpressed fears of becoming fat usually become evident as they begin to gain weight and exhibit a resistance to gaining more weight. Patients with anorexia nervosa may have a body image disturbance so severe that it seems psychotic (i.e., a patient may claim that she is fat when she is actually extremely emaciated). However, a psychotic disorder should not be considred in these patients unless the psychosis extends into other areas of their lives. ➧ One underweight patient with a fear of gaining weight believed that God would not be able to lift her into heaven if she weighed more than 88 pounds. Because her body image disturbance existed in the context of a larger delusion, she was diagnosed as having a psychotic disorder rather than an eating disorder. ◀

The differential diagnosis of bulimia nervosa includes rare medical causes, such as genetic disorders (e.g., Prader-Willi syndrome) and ventromedial hypothalamic tumors, or trauma. Atypical depression can present with overeating and weight gain. In all of these cases, patients usually do not meet the criteria for bulimia nervosa, either because their overeating does not take the form of discrete eating binges or because they do not attempt to compensate for binge eating by purging, fasting, or vigorous exercising.

MEDICAL EVALUATION

Patients should have a complete physical examination. Laboratory tests should include serum electrolytes, magnesium, and phosphate; blood urea nitrogen, creatinine, and liver enzymes; and a complete blood count. Given the coexistence of eating disorders and substance abuse, urine toxicologic screening is often useful. An ECG should be part of the baseline workup for patients who are seriously underweight, have significant electrolyte disturbances, or have a history of abuse of syrup of ipecac. Other laboratory tests may be suggested by the history or physical examination (e.g., a chest x-ray is indicated in patients with evidence of pulmonary congestion or pleural effusion on physical examination, and bone density studies may be useful in chronically underweight patients with a history of bone fractures).

ETIOLOGY

The factors that predispose an individual to developing an eating disorder, trigger the onset of the illness, and sustain the disorder once it is established are as yet incompletely understood. Several of the features of eating disorders discussed above provide clues to their etiology. Eating disorders are also more prevalent in some cultures than in others. Biological factors may predispose certain individuals but they are not sufficient to explain these disorders completely. As with many psychiatric syndromes, interaction among biological, psychological, and cultural factors clearly contributes to the onset and continuance of the illness. Any coherent theory of causation must take this observation into account and attempt to explain why the eating disorders are much more common in women than in men.

The etiology of the eating disorders can be considered from two different perspectives. One perspective focuses on the disturbed biological states found in patients with these disorders and the degree to which these states give rise to the characteristic abnormal behaviors. From another perspective, these disorders are seen as attempts by individuals to solve problems in their lives by developing, either consciously or unconsciously, disturbed behaviors that ultimately have physiological consequences.

Biological Theories

Patients with anorexia nervosa are suffering from, among other things, starvation, and they have most of the expected biological (and psychological) sequelae. Patients with bulimia nervosa, although usually of normal weight, also have some of the physiological signs of starvation, probably because of the pattern of dieting and undereating on which their intermittent binges are superimposed. It is important to distinguish between biological factors that *give rise to* eating disorders and biological abnormalities that *result from* the illness. The latter do not contribute to the onset of the eating disorder, but may, in some cases, contribute to its continuance.

Genetic Factors

Family and twin studies suggest that there is a genetic diathesis for both anorexia nervosa and bulimia nervosa. In anorexia nervosa, there is a 50% concordance in monozygotic twins and 7% in dizygotic twins; in bulimia nervosa, there is a 23% concordance in monozygotic twins and 9% in dizygotic twins. For both disorders, first-degree relatives of probands are at increased risk for eating disorders, affective disorders, and substance abuse. Patients with anorexia nervosa binge-eating/purging are more likely to have relatives with bulimia nervosa and substance abuse disorders. Although these studies suggest that certain individuals may be genetically predisposed to eating disorders, the mechanism is not yet understood. A genetic predisposition does not mean that a person is predestined to develop an eating disorder but rather that a person is at increased risk if the right cultural and psychological milieu is present. Given what is known about the different rates of the eating disorders in different cultures and historical periods, it is unlikely that a person is destined from birth to suffer from these disorders. It is more likely that a predisposition is inherited, which may or may not be expressed in the course of a person's lifetime. A person with a predisposition to obesity who is living in a culture that overvalues thinness might restrict her eating, which would put her at increased risk of developing a full-blown eating disorder. A person with a genetic predisposition to dysphoria and low self-esteem might react to cultural influences by manipulating her body shape and weight in an attempt to feel better about herself. The biological changes resulting from an eating disorder might also in some way counter the dysphoria. Further sophisticated genetic epidemiological studies will be needed in order to discriminate between competing hypotheses concerning the nature of genetic risk.

Neurotransmitters and Neuropeptides

Neurotransmitters such as norepinephrine and serotonin regulate the appetite, feelings of satiety, and emotional moods. It is tempting to speculate about the influence of abnormal levels or imbalances of neurotransmitters on the behavior of patients with eating disorders. Abnormal levels of neurotransmitters and their metabolites have been found in the central nervous system and the peripheral circulation in patients with eating disorders and in some patients who have recovered from these disorders. Longitudinal data that would definitively distinguish preexisting abnormalities (that might have triggered the disorder) from abnormalities resulting from behavior related to the disorder (and that may also play a role in maintaining the disorder) are as yet lacking. Some interesting patterns have emerged, however. In patients with anorexia nervosa and bulimia nervosa, the **noradrenergic pathways** may be underactive. Serotonergic systems, which are involved in regulating feelings of satiety (and are also implicated in the production of depressive and obsessive symptoms), also appear to be underactive in patients with eating disorders. This abnormality may reverse in patients who have recovered from eating disorders, and serotonergic activity may actually be increased in long-term recovered patients. Recently identified appetite-stimulating neuropeptides, such as peptide YY, have been implicated in the maintenance of binge eating in patients with bulimia nervosa.

Neuroendocrine Factors

The neuroendocrine system (i.e., the hypothalamus, pituitary gland, and endocrine glands) has been regarded for many years as a "window" through which the functioning of the brain can be observed. The many neuroendocrine abnormalities that have been described in anorexia nervosa were at one time thought to be potential causes of the illness. It is now clear that, for the most part, they are consequences of starvation rather than preexisting trait markers. The fact that some of these abnormalities exist in women with bulimia nervosa who are of normal weight suggests that, in some cases, intermittent dieting and binge eating can have biological consequences similar to those of semistarvation.

Most of the neuroendocrine abnormalities seen in patients with eating disorders are thought to be secondary to starvation or, in the case of bulimia nervosa, to intermittent strict dieting. In some cases, these abnormalities may reinforce the illness, setting up a positive feedback cycle that is difficult to interrupt. **Corticotropin-releasing hormone** is elevated in patients with anorexia nervosa, probably as a result of malnutrition. When this hormone is injected into the cerebral ventricles of laboratory animals, it may produce an anorexia nervosa–like syndrome characterized by decreased feeding, diminished sexual activity, and increased physical activity. Thus, elevated levels of this hormone result from and may contribute to the behavior of patients with anorexia nervosa.

Another example of bidirectional feedback between illness-related behavior and neuroendocrine abnormalities involves the hypothalamic-pituitary-gonadal axis. In patients with anorexia nervosa, the abnormal secretion of luteinizing hormone is the underlying cause of amenorrhea. The pattern of secretion regresses to a prepubertal state. Recovery from starvation is associated with the recurrence of mature patterns of secretion of luteinizing hormone and the resumption of menstruation. This physiological regression, which also occurs in patients who are undernourished for other reasons, is often reinforcing in patients with anorexia nervosa who have a fear of sexual maturity.

Gastrointestinal Factors

Studies of eating behavior suggest that patients with bulimia nervosa have a deficit in the satiety response to eating (i.e., after eating a normal amount of food, they do not feel "full" or wish to stop eating). Although this may reflect abnormalities in the way the brain processes signals of hunger and satiety, it may also reflect abnormalities in the signals themselves. Preliminary evidence exists that gastrointestinal abnormalities mediate this deficit. Following a test meal, patients with bulimia nervosa secrete subnormal amounts of the hormone **cholecystokinin,** which, among other functions, acts as a mediator of satiety. This abnormality in peripheral satiety signals is thought to result from repeated binge eating and purging. Once the blunted release of cholecystokinin has become established, it leads to further blunting of the satiety response following meals. In this way, a positive feedback cycle develops in which the illness causes a biological abnormality that becomes a factor in sustaining the binge eating. Further research is needed to clarify the role of this and other gastrointestinal mechanisms in the pathophysiology of eating disorders.

Psychosocial Theories

The classic patient with anorexia nervosa (particularly the restricting subtype) is described by Hilde Bruch in *The Golden Cage* (1978) as a "sparrow in a cage." She is an adolescent growing up in a privileged family that responds to her material needs but not her emotional needs. Her parents place excessive demands on her to conform to their expectations, and, as a result, she feels that none of her achievements are good enough. She seizes upon food restriction and excessive exercise as ways to feel successful and alter an intolerable family situation. Typical family characteristics that have been observed include enmeshment and overintrusiveness of family members, overprotectiveness of parents toward children, rigid adherence to roles within the family, and avoidance of overt conflict. The eating disorder often serves in some way to keep family conflict at bay. The self-induced starvation represents, among other things, compliance and rebellion, since the patient is engaging in the "healthy" behaviors of dieting and exercising but to a degree that brings her into conflict with the family. In addition, the patient may have an unconscious conflict between dependence and separation or individuation. By refusing food, which would nurture her physical body, the patient undercuts her ability to become an independent adult woman. Starvation also causes the cessation of menstruation and retards the development of secondary sexual characteristics, which may serve to alleviate anxiety in an adolescent who finds the prospect of womanhood threatening. This formulation is simplistic, but it applies, to a greater or lesser degree, to many patients with anorexia nervosa.

The psychological factors involved in bulimia nervosa vary greatly from individual to individual. Binge eating is often experienced as a temporary escape from rigid control both in the realm of eating and in other areas of life. Purging becomes the means of undoing this lapse and regaining a sense of control. Many patients with bulimia nervosa use binge eating and vomiting to divert feelings that they are unable to express because they are unacceptable to themselves or to others. Episodes of binging and purging are often triggered by situations in which the patient's self-esteem, which is often closely tied to body image, has been threatened (e.g., if a perceived slight from a boyfriend causes the patient to think she is fat and unattractive and to feel angry, despondent, and empty). Paradoxically, although patients with bulimia nervosa often feel at first that they have found the ideal way of controlling their intake, they eventually feel that they have lost control and have little idea of how much they are eating and how much they are keeping down. As the patient becomes more involved in the eating disorder, she tends to become increasingly isolated, often refusing social opportunities because she feels fat and instead staying home to engage in binge eating and purging. From a psychodynamic perspective, a patient's conflicted need for and fear of greater independence may give rise to binging and purging episodes that simultaneously express her needs to assert herself and to maintain her dependent position.

For patients with chronic forms of anorexia nervosa and bulimia nervosa, the illness may be a way of avoiding difficult interpersonal or career issues. Patients recovering from severe eating disorders face the challenge of rebuilding a life in which important decisions and pursuits have been deferred, sometimes for several years.

According to the **cognitive model,** patients with bulimia nervosa are driven to binge and purge by strict dietary rules that periodically break down. This dieting is in turn driven by an excessive concern with body shape and weight that has its basis in poor self-esteem. The system is self-reinforcing at many levels. Binge eating and purging further damage self-esteem, which increases the concern with body weight and shape, leading to further dieting, binge eating, and purging. The cognitive model of anorexia nervosa is similar, except that uncontrolled starvation rather than binge eating and purging is the behavioral component of the vicious circle.

The **behavioral model** views binge eating and vomiting as being positively reinforced by the sensations associated with the consumption of highly palatable "forbidden foods" and, for some patients, by the reduction of anxiety they experience after vomiting. In patients with anorexia nervosa, reinforcement may be derived from the physiological responses to starvation and, in the early stages of the illness, from praise received for their thinness.

Viewed from an **interpersonal perspective,** eating disorders are maintained by disturbances in relationships (e.g., difficulty in negotiating major role transitions such as leaving the family and taking on an adult role). Other disturbances include interpersonal disputes, unresolved grief reactions, and pervasive interpersonal deficits.

Cultural Factors

Only a modern-day Rip van Winkle could fail to notice and be affected by the cultural preoccupation with body image in the United States. Young women at risk for developing eating disorders are assailed daily by images of perfect bodies, with the implication that it is this and only this which guarantees happiness and fulfillment.

For women, the ideal image has changed in recent decades. This shift has been documented by studies of women who have posed for the centerfold in *Playboy* magazine or won the Miss America title. On the average, these women have become substantially thinner over the past 30 years, while the percentage of American women who are overweight has increased. Therefore, the gap between actual weight and the culturally ideal weight has progressively widened. The perception that one is 20 pounds overweight compared with the culturally sanctioned body type is more likely to lead to drastic attempts at weight control, such as vomiting or laxative abuse, than is the perception that one is 5 pounds overweight. As these cultural factors have promoted greater degrees of food restriction, the risk of eating disorders may have been increased.

Over this same period of time, the role of women in westernized societies has changed markedly. The **feminist model** views eating disorders as resulting from the rapid change, in recent decades, in social roles and appearance norms for women in westernized societies. Binge eating is seen as symbolic of attempts to fulfill unmet needs; starvation results from the need to succeed within the system; and purging expresses guilt associated with the leaving behind of traditional social roles (i.e., that young women are allowed and expected to achieve more than their mothers did).

Some believe that eating disorders are a form of resistance on the part of individuals and society as a whole to the empowerment of women.

An important epidemiological feature of the eating disorders is that they appear to be bound to certain cultures, occuring primarily in the developed countries of North America and Europe, as well as Australia, New Zealand, South Africa, and Japan. The risk of illness may be related to the degree of assimilation of a person into the dominant culture within a country. Although eating disorders are commonly thought of as illnesses of middle and upper class white women, studies have increasingly documented their occurrence among minority women and women from various social classes.

Interestingly, anorecticlike syndromes in different cultures may present somewhat differently. In Hong Kong, patients usually do not display a fear of obesity and distorted body image but rather tend to attribute undereating to a somatic disturbance, such as abdominal bloating. It is debatable whether this syndrome, which occurs in young women and has physiological features similar to those of anorexia nervosa but a different psychological context, should be excluded from the diagnosis of anorexia nervosa or whether the criteria for anorexia nervosa should be broadened to accommodate it.

TREATMENT
Anorexia Nervosa

The fundamental principle of treatment for anorexia nervosa is that it cannot proceed in a meaningful way in the absence of **weight gain.** The first order of business is to evaluate the patient's nutritional status and medical stability. Patients with severe electrolyte disturbances, abnormal findings on ECG, or other abnormalities may require medical hospitalization. When patients are medically stable, they may be treated on a psychiatric inpatient unit or in outpatient treatment. Some patients, especially those with solid support systems, do well with outpatient treatment, but many others, especially those who are extremely underweight, require inpatient treatment.

Behavior Treatment

Treatment for anorexia nervosa is usually multimodal. Inpatient treatment is most often based on **behavior modification,** with contingencies constructed to promote weight gain. A minimum acceptable weight is set by the physician (usually 85–90% of the ideal body weight). The physician prescribes a diet (consisting of variable amounts of food and a calorically dense liquid nutritional supplement) that will enable the patient to gain weight at the desired rate. The patient's weight is monitored on a regular basis (e.g., once per week), so that the physician and patient can detect any upward or downward trends and decide how to manage them. As the patient's weight increases, she is given more privileges and has more freedom to leave the hospital.

The caloric requirements increase as the patient gains weight. It is not unusual for a patient to require as many as three thousand calories per day during the later phases of refeeding, in order to continue to gain weight. This requirement usually drops when the patient has achieved her target weight and needs only to maintain it. Most patients are able to achieve their minimum weight during hospitalization, but it is often difficult for them to maintain this weight and expand their food choices.

Patients in inpatient behavior weight control programs are especially likely to engage in power struggles with the treatment team over exactly how much weight must be gained, how much food must be consumed, and how many concessions will be made to accommodate patients' idiosyncratic needs and preferences. Patients often wish to ingest all of their calories in only one or two "safe foods" and will struggle mightily if a meal deviates even slightly from their set plan.

Patients who are superficially compliant should be encouraged to discuss their ambivalence about gaining weight. Some resolve to gain weight only so they can leave the hospital and lose it again. The therapist must walk a tightrope with these patients while gently but firmly setting limits, on the one hand, and, on the other hand, letting patients know that the treatment is ultimately in their control and cannot take place without their cooperation. Some patients may decide to end the treatment but will later reenter treatment when their motivation is stronger.

Occasionally, a patient has deteriorated so much that she must be fed against her will. This situation is difficult to manage on a psychotherapeutic level. Unless the patient comes to realize that she needs ongoing treatment, the gains made will be only temporary. These patients are often hospitalized repeatedly and fed involuntarily but lose the weight they have gained soon after discharge.

While this behavioral protocol is being followed, patients are involved in individual and group psychotherapy and family therapy when appropriate. They also receive nutritional, vocational, and leisure counseling.

Patients who are treated on an outpatient basis cannot be supervised to the same degree as those in an inpatient setting. The physician often sets a minimum weight that patients must maintain and tells them that if they cannot maintain this weight, they will be hospitalized.

Psychotherapy

There is relatively little systematic information concerning the efficacy of different forms of psychotherapy in treating patients with anorexia nervosa. Psychodynamic, interpersonal, and, especially, cognitive-behavior psychotherapies are often used (see Bulimia Nervosa, below). Also, there are some indications that family therapy is helpful, especially for younger patients.

Psychopharmacological Treatment

Drug treatment with antipsychotics, cyproheptadine (an antihistaminic and antiserotonergic drug that is used to treat allergies and tends to promote weight gain), or antidepressants has not significantly improved the outcome of anorexia nervosa. There is preliminary evidence that the antidepressant fluoxetine may be useful in avoiding relapse in patients who have been successfully refed and are leaving the hospital. Patients with symptoms of depression or anxiety that do not resolve with refeeding and weight gain may benefit from appropriate psychopharmacological interventions (see Chapter 3, Mood Disorders, and Chapter 6, Anxiety Disorders).

Bulimia Nervosa

Treatments that appear to have little in common with one another, such as antidepressant medication, cognitive-behavior therapy, and interpersonal therapy, are all effective in bulimia nervosa. This fact underscores the difficulty of making inferences about the etiology or pathophysiology of the disorder on the basis of treatment response. Carefully designed treatment studies may shed some light on the processes by which the illness arises and is maintained and may ultimately allow physicians to make better-informed decisions when they recommend particular forms of treatment.

Patients with bulimia nervosa are most often treated on an outpatient basis. Indications for inpatient treatment include medical instability (usually, extreme electrolyte imbalance), severe bulimic symptoms (i.e., binge eating and vomiting a number of times per day), significant coexisting disorders, or insufficient response to adequate trials of outpatient treatment. Hospital treatment is usually multimodal and similar to that for anorexia nervosa. Antidepressant medications and structured psychotherapy have been effective for this disorder. As with patients with anorexia nervosa, the physician should monitor the patient's weight on a regular basis (e.g., once per week), so that any upward or downward trends can be managed.

Psychotherapy

Although psychotherapy for bulimia nervosa usually takes place in an outpatient setting in which the therapist has less control over what and how the patient eats, power struggles sometimes ensue. It is useful to create a collaboration with the patient in which both parties agree that the patient will make certain provisional changes in her eating (e.g., trying particular new foods in the coming week) and that the patient and therapist together will monitor the results and decide on further changes. The patient may consciously or unconsciously use binge eating and purging as a way to gain the therapist's approval (i.e., may decrease or stop bulimic behaviors), ensure the therapist's ongoing presence and concern, or divert the therapist's attention from other anxiety-provoking issues. Decisions about whether, when, and how to address such patterns must be made on an individual basis. ➡ One patient who had stopped binge eating and vomiting early in treatment enthusiastically praised the therapist's skill in "curing" her. On closer examination, the therapist realized that the patient was eating only salads and fruit. It was imperative for the therapist to support the patient's efforts but also to reinforce the importance of developing a more normal eating pattern and dealing with the anxiety and discomfort involved in doing so. ◄▮▮

The physician must acknowledge the patient's subjective experience and gradually begin to challenge it. The physician should then help the patient to modify her coping strategies, be more flexible in evaluating her body, and develop a more complete, better integrated view of herself. ➡ The patient who was obsessed with her "fat thighs" (see above) made little progress in altering this perception but was more successful in identifying and challenging the assumptions that stemmed from the perception (e.g., the idea that others were looking at her thighs disapprovingly and the thought that her overall appearance was ruined by this one feature). ◄▮▮

Cognitive-behavior psychotherapy emphasizes patients' self-monitoring of eating and of thoughts, feelings, and circumstances surrounding eating binges in an attempt to identify patterns and triggering factors of binge eating and vomiting. In sessions with the physician and at home, the patient begins to identify dysfunctional thought patterns, such as all-or-nothing thinking ("I've blown my diet by eating this cookie, so I might as well go ahead and binge") or jumping to conclusions ("My boyfriend isn't paying attention to me because he thinks I'm too fat"). The next step is to develop rational responses to these thoughts. In situations likely to trigger binge eating, the patient systematically identifies dysfunctional thoughts and responds to them in ways other than binge eating and purging. The patient who feels that eating an extra cookie has "blown" her diet is encouraged to challenge this thought, marshal the arguments for and against it, and come up with a more reasonable, balanced response to the situation. Behavioral techniques such as systematically delaying binge eating and vomiting or using behavioral alternatives to binge eating and purging are also introduced and practiced. Alternative behaviors may be calling a friend, going for a walk, or reading a magazine. They must be appropriate to the specific situation, rewarding, and easy to execute. Finally, the patient is encouraged to develop her own ongoing treatment plan, including strategies for preventing relapse.

Controlled studies of this therapy in individual and group formats have revealed rates of improvement that are somewhat higher than those reported for drug treatment. Studies comparing psychotherapy with antidepressant treatment for bulimia nervosa have found psychotherapy to be more effective. Antidepressant treatment is clearly helpful for some patients, however, either alone or in combination with psychotherapy.

Other forms of psychotherapy have also been useful in the treatment of outpatients with bulimia nervosa. **Interpersonal therapy** focuses on the interpersonal disturbances that may underlie and reinforce bulimic behaviors. **Exposure with response prevention** is a behavioral technique also used in obsessive-compulsive disorder. During the therapy session, the patient consumes the foods that she would normally eat when bingeing and discusses the ensuing feelings of anxiety with the physician. **Psychodynamic psychotherapy** has not been well studied but may be particularly useful for patients presenting with coexisting personality disorders.

Psychopharmacological Treatment

Cyclic antidepressants, selective serotonin reuptake inhibitors (SSRIs), monoamine oxidase inhibitors (MAOIs), and atypical antidepressants have been effective in more than a dozen randomized controlled clinical trials. Only a few patients attain full remission when treated with drugs alone, however. There is little information concerning the long-term efficacy of these drugs, but they may be useful for many patients. Information about the interaction of drugs and psychotherapy and about factors that predict a successful response to a particular intervention is needed.

The usefulness of antidepressant drugs is not limited to patients with bulimia nervosa who are depressed. Trials of these drugs were originally stimulated by theories about the relationship between eating disorders and affective disorders. It is now known that the neurotransmitter systems targeted by these drugs also mediate feelings of hunger and satiety. Therefore, the mechanism of action of the drugs in bulimia nervosa may be largely independent of their antidepressant effects. In spite of the similarities between bulimia nervosa and anorexia nervosa, antidepressant medications are effective for the former but not the latter. This suggests that starvation may in some way interfere with their actions.

Binge-Eating Disorder

Little is known about the treatment of binge-eating disorder and other eating-related syndromes. Preliminary studies of patients with symptoms similar to those of binge-eating disorder suggest that both antidepressant medication and cognitive-behavior psychotherapy may be beneficial.

Another approach to the treatment of binge eating and overeating is the **12-step method,** which is widely practiced but little studied. This approach is based on the method used at Alcoholics Anonymous and grounded in the **addiction model** of eating disorders (i.e., the patient is viewed as a food addict whose experience and behavior parallel that of alcohol- or drug-addicted individuals). One limitation

BOX 9–1. An Historical Perspective on Eating Disorders

Descriptions of syndromes that resemble anorexia nervosa date back to medieval times, when the psychological context of the illness had more to do with spiritual beliefs than with the aesthetic aspects of emaciation. Narratives of self-starvation can be found in accounts and writings of several saints. The "fasting girls" of the nineteenth century attracted the attention of both religious admirers and skeptical physicians. One of the earliest medical descriptions of an anorexialike syndrome is that of Mr. Duke's daughter, written by Richard Morton in 1689:

> In the month of July, she fell into a total suppression of her monthly Courses from a multitude of Cares and Passions of her Mind, but without any symptoms of the Green-Sickness following upon it. From which time her Appetite began to abate, and her Digestion to be bad; her flesh also began to be flaccid and loose, and her looks pale . . . she was wont by her studying at Night and continual poring upon Books to expose herself both Day and Night to the Injuries of the Air . . . I do not remember that I did ever in all my practice see one that was conversant with the Living so much wasted with the greatest degree of Consumption (like a Skeleton only clad with Skin).

The term *anorexia nervosa* was coined in the nineteenth century by Sir William Gull. Anorexia, meaning lack of appetite, is now thought to be a misnomer, because patients with anorexia nervosa are often quite preoccupied with food but deny, to a greater or lesser extent, the experience of hunger and refuse to act upon it.

In contrast to anorexia nervosa, which has been discussed in the medical literature for more than a century, bulimia nervosa did not appear in the literature until quite recently. Although the practice of occasional excessive eating followed by purging has precedents extending as far back as ancient Rome, the first recognition of bulimia nervosa as a psychiatric syndrome occurred in the 1970s in the United States, Japan, and Great Britain, where the term bulimia nervosa was coined. It is not clear whether the syndrome has truly originated in our current cultural climate or whether it has existed as an unrecognized entity for decades or even centuries. Certainly, there has been a rapid escalation in research and popular interest in eating disorders. During the past decade, they have been the subject of television movies, feature films, medical journals, and many books.

of this approach is that abstinence from food is neither possible nor desirable, and many physicians believe that patients' attempts to severely restrict eating actually contribute to the maintenance of the illness. However, the concept of abstinence may be broadened to include avoidance of particular types of eating (e.g., eating in response to stress, eating large amounts of a particular food) or even avoidance of particular thinking patterns that have been recognized as deleterious. Systematic study is needed to assess the effectiveness of this approach, its possible risks, and the characteristics of patients who might benefit from it.

Selected Readings

American Psychiatric Association. Practice Guidelines for Eating Disorders. American Journal of Psychiatry 150:207–228, 1993.

Bruch, H. Eating Disorders: Obesity, Anorexia Nervosa, and the Person Within. New York, Basic Books, 1973.

Bruch, H. The Golden Cage: The Enigma of Anorexia Nervosa. Cambridge, Harvard University Press, 1978.

Brumberg, J. J. Fasting Girls: The Emergence of Anorexia Nervosa as a Modern Disease. Cambridge, Harvard University Press, 1988.

Cauwels, J. M. Bulimia: The Binge-Purge Compulsion. New York, Doubleday and Company, 1983.

Fairburn, C. G., and G. T. Wilson (editors). Binge Eating: Nature, Assessment, and Treatment. New York, Guilford Press, 1993.

Fallon, P., M. A. Katzman, and S. C. Wooley (editors). Feminist Perspectives on Eating Disorders. New York, Guilford Press, 1994.

Franklin, J. C., et al. Observations on human behavior in experimental semistarvation and rehabilitation. Journal of Clinical Psychology 4:28–45, 1948.

Garner, D. M., and P. E. Garfinkel (editors). Handbook of Psychotherapy for Anorexia Nervosa and Bulimia. New York, Guilford Press, 1985.

Hsu, L. K. G. Eating Disorders. New York, Guilford Press, 1990.

Kaplan, A. S., and P. E. Garfinkel (editors). Medical Issues and the Eating Disorders: The Interface. New York, Brunner/Mazel, 1993.

Kendler, K. S., et al. The genetic epidemiology of bulimia nervosa. American Journal of Psychiatry 148:1627–1637, 1991.

Nogami, Y., and F. Yabana. On kibarashi-gui (binge-eating). Folia Psychiatrica et Neurologica Japonica 31:159–166, 1977.

Russell, G. Bulimia nervosa: an ominous variant of anorexia nervosa. Psychology and Medicine 9:429–448, 1979.

CHAPTER TEN

SOMATOFORM AND FACTITIOUS

DISORDERS

STEVEN E. HYLER, MD

Patients with somatoform and factitious disorders suffer from physical symptoms and are generally seen first by nonpsychiatric physicians. Individuals with **somatoform disorders** have physical complaints for which no general medical etiology is present. Associated unconscious psychological factors contribute to the onset, exacerbation, or maintenance of the physical symptoms. In the past, the somatoform disorders were grouped under the broad category of hysteria or hysterical neurosis. **Factitious disorders** are those in which the patient intentionally simulates or produces symptoms of illness for the purpose of achieving the "sick role" of being a patient. (See Table 10–1 for a comparison of these disorders.)

These disorders may be conceptualized as being along a continuum that progresses from the somatoform disorders, in which the symptom production is unintentional, i.e., unconscious with no obvious, recognizable environmental goal, through the factitious disorders, in which an individual intentionally produces symptoms but has no obvious, recognizable environmental goals, to **malingering,** in which the symptom production is intentional and is motivated by a recognizable environmental goal, e.g., financial gain or drugs. Unlike the somatoform and factitious disorders, malingering is not considered to be a psychiatric disorder. Treatment is rarely indicated because patients who engage in malingering are not usually motivated to change their behavior.

SOMATOFORM DISORDERS

All patients who see a physician present with symptoms and signs suggestive of physical illness. In the vast majority of cases, the physician takes a careful history, performs a physical examination, orders ancillary tests, and develops a diagnosis (or differential diagnosis) that explains the symptoms. This diagnosis then determines the treatment plan and yields information about the course of the illness and the prognosis. If, after the physician has performed a careful medical workup, the diagnosis remains unde-termined, either the physical illness is of undetermined etiology or the presentation of symptoms is related not only to possible physical factors but also to psychological factors. In patients with a somatoform disorder, the physical symptoms are genuine: They are unconsciously, not intentionally, produced, are distressing to patients, and lead to functional impairment in many areas of patients' lives. The etiology of these disorders is to be found, however, in the patient's internal emotional life, in the psychological stressors and conflicts that initiate, exacerbate, and maintain symptoms.

In general, these disorders tend to run in families and are diagnosed far more commonly in women than in men. Men may have these illnesses as often as women do, but they do not seek medical advice as often for them; when they do see a physician, it is usually in reaction to minor but real physical illnesses. (Epidemiological information on all somatoform disorders is presented in Table 10–2.)

DIAGNOSTIC AND CLINICAL FEATURES

In the DSM-IV, the somatoform disorders include somatization disorder, conversion disorder, pain disorder, hypochondriasis, and body dysmorphic disorder.

Somatization Disorder

Somatization disorder is polysymptomatic and generally begins before individuals are 30 years old and lasts for many years. Patients with somatization disorder experience **multiple, unexplained somatic symptoms.** If they have a general medical condition, the subjectively experienced extent of the problem is out of proportion to the objective findings. Often, the symptoms are related to **pain** at several different sites of the body, e.g., the back, a joint, the abdomen; **gastrointestinal disturbance,** e.g., diarrhea, bloating, or vomiting; a multitude of various symptoms pertaining to the **sexual or reproductive system;** and **neurological or pseudoneurological** disturbance,

TABLE 10–1.   Somatoform and Factitious Disorders

	Somatoform Disorders	Factitious Disorders
Presenting Complaints	Acute or chronic; consistent	Acute and dramatic; shifting
History	Evidence of psychosocial stressor	Evidence of prior treatment
Request for Treatment	Outpatient or inpatient	Hospital admission with invasive or painful procedures
Symptom Production	Unconscious	Intentional
Motivation	No external gain	No external gain

e.g., pseudoblindness or pseudodeafness, coordination disturbance, or pseudoweakness or pseudoparalysis (Table 10–3). Patients with somatization disorder voice their complaints in a vague ("la belle indifférence") manner, e.g., "I guess I couldn't move my arm"; in a dramatic and exaggerated fashion, e.g., "The pain was so bad I nearly died"; or in a vague and shifting manner that jumps from symptom to symptom without good description, e.g., "My head was numb, my stomach just wasn't right, nothing felt like it should." These patients are usually seen first by internists, general practitioners, or gynecologists rather than by psychiatrists. Often, they have seen many different physicians and have received a variety of medical diagnoses and treatments. The prototypical patient spends several hours a week at doctors' appointments and is treated symptomatically with a variety of over-the-counter and prescribed medications, which provide only temporary relief. None of the illnesses diagnosed is serious, nor does there seem to be a physiologically based connection between the various organ systems apparently affected. Also, despite having many symptoms, the patient does not seem to be overly concerned about any specific diagnosis. The center of these patients' lives is their symptoms and treatments, and they are not aware of having any psychological, emotional, or interpersonal difficulties, even though the extraodinary amount of time they spend in seeing physicians precludes the possibility of employment or the enjoyment of a social and family life. This is a serious psychiatric illness. Many of these patients have concurrent anxiety, depressive, or personality disorders and may sometimes make suicide threats or attempts.

TABLE 10–2.   Epidemiology of Somatoform Disorders

	Somatization Disorder	Conversion Disorder	Pain Disorder	Hypochondriasis	Body Dysmorphic Disorder
Prevalence	0.2–2% of females	11–300/100,000 persons; 1–3% of outpatients	Relatively common	Unknown in general population; 4–9% of patients seen in general medical practice	Unknown
Age of Onset	Adolescence	Late childhood	Any age	Early adulthood	Adolescence
Gender	Usually occurs in females	More frequent in females (2:1–10:1)	More common in females than males	Equally common in females and males	Equally common in females and males
Course	Chronic, fluctuating	Remits within 2 weeks, but recurrence is common	Wide variation	Chronic	Chronic
Familial Pattern	Observed in 10–20% of female first-degree biological relatives of female patients	Occurs more frequently in relatives of patients; increased risk in monozygotic twins	Depressive disorders, alcohol dependence, chronic pain are more common in first-degree relatives of patients	Unknown	Unknown

Source: American Psychiatric Association. Diagnostic and Statistical Manual of Mental Disorders, 4th ed. Washington, D. C., American Psychiatric Association, 1994.

TABLE 10-3.   DSM-IV Diagnostic Criteria for Somatization Disorder

A. A history of many physical complaints beginning before age 30 years that occur over a period of several years and result in treatment being sought or significant impairment in social, occupational, or other important areas of functioning.

B. Each of the following criteria must have been met, with individual symptoms occurring at any time during the course of the disturbance:
   (1) four pain symptoms: a history of pain related to at least four different sites or functions (e.g., head, abdomen, back, joints, extremities, chest, rectum, during menstruation, during sexual intercourse, or during urination)
   (2) two gastrointestinal symptoms: a history of at least two gastrointestinal symptoms other than pain (e.g., nausea, bloating, vomiting other than during pregnancy, diarrhea, or intolerance of several different foods)
   (3) one sexual symptom: a history of at least one sexual or reproductive symptom other than pain (e.g., sexual indifference, erectile or ejaculatory dysfunction, irregular menses, excessive menstrual bleeding, vomiting throughout pregnancy)
   (4) one pseudoneurological symptom: a history of at least one symptom or deficit suggesting a neurological condition not limited to pain (conversion symptoms such as impaired coordination or balance, paralysis or localized weakness, difficulty swallowing or lump in throat, aphonia, urinary retention, hallucinations, loss of touch or pain sensation, double vision, blindness, deafness, seizures; dissociative symptoms such as amnesia; or loss of consciousness other than fainting)

C. Either (1) or (2):
   (1) after appropriate investigation, each of the symptoms in Criterion B cannot be fully explained by a known general medical condition or the direct effects of a substance (e.g., a drug of abuse, a medication)
   (2) when there is a related general medical condition, the physical complaints or resulting social or occupational impairment are in excess of what would be expected from the history, physical examination, or laboratory findings

D. The symptoms are not intentionally produced or feigned (as in Factitious Disorder or Malingering).

Conversion Disorder

Conversion disorder is a monosymptomatic somatoform disorder that specifically affects either the individual's **voluntary motor system** or **sensory functions.** In the classic cases of conversion disorder, patients experience blindness, deafness, paralysis, inability to speak, seizures, or an inability to walk or stand. Although the symptoms, or deficits, suggest a physical condition, their etiology is psychological. Emotional conflicts or stressors are responsible (Table 10-4). The symptoms typically are symbolic representations that relieve an underlying emotional conflict. ➡ For example, a man who discovered his wife was unfaithful became enraged and developed a conversion paralysis of his right arm, which prevented him from acting out murderous impulses toward his wife. This prevention was the primary gain of his symptom. The secondary gain was the disability benefits the patient received because his paralysis prevented him from being able to work. ⬅

The symptoms often reflect patients' conceptions of what neurological disorders should be rather than any known neurological or muscular distribution. Thus, conversion paresthesia may show a "glove and stocking" distribution, or a vision loss may be of a "tunnel vision" variety, neither of which is neurologically possible. The diagnosis of conversion disorder is generally considered only after the results obtained from appropriate examination and testing have been used to rule out all medical conditions.

Conversion symptoms may also coexist with documented medical illness, e.g., an individual with epilepsy may also have conversion seizures, which are called pseudoseizures. ➡ For example, a 42-year-old man complained to his general internist about facial numbness, demonstrating the complaint by pinching his own cheeks and pushing his face very close to the physician's face. According to the patient, the distribution of the numbness was circular, running around the circumference of his face, along the hairline and under the jaw and chin. Because the sensory nerve distribution of the face does not follow such a pattern and instead is segmental and overlapping, the internist concluded that the symptom was psychogenic in origin. Upon inquiry, the patient showed many signs of major depression but attributed them to his facial numbness. Because of the depression, the internist prescribed an antidepressant. When this resulted in moderate but incomplete improvement, the patient was referred to a psychiatrist. In taking the psychosocial history, the psychiatrist soon discovered that the patient was in a public fight with a boss at work who the patient experi-

TABLE 10-4.   DSM-IV Diagnostic Criteria for Conversion Disorder

A. One or more symptoms or deficits affecting voluntary motor or sensory function that suggest a neurological or other general medical condition.

B. Psychological factors are judged to be associated with the symptom or deficit because the initiation or exacerbation of the symptom or deficit is preceded by conflicts or other stressors.

C. The symptom or deficit is not intentionally produced or feigned (as in Factitious Disorder or Malingering).

D. The symptom or deficit cannot, after appropriate investigation, be fully explained by a general medical condition, or by the direct effects of a substance, or as a culturally sanctioned behavior or experience.

E. The symptom or deficit causes clinically significant distress or impairment in social, occupational, or other important areas of functioning or warrants medical evaluation.

F. The symptom or deficit is not limited to pain or sexual dysfunction, does not occur exclusively during the course of Somatization Disorder, and is not better accounted for by another mental disorder.

Specify type of symptom or deficit:
   With Motor Symptom or Deficit
   With Sensory Symptom or Deficit
   With Seizures or Convulsions
   With Mixed Presentation

enced as excoriating and humiliating. When talking about the boss, the patient became agitated and said "he is constantly in my face." Increasing the antidepressant and discussing the public humiliation that he felt enabled the patient to feel still better and to request and receive a change in job assignment. The remainder of the "shamefaced" numbness symptom faded away. ◂

Some patients with conversion disorder may show "la belle indifférence," i.e., appear relatively unconcerned about the severity of their symptoms and resultant disability.

The majority of cases of conversion disorder are seen in the context of the general hospital rather than in psychiatric facilities. Estimates suggest that from 5% to 20% of patients seen by psychiatrists in consultation in general hospitals can be given a diagnosis of a conversion disorder.

The majority of patients with conversion disorder of the more flagrant type such as hysterical blindness, deafness, or paralysis are young women, generally from low socioeconomic groups and with little formal education. However, less dramatic conversion sensory symptoms of pain, dysesthesia, or absent sensation are seen in men and women across all socioeconomic groups.

Pain Disorder

Pain is one of the most common symptoms found in all medical and psychiatric disorders. Pain disorder is characterized by pain, the presence of which causes the patient significant impairment or distress in important areas of functioning (Table 10–5). In patients with pain disorder, as in those with conversion disorder, the etiology of the symptoms or a partial cause of the exacerbation or maintenance of the symptoms is found in psychological factors. In patients with pain disorder, no organic pathology or pathophysiological mechanism that sufficiently accounts for the degree or location of pain can be identified. When organic pathology is present, the pain the patient associates with it is in gross excess of what the physical findings would suggest and results in significant occupational or social impairment. Confirmation of the psychological origin can be found by the physician obtaining enough information from the patient to establish a temporal relationship between the occurrence of a known preceding psychosocial stressor (or conflict) in the patient's life and the subsequent occurrence of pain symptoms. In one case, a woman who was having problems at her job with a particular supervisor found that her back pain returned after each time she was criticized by that supervisor. When the supervisor was away on vacation, she did not have back pain.

The pain often results in secondary gain, e.g., increased attention and sympathy from others or financial compensation for the disability. (See Chapter 12, Psychological Factors Affecting Medical Conditions.)

The symptoms with which patients with pain disorder present vary widely and include musculoskeletal (back), arthritic (joint), and cardiovascular (anginal) pain. Patients often visit a large number of physicians, seeking relief and time off from work. Analgesics, of all sorts, are prescribed to them and may be temporarily effective; however, the pain in-

---

TABLE 10–5. DSM-IV Diagnostic Criteria for Pain Disorder

A. Pain in one or more anatomical sites is the predominant focus of the clinical presentation and is of sufficient severity to warrant clinical attention.

B. The pain causes clinically significant distress or impairment in social, occupational, or other important areas of functioning.

C. Psychological factors are judged to have an important role in the onset, severity, exacerbation, or maintenance of the pain.

D. The symptom or deficit is not intentionally produced or feigned (as in Factitious Disorder or Malingering).

E. The pain is not better accounted for by a Mood, Anxiety, or Psychotic Disorder and does not meet criteria for Dyspareunia.

Code as follows:

Pain Disorder Associated With Psychological Factors: psychological factors are judged to have the major role in the onset, severity, exacerbation, or maintenance of the pain. (If a general medical condition is present, it does not have a major role in the onset, severity, exacerbation, or maintenance of the pain.) This type of Pain Disorder is not diagnosed if criteria are also met for Somatization Disorder.

Pain Disorder Associated With Both Psychological Factors and a General Medical Condition: both psychological factors and a general medical condition are judged to have important roles in the onset, severity, exacerbation, or maintenance of the pain. The associated general medical condition or anatomical site of the pain (see below) is coded on Axis III.

Specify if:
Acute: duration of less than 6 months
Chronic: duration of 6 months or longer

Note: The following is not considered to be a mental disorder and is included here to facilitate differential diagnosis.
Pain Disorder Associated With a General Medical Condition: a general medical condition has a major role in the onset, severity, exacerbation, or maintenance of the pain. (If psychological factors are present, they are not judged to have a major role in the onset, severity, exacerbation, or maintenance of the pain.) The diagnostic code for the pain is selected based on the associated general medical condition if one has been established or on the anatomical location of the pain if the underlying general medical condition is not yet clearly established—for example, low back, sciatic, pelvic, headache, facial, chest, joint, bone, abdominal, breast, renal, ear, eye, throat, tooth, and urinary.

evitably returns over time. Patients may seek out potentially dangerous invasive procedures or surgeries, which grant them little lasting relief. They generally do not recognize, or refuse to consider, the contribution of psychological factors to the pain.

Depending on how the diagnosis of pain disorder is defined, the prevalence varies. In as many as 40% of patients who present with pain, the pain is related to psychological factors. Women are twice as likely as men to receive this diagnosis. There is some evidence of a familial pattern of relatives of individuals with the disorder having an increased prevalence of depression, alcohol dependence, or other pain related illnesses, as compared to the general population. The disorder usually occurs at ages 30–50 during the most productive years of employment.

Hypochondriasis

Patients with hypochondriasis are preoccupied with the **fear or belief that they have a serious disease.** Their misinterpretations of normal bodily functions are generally to blame. For example, an individual may be convinced that his bowel sounds indicate that he has an intestinal cancer. They are often preoccupied with a specific disease or organ, e.g., heart disease (cardiac neurosis) or cancer. Or they may believe that they have an illness but do not have any symptoms. For example, an individual who had paid a lot of attention to media coverage of AIDS became convinced that he had the disease even though he had no symptoms of the illness and had not engaged in any behaviors that might have put him at risk for developing the infection (Table 10–6). These patients are most often seen by physicians in general medical practice. Despite thorough physical examinations and reassurances that they are not ill, they are not convinced and so they "doctor shop," hoping to find a physician who will discover the cause of their prob-

lem. Patients with hypochondriasis differ from those who have somatization disorder in that they worry that they have a *disease* whereas patients with somatization disorder focus on having a variety of *symptoms* rather than a specific disease.

⟹ In one case, a 33-year-old academic physician, in a very competitive grant-seeking phase of his academic career, tripped on the street while running to catch a bus and worried that he tripped because his foot dropped, which meant that he had a nerve palsy in his right leg. Over a period of weeks, the man's worry progressed to a fear of multiple sclerosis. He visited his friend, a neurologist, who took a careful history, performed a complete neurological examination, demonstrated, in particular, that all of the man's reflexes and strength testing were normal in the right lower extremity, and attempted to reassure his friend. The man felt better immediately, experienced great relief, thanked the neurologist and rushed back into his busy academic life only to find that within several days, and increasing over the next several weeks, his fear of multiple sclerosis returned. The physician patient began to repeatedly test his Achilles tendon reflex throughout the day and found, as is typical in testing one's reflexes, that sometimes he elicited a brisk response and sometimes no response at all. His friend the neurologist saw him in the hall during this time and asked how he was doing. When the neurologist heard that his patient was still worried and was testing his own reflexes, the neurologist told him that despite his obvious concern, no trace of the illness had been found and that whenever the patient had the urge to test his reflexes, he wanted to see him, even if it was every day or several times a day, in order to effectively test the reflex. The neurologist then suggested that the physician patient was worried that he would not effectively meet the competitive challenges in which he was engaged and that his temporarily crippled confidence was being reflected in his worry that he had a crippling disease. He encouraged his friend to take some time off, consider his career and the difficulties ahead, and see if he could make realistic and worry-easing plans to confront and meet the challenges facing him. He asked the patient to call him in a week to tell him what those plans would be. The physician-patient thanked his friend, took two days off to consult with mentors and experts in his field, drew up an action plan for himself, and found that he did not need to have the neurologist check his reflexes. His fear slowly disappeared over the next few weeks. Of interest was the neurologist's elicitation while taking the patient's initial past medical history of his having had two previous episodes involving hypochondriacal reactions, one in college when applying to medical school and one during the first year of medical school, which was the most difficult time for this patient. ⟸

About 10% of patients seen by physicians have hypochondriasis. Though seen in all age groups, it is most likely to occur in patients who are in their 40s or 50s. Men and women are about equally likely to have hypochondriasis.

TABLE 10–6. DSM-IV Diagnostic Criteria for Hypochondriasis

A. Preoccupation with fears of having, or the idea that one has, a serious disease based on the person's misinterpretation of bodily symptoms.
B. The preoccupation persists despite appropriate medical evaluation and reassurance.
C. The belief in Criterion A is not of delusional intensity (as in Delusional Disorder, Somatic Type) and is not restricted to a circumscribed concern about appearance (as in Body Dysmorphic Disorder).
D. The preoccupation causes clinically significant distress or impairment in social, occupational, or other important areas of functioning.
E. The duration of the disturbance is at least 6 months.
F. The preoccupation is not better accounted for by Generalized Anxiety Disorder, Obsessive-Compulsive Disorder, Panic Disorder, a Major Depressive Episode, Separation Anxiety, or another Somatoform Disorder.

Specify if:
  With Poor Insight: if, for most of the time during the current episode, the person does not recognize that the concern about having a serious illness is excessive or unreasonable.

Body Dysmorphic Disorder

In patients with body dysmorphic disorder (BDD), the essential feature is a **preoccupation with an imagined defect in physical appearance.** If a slight physical defect exists, the person's complaints are grossly out of proportion to the objective findings (Table 10–7). The defects most often complained about concern the face (e.g., nose size or shape, spots, bumps, and excessive facial hair). More rarely, patients complain about their extremities, back, breasts, genitals, buttocks, or other parts of the body. Although patients generally focus on a specific perceived anomaly, they may also see several defects simultaneously or their perception may shift, over time, from one body part to another. Individuals with BDD are far more likely to be seen initially by plastic surgeons or dermatologists than by psychiatrists, are generally self-conscious, and believe that others are mocking their appearance. They frequently check their appearance in mirrors and spend an excessive amount of time in grooming rituals. Depression is a common accompaniment of BDD; other conditions that also occur in patients with BDD are obsessive-compulsive disorder, social phobia, and various personality disorders and psychoses. ➡ In one case, a 36-year-old woman went from one plastic surgeon to another complaining that her eyes were swollen. Examinations by the plastic surgeons did not show any swelling, and the woman was unclear about the exact location of the swelling. Finally, she was sent for psychiatric consultation. Psychiatric history revealed most of the criteria for a major depressive episode. A parallel psychosocial history revealed a long-standing engagement that broke up when the man "ran off with a younger woman." The patient, while reporting the story, focused on the age difference as being particularly humiliating. The psychiatrist prescribed antidepressant medication and discussed with the patient her sadness, humiliation, disappointment, and rage. The discussion of her humiliation and her rage produced several very tearful sessions, after which the patient's preoccupation with her swollen eyes slowly faded. In this case, the concern about swollen eyes symbolically represented tearful affect blocked by wounded pride and feelings of humiliation. ◄

The actual prevalence of BDD is not known. The initial onset is typically in adolescence or early adult life.

**TABLE 10–7.   DSM-IV Diagnostic Criteria for
Body Dysmorphic Disorder**

A. Preoccupation with an imagined defect in appearance. If a slight physical anomaly is present, the person's concern is markedly excessive.
B. The preoccupation causes clinically significant distress or impairment in social, occupational, or other important areas of functioning.
C. The preoccupation is not better accounted for by another mental disorder (e.g., dissatisfaction with body shape and size in Anorexia Nervosa).

Course of Illness

Somatization disorder is a chronic condition that has a **fluctuating course of exacerbations and temporary remissions.** In spite of their multitude of physical complaints, patients with this disorder do not show a significantly increased mortality rate. Some increased morbidity may be caused by the many contacts with numerous physicians and diagnostic procedures. **Concomitant substance abuse** of prescribed medications is not uncommon nor is the risk of **unnecessary surgery.** When accompanied by substance abuse, an increased risk of **suicide** exists. Often, the interpersonal relationships of these individuals are stormy and chaotic.

The course of uncomplicated conversion disorder (i.e., conversion symptoms not seen as part of a more pervasive disorder, such as somatization disorder, depression, or schizophrenia) is generally of **short duration with full resolution.** Good premorbid functioning, abrupt onset of symptoms, and the presence of recognizable environmental stressors are all good prognostic indicators. ➡ A 30-year-old married female attorney, for example, with no psychiatric history observed a car accident in which a close friend was killed. When she saw her friend's body, she fainted and upon awakening had lost her vision. Within 24 hours, this conversion disorder resolved. ◄ Patients with conversion symptoms occurring in the context of other physical disorders (e.g., conversion seizures in a patient with a preexisting seizure disorder) generally have a poor prognosis. Any patient who has recurrent conversion disorder or symptom-contingent secondary gain will also show a poorer outcome. ➡ Thus, a 42-year-old single mother, with a history of abuse as a teenager, suffering from chronic back pain, developed recurrent right arm and leg weakness that prevented her from going to work and provided her with attention and help from her siblings. ◄

The course of hypochondriasis is generally **chronic** but interspersed with **remissions** and **relapses.** In some instances, a spontaneous recovery occurs. The onset is usually sudden and increases in severity over time. The patient has usually seen several other physicians and received various courses of medication and physical therapies before being referred for psychiatric evaluation.

BDD generally persists for years. In some instances, the symptoms worsen and become delusional in intensity. In other instances, the perceived defect may shift from one area of the body to another. Spontaneous remissions are rare.

Little is known about the course and ultimate outcome of individuals with pain disorder.

THE INTERVIEW

Developing a working alliance with patients with somatoform disorders poses unique problems for physicians. These patients are not easy to interview. They often have multiple, seemingly unrelated complaints. Their stories range from being incredibly detailed to overly vague. At times, they may not seem terribly concerned with the examination, and they frequently do not comply with medical recommendations. Their dissatisfaction with physicians leads to "doctor shopping," and they are often being seen simultaneously by several physicians. To work effectively with such patients, physicians must develop a good rapport with them. They need to be good listeners as well as good detectives in order to sort out the information provided by patients and to determine effective treatment plans. (See Interviewing Guidelines box.) Because patients' somatic complaints may mask major depressive or dysthymic disorders, general physicians and psychiatrists who see such patients must become very familiar with the differential diagnosis of the various mood disorders, which should always be explored as possible diagnoses.

Somatization Disorder

Individuals with **somatization disorder** may recount their history in a vague manner or, conversely, in a dramatic, overly detailed, exaggerated manner. Referral to a psychiatrist is usually made by a pri-

mary care physician (e.g., internist or gynecologist) after a workup for organic etiology has produced negative results.

These patients are frustrating to both their primary clinicians and psychiatrists. Physicians should be aware of any negative emotional reactions that might lead them to overprescribe, order unnecessary diagnostic tests and surgical procedures, or ignore these patients. Conversely, physicians should guard against attributing any and all new symptoms that develop in these patients to their somatization disorder lest they miss the presence of treatable medical conditions. They should recognize that patients with somatization disorder use their physical complaints as a form of communication. These patients are not able to relate their problems in terms of stress, affect, or conflict; instead, they express themselves through their multiple somatic complaints. Other aspects of patients' lives should be explored gently by physicians in order to uncover any occupational or interpersonal problems. This **parallel psychosocial history** is taken alongside the medical history and does not require that patients see a cause-effect relationship. These causal relationships will be obvious to physicians and to patients' significant others.

Conversion Disorder

Individuals with conversion disorder are often seen initially in a consultation that has been requested by a neurologist, orthopedic surgeon, or other nonpsychiatric physician. While some patients may show "la belle indifférence," others may be very troubled by their symptoms. Many patients with conversion disorder show little psychological mindedness or understanding of the relationship between their onset of symptoms and any environmental stressors that might have brought them about. They tend to be particularly obtuse about emotional reactions to stress. They do not feel affect easily and do not relate affect to reality triggers. Again, by taking a parallel psychosocial history, the physician usually makes such stressors readily apparent. The corresponding affect, of which the patient may be unaware, is often clear from the manifest content of the story. It is sometimes helpful to point out the affect that would be appropriate. ➠ In one case, it was necessary for the physician to make the empathic comment that "many people would be quite sad for a number of weeks after their mother died." The patient to whom this was said was startled because he knew that the physician was pointing out the obvious and yet he did not feel sad. Instead, he had numbness in a nonneurological distribution over his abdomen and thighs. He first noticed this when told of his mother's death. The symptom became much worse during the funeral and persisted for several weeks, at which point he saw his general physician. The history of his mother's death was elicited by the physician while taking a parallel psychosocial history. The missing emotional response of anxiety and

---

Interviewing Guidelines

Somatoform Disorders
- Note whether the patient exhibits "la belle indifférence."
- Try to ascertain whether the patient is receiving secondary gain from the symptoms.
- Reassure the patient that the symptoms are being taken seriously.
- Discourage "doctor shopping."
- Note whether the patient has insight into psychological functioning.
- Take a parallel psychosocial history.
- Search for depression.

Factitious Disorder
- Maintain a high level of suspicion if the patient's symptoms and signs seem to be "textbook perfect."
- If the patient is lying about the medical history, he or she is probably lying about other aspects of the history.
- Note whether the patient uses medical jargon.
- Observe whether the patient is visited in the hospital by family or friends.
- Examine for evidence of a personality disorder.
- Try to obtain corroborative information about the patient's history.
- Keep in mind that the patient will probably flee once confronted with the physician's suspicions.

sadness was displaced by the patient to the symptom of numbness, to which he felt an emotional reaction rather than to the traumatic event. ←

Pain Disorder

Patients with pain disorder have usually seen a variety of other medical physicians prior to their referral for psychiatric consultation. Many are reluctant to see a psychiatrist because they view the referral as a sign that their physicians either have given up on them or disbelieve them. Patients referred for psychiatric evaluation may, therefore, initially be defensive. The manner in which the treating physician makes the referral to the psychiatrist is important in obtaining patients' acceptance of the referral. Patients should be reassured that their physicians are not giving up on them, neither do they believe the patients are just "sick in the head." Psychiatrists should acknowledge the suffering of these patients and assure them that their primary care physicians are not abandoning them but that a psychiatrist is needed as well to help with their emotional suffering.

It is preferable for a psychiatric referral to be made earlier rather than later in the diagnostic evaluation process. Psychiatric examinations of these individuals often reveal that they are not in touch with and do not openly display their emotions. Although they are genuinely suffering, they are unable to recognize the contribution of stressors, conflicts, or emotional trauma. They often need reassurance from the psychiatrist that they are not crazy. As with conversion disorder, the presence of secondary gain (e.g., financial compensation) greatly complicates the treatment of these patients. It is useful, although not always possible, for physicians to encourage patients to expedite any pending litigation (e.g., accepting a lump sum settlement) to remove any financial incentive to maintain the pain.

Hypochondriasis

Patients with hypochondriasis are usually first seen by nonpsychiatric physicians in general medical practice. Consultation with a psychiatrist is indicated to make the correct diagnosis of the hypochondriacal complaints (see Differential Diagnosis, below). Primary care physicians of such patients should develop a positive alliance with them in order to minimize their tendency to "doctor shop." It may be useful to schedule regular appointments with patients and allow sufficient time during each visit for patients to discuss their problems. Once the diagnosis of hypochondriasis is made, it is also important to minimize the number of invasive procedures patients undergo that can lead to iatrogenic complications. Physicians should recognize that they may not be able to eliminate these patients' complaints, but instead should attempt to reassure them that they have been carefully examined and that they are not seriously ill. Physicians can then encourage these patients to accept psychiatric referral.

Body Dysmorphic Disorder

As mentioned above, it is far more likely for individuals with body dysmorphic disorder to be seen initially by dermatologists or plastic surgeons than by psychiatrists. Being familiar with this disorder helps physicians prevent unnecessary cosmetic surgery. Cosmetic surgery rarely succeeds in satisfying these patients, and attempting to cure patients with this condition by multiple attempts at cosmetic surgery is more likely to result in a lawsuit against the physician than in any long-term patient satisfaction with the change in appearance.

DIFFERENTIAL DIAGNOSIS

Genuine **physical disorder** should always be placed first in the hierarchy of differential diagnosis for patients with somatization disorder. Disorders with an inconsistent and often confusing array of physical symptoms such as systemic lupus erythematosus, multiple sclerosis, and Lyme disease may present similarly. **Schizophrenia** or **mood disorders** with prominent somatic delusions should be ruled out. Individuals with panic disorder may have many of the same cardiovascular symptoms (e.g., chest pain, dyspnea, palpitations); however, the symptoms occur in the context of the panic attacks. Individuals with **factitious disorder** may intentionally simulate the symptoms of physical illness, and **malingerers** usually have a recognizable environmental goal for illness fabrication.

The mere presence of physical symptoms that are not explained by known or recognized medical illness is not sufficient for the diagnosis of conversion disorder. There needs to be, in addition, some recognizable environmental stressors that produce, exacerbate, or maintain the symptoms. In as many as 30–50% of cases in which the diagnosis of conversion disorder has been made, there may be an unrecognized medical illness. Medical illnesses that can be confused with conversion disorder include neurological syndromes (e.g., multiple sclerosis, collagen vascular disease, systemic lupus erythematosus) and muscular abnormalities (e.g., muscular dystrophy).

As with the other somatoform disorders, the first differential diagnosis to rule out with hypochondriasis is true general medical condition. In patients whose medical condition predates their hypochondriacal complaints, this can be quite difficult. In the absence of physical or laboratory findings that account for the current symptoms, hypochondriasis may coexist with the original disease. In individuals without any previous diagnosable general medical condition, consideration should be given to the possibility that the symptoms represent an early stage of difficult-to-diagnose disorders that have an intermittent course or variable findings (e.g., multiple sclerosis, collagen vascular disease, or endocrine disorders). If the hypochondriacal beliefs are of delusional intensity, a psychotic disorder such as **major depression** with psychosis, **schizophrenia**, or **delusional disorder** should be considered. Many individuals with hypochondriacal symptoms have physiological symptoms of anxiety; therefore, **anxiety disorders** such as panic disorder or generalized anxiety disorder should be ruled out. In patients with obsessive ruminations of illness, the diagnosis of **obsessive-compulsive disorder** should be considered in the differential.

As with other somatoform disorders, the mere complaint of pain that is unexplained by known organic etiology is not sufficient to warrant the diagnosis of pain disorder. The pain, or the social or occupational impairment, must be grossly out of proportion to the physical findings. In addition, some evidence of stressors or conflicts should be present that either preceded the onset of the pain or, by its continued presence, has exacerbated or maintained the pain symptoms. Complaints of pain may also occur in the context of other mental disorders, e.g., **schizophrenia, major depression,** or **somatization disorder.** In instances of malingering, the individuals' complaints of pain become understandable given the environmental circumstances. A person with a heroin addiction who complains of pain to obtain analgesics should not be given the diagnosis of pain disorder. Overconcern and perceived defects in appearance may occur during the course of **normal adolescence.** It may also be part of a more pervasive disorder such as **anorexia nervosa.** Taken to an extreme, it may be delusional in intensity and diagnosed as a **delusional disorder.** It may also occur in the context of **schizophrenia, major depression, social phobia,** or an **avoidant** or **schizotypal personality disorder.** Given the often excessive rumination and anxiety, the diagnosis of **obsessive-compulsive disorder** should be considered in the differential.

Borderline narcissistic, obsessive-compulsive, and histrionic personality disorders may all form the context for, and be comorbid with, one of the somatoform disorders.

MEDICAL EVALUATION

A thorough medical evaluation that includes laboratory investigations is vital for patients with somatoform disorders. Because presenting complaints are suggestive of physical illness, it is crucial to rule out the presence of any underlying medical illness that might explain the symptoms. Investigators who followed patients originally given the diagnosis of conversion hysteria found that, over time, many of the patients developed genuine and serious medical conditions, including brain tumors, ulcerative colitis, collagen diseases, and degenerative disc diseases. In such cases, the worry is that the physical discomfort was the first and only sign of the developing physical illness. In addition to careful history taking, it may be necessary to perform various diagnostic tests including brain scans, CT scans, MRIs, and EEGs for, say, unexplained headache pain. Consultation with a specialist in neurology, orthopedic surgery, or neurosurgery would be necessary for someone presenting with an unexplained paralysis. As a rule of thumb,

once the diagnosis of a somatoform disorder is considered, the physician should avoid any diagnostic procedure that is invasive and puts the patient at risk for additional pain or complications. Psychiatric consultation should usually be obtained at this point. Even after the psychiatric evaluation confirms the diagnosis of a somatoform disorder, the physician should continue to regularly assess the patient for physical illness that requires early intervention. There is no reason why a person with documented hypochondriasis cannot develop a carcinoma or die suddenly of a myocardial infarction.

ETIOLOGY

The familial pattern of **somatization disorder** suggests contributions from genetic and environmental factors. Children of affected mothers may learn to express themselves through physical symptoms, i.e., to somatize anxiety or depression.

Conversion disorder is one of the few disorders in the DSM-IV that incorporates a psychodynamic etiology into its diagnostic criteria. Conversion symptoms usually serve the purpose of resolving an emotional conflict without the conscious awareness of the patient. An exploration of environmental stressors or changes in life situation often reveals the etiology of the symptoms. Once the symptoms have appeared, the patient may reap secondary gains of sympathy, attention, and support that might otherwise not be forthcoming. These secondary gains (although not of etiological significance) may serve the purpose of maintaining or prolonging the conversion symptoms. For example, a person who during the course of a hospitalization received attention from relatives or coworkers that was usually not forthcoming.

Often the individual with **hypochondriasis** has a previous experience with an organic disease. Those who recover from a serious disease (e.g., heart attack or cancer) may become fearful of relapse and interpret normal somatic sensations (e.g., muscle aches or gas pains) as evidence of illness. Sometimes, true physical illness does occur in a family member. Hypochondriasis may begin in response to stressors, such as marital conflict, occupational dissatisfaction, or unemployment. Having an illness may allow the patient to obtain sympathy or avoid an unpleasant family or occupational situation.

In the majority of cases of **pain disorder,** the pain is preceded by a physical injury or trauma. Often, a relationship exists between the onset of the pain and the presence of a recognizable environmental stressor or conflict. Individuals who may be predisposed to developing pain disorder are those who perform dangerous or physically strenuous jobs. They usually have good work histories and have held their jobs for many years. Psychodynamic theory suggests that individuals with pain disorder have difficulty in directly expressing emotions, e.g., anger, depression, anxiety and, when faced with a stress or conflict, may express their "pain" (mental anguish) indirectly by somaticizing and presenting with physical pain.

The etiology of **body dysmorphic disorder** is complex and probably multidetermined. The onset may be triggered by an innocuous comment about appearance or by childhood teasing. From a psychodynamic perspective, the etiology may be uncovered over the course of therapy. The displacement of an underlying anxiety into morbid overconcern about appearance may permit the person to avoid issues of intimacy or sexuality. Alternatively, the focus on perceived faults in appearance leading the individual to avoid social contacts may protect against a fear of rejection. Rather than consider any psychological shortcomings, such as low self-esteem, the individual can avoid social interactions and blame the avoidance on defects in his or her appearance. Patients then feel justified in focusing on finding "medical cures" (e.g., through cosmetic surgery) rather than embarking on an exploration of the psychological causes.

TREATMENT

Patients with somatoform disorders often require multiple therapeutic modalities, including psychotherapy for their interpersonal and psychological problems, in particular, the dissociation of affect from life events that they tend to have. Medication to treat an underlying depressive disorder may also be required. Coordination of care between the psychiatrist and the other physicians—and sometimes the family—is also most beneficial. Some medical practices and clinics have found group therapy for these patients to be very helpful. Because successful treatment depends on an accurate differential diagnosis, the physician must diagnose and treat any associated psychiatric illnesses.

Treatment planning must be individually prescribed to address specific illnesses and their degree of severity in order to maximize patients' chances of recovery. As with all other psychiatric disorders, patients' specific emotional conflicts vary as do their aptitudes for psychotherapy. In addition, the intensity of their symptoms varies and may shift along an axis that ranges from neurotic to near psychotic. These locations and shifts in severity dramatically alter the type of treatment that should be planned.

One of the main difficulties in designing treatment plans for patients with somatoform disorders is the variety of psychiatric illnesses, including depression or personality disorders, that may coexist. General principles of treatment planning for patients with somatoform disorders include the taking of a careful history for depression and bipolar illness, schizophrenia, cognitive syndromes, and personality disorders. As with personality disorders, medication is useful in patients with comorbid conditions (e.g., antidepressants for mood disorders) and for symptomatic relief during the course of treatment (e.g., benzodiazepines for severe anxiety). In addition, a careful medical and parallel psychosocial history must be taken to uncover exacerbating events, ameliorative situations, and the state of the patients' relationships with their primary care physicians. These lines of exploration reveal the variables that treatment planning can then address. As mentioned above, combination treatments are usually recommended. The exact mix of therapies depends on the patient's illness profile and personality type and strengths.

Somatization Disorder

The psychiatrist, acting concurrently as a consultant with the primary care provider, usually suggests that the patient maintain ties with only one primary physician and avoid contact with other physicians not familiar with the patient. This limitation should minimize overprescribing, overinstrumentalization, and unnecessary surgery. Conceptually, somatization disorder is similar to a type of personality style that is pervasive, long-standing, and not likely to be affected by any "quick fixes." All physicians working with these patients need to be aware of the chronic pervasive nature of their illnesses and to be prepared for long-term involvement with them. One goal for the psychiatrist is to help patients cope with symptoms and learn ways in which they can deal more effectively with their psychological and interpersonal problems. Medication treatments should be closely monitored because noncompliance is a common problem and because with chronic usage there is the danger of possible interactions with over-the-counter medications and medications prescribed by other physicians.

Conversion Disorder

Treatment of the patient with conversion disorder involves a joint undertaking by the referring medical specialist and the psychiatrist. It is important that a thorough medical workup be completed. In the absence of demonstrable organic pathology that accounts for the patient's symptoms, the patient should be confidently reassured that no serious illness has been found. When a relationship between trauma, conflict, or stressors is discovered by the psychiatric consultant, a course of psychotherapy should be suggested. Therapy should be directed toward helping the patient understand and accept the intense conflicts and emotions that are producing or maintaining the symptoms. Once insight is gained into these psychological factors, the patient's symptoms should subside. Some patients may respond better to the relaxation techniques employed in a behavioral approach than to more psychodynamic approaches. Brief treatment with anxiolytic medications can be a useful adjunct that facilitates the psychotherapeutic process. The longer the symptoms persist, the more difficult it becomes to treat the disorder successfully. Successful treatment is problematic in patients who have secondary gain issues, e.g., disability or workers' compensation. Ideally, the psychiatrist would suggest a quick settlement of compensation issues; however, given the adversarial nature of some proceedings, this is often impossible. These situations are often frustrating for psychiatrists because while they are trying to help patients recover from their symptoms, they are concurrently being asked by patients for letters supporting their disability claims or by attorneys insisting on their appearance in court.

Pain Disorder

In most instances, the psychiatrist's role in the treatment planning of patients with pain disorder is to collaborate with the referring physician to alleviate (rather than eliminate) the patient's pain and to minimize its social and occupational consequences. The psychiatrist should be familiar and comfortable with a variety of treatments, including behavior, interpersonal, and psychodynamic psychotherapy, biofeedback, and pharmacological. Tricyclic antidepressant medications, particularly those that most affect the noradrenergic system (e.g., desipramine), seem to provide significant pain relief even in patients who do not have a depressive syndrome. The use of analgesics that are physically addicting should be discouraged. In some instances, time-limited use of antianxiety medication may be appropriate. Many of these patients respond to the multimodal therapies provided at pain-control centers. Inpatient treatment may be necessary for detoxification of patients addicted to narcotics or tranquilizers. Outpatient regimens might include group therapy, educational instruction, physical therapy, relaxation, nerve blocks, and transcutaneous nerve stimulation (to block the nerve impulses).

Hypochondriasis

The treatment of hypochondriasis is generally managed by the primary care physician. Treatment planning should include regular appointments with adequate time allowed for discussing aspects of the patient's life other than the physical complaints. It may be helpful to conduct a brief physical examination of the patient at each visit to reassure him or her that a condition has not worsened. Psychotropic medication may be indicated when a coexisting mental disorder, e.g., major depression, would respond to medication. Depending on the physician's interest and familiarity with psychotropic medications, he or she may choose to manage the medication or to refer the patient to a psychiatrist for management. Antianxiety medication and sleep medication should be used with caution because of its potential for abuse and dependence. It is possible that a patient may continue taking an antianxiety medication (e.g., by borrowing medication from a relative) without revealing this to the original prescribing physician. In time, the patient may see another physician and be started on a similarly acting medication that he or she continues in addition to the originally prescribed medication. By the time a physician realizes

the extent and true doses that the patient is taking, discontinuing the medications may be difficult and dangerous.

When a patient with hypochondriasis is amenable to psychotherapy, the goal should be to support and maximize his or her functioning in spite of the physical complaints. In addition, the patient should be instructed in how to develop more adaptive coping skills to stress that can substitute for the less adaptive coping mechanism of adopting the "sick role." For example, if a patient's overconcern about his or her heart worsens regularly with job-related stress, the patient may benefit from stress management exercises or relaxation training. When a patient with a chronic illness develops hypochondriacal symptoms, he or she should be educated about the illness and taught to adjust to limitations and disabilities. The post myocardial infarction patient who fears that every instance of chest pain indicates a new attack may benefit from learning the difference between angina and infarction. These patients should also be taught how to differentiate activities that are potentially dangerous (e.g., shoveling snow in extremely cold weather) from those that are not (e.g., sexual relations with a spouse). Recent evidence suggests that the serotonin reuptake inhibitors may be helpful for patients with hypochondriasis even when there is no coexisting mood disorder.

Body Dysmorphic Disorder

Once this diagnosis is made, the patient should avoid all cosmetic surgery because it is unlikely that any surgical cosmetic change in appearance will result in a long-lasting change in his or her thinking. Patients are likely to be unsatisfied with any result and seek additional surgeries. Although much has been written on the psychodynamic etiology of this condition, attempts to engage these patients in therapy and treat their symptoms have had limited success. The efficacy of other therapies, such as behavior (e.g., desensitization and exposure), confrontational, and supportive, is mixed.

Although no controlled case studies have been conducted on the use of psychotropic medications to treat patients with body dysmorphic disorder, several case reports support the efficacy of a trial of antidepressants. The best results have been found using serotonin reuptake blockers, e.g., clomipramine and fluoxetine. Pimozide is the one antipsychotic medication that seems to have particular efficacy for these patients. Treatment with other antidepressants, antipsychotics, benzodiazepines, and lithium carbonate has been largely unsuccessful.

FACTITIOUS DISORDERS

Episodes of patients simulating physical illness are not uncommon. Such patients, the majority of whom are women, are often seen within the hospital setting. Men make up the majority of patients who have Munchausen's syndrome, the fairly rare but more chronic form of factitious disorder, which is characterized by patients' continuing odysseys of hospitalization followed by rehospitalization. These patients travel widely and, because of their flamboyant style, intriguing histories, and outrageous behaviors, are probably overreported in medical literature, in respect to their actual numbers. (Often, a single patient is the subject of many physicians' reports that appear in a number of journals in a variety of medical specialties.) The disorder typically begins in early adulthood, often following a hospitalization for true physical illness.

Although little information exists concerning the epidemiology, course, and etiology of factitious disorder with predominantly psychological symptoms, the production of factitious symptoms in individuals with another, more pervasive mental disorder (e.g., schizophrenia or borderline personality disorder) may occur in response to environmental stress or emotional conflicts.

Patients with factitious disorder intentionally simulate or produce symptoms of illnesses for the purpose of achieving the "sick role" of a patient. These disorders fall midway between somatoform disorders, in which symptom production is not intentional, and malingering, in which the goals are recognizable given an understanding of the circumstances. The patient with a factitious disorder consciously simulates illness for psychological purposes. ➡ For example, a patient had been producing symptoms and signs of hypoglycemia by surreptitiously injecting himself with insulin with syringes that he had taken with him to the hospital. Following a confrontation by his physician (who found the insulin and syringes in a search of the patient's belongings), the patient left the hospital. Later that evening, he was admitted via the emergency room to another hospital less than a mile away from the first hospital for hypoglycemic delirium. It was clear from the patient's behavior that he knew he was causing the symptoms. There was no clear-cut goal for the behavior other than to assume the psychological role of "patient." ➡

Patients with factitious disorder may have physical symptoms, psychological symptoms, or a mixture of the two. The DSM-IV allows for the coding of three subtypes of the disorder: factititous disorder with predominantly psychological signs and symptoms, factitious disorder with predominantly physical signs and symptoms, or factitious disorder with combined psychological and physical signs and symptoms (Table 10–8). The best known factitious disorder is that with predominantly physical signs and symptoms, popularly called Munchausen's syndrome. In this most severe and chronic form of factitious disorder, patients spend the majority of their time either in the hospital or in seeking admission to a hospital. ➡ One patient had over 200 documented hospitalizations over a 7-year span. The patient's odyssey had taken him from the coast of Maine to Boston, then to Albany, NY, and New York City, then

---

TABLE 10–8.   DSM-IV Diagnostic Criteria for Factitious Disorder

A. Intentional production or feigning of physical or psychological signs or symptoms.
B. The motivation for the behavior is to assume the sick role.
C. External incentives for the behavior (such as economic gain, avoiding legal responsibility, or improving physical well-being, as in Malingering) are absent.

Code based on type:
   With Predominantly Psychological Signs and Symptoms: if psychological signs and symptoms predominant in the clinical presentation
   With Predominantly Physical Signs and Symptoms: if physical signs and symptoms predominate in the clinical presentation
   With Combined Psychological and Physical Signs and Symptoms: if both psychological and physical signs and symptoms are present but neither predominates in the clinical presentation

---

to Philadelphia, and then Pittsburgh. His last documented hospitalization occurred in West Virginia. ➡ Though no systematic studies of outcome exist, it seems likely that some patients succumb either to the medical complications of their self-induced illnesses or to adverse effects of various invasive procedures.

DIAGNOSTIC AND CLINICAL FEATURES
Factitious Disorder With Predominantly Physical Signs and Symptoms

The symptoms of patients with a factitious disorder with predominantly physical signs and symptoms are suggestive of a physical disorder that they intentionally produce. The only obvious motivation for the deception is to assume the sick role. The simulation of almost every medical illness is possible. Only patients' imagination, medical sophistication, and daring limit the physical symptoms they can produce. They can convincingly support their physical complaints, and they can even induce some laboratory abnormalities, such as increased body temperature. ➡ For example, one man who presented to his physician complaining of weakness and dizziness had a rapid, weak pulse and low blood pressure with significant orthostatic changes on physical examination. Laboratory tests indicated that he had low serum potassium. The man was then admitted to a hospital. A consulting nephrologist and endocrinologist helped formulate a working diagnosis of idiopathic familial hypokalemia. The man had been surreptitiously ingesting potassium-losing diuretics.

In another instance, a patient presented in a highly agitated and delirious state. Routine laboratory tests revealed a blood sugar of less than 50 mg/dL. The patient had no history of diabetes. The working diagnosis was an insulin-producing tumor of the pancreas. The actual cause of the symptoms was the patient's surreptitious injection of insulin, which was discovered only when vials of insulin and syringes were discovered accidentally among the patient's belongings. ➡

Other presenting conditions that often turn out to be factitious are bleeding caused by the ingestion of anticoagulant medication, endocrine abnormalities caused by the ingestion of thyroid hormone, abscesses caused by subcutaneous injection of saliva or feces, hyperthermia caused by manipulating the thermometer, and voluntary limb dislocation.

Certain behavioral features are associated with patients with factitious disorder. Pathological lying about various aspects of history and background sometimes occurs. Patients may claim to be related to rich, famous, powerful individuals. One patient was treated royally by the hospital staff, who had been led to believe that he was a prince of a central African country. Another patient reported being related to the senator of an adjoining state. These patients often wander from city to city, state to state, or country to country in search of treatment for their symptoms. In addition, patients with factitious disorder may complain of new physical problems related to different organ systems as soon as one set of symptoms is under control. When hospitalized, many of these patients have no visitors. Some patients have collaborators who bring paraphernalia (syringes, medications) when they visit so that these patients can continue their charades. Patients with factitious disorder often have an extensive knowledge of medical terminology and procedures, and they often do not object to potentially dangerous invasive procedures and operations. When these patients are confronted with evidence of their fabrication, they quickly leave the hospitals, usually against medical advice. Physicians encountering patients who have a bewildering array of shifting complaints, which they present dramatically but whose medical history cannot be verified, should always consider factitious disorder in the differential diagnosis.

Factitious Disorder With Predominantly Psychological Signs and Symptoms

People with factitious disorder with psychological symptoms simulate mental rather than physical illnesses. They either falsify their history or feign symptoms of mental illness. The presenting symptoms often reflect the individual's conception of mental illness rather than any recognized disorder. Such patients may present with a combination of psychotic, affective, and cognitive findings. ⇒ In one case, a patient went to an emergency room and complained of hearing voices and seeing visions. Psychiatric examination revealed a positive history for symptoms of mania, depression, and dementia, as well as panic attacks, conversion symptoms, and dissociative experiences. Since it is highly unlikely that any patient would have simultaneous presentation of all of these disorders, the psychiatrist extended the examination. Upon doing so, it became evident that the patient wanted to ensure his hospitalization. ⇐

These patients try to please the physician by presenting signs and symptoms of illnesses that suggest acute and often rare or interesting medical conditions so that physicians will take an interest in them and admit them to their service. In the past, some of these patients were diagnosed with pseudopsychosis, hysterical psychosis, pseudodementia, or Ganser's syndrome (the syndrome of approximate answers), which is often indistinguishable from malingering. The patient with Ganser's syndrome feigns illness by responding to questions in a manner that indicates a knowledge of the answer or task, but is off by a bit. This was frequently seen in prisoners who would answer "five" when asked to add "two plus two." Physicians are most likely to see these patients in emergency rooms or in other hospital settings.

Factitious symptoms may arise in patients who have preexisting genuine mental disorders, but the new symptoms are not consistent with the patients' diagnoses. ⇒ For example, one patient who was diagnosed with major depressive disorder and dependent personality disorder and who never claimed to see and hear spirits, began to voice these complaints just before he was to be transferred to a day hospital. As with factitious disorder with physical symptoms, no obvious recognizable goal explained the psychological findings. His physicians concluded that the patient was "dependent" on his present facility and frightened of leaving a familiar environment and of getting used to new surroundings. These psychological explanations indicated that the new, feigned symptoms were factitious rather than malingering. The man's original diagnosis remained the same, and the newly feigned symptoms supported an additional diagnosis of factitious disorder with psychological symptoms. ⇐

Patients who are known to the staff at a hospital may present with factitious psychological symptoms to gain admission to an inpatient unit when their usual symptoms would not warrant admission. Such patients may present with auditory hallucinations commanding them to kill themselves even though their chronic suicidal ideation has in the past not included the presence of any hallucinations.

THE INTERVIEW

With such patients, the medical physician must exhibit the wisdom of Solomon, the patience of Job, and the detective work of Sherlock Holmes (or Columbo). These patients stir up feelings of impotence, righteousness, and even rage in their physicians. Physicians must be aware of these feelings in order to avoid unconsciously punishing the patients by ordering a host of painful and potentially dangerous diagnostic or therapeutic procedures. Psychiatrists are usually called in to evaluate patients with factitious disorder during a medical or surgical hospitalization when patients are either behaving bizarrely, creating a disturbance on the ward, or are discovered—or recognized—to be simulating their illnesses. The psychiatrist is often put into the difficult position of being the first professional to confront and "unmask" patients and then treat them. If possible, the psychiatrist should suggest that any unmasking of patients be done by the treating staff, then the psychiatrist can be called in to assist the patient as an ally rather than as an adversary. In many instances, the patient will leave the hospital after being informed that a psychiatrist is being called to consult. When the psychiatrist does get the opportunity to examine the patient, the patient may be guarded or vague about details. When asked to discuss previous physicians or hospitalizations, these patients may report that they have forgotten the names of the physicians or hospitals. They may say that they would rather that the psychiatrist not contact them because they have had significant disagreements about the care that they received. Alternatively, the history may be presented with great dramatic flair in a manner designed to intrigue the psychiatrist similar to the way the medical staff may have been captivated by the story. The patient may tell a tale full of, perhaps, Freudian significance such as vivid dreams and present a textbook case of childhood sexual seduction. With these patients, it is important to obtain confirmatory evidence whenever possible to find the facts within the fiction.

The topic of confrontation is controversial. Many patients will flee but some investigators believe that this is the only way to get these patients in touch with their underlying motivation. Depending on the patient's needs and the underlying illness the patient may be either guarded and vague or overly cooperative and compliant. During a mental status examination, the patient may present with "voirbereden," i.e., inexact answers or talking past the point. A patient who is asked the name of the current president may reply "Lincoln." This indicates that the patient has understood the nature of the task and is giving inexact answers to the questions. Whereas a single instance may be merely a mistake, such repeated answers indicate a deliberate intent to simulate. Some clinicians report success with Amytal interviews in determining what the new symptoms mean. Probably the most reliable method for understanding these patients is to observe them over time and to consider reports from staff on other shifts who may be in a better position to observe the patient's symptoms and behavior. Once these patients feel that their problems are understood and begin to understand their own motivation, they may no longer have to feign new symptoms.

DIFFERENTIAL DIAGNOSIS

Because of the nature of their illness, many patients with factitious disorder do, in fact, need treatment for genuine physical illnesses. For example, a patient who surreptitiously injected saliva and fecal material into his skin did have genuine infections, fevers, and septicemia that were life threatening and required medical intervention (intravenous antibiotics). However, until the factitious etiology of the abscesses is uncovered, the treatment may be very problematic. A high level of suspicion should be aroused in a physician when a patient has (1) a dramatic presentation, (2) extensive evidence of prior treatment (e.g., a gridiron abdomen, burr holes, cutdown sites), (3) a sophisticated medical knowledge and vocabulary, (4) traveled widely, (5) complaints and signs that rapidly shift from one organ system to another, (6) few visitors, and (7) discharges against medical advice from prior hospitalizations.

People who **malinger** usually have an obvious, recognizable environmental goal, such as drug seeking or financial compensation, that accounts for the simulation of illness. Factitious disorder should be considered when no such goal can explain the symptom production.

In **somatoform disorders** such as somatization disorder or hypochondriasis, patients may have a variety of complaints; however, they are not intentionally producing (or simulating) their illness. Because of these patients' admittedly bizarre life-styles and strange affects (e.g., flat or inappropriate), some of these patients have been diagnosed with schizophrenia. However, psychiatric examination generally reveals the absence of schizophrenic criteria. Some of the patients with episodic factitious disorder have major depression with psychotic features. A man with factitious disorder may have a history of repeated conflicts with the law or evidence of frequent problems pertaining to substance abuse. The diagnosis of **antisocial personality disorder** should be made only when the full criteria are met. In both women and men who display features that meet criteria for **borderline personality disorder** (see Etiology, below), both diagnoses should be reported.

The major differential diagnosis for factitious disorder with predominantly psychological symptoms is a true mental disorder. This diagnosis is even more difficult to establish with certainty than is factitious disorder with physical symptoms because, in most cases, no confirmatory laboratory findings exist. In a majority of instances, physicians use their experience, intuition, or educated guesses to determine whether certain new symptoms are inconsistent with the original diagnosis and have been produced by patients in an attempt to cope with stressors that they cannot communicate well to their physicians.

Another important differential is the presence of a **new physical disorder** that may be caused by side effects of medication, such as a dystonic reaction, or disguised physical illness that patients may not be able to communicate well because of the nature of their original mental disorder. For example, a patient who had been hospitalized for many years for chronic schizophrenia suddenly became dysphasic. Although he had a factitious disorder, he had also experienced a cerebrovascular accident.

Patients with serious character pathology such as borderline personality disorder or antisocial personality disorder may feign symptoms of mental illness for psychological reasons of attention, dependency, or indirect expression of anger. In these instances, both diagnoses should be made.

MEDICAL EVALUATION

Once the diagnosis of factitious disorder is considered, any additional invasive or traumatic procedures or treatments with a likelihood of serious adverse side effects should be avoided. These procedures may lead to additional factitious symptoms and signs. For example, one patient who had an intravenous pyelogram developed an "allergic" reaction to the dye and went into feigned respiratory arrest. Another patient who had a biopsy showed excess bleeding from the site because the coagulum was disrupted. Of course, the physician should realize that, even though the etiology of the symptoms is factitious, the patient may, in fact, be physically ill and need treatment. A patient who has surreptitiously bled himself can develop a genuine anemia from the blood loss and need immediate attention. The physician should obtain psychiatric consultation whenever feasible and should be prepared for patients to take this recommendation as their cue to sign out.

ETIOLOGY

Factitious disorders are thought to represent a final common pathway that is multidetermined. During their childhood, many of these patients or a close family member experienced a serious physical illness. Some patients report having a grudge against the medical profession, often the result of some real or perceived medical mismanagement. An occupational association may exist since many patients report having worked as nurses, laboratory technicians, and other health professionals. However, it is difficult to differentiate between cause and effect. Patients with factitious disorder frequently report that they have had an important relationship with a physician, and some report that they were seduced by a physician. (Obtaining confirmatory information of these reports, although important, may be difficult if not impossible.)

One newly recognized etiological factor involves the relationship between factitious disorder and **factitious disorder by proxy.** In factitious disorder by proxy, an adult (usually, the parent) fabricates illness in a child, who then receives unnecessary medical interventions and hospitalizations. These parents may do this either to ensure that the child gets appropriate medical attention or to gain attention or admiration for themselves by playing the role of caring or grieving parent. It seems likely that these children, upon reaching adulthood, may continue the factitious disorder by simulating illness themselves.

Other investigators have reported that patients with factitious disorder have a **borderline personality disorder.** However, rather than be hospitalized in a psychiatric facility for committing impulsive or self-destructive acts, these patients "act out" by simulating physical illness, which mobilizes caregivers and gains them admission to medical hospitals. Many of the underlying dynamics found in patients with facti-tious disorder, including constant anger, chronic feelings of emptiness and boredom, intolerance of being alone, idealization and devaluation, and poor impulse control, are consistent with the criteria for borderline personality disorder, as well.

THERAPY

There is no specific effective treatment for patients with factitious disorder. Most psychiatric interventions have not been found to be effective, but since treatment tends to be terminated prematurely by the patient's departing after he or she learns that a psychiatrist has been called in for consultation, it is impossible to conclude what effect a full course of treatment would have had. The overall goal of a consultation psychiatrist is to prevent patients from undergoing unnecessary and potentially dangerous or invasive procedures. Another goal is to sufficiently engage patients so that they receive care in only one facility, where staff members can become familiar with them and follow them over time. This strategy may prevent factitious disorder from progressing into persistent Munchausen's syndrome. One way in which the psychiatrist can achieve this is by acknowledging to patients that their need to feign illnesses means that they are indeed very seriously ill with a psychiatric disorder. The psychiatrist then helps the entire medical staff regard these patients as being really very ill and in need of intensive psychiatric care. The patients may be able to accept their true diagnosis when it is given within the context of an already begun supportive and exploratory treatment for a serious illness, although not the particular one with which they presented.

In cases of Munchausen's syndrome by proxy, it is important to involve the appropriate agencies responsible for the welfare of children because the traumas inflicted upon children through the parents' feigning of illness are tantamount to child abuse. In severe instances, it may be necessary to remove the child from the care of the offending parents.

Selected Readings
Somatoform Disorders

Barsky AJ, Klerman GL: Overview: hypochondriasis, bodily complaints, and somatic styles. American Journal of Psychiatry 140:273–283, 1983.

Barsky AJ, Wyshak G, Latham KS, et al: The relationship between hypochondriasis and medical illness. Archives of Internal Medicine 151:84–88, 1991.

Ford CV: *The Somatizing Disorders: Illness as a Way of Life.* New York, Elsevier, 1983.

Ford CV, Folks DG: Conversion disorders: An overview. Psychosomatics 26:371–383, 1985.

Golding JM, Smith GR, Kashner TM: Does Somatization disorder occur in men? Clinical characteristics of women and men with multiple unexplained somatic symptoms. Archives of General Psychiatry 48:231–235, 1991.

Guze SB: The validity and significance of the clinical diagnosis of hysteria (Briquet's syndrome). American Journal of Psychiatry 132:138–141, 1975.

Hyler SE, Spitzer RL: Hysteria split asunder. American Journal of Psychiatry 135:1500–1503, 1978.

Kellner R: Hypochondriasis and somatization. Journal of American Medical Association 258:2718–2722, 1987.

Kellner R: *Somatization and Hypochondriasis.* New York, Praeger, 1986.

Kenyon FF: Hypochondriacal states. British Journal of Psychiatry 129:1–14; 1976.

Merskey H: Psychiatry and chronic pain. Canadian Journal of Psychiatry 34:329–336; 1989.

Phillips KA: Body dysmorphic disorder: the distress of imagined ugliness. American Journal of Psychiatry 148:1138–1149; 1991.

Smith GR, Monson RA, Ray SC: Psychiatric consultation in somatization disorder. New England Journal of Medicine 314:1407–1413; 1986.

Thomas CS: Dysmorphophobia: A question of definition. British Journal of Psychiatry 144:513–516; 1984.

Factitious Disorders

Asher R: Munchausen's syndrome. Lancet 1:339; 1951.

Bursten B: On Munchausen's syndrome. Archives of General Psychiatry 13:261; 1965.

Cramer B, Gershberg RR, Stern M: Munchausen's syndrome: Its relationship to malingering, hysteria, and the physician-patient relationship. Archives of General Psychiatry 24:573; 1971.

Feinstein A, Hattersley A: Ganser syndrome, dissociation, and dysprosody. Journal of Nervous and Mental Diseases 176:692–693; 1988.

Hollender RH, Hersh SP: Impossible consultation made possible. Archives of General Psychiatry 23:343; 1970.

Hyler SE, Sussman N: Chronic factitious disorder with physical symptoms (the Munchausen syndrome). Psychiatric Clinics of North America 4:365–377; 1981.

Meadow R: Munchausen syndrome by proxy: The hinterland of child abuse. Lancet 2:343; 1977.

Pope HG, Jonas JM, Jones B: Factitious psychosis: phenomenology, family history and long term outcome of nine patients. American Journal of Psychiatry 139:1480–1483; 1982.

Reich P, Gottfried LA: Factitious disorders in a teaching hospital. Annals of Internal Medicine 99:240–247; 1983.

Spiro HR: Chronic factitious illness. Archives of General Psychiatry 18:569; 1968.

Taylor S and Hyler SE: Update on factitious disorders. International Journal of Psychiatry in Medicine (1993), 23:81–94.

CHAPTER ELEVEN

SUICIDE AND VIOLENCE

ROBERT E. FEINSTEIN, MD

Suicide and violence are major public health issues. Suicide is the ninth leading cause of all deaths in the United States and is frequently associated with a psychiatric disorder. The exact magnitude of suicide and psychiatric violence is difficult to estimate. The reported incidence and prevalence vary widely, because law enforcement agencies, social service agencies, and health care providers often have different definitions of these behaviors. Many suicidal and violent behaviors are not reported at all, and many deaths caused by these behaviors are reported as accidents. Hence, the following epidemiological information may not reflect the true incidence of these dangerous behaviors.

Approximately 30,000 persons, or about 12 in every 100,000 persons, kill themselves each year. Ten times that number of people make suicide attempts. Suicide occurs in all age groups, with the peak incidence in persons 20–24 years old. Suicide is the leading cause of death in persons under the age of 35 years. Of particular concern are the dramatically increased rates of suicide since 1980 in persons 5–19 years old and in persons 65 years or older. Men are three times more successful in their suicide attempts than are women, although women are ten times more likely to attempt suicide (Table 11–1).

Violence is a social problem that is not always within the province of psychiatry, but a number of common psychiatric disorders can be complicated by varying degrees of violent behavior. Violent behavior due to a psychiatric disorder is most likely to be seen in persons with brain injuries or in those who use illegal drugs (Table 11–2). Approximately one million cases of brain injury result each year from trauma, cerebrovascular accidents (strokes), and tumors; approximately 70% of people with traumatic brain injury become irritable and aggressive within months. Dementia causes 25% of all agitated or aggressive behavior seen in nursing home patients. Mentally retarded patients and patients with psychoses, particularly those with command auditory hallucinations, also have a high incidence of violent behavior.

According to the US Department of Justice, 24% of homicides committed in many major cities are related to the use of illegal drugs. Of persons injured by a violent act, 12% report that their assailants were under the influence of drugs. About 33% of the inmates in state prisons have said that they were under the influence of drugs at the time they committed the offenses for which they have been imprisoned.

Although individuals with suicidal behavior frequently do not suffer from the same psychiatric disorders that individuals with violent behavior do, both groups experience similar destructive feelings, thoughts, fantasies, and behaviors, and a significant number of these patients have both suicidal and violent symptoms. The intensity of their suicidal or violent symptoms varies from low risk to life threatening. These patients are among the most challenging for physicians and are capable of evoking anxiety even in the most experienced clinicians. In order to prevent suicidal or violent patients from causing serious injury or death to themselves or others and to provide them with effective treatment, the physician must take an approach that is calm, thoughtful, and informed by a biopsychosocial understanding.

DIAGNOSTIC AND CLINICAL FEATURES

The definition of suicide is deceptively simple: the taking of one's own life. It can, however, be quite difficult to determine whether or not a death was suicide. For the purposes of basic scientific research and legal verification, a death is considered **suicide** only when physical and behavioral evidence indicate that the death was both intentional and self-inflicted. A broader perspective suggests that it is often difficult to accurately assess intent after death has occurred because the concept of intent includes unconsciously motivated thoughts, feelings, and behaviors.

Patients with **suicidal symptoms** commonly say that they feel frustrated, helpless, or hopeless. They tend to become extremely pessimistic when their repeated attempts to solve problems appear to have failed. These individuals often have a style of thinking that can be described as tunnel vision, which leads them to believe that suicide is the only solution to their problems. They are frequently angry, self-punishing, and harshly self-critical. They may describe themselves as stupid or worthless and say that they deserve to die. Some covertly use their symptoms or threats of suicide to control other persons, saying, in effect, "Do what I want or I'll kill myself."

Violence is operationally defined as an individual's use of verbal threat, intimidation, or physical

TABLE 11–1.   Characteristics of Patients Who Commit Suicide

Mean age for suicide
  30 years.
Most common means
  Men: Gunshot.
  Women: Ingestion of pills or slashing of wrists.
Racial statistics
  Non-Hispanic whites are twice as likely to commit suicide as people of color.
  Native Americans have a higher rate than the national average.
Religious statistics
  Protestants and atheists have the highest rates.
  Catholics and Orthodox Jews have the lowest rates.
Demographic statistics
  Urban residents have higher rates than suburban or rural residents.
Marital status
  Ranked from the highest to the lowest rates: divorced persons, widowed persons, single persons, married persons.
Risk factors for suicide
  Poor health, living alone, a history of previous attempts, recent loss, alcohol or drug abuse, mood disorder, psychosis.
Contact with physician
  Of patients who commit suicide, 53% have seen a physician within the previous 6 months.
General hospital suicides
  Most common means is jumping from a dangerous height.
  Most common psychiatric syndrome is psychosis.
  Most common nonpsychiatric diagnoses are cancer, chronic obstructive pulmonary disease, and chronic pain.
  Patients undergoing renal dialysis have a suicide rate 400 times that of the general population.

force with the intent to cause property damage, personal harm, or death to another person. Violence is considered to be a psychiatric problem only when it is clearly associated with certain psychiatric illnesses, such as psychotic disorders and substance-related disorders. Violence as a psychiatric symptom is distinguished from the commission of violent crimes and institutionalized violence such as war or terrorism. This distinction is made because psychiatrists do not have an effective treatment to offer violent individuals who do not suffer from a specific psychiatric disorder. Obviously, this distinction also has important implications for those individuals who might try to absolve themselves of responsibility for their crimes.

Patients with **violent symptoms** often say that they feel frustrated, impatient, chronically irritable, or angry. They tend to challenge authority, have verbal or physical outbursts or temper tantrums, and criticize others harshly. They often enjoy gaining power and control through threats, saying, in effect, "Do what I want or I will hurt or kill *you.*" They may get sadistic pleasure from scaring other people, making them beg for mercy, or putting them in a weakened position. They commonly demand special treatment, making statements such as, "I want to be seen *now!*" They often angrily attack or devalue anyone who confronts them (e.g., physicians) with the result of their violent actions or suspected dishonesty. They may also resort to other psychopathic manipulations, such as deception, lying, cheating, or stealing.

Despite their aggressive appearance and behavior, violent patients are frightened people who feel weak and powerless. They fear being humiliated and scorned and are tired of feeling controlled, manipulated, or demeaned by others. They commit violent acts in an effort to bolster or hide their low self-esteem or because they feel that they have no other means by which to protect themselves from perceived threats and survive in a frightening world.

Phases of Behavior

As the intensity of their symptoms increases, suicidal and violent persons usually go through four different phases of behavior, ranging from the least to the most dangerous: calm, psychomotor agitation, verbal, and acting-out phases (Table 11–3).

Calm Phase

The lowest level of immediate risk is associated with patients who are in the calm phase. They appear calm, have maintained a level of good self-care, are alert and fully conscious, and are engaged in normal social interactions. Patients develop a slightly greater risk for suicidal or violent behavior as they move into a psychomotor agitation phase.

Psychomotor Agitation Phase

The psychomotor agitation phase is signalled by an increase in the patients physical activity, e.g., tapping his or her feet, rapidly leafing through a magazine, smoking compulsively, or pacing. Accompanying the **physical hyperactivity** is a **psychic agitation,** which is experienced by patients as anxiety, diffuse uneasiness, increased tension, or confusion. These internal states can be observed in the patients' anxious, angry, or sad facial expressions.

Subjectively experienced psychic agitation in suicidal patients is sometimes not accompanied by obvious external signs. Some patients may sit alone in an isolated area with a lowered head and avoid eye contact with other persons. They may not want to

TABLE 11–2.   Factors Contributing to Violent Behavior

Intoxication (most common)
Alcohol, cocaine, phencyclidine (PCP)
Withdrawal
Delirium tremens, methadone and opiates, barbiturates
Cognitive disorders due to general medical conditions
Traumatic brain injury
Alzheimer's disease, multi-infarct dementia, delirium, seizures, Down's syndrome
Mood disorder
Manic episode
Psychotic disorders
Paranoid schizophrenia; delusional disorder, persecutory type
Severe personality disorders (least common)
Paranoid, borderline, histrionic, antisocial

TABLE 11–3.   Acute Management of Suicidal or Violent Patients

Phase	Observed Behavior	Suggested Intervention
Psychomotor Agitated Phase (Slight Risk)	Suicidal patients: Secrecy, high anxiety, impulsive behaviors, ambivalent statements about suicide, evasiveness, oppositionalism.	Observation. Explain waiting time and evaluation process. Express empathy for the patient. Use a caring and supportive approach.
	Violent patients: Increased activity, threatening looks, mild approach-avoidance behaviors.	Offers of food, drink, or medication. Body search and restraint are rarely, if ever, required at this stage.
Verbal Phase (Increasing Risk) Early	Uses language to question authority and make demands.	Caring, supportive approach.
Late	Curses, shouts, marked increase in approach-avoidance behaviors.	Directive or counterprojective statements, slumped posture, show of force, involuntary medication, physical restraint. Violent patients: Time outs, offer of food, juice, medication. Suicidal patients: If verbal, same as above. If nonverbal, inquire about suicidal feeling, consider body search, constant observation in holding area.
Acting-Out Phase (Highest Risk)	Suicidal acts. Violent episodes.	Physical restraint. Medication: Haloperidol for psychosis; lorazepam for severe anxiety, acute alcohol withdrawal. Or alternate haloperidol with lorazepam.

talk about their feelings. Physicians should always suspect suicidal feelings in such sad, nonverbal patients and ask them directly, "Are you thinking of hurting or killing yourself?" Patients are usually reassured by such direct inquiry and may nod "yes" or begin to talk. If the physician cannot determine a patient's risk of committing suicide, the safest course of action is to place the patient under constant observation in a holding room or psychiatric hospital.

Suicidal patients with more obvious signs of agitation are likely to be on the verge of carrying out their intentions. Patients who are imminently suicidal may give the following clues: There is a sudden increase in their impulsive behavior, they make conflicting and ambivalent statements about killing themselves, they exhibit a general evasiveness; or they refuse to accept acute treatment recommendations. When patients exhibit these behaviors, the physician must consider having them placed in a safe environment where, if necessary, they can be under constant observation, searched, offered appropriate medication, or even restrained, when necessary.

Violent patients in the psychomotor agitation phase usually exhibit **approach-avoidance behavior.** They may walk up to another person and glare in a hypervigilant or paranoid manner and then walk away. Increased frequency and intensity of such "stalking" behaviors are often the cardinal signs of a person who is about to commit a violent act. ⟹ For example, one man was brought to the emergency room by police officers after he had gone on a cocaine binge, beat his wife, and wrecked their apart-

ment. For a short time, he sat fidgeting in a waiting room chair. Then, with an intent look on his face, he got up and approached the front desk. He scanned the area, stared at a staff member, and then circled around to the other side of the room and paced. The staff felt that he was preparing for an assault and intervened by offering him medication before anyone could be hurt. ⟸

Verbal Phase

Patients who progress from the psychomotor agitated phase to a verbal phase have an increased risk for imminent violence. This phase typically begins when a patient starts to question authority and becomes increasingly insistent and demanding. In this early verbal phase, a patient might ask, "How much longer do I have to wait?"; "What's taking so long?"; or "Who is in charge?" One patient, who had started cursing and glaring menacingly as he approached the nursing station, banged his hand on the counter and yelled, "Who's the head doctor? I want to be seen now!" He then walked to the back of the waiting area. His threatening behaviors were a clear warning that a violent attack was imminent.

Patients who are imminently suicidal may or may not go through a verbal phase before attempting suicide. Many are quiet, withdrawn, or secretive about their suicidal feelings. Loud, talkative patients who are openly threatening to kill themselves are likely to be intoxicated or suffering from agitated depression or a personality disorder. One such patient, suffering from borderline personality disorder, threatened to take pills if she were not seen immediately.

Acting-Out Phase

The behavior of some patients continues to escalate to the acting-out phase, in which they attempt suicide or commit violent acts. Once they have entered the **post acting-out phase,** physical restraint and psychopharmacological intervention are usually imperative.

THE INTERVIEW

When interviewing a suicidal or violent patient, the physician should follow a particular sequence in order to systematically assess the patient's risk for destructive behavior. Assessment of this risk is an essential goal for these evaluations.

Establishing A Safe Environment

Patients with acute violent or suicidal impulses are typically experiencing a turbulent emotional crisis, which leaves them fragile, volatile, and determined to take action. If they feel apprehensive or if the physician is afraid of them, the physician will not be able to conduct a psychiatric interview. In order to work toward an understanding of the patient's problem and to plan appropriate treatment, both physician and patient must feel safe and calm.

As mentioned above in Diagnostic and Clinical Features, before beginning the interview, the physician should observe the patient's appearance and behavior for a sufficient amount of time to determine the patient's status and risk for imminently dangerous behaviors. A potentially suicidal patient should be rapidly evaluated and never left alone but, rather, immediately escorted to a safe location, such as the holding area in an emergency room or the quiet room in an inpatient psychiatric service. Potentially violent patients should be evaluated to determine whether they need medication or physical restraint. Ensuring that patients will not harm themselves or others is crucial.

The physician should display an **empathic, nonconfrontational attitude** when approaching a patient who is in the psychomotor agitation phase. The patient may be calmed, for example, by the physician's saying, "How can I help?" or "You seem a bit upset." The patient may then be able to talk. When medically appropriate, a patient who is potentially violent can be directed to take a few minutes of quiet time to think things over and be offered cool liquids or medication. The offering of food or juice may help the patient calm down and prevent his or her behavior from escalating to a more dangerous phase.

The physician's supportive, caring attitude and reassurance that help will be available soon can also be used to manage patients who have progressed to the early verbal phase and have begun making insistent demands. The physician might say, "You are the next patient to be seen, and it may take half an hour. Is there something I can do to help you wait comfortably?"

For patients in the late verbal stage, supportive verbal interventions are usually not effective. Violent behavior can be prevented and control reestablished by the physician's use of **directives.** For example, at the height of a patient's agitation, the physician may use short, firm, nonthreatening commands such as, "Stop cursing! I can't help you like this!" or "Calm down! Sit down! And tell me what is bothering you."

In other circumstances, **counterprojective statements** made by the physician can prevent violence by turning the focus of the patient's intense affect (usually anger) away from the physician and directing it to someone or something "out there." Such statements, which should reflect the patient's feelings about the problematic situation, call attention to other people who are not present but who may have caused the patient's anger. ➡ In one instance, an intoxicated woman was handcuffed by police officers and brought to the emergency room after she assaulted her sister, who was having an affair with her husband. When the physician walked into the holding room, she screamed, "You are killing me, you f—ing idiot! Get me out of these damn cuffs, now!" A counterprojective reply might be, "You're p—ed off at the police who cuffed you, your sister who hurt you, and your husband who betrayed you. You're feeling enraged, caged, and helpless. Let's try to figure out this mess together. If you are able to stay calm and talk with me, we will be able to remove the handcuffs." ⬅

As they talk with patients, physicians can appear less threatening by slouching their shoulders, turning their bodies to one side, and keeping their hands visible at all times. However, even these measures may not prevent a patient from becoming increasingly agitated or hostile during the interview. When it appears that patients are about to lose control, it is extremely important for the physician to stay a safe distance away from them, usually one and one-half leg lengths. This distance not only prevents patients from feeling threatened but also keeps the physician out of reach of explosive kicks or punches. Should the physician become afraid at any time, the interview should be terminated.

When a patient is on the verge of acting violently, the physician should use verbal commands to prevent the dangerous behavior. If this is unsuccessful, other staff members may need to be called upon to produce a **show of force,** administer **involuntary medication,** or **physically restrain** the patient to help establish a safe environment. ➡ A patient who reported hearing voices commanding him to hurt others did not respond to verbal interventions. A "code blue" was announced, which brought five specially trained staff members to the area. With the others standing beside her, one staff member announced, "I've brought all these staff members together to help you regain control of yourself and make sure nobody gets hurt. Would you like to take some medication by mouth, or would you prefer an injection?" This show of force enabled the man to calm down and take the drug orally, thereby avoiding an injection and physical restraint. Patients may be offered nonsedating, calming drugs such as lorazepam at any time before, during, or after the interview. ◂▥

Acute Management

With acutely suicidal and violent patients, the physician's first task is to establish a safe, calm atmosphere. To accomplish this, the patient may need physical restraints or medication.

Physical restraint should be used when the physician has little or no information about an actively violent patient. The goal of restraining is to help the patient gain control of the aggressive impulses so that no one is hurt. Every hospital has a protocol for using restraints that, ideally, is carried out by four staff members who have been specially trained to use restraints and drugs as part of a therapeutic encounter.

Once the patient has been restrained, the staff has time to gather information about the patient and decide which drug would be most effective during this acute stage. The goal is to have the patient lightly sedated but easily arousable. The drug should target the underlying disorder that is causing the patient to act in a dangerous manner. A violent attack precipitated by a psychosis, for example, should be treated with a relatively nonsedating antipsychotic drug such as haloperidol. A patient who has made a suicide attempt that was precipitated by alcohol withdrawal and depression may be acutely managed with chlordiazepoxide or lorazepam.

After a violent episode or suicide attempt, most people feel guilty about losing control, are afraid that they will be punished or suffer retaliation in the immediate future, or experience a loss of self-esteem. These patients need to be reminded that restraint or medication was used to help them regain self-control. Reassuring them that they will suffer neither punishment nor retaliation will alleviate their fears, decrease the chance of repeat episodes, and may also prevent patients from developing a grudge against staff members who were involved in restraining them.

When the patient has been calm, composed, and reasonable for 20–60 minutes, restraints should be removed. This release helps to restore the patient's dignity and self-esteem. The restraints can gradually be removed (e.g., first from the legs and then from one arm at a time). After several hours have passed, it is important to review the episode, discuss the patient's feelings of embarrassment or shame about losing control, and make specific plans to prevent future episodes.

▸ In one case, a psychotic patient who assaulted a security guard was restrained, given haloperidol, and placed under constant observation in an emergency holding room. After two hours had passed, the physician began to talk with the patient about the events that had led up to the assault. The patient said that he had heard loud voices, felt frightened, and thought the guard was going to hurt him. He added that he knew he could remain calm now that the voices were softer. The physician agreed to remove the restraints over the next hour, first from the feet and then from one hand at a time. When he had been freed from the restraints and was talking with the physician in his office, the patient became worried that the staff would be angry at him. He said he felt bad about striking the guard. The physician reassured him that the guard was not seriously hurt and suggested that the patient might later apologize. The physician added that the staff members had no interest in holding a grudge and were very interested in helping the patient deal with his voices and avoid future violence. The physician asked the patient if he would be willing to ask for help or medication, or both, the next time he heard a voice. The patient agreed to do this and was admitted to the inpatient psychiatric unit, in a nonviolent state, for further treatment. ◂▥

Beginning the Psychiatric Interview

The psychiatric interview can begin once the patient no longer feels the need to take action and is able to participate in a thoughtful discussion. Only then can the physician and patient explore the events that incited the dangerous impulses or behaviors and try to understand their significance to the patient. The physician should explain that the main purpose of the interview is to find out what drove the patient to desperation (see Interviewing Guidelines box). It is often helpful to ask, "Why are you feeling violent or having suicidal impulses *now?*"

During the interview, the physician should remember that many patients who have attempted suicide are defensive and tend to deny or minimize their intentions. Although some attempts are less life threatening than others, the physician must be careful not to collude with the patient's denial that the attempt was not serious. A 16-year-old girl's attempted suicide by ingesting six acetaminophen tablets was not pharmacologically dangerous. She later said, "I wasn't suicidal. I was just getting rid of a headache." From a clinical point of view, this suicide attempt is a warning sign that should be taken as seriously as an ingestion of 50 antidepressant pills. The denial must be confronted, and the meanings of the patient's suicidal crisis must be vigorously explored. The physician should encourage the patient to describe all of his or her feelings before, during, and after the attempt by asking questions such as "Can you describe what happened and how you were feeling the day before you took the pills? Where were you when you decided to take the pills? Who was there? How did you take the pills? One at a time? All together? With water? What were you thinking and feeling at the time? After you took the pills, what happened? Who did you tell? How did they find you? How did you get here for medical treatment? How did you feel when you didn't die? What do

Interviewing Guidelines

- Do not attempt to interview a suicidal or violent patient until a safe environment has been established.
- Interview the patient in a private setting and maintain a calm atmosphere. Respect the patient's right to confidentiality, unless it would be dangerous to the patient or other persons to do so.
- Begin the interview by focusing on the recent crisis. Ask the patient, "Why are you feeling suicidal or violent *now?*"
- Identify factors that may have immediately precipitated the suicidal or violent symptoms.
- Explore the meaning of the symptoms and the way in which they have evolved over the past six weeks. Create a timeline showing this development.
- Ask the patient to describe past suicidal or violent symptoms. Use this information to create a focal past history that may illuminate the present symptoms.
- Be aware of the common reactions of physicians to suicidal patients (e.g., having fantasies of rescuing the patient that may lead to inappropriate treatment, wishing that a difficult patient would die).
- Confront the suicidal patient's denial by asking the patient to describe the feelings and events surrounding the suicidal behaviors.
- Be aware of the common reactions of physicians to violent patients (e.g., wishing for revenge or retaliation against them, feeling strong anger or hatred, wanting to offer moral judgments regarding their actions).
- Be an ally in the patient's desire to regulate his or her anger or violent impulses. Direct the patient to calm down or take a time-out. Use counterprojective techniques and drug therapy to diffuse violent behaviors.
- If the interview with the patient is not satisfactory, interview the patient's family. Ask them for information about the patient. Assess the emotional status of the family members and their capability for assisting in treatment. If other family members are violent, interview them only when they are calm or when the patient would benefit from treatment of the entire family.
- Gradually direct the focus of the interview toward risk assessment and treatment recommendations.

you wish had happened? Why did you or do you want to die?"

If the patient is still unable to gain access to his or her feelings and make sense of the events, the physician should consider changing from an individual approach to a **crisis-systems-family model,** in which family members are invited to tell their versions of the events. This approach may be effective in breaching the blockade of the patient's denial and allowing the open expression of feelings. ➡ In the case of the 16-year-old girl described above, the patient's mother was brought in and asked, "What would you have felt if your daughter had died?" This question made the mother cry profusely, which caused the patient to cry. The patient was then able to describe the conflicts she had with her mother and the meaning of her suicidal gesture. She expressed the anger she felt toward her mother for trying to break up her relationship with a married man. The mother had threatened to call the man's wife and tell her about the affair. Stemming from her vengeful anger toward her mother and in an effort to prevent the mother's interference, the daughter took the overdose and then told her mother what she had done. ⬅

When interviewing a violent patient, the physician should express the desire to become an ally who will help the patient resolve his or her anger and develop an understanding of the violent crisis. Any intervention that prevents violence should be considered successful. Calm questioning by an unruffled, confident physician helps agitated patients to remain engaged and in control. If the patient is not able to remain calm, the physician can break off the interview at any time.

➡ An adolescent male was brought to an emergency room by police officers after he threatened a candy store operator and also threatened to kill his father. The patient said he made the threats 5 minutes after his father called him "a lousy, stupid, lazy bum who couldn't hold a job if he tried." During the evaluation by the physician, the patient got angrier and again became threatening. The physician directed him by saying, "Calm down. I am here to help you talk over your problems with violence. I'm not here to relive them with you." He added, "Take a time-out for a few minutes, get a soda from the nurse, and come back and let me help you find a way to talk to your father and tell him how you feel when he criticizes you." The patient returned with the soda in hand and felt calmer, and the evaluation proceeded. Like most violent patients, he needed to be encouraged to talk about his pain and not act it out in violence, and he needed help in expressing his rage and thinking about how he might best talk with his father. ⬅

With violent patients, as with suicidal patients, interviewing members of the patient's family may be helpful. ➡ During a later stage in the evaluation of the patient described above, the patient's father was brought in to be interviewed. He immediately began to condemn his son, who became angry and threatened violence. The physician again asked the patient to take a time-out and return when he was calmer to tell his father how he felt when his father put him down. The physician also asked the father to listen to his son without responding. An important dialog began between father and son, who both subsequently accepted a referral for crisis family treatment. ◄▥

In some cases of violence, such as spousal abuse, child abuse, or incest, physicians need to exclude family members who would threaten patients or provoke them to violence. Social agency personnel or police officers have the initial responsibility of intervening in these cases and keeping everyone involved safe and alive. In these cases, nonviolent, supportive family members can be brought in to help resolve the crisis.

Obtaining the History

It is often helpful to approach suicidal and violent patients from the perspective that they are persons "in crisis." Eric Lindemann discovered that everybody experiences a severe emotional upheaval when given enough stress. Using grief as a prototypical emotional storm, he defined **crisis** as intense emotional pain, confusion, and anxiety that temporarily interrupt daily functioning. He was the first researcher to recognize that a crisis usually lasts for six weeks. He also found that the psychological trauma caused by a crisis is closely related to the severity of the stressor, the person's reaction to the trauma, and the effect the trauma has on the person's support network of family and friends. Crisis intervention theory suggests that the following factors should be considered in developing a formulation of the crisis: precipitants or stressors leading to the event; the specific, unique meaning of the suicidal or violent symptoms; evaluation of the patient's psychological state, including predominant defense mechanisms and capacity for reality testing, distortions in object relations, and typical coping styles. (See also Treatment, below.) Current medical or psychiatric diagnoses and problems that are causing or contributing to the dangerous symptoms must be identified as well. The wheel-and-spoke diagram shown in Figure 11–1 can be useful for visualizing the categories necessary to construct a crisis formulation. Similarly, a written narrative and the wheel-and-spoke diagram help the physician identify and formulate the problems, set the priorities for resolution, and suggest treatment approaches.

Assessment of the patient's risk for dangerous behavior in the future is a crucial part of the overall evaluation of the suicidal or violent patient. Most physicians who have studied suicidal and violent behavior agree that long-term forecasting of dangerous events is not possible but that short-term forecasting can be done by weighing a number of risk factors, which include the patient's ideation, recent and past history (including substance abuse history), support system, stressors, and ability to cooperate with treatment. The physician's intuitive feelings, which

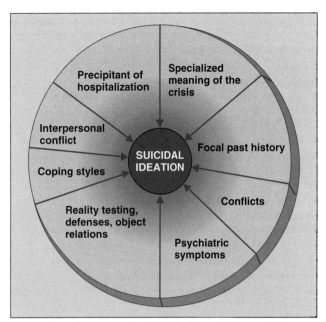

FIGURE 11–1. At the center of the wheel is the primary focus of the treatment, the suicidal or violent behavior. The spokes are the causal or contributing factors.

have developed during the clinical interview, about the patient's risk should be taken into account. Assessment scales can also be used (one is shown in Table 11–4). Another important factor in making a complete risk assessment is the patient's psychiatric diagnosis (see Differential Diagnosis, below).

Stressors

Under normal circumstances, a person has a stable internal psychological equilibrium and receives emotional and other kinds of support from a network of relatives, friends, and other persons, which permits the individual to be involved in and enjoy the normal activities of daily living. Violent or suicidal symptoms usually develop when a stressful event disturbs this equilibrium. The patient is often not aware of these stressors or may deny that they exist. They can usually be identified by asking the patient to describe, in minute detail, the interactions and events that occurred immediately preceding, during, and after the suicidal or violent behavior. These questions may also help a patient to become calmer and willing to enter into a discussion with the physician.

Stressors can be psychological events, such as a disturbing dream, hallucination, surge of anger, sudden feeling of hopelessness, or feeling of disappointment over the loss of love. Interpersonal conflicts, such as a fight with a spouse, may play a role. Developmental changes, such as the challenges of adolescence, the loss of grown children who are leaving home for the first time, or retirement, may be stressors. External life events, such as the loss of a job, may also precipitate a suicidal or violent episode.

TABLE 11–4. Violence and Suicide Assessment Scale

Current violent thoughts (during interview)
4 Expresses intense wish to kill a particular person.
3 Reveals command hallucinations to injure someone.
2 Expresses ambivalent wish to kill a particular person.
1 Expresses nonspecific feelings of rage and belligerence.
0 Reveals no homicidal ideas.

Recent violent behaviors (during the past several weeks)
4 Made serious assault on another person (e.g., attempt to strangle, stab, or shoot the person).
3 Beat another person badly (e.g., broke bones or caused injury requiring hospitalization).
2 Slapped, pushed, or punched someone but did not cause serious injury.
1 Broke objects in the house or elsewhere.
0 Showed good control over his or her behavior.

Past history of violent, antisocial, or disruptive behaviors (lifetime history)
4 Has committed violent acts in the past (e.g., beat other persons).
4 Has been arrested for assaultive behavior.
3 Carries weapons (e.g., knife, gun, chain, razor).
3 Has access to weapons.
2 Has been arrested for automobile infractions.
2 Has a criminal record.
2 Has chronic problems with authority (e.g., truancy, running away from home, family fights).
2 Has history of impulsive or unpredictable behavior (e.g., loses temper easily, overeats, is sexually promiscuous).
2 Has childhood history of frequent changes in living situation.
0 Has no past history of violence.

Current suicidal thoughts (during interview)
4 Expresses intense wish to kill self and has made a plan to do so.
4 Reveals psychotic or delusional ideation or hallucinations involving killing or injuring self.
3 Expresses intense wish to kill self but has made no plan to do so.
2 Expresses ambivalent wish to kill self.
0 Reveals no suicidal ideas.

Recent suicidal behaviors (during the past several weeks)
4 Made a serious attempt to kill self (e.g., by gunshot, ingestion of poison, hanging, or jumping from a dangerous height).
3 Made a suicidal gesture (e.g., cut wrist superficially or ingested two pills).
3 Made a specific plan to kill self.

3 Made a suicide attempt with little chance of discovery by other persons.
2 Had no interest in or hope for the future.
0 Had made no suicidal plans or attempts.

Past history of suicidal behaviors (lifetime history)
4 Mother, father, or sibling has committed suicide or made a suicide attempt.
3 Has or had a diagnosis of major affective disorder or psychosis.
3 Has made one or more previous suicide attempts.
2 Current attempt is a reaction to a meaningful "anniversary." such as the death of a loved one.
2 Has a serious medical illness or disability.
0 Has no past history of suicidal ideas or attempts.

Support systems and stresses
3 Has no family, friends, social agency, or psychiatrist available.
2 Has tenuous connection with family, friends, social agency, or psychiatrist.
2 Has had many recent life stresses (e.g., job, family, children, health).
1 Has family that is marginally willing or able to help.
0 Has family strongly committed to and capable of helping.

Ability to cooperate
3 Refuses to cooperate with interview and treatment plan.
2 Is unable to cooperate with interview and treatment plan.
1 Wants help but has weak motivation.
0 Actively seeks treatment and is willing and able to cooperate.

Substance abuse
3 Is currently intoxicated.
3 Is currently in withdrawal.
3 Is a compulsive, long-term abuser of drugs or alcohol.
2 Is an occasional abuser of drugs or alcohol.
0 Does not abuse drugs or alcohol.

Reactions during interview
4 Shows assaultive behavior toward a person or object in the environment.
3 Challenges authority (e.g., curses, yells, screams).
2 Shows approach-avoidance behavior toward interviewer.
1 Shows motoric activity (e.g., pacing, smoking, fidgeting).
1 Seems very impatient.
0 Is calm, remains seated, is responsive to questions.

Scoring
If the score is higher than 11, consider admission to hospital or extensive outpatient plan. If the score is less than 11, consider outpatient treatment.

Reproduced, with permission, from Feinstein, R. E., Plutchik, R. Violence and suicide risk assessment. Comprehensive Psychiatry 31(4):337–343, 1990.

Using a timeline or focal past history often helps identify the stressors and their significance to the patient.

Timeline

A timeline begins with the patient's most recent suicidal or violent crisis and goes back, in reverse chronological order, through the six weeks immediately preceding the event. (The usual psychiatric history goes from past to present.) Focusing on recent stresses helps the patient and the physician address the acute life-threatening problem before going on to explore long-standing difficulties. The timeline is based on crisis theory, which suggests that an acute crisis rarely lasts for more than six weeks. After that amount of time has passed, a person will cope with the situation in some way.

Focal Past History

A history is a record of seminal events from the past that have influenced the patient's recent symptoms and behaviors. It is not a comprehensive, open-ended exploration of the patient's life. The focal past history usually centers on previous suicidal or violent events (including the timing and specific circumstances of suicide attempts or hospitalizations), suicide or violence in the patient's family, significant anniversaries related to the current symptoms, drug use, losses experienced, prior depressions, and serious chronic medical illnesses.

➡ A focal past history was valuable in treating a 15-year-old patient who made a suicide attempt shortly after she became pregnant. This history revealed that her mother had also made a suicide attempt when she was 15 years old and pregnant with the patient. ◀▥ Working with the patient to develop focal connections from past events to current symptoms can be a powerful tool in understanding the meaning of the symptoms and developing treatment.

The physician must try to understand the dynamic personal meaning underlying the patient's suicidal or violent symptoms. An event may affect different individuals in different ways, depending on their interpretation and the significance they attribute to the event.

▥▶ A 34-year-old man had suffered his first psychotic break at age 24 years, while he was a second-year medical student. After this event, the patient became chronically psychotic and was hospitalized several times but had never made a suicide attempt. His last period of inpatient treatment occurred when he suffered an exacerbation of his psychotic symptoms after losing his job and stopping medication. Admitted to a teaching hospital, he was interviewed by third-year medical students who were doing their psychiatric clerkships. He seemed to enjoy these conversations and even sought out the medical students, spending time talking to them. His thinking became logical, he expressed no suicidal ideas, and he began to write and draw in a personal diary. In preparation for discharge, he was allowed to leave the hospital on a day pass to visit his mother. On that day, he leapt to his death from the roof of his 20-story apartment building. The drawings in his diary from the last two weeks of his life revealed a change in mood. The sketches made during the first week were animated drawings in color filled with people and smiling faces. The sketches made during the final week were few in number, were drawn in black chalk, and depicted gloomy, robotic, violent people. The genderless figures were depicted as crying "hopeless," "death," and "lonely." The patient's contact with the medical students during this period of treatment was the first such contact he had had since he had dropped out of medical school 10 years earlier. They may have been a painful reminder of his failed hopes to become a physician and made him acutely aware of the loss of his talents because of schizoaffective illness. ◀▥ Figure 11–2 shows the wheel-and-spoke diagram of this case.

Even mild stress may induce dangerous symptoms if it has effects that are significant to a person. ▥▶ A 30-year-old mentally retarded man with no history of violence had a rigid daily routine of eating a certain favorite hot cereal for breakfast. He had not changed this routine even once in 10 years. He had invested this cereal with the special meaning that it gave him his prized physical strength. During a winter snowstorm, his mother was unable to obtain his cereal. This seemingly trivial stressor had special significance for him. He felt that his mother was robbing him of his strength-giving food, and he experienced this loss as a catastrophe. He had an angry, violent outburst during which he wrecked the house and assaulted his mother. To prevent future violence, he needed help in understanding that the cereal had no special power to give him physical strength. ◀▥

Sometimes, events that appear to be positive can contribute to the development of suicidal or violent thoughts. ▥▶ For example, a 34-year-old woman became depressed and suicidal after she gave birth to her first son and moved to a new home. In a therapy session, she said that she had named her son after her father, who had killed himself when she was 4 years old. She suddenly realized, during the session, that it was the thirtieth anniversary of her father's suicide and that she had unconsciously chosen a home overlooking a cemetery because she was looking for her father. ◀▥

Suicidal or Violent Ideation

Self-destructive or violent ideation (i.e., thoughts) range from those involving the deliberate planning of a destructive act (these are the most dangerous) to those that are ambivalent and fleeting, to those that involve fantasies but with no intention of action (least dangerous).

An intense wish to kill oneself as a specific solution to a specific problem suggests a high risk of suicide. In one case, a man wanted to kill himself because he was deeply in debt and hoped that his family could benefit from his life insurance. Because he was dealing with a specific problem and had made a definite plan, he would be extremely likely to complete the suicide. Psychotic patients who are suicidal in response to command auditory hallucinations or delusions are probably also at high risk. Patients who have not made a plan and are ambivalent about hurting themselves have a lesser risk. For example, a person who takes an overdose of six acetaminophen pills and immediately tells a family member about it is probably ambivalent about committing suicide. When a patient has no suicidal thoughts or fantasies, the risk of suicide is quite low.

Violent persons are most likely to commit a dangerous act in the near future if they have an intense desire to kill a specific person (e.g., a drug dealer who wants revenge against another drug dealer). Patients suffering from command auditory hallucinations or delusions involving killing or hurting someone and patients whose impulsive thoughts involve violence are also at high risk (e.g., a patient who has command hallucinations that "Jesus wants me to kill" and a history of impulsivity). Patients with a nonspecific wish to hurt or kill someone are at lower risk (e.g., a patient who wants to kill all homosexuals or AIDS patients). Ambivalent wishes to hurt someone or something or nonspecific feelings of hostility may be associated with a lesser risk (e.g., an intoxicated patient who is angry at the world and wrecks the house). Patients who have no thoughts of violence or homicide have the least risk.

Recent Dangerous Behaviors

When patients' thoughts about suicide or violence are translated into action, the risk for loss of life increases. Recent events are those that have oc-

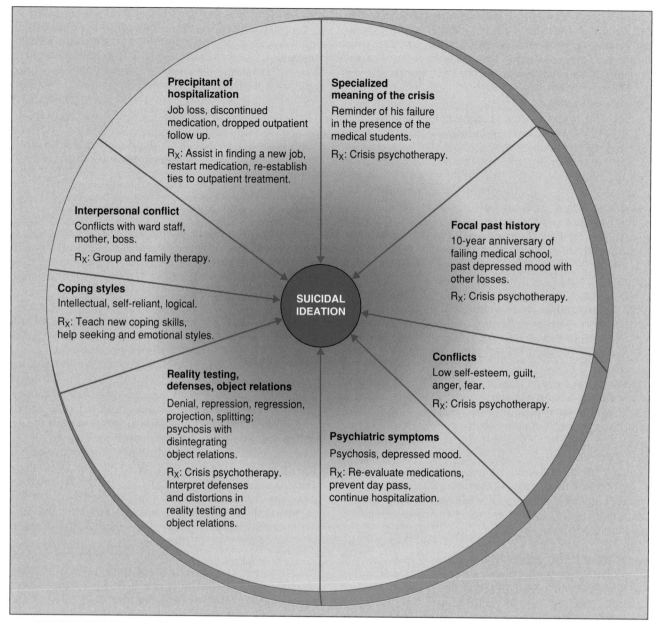

FIGURE 11–2. This wheel-and-spoke diagram represents the formulation of the hospitalized patient who committed suicide.

curred during the past few weeks that may predispose patients to commit a suicidal or violent act.

Suicidal behaviors, from those with the highest to the lowest risk, are a serious attempt by lethal means (e.g., using a gun, ingesting poison, hanging by the neck, or jumping from a dangerous height) or a specific plan to commit suicide; an attempt made with little chance of discovery; a suicidal gesture (e.g., superficially cutting the wrists or ingesting a few pills when there is a great likelihood of being discovered); leaving suicide notes or nonverbal messages such as writing a will, giving away prized possessions, or purchasing a handgun; and a change in attitudes toward life and death (e.g., a sudden change in religious practices or beliefs). From a clinical point of view, such behaviors should be taken seriously as an increased risk for suicide.

Violent behaviors may occur impulsively or be the result of a deliberate plan. A specific **external trigger** or **internal precipitant** typically exists. A child's crying is a common external trigger for child abuse, and an angry thought or fantasy may be an internal precipitant for a violent act. The assessment of recent violent acts involves uncovering the specific pattern or sequence of events that culminated in the act. ⇒ In one case, a middle-aged man was continually suspicious that his wife was having an affair. He saw her talking to a neighbor, and this event triggered dangerous behavior. He accused his wife of inviting the neighbor into the house. When she denied having done so, he hit her and said, "Does it give you that much pleasure to humiliate me?" As soon as this sequence of events was known, the physician could immediately suggest that in order to avoid violence in the future, the patient would have to develop an understanding of his paranoia, pathological jealousy, and fear of humiliation and that therapy for the man and his wife would be appropriate. ◄

The nature of recent violent behavior may also indicate the risk of more violent behavior during the next several weeks. Patients who have committed recent impulsive or planned assaults with weapons have the highest risk for imminent violence. Patients who are impulsive or have planned a physical assault without weapons that has caused serious physical injuries to the victim may also be highly likely to commit violence in the near future. Recent impulsive, less physically damaging assaults such as slapping, pushing, or hitting probably indicate a moderate risk for future violence. Patients who have damaged property but not people are less likely to commit violence against others. Those who are verbally abusive but not physically abusive may have less risk for future physical violence, since they have not crossed the boundary between words and acts. There is little risk of imminent violence in patients who are not impulsive and can carry on normal social interactions.

Past History of Suicide Attempts or Violence

Patients' past histories may be the single best predictor of dangerous acts in the near future, although it is not a basis for predicting when these acts will occur. The nature and context of prior suicide attempts may help in assessing the short-term risk for suicide and in planning for acute suicide prevention. The physician should take into account the factors that precipitated the attempts, the lethality of the means used, and the motives for, frequency of, and timing of the attempts. ➡ A 25-year-old woman felt suicidal and was thinking of taking an overdose after her boyfriend said he needed "more space to see others." The focal past history obtained during the acute evaluation revealed that she had made two suicide attempts by taking pills after breaking up with previous boyfriends. Her mother had committed suicide 10 years earlier, when her father had left her for another woman. ◄

A detailed history of the **lifetime pattern** of violence is essential for understanding the patient's potential for imminent assault. The precipitating factors, intensity, frequency, nature, and context of the violent acts deserve special inquiry. ➡ For example, a 40-year-old man regularly became violent after his wife left on business trips. Feeling lonely, he would go to the local bar, become intoxicated, and accuse a man in the bar of having an affair with his wife. This inevitably led to a brawl. In order to avoid future violence, the patient would need help in dealing with separation, so that he could avoid alcohol and bars when his wife was away, and both partners would need crisis treatment to discuss and resolve the husband's jealousy. ◄

Patients who have learned to use violence as a method of coping usually continue to use violence to solve problems in the future. One man cursed at, threatened, and beat his wife whenever she did not respond quickly to satisfy his wishes. He created an atmosphere of terror and domination in his home.

A past history predictive of violence includes an arrest record for criminal offenses, a history of driving infractions, or frequent involvement in lawsuits. Other risk factors include a childhood history of abuse, disruptive changes in caretakers, family violence, or cruelty to animals; an adolescent history of problems with authority (e.g., truancy, running away, temper tantrums); and sexual promiscuity.

Support System

A support system is the social network on which the patient can rely. It may consist of members of the patient's immediate family, other relatives, friends, members of a religious group or community organization, health care personnel, and social welfare personnel. A large, stable, and helpful support system usually serves as a buffer against the stresses that cause suicidal or violent symptoms. Some support systems are so strong that no member ever becomes suicidal or violent (e.g., closely knit families, some religious communities). Patients who do not have a network of family or friends are at higher risk for suicidal or violent symptoms and may need to rely on the social welfare system for support. The physician must evaluate the effectiveness of the support system. In order to be helpful, it must be competent, interested in the patient, and accessible to the patient.

A competent support system includes persons with appropriate skills who can directly assist the patient in resolving stressful problems, such as emotional, psychological, intellectual, legal, or financial difficulties. An interested support system has a personal investment in the patient's welfare. Family members may lose interest in helping the patient because they have exhausted their abilities to help or because they feel angry at the patient. An accessible support system is located geographically near the patient and has the time and energy to help. Family members may have to be available on a continuous basis to provide support.

A healthy support system can be of great help to the patient. ➡ In one case, a police officer took an overdose of pills after his wife had had an affair. His father, grandfather, and three brothers, all of whom were or had been police officers, were highly motivated to form a strong support network on his behalf. They eagerly agreed to organize a nonstop suicide watch while the patient attended two weeks of intensive outpatient crisis treatment. ◄

A disinterested support system may develop when family members become exhausted from dealing with the patient's problems or are angry at the patient. Once they have been reassured that the physician understands their feelings and will not ask them for help that they cannot give, these ambivalent family members can often be engaged in treatment and may be willing to provide information about the current crisis or past events. Some may even be able to renew their efforts on the patient's behalf.

In some cases, the patient has an underutilized support system because he or she is reluctant to ask for its help. The physician should discuss the patient's fears in this regard and then encourage the patient to approach family members or friends who are likely to provide whole-hearted support. The physician may also ask for help on the patient's behalf.

For a patient with no support system, outpatient crisis treatment is still possible if social agencies can provide the support. If no community support is available, as with a homeless suicidal patient, it may be necessary to hospitalize the patient even if he or she is at low risk for further suicidal or violent thoughts or behaviors.

Some members of the support system may be able to facilitate psychiatric, family, or substance abuse treatment or help the patient negotiate the social welfare system. Community organizations or religious groups may support the patient by providing a sense of belonging.

The physician or the patient should contact members of the potential support system. Members who have no interest in the patient or who may be harmful to the patient should not be enlisted to assist in treatment. Unfortunately, not all systems are truly helpful, and it is important for the physician to carefully weigh the amount of support that the system can offer the patient. If the support system is not competent, interested in, or accessible to the patient, he or she is at increased risk for recurring suicidal or violent symptoms.

At one extreme is the **toxic support system,** whose members may covertly want the patient to commit suicide or violence. ➡ A 32-year-old single woman made a serious suicide attempt and began to discuss it with her mother and her physician. Her mother said, "You can't do anything right. You can't even kill yourself!" The mother's extreme anger was toxic to the patient and could cause her to kill herself. The patient had to be hospitalized because she was at high risk for suicide, and her mother had to be excluded from participating in the initial treatment. ⬅

In some cases, a dysfunctional network that is contributing to the patient's problems must be engaged in treatment in order for the treatment to be effective. ➡ An 18-year-old man had brutally assaulted a friend for the second time when the police brought him in for a psychiatric evaluation. He revealed that his father called him a "sissy" and humiliated and beat him. During the family interview, the father said, "You have rights. Don't ever let your friends push you around. You should have killed that bastard. Sometimes, I don't know why I talk to you any more. I told you, there is no room in my house for sissies." His father was inciting the son to violence and preventing the treatment from being effective. After the father was drawn into a discussion of why he was so angry, needed to fight, and needed to provoke the patient to fight, the father revealed his own father's brutality and began to cry. The patient also began to cry

and expressed regret for the latest assault on his friend. This session permitted father and son to share their pain and discuss alternatives to violence. They accepted a family referral for ongoing violence prevention treatment. ⬅

➡ In the case of the adolescent woman and her mother described above, the mother expressed fear and anger that her daughter would get pregnant and drop out of school. She worried that the married boyfriend would abandon her daughter. When the patient was reminded that she had been born out of wedlock, she was more able to appreciate her mother's criticism. She agreed to get contraceptive counseling if the mother would stop trying to speak to the boyfriend's wife. Both agreed to accept further crisis counseling to resolve more fully the problems in their relationship. ⬅

Motivation for Treatment

The physician must determine whether the patient is capable of following through with treatment. Some high-risk suicidal or violent patients are incapable of engaging in therapy because the severity of their symptoms impairs their ability to think, plan ahead, and take action to help themselves. Other patients may lack the motivation to follow through. The physician should observe the patient's thoughts, feelings, and actions to assess his or her motivation for change.

During treatment planning, a patient may agree willingly to take a medication or participate in outpatient treatment, but when the time comes to take the first pill or make the first appointment, he or she may be hesitant, ambivalent, or reveal in other ways a lack of motivation for treatment. If the patient is engaged in treatment in an outpatient setting, the physician can increase the level of supervision. The physician can also explore potential reasons for the patient's reluctance, which include fears of what is involved in treatment, dread of the stigma associated with psychiatric treatment, or worry about the cost of treatment.

If all attempts to encourage or help the patient are unsuccessful, conservative management with more frequent consultations, acute voluntary hospitalization, or involuntary commitment to a psychiatric hospital should be made available.

Physician Reactions

While working with a suicidal or violent patient, the physician may have a strong reaction to the patient. The physician should be aware of these feelings so they do not interfere with the treatment process.

During the interview with a violent or suicidal patient, the physician may also develop intuitive feelings about the patient's risk for dangerous behavior. These feelings may be difficult to verbalize but are important nonetheless. For instance, the physician may notice that the patient is becoming more active physically, with increased feelings of frustration or impatience, challenging the physician's authority more frequently, or exhibiting increased approach-avoidance behaviors. These changes usually mean that further evaluation is necessary before the patient can be safely discharged.

The physician's reactions to a suicidal patient include feelings of helplessness and hopelessness, excessive worry that the patient might die, and fear that his or her medical career might be ruined if the patient commits suicide. Physicians often feel **angry** at manipulative patients and find themselves wishing that these patients *would* actually die and stop "torturing" everyone.

Some physicians imagine that they can keep suicidal patients alive through heroic measures. Such rescue fantasies have led to misguided decisions to hospitalize a patient for a long period or have a patient undergo unnecessary electroshock treatments. When patients do make suicide attempts or succeed in committing suicide, physicians may feel **guilty** and responsible. Physicians need to avoid the trap of ignoring or minimizing their patients' recurrent symptoms. They must also avoid giving the symptoms undue attention, which may prevent patients from discussing the reasons for and meanings of their symptoms.

Physicians who deal with violent individuals often feel intimidated, bullied, threatened, and afraid. If the physician feels used, exploited, or deceived, he or she may adopt a **punitive attitude.** Sometimes a physician is provoked to express such a degree of anger or hatred that a patient will develop revenge fantasies. When a patient gets to the point at which he or she can express remorse for violent acts, the physician should neither be overly sympathetic to the patient nor gleeful about the patient's suffering.

Some violent patients discuss their symptoms so rationally and with such perception that the physician may feel moved to protect them from the criminal justice system. Others seem so despicable that the physician may unconsciously retaliate against them by secluding them, keeping them waiting, or giving them intramuscular medication when oral medication could have been prescribed.

DIFFERENTIAL DIAGNOSIS

Suicidal symptoms are almost invariably associated with psychiatric disorders. Depression combined with a feeling of hopelessness is a major risk factor for completed suicide. Suicide is less likely to be attempted when the patient is in the depth of the depression and is more likely to be attempted when the patient appears to be recovering. **Major depression** in conjunction with **anxiety symptoms** or **panic disorder** may also dramatically increase the likelihood of suicidal behaviors. Patients with a **major depressive episode with psychotic features** are at particularly high risk for suicide, even if they deny suicidal ideation. From 10–25% of patients with significant suicidal risk are suffering from **alcohol abuse, intoxication, or withdrawal;** another 10–20% are **schizophrenic.** In the latter group, suicide, if it occurs, most often happens before the age of 40. By this age, many patients feel discouraged that their illness has no cure. Less common diagnoses associated with suicide risk include borderline, histrionic, or antisocial personality disorders. Patients who have more than one disorder associated with suicide, such as a severe personality disorder and substance abuse, have the highest risk for dangerous behaviors.

The potential for violence is greatest when the patient is **intoxicated** or in **withdrawal from alcohol or other drugs.** Disorders causing brain damage are commonly associated with violence; therefore, **neuropsychiatric conditions** must be carefully considered (see Medical Evaluation, below, and Chapter 5, Cognitive and Mental Disorders Due to General Medical Conditions). **Manic patients** often become assaultive as a result of their irritable, labile moods and impulsivity. Patients with **psychotic symptoms** (usually paranoid delusions or command auditory hallucinations, or both) have a high risk of escalating to violence. Patients with **borderline** or **antisocial personality disorders** or **posttraumatic stress disorder** are at risk for violence, as well. In the absence of these conditions, **intermittent explosive disorder** should be considered (Table 11–5).

MEDICAL EVALUATION

A thorough assessment of suicidal and violent patients should include a medical and neurological evaluation to determine whether a medical illness is causing or exacerbating their symptoms (see Chapter 5, Cognitive and Mental Disorders Due to General Medical Conditions).

There is an increased risk of suicide in patients with chronic diseases such as diabetes mellitus, renal disorders requiring dialysis, acquired immunodeficiency syndrome (AIDS), or chronic obstructive pulmonary disease. Diseases that cause depression (e.g., thyroid disease) or drugs that cause depression may also contribute to suicidal symptoms. Common medical disorders associated with violence include mental retardation, traumatic brain injury, delirium, demen-

---

TABLE 11–5.   DSM-IV Criteria for Intermittent Explosive Disorder

A. Several discrete episodes of failure to resist aggressive impulses that result in serious assaultive acts or destruction of property.

B. The degree of aggressiveness expressed during the episodes is grossly out of proportion to any precipitating psychosocial stressors.

C. The aggressive episodes are not better accounted for by another mental disorder (e.g., Antisocial Personality Disorder, Borderline Personality Disorder, a Psychotic Disorder, a Manic Episode, Conduct Disorder, or Attention-Deficit/Hyperactivity Disorder) and are not due to the direct physiological effects of a substance (e.g., a drug of abuse, a medication) or a general medical condition (e.g., head trauma, Alzheimer's disease).

tia, and seizures. Violence may also occur if a patient has a disturbed reaction to a prescribed or illicit drug.

ETIOLOGY

Suicidal and violent symptoms have many causes. They are associated with a range of psychiatric disorders and different life circumstances. A biopsychosocial approach takes into consideration the neurobiological and psychosocial factors that may contribute to these symptoms.

Neurobiological Causes

Ongoing research is being conducted into the complex neurobiological process that underlies suicidal and violent behavior. Although the precise mechanism is not yet adequately understood, the leading theory suggests that the neurotransmitter **serotonin** plays a role in modulating these impulsive behaviors.

Many studies show that persons who attempt suicide have significantly decreased amounts of the serotonin metabolite 5-hydroxyindoleacetic acid (5-HIAA) in the cerebrospinal fluid. Studies have also found an increased number of 5-hydroxytryptamine (5-HT) receptors in suicidal patients, suggesting serotonin deficiency. Patients who have committed suicide often have lower concentrations of 5-HT or 5-HIAA, or both, in the subcortical area, brain stem, or raphe nuclei. Cortical levels of these substances are unchanged. These studies were not controlled for the various methods of suicide.

Most studies suggest that lower levels of serotonin and its metabolites are also associated with violent behavior. Early studies showed that levels of 5-HIAA in the cerebrospinal fluid were lower in some violent patients than in control subjects. More recently, it has been shown that violent offenders with a personality disorder and impulsivity have lower levels of 5-HIAA than those without impulsivity. Arsonists with impulsivity had even lower levels of 5-HIAA than did other violent offenders.

The results of these studies suggest some of the biological mechanisms of aggression. Suicidal and violent persons have clear evidence of dysregulation of the serotonergic systems when they are compared with control subjects. The underlying biological factors for suicidal patients are probably somewhat different from those for violent patients. Current research suggests that the *direction* of the aggression (i.e., whether aggression is directed inward as in suicidal patients or outward as in violent patients) is more significantly mediated by environmental and psychological factors.

Psychosocial Influences
Familial Patterns

When it occurs in multiple family members, suicidal ideation or behavior may serve as a means of communication between family members, or as a sign of serious underlying family problems.

As a form of communication between family members, suicidal and violent expressions operate on many levels. The pattern may include verbal threats, nonverbal threats communicated by facial expressions or body language, or overt actions.

It is often useful to look for the **dyadic (second) person** against whom the suicide or violence is primarily directed. The dyadic person is frequently, but not always, the one who precipitated the act. ➡ In the case of an adolescent girl who tried to kill herself after breaking up with her boyfriend, it appeared on the surface that the dyadic conflict was between the patient and her boyfriend. However, there was a more serious underlying dyadic conflict between the patient and her mother. The mother disapproved of the boyfriend and was extremely angry about the relationship. When the daughter broke up with her boyfriend, she saw no alternative other than suicide. ⬅

Threats of violence or suicide are often used to gain power and control over other family members. A man may use anger, threats, or beatings to control his wife and children, establish himself as an authority figure, or coerce the family into satisfying his needs or wants. Similarly, a woman may use threats of suicide to control her husband and children.

Children learn violent and suicidal patterns of coping by modeling themselves after their parents or as a way of solving problems that seem to have no other solution. An adolescent may threaten suicide to stop his parents from divorcing. When his behavior keeps the parents talking and causes the family to seek treatment, the possibility of marital reconciliation is kept alive.

Suicidal or violent symptoms may be a sign of serious underlying family problems. ➡A woman had repeatedly attempted suicide by slashing her wrists and taking overdoses of pills. These attempts began when she was 15 years old and continued until she was 25 years old. Family therapy revealed that the attempts occurred after episodes of sexual abuse by her father. ⬅

Societal Influences

The complex relationships among various sectors of society may play a role in the development of suicidal or violent symptoms.

Cultural influences vary widely and can greatly affect attitudes toward suicide and violence. Citizens of Japan traditionally have viewed suicide as an honorable solution to a disgraceful situation, whereas members of the Roman Catholic church consider it a sinful act. Criminals consider violence to be acceptable and even normal. The media (i.e., television, motion pictures, and popular music) has become increasingly violent in content and has been accused of encouraging the likelihood of violence and suicide in its devotees. In the 1980s, for example, publicity by the news media about sexual asphyxia and suicide caused by inhaling automobile exhaust fumes may have contributed to a rash of copycat deaths.

Economic factors can affect the incidence of suicide and violence. Both behaviors are reported with greater frequency among the poorer socioeconomic classes. Rates of suicide and violence increase during times of economic prosperity and decrease during times of economic collapse.

TREATMENT

The first step in the treatment of suicidal or violent patients is to make sure they are stable and will not harm themselves or other persons. Next, the physician must decide what type of ongoing treatment is appropriate (e.g., hospitalization versus outpatient treatment). An integrated approach, for example, using a combination of crisis intervention, individual and family psychotherapy, and drug treatment, is often recommended.

Outpatient treatment of a suicidal or violent patient should be attempted only when the physician is certain that the patient wants help and has a fully available support system. The potential for an acute reemergence of suicidal or violent symptoms must be discussed with the patient. A detailed contract and plan for the prevention of future dangerous acts should be negotiated with the patient and the support network. The safest approach is to use crisis intervention combined with family monitoring of the patient. Daily outpatient sessions can be conducted with a crisis practitioner who would visit the home or summon the police should a life-threatening situation develop. Psychiatric hospitalization should be readily available if the outpatient treatment fails.

Building on Lindemann's work, Gerald Caplan formulated modern **crisis intervention treatment** in the 1960s. He demonstrated that a crisis implies both potential for danger and opportunity for growth. He confirmed the observation that most crises resolve in about six weeks, with one of four possible outcomes: improved functioning; functioning that is restored to precrisis levels; functioning that is incompletely restored, resulting in susceptibility to the development of future crises; or functioning that is severely impaired but stable. He developed a crisis treatment protocol that fosters the development of flexible, imaginative styles of coping or solving problems.

Crisis intervention may be effective in preventing suicide and violence, especially in patients who are intensely ambivalent about hurting themselves or others. During crisis treatment, the physician focuses on precipitants or stressors leading to the event; explores with the patient the specific, unique meaning of his or her suicidal or violent symptoms; develops a timeline of etiological or contributing events over the previous six weeks; uses the focal past history of violence or suicide to reach a deeper understanding of the current dangerous symptoms; and assesses and solicits help from the support network.

Hospitalization provides interventions, such as one-on-one continuous supervision, seclusion of the patient, and the use of physical restraint or medications, if necessary, which are not available in most outpatient treatment programs. The hospital is an ideal place for patients with extremely complicated psychiatric, medical, and psychosocial issues that require coordinated, integrated interventions.

For many patients, a hospital is the only setting where treatment can proceed safely. When suicidal or violent symptoms are so severe that a patient cannot be treated in any other setting or when outpatient treatment has failed, hospitalization may be necessary to protect the patient or other persons. Once a patient has been admitted, an extensive assessment is made to determine the biopsychosocial diagnosis, medical status, and quality of the occupational, family, and social support system.

Individuals who request or accept inpatient hospitalization are often easier to engage in treatment. Patients who must be involuntarily committed may also become engaged in the treatment process once they realize it is helping them. Patients who cannot or will not engage in treatment are often transferred for long-term stays in other psychiatric facilities.

Most suicidal patients who are hospitalized need continual observation for hours and sometimes days. They must be searched for pills, razor blades, and knives, and their belts and shoes must be removed. Antianxiety or antipsychotic drugs may be given to decrease agitation.

PSYCHOTHERAPY
Individual Psychotherapy

Psychotherapy can be extremely effective treatment for patients with suicidal and violent symptoms. Psychotherapeutic techniques, such as confrontation, clarification, and interpretation, as well as the formation of an empathic therapeutic alliance, can alleviate suicidal or violent symptoms and are relevant for outpatients, inpatients, patients in ongoing treatment, and even for patients being evaluated cross-sectionally (i.e., at one moment in time).

After a brief period of focusing on the patient's suicidal or homicidal symptoms, the physician should begin to respond with **empathy** to the patient's emotional pain, for example, by suggesting that the symptoms are the result of an internal conflict and an effort to find a solution to a deeper problem. The patient should be asked to join the physician in an **alliance,** through which they will work together to reach an understanding of all aspects of the conflict and find a new and better solution to the problem.

A **confrontation** is an observation by the physician that draws attention to discrepancies or contradictions in the patient's perceptions or behaviors that are interfering with his or her stated goals of treatment. The physician might say, "I know that you don't enjoy feeling suicidal, but your refusal to tell me what happened and how you are trying to kill yourself makes it likely that you will stay suicidal for some time." This technique is confrontational because it forces the patient to examine his or her contradictory behavior. A confrontational tone should not, however, be used when applying this technique.

A **clarification** is a request for the patient to supply additional information or perspective on the situation when the physician does not fully understand what the patient is trying to say or finds what is said vague and confusing. When clarification is needed, the physician might ask, "When you heard your mother say you should hurt yourself, what did you think was happening to you? Why would she want you to hurt yourself?" In addition to open-ended questioning, the physician might suggest a hypothesis as another means of clarification. To obtain a detailed understanding of suicidal and violent patients' symptoms, frequent clarification is often needed.

An **interpretation** deepens patients' understanding by integrating their suicidal or violent behavior with the information obtained from confrontation and clarification. ➡ One woman was offered the following sequence of comments: "I think you do not enjoy feeling suicidal. Yet your refusal to tell me what has happened means you may continue to be a danger to yourself for some time (confrontation). When I say this to you, it makes you angry with me, and this has resulted in your ending our last meeting abruptly (clarification). Your anger at me helps you avoid the pain of your suicidal thoughts and relives with me the battles with your mother that I believe are contributing to your current suicidal feelings (interpretation)." ⬅

Confrontation, clarification, and interpretation can be used to modify patients' pathological psychological defenses, improve their reality testing, uncover and treat pathological object relations that are driving the suicidal or homicidal impulses, and help patients develop more adaptive coping styles.

Reality Testing

Distorted perceptions of reality may be prevented by encouraging the patient to test his or her perceptions before taking actions based on them. Patients can do this by asking the therapist or another trusted person whether their perceptions of a situation are similar. A suicidal person who feels rejected or abandoned by other people can learn to ask, "Are you really rejecting me? Is there something I have done? Is there a problem between us?" or "Are you really abandoning me or is there something else you need to take care of?" Patients should also be asked not to use substances such as alcohol or drugs that may foster transient breaks in reality. These psychotherapeutic approaches can be supplemented by medication and hospitalization. For example, if a patient experiences frequent transient breaks in reality or a psychotic episode, antipsychotic drugs can be given. These drugs should always be considered for suicidal or violent symptoms when breaks in reality testing are observed.

Pathological Defenses

The physician must identify the patient's predominant psychological defenses and use therapeutic techniques to modify their pathological functioning. The psychological defense mechanisms associated with suicide are repression and regression. The defenses associated with violent behavior are projection and displacement. The defense mechanisms of acting out, denial, splitting, idealization, omnipotence, devaluation, and projective identification are associated with both suicidal and violent behavior. (These defense mechanisms are described in Chapter 2, The Psychiatric Interview.)

A physician might use the following interpretation of a violent man's tendency to project his aggression onto others: "You think others are mad at you, when, in fact, you are angry at them. Seeing others as angry with you lets you feel like the victim so you don't have to acknowledge the fact that your violence hurts others." For a patient who has attacked his boss, the physician might use this interpretation: "When you hit your boss, I know you were angry at him. However, I think you gave him the fury that was directed at your father from the argument you had last night."

Object Relations

Psychological perceptions of one's self and other people are modeled on past relationships with significant individuals. Suicidal or violent symptoms may be acutely reduced and occasionally eliminated if the physician can link them to the patient's past relationships. The following interpretation, for example, might be used for a violent husband: "You begin to beat your wife when you see her as controlling, demanding, and incapable of being satisfied and when you see yourself as helpless to change the situation. This perception of your wife is distorted and confused with an image of your mother, who was that way with you. With your wife, you are not a helpless boy but a man who has many alternatives to violence."

The basic technique is to elicit patients' perceptions of and feelings about themselves and other persons prior to, during, and after the onset of the symptoms. Patients may express intense affects, such as rage, anger, helplessness, fear of being threatened or losing control, inferiority, or worthlessness. The physician and patient can trace the path by which a precipitant caused the patient's view of self and others to shift and create the powerful suicidal or violent impulses.

➡ One woman made a suicide attempt after discovering that her boyfriend had slept with her sister. Before she learned of the affair, she had felt valued, safe, and loved by her boyfriend, whom she saw as extremely loyal, kind, and trustworthy. She also loved her sister but had felt competitive with her. After she learned of the affair, the woman's feelings toward herself and the others involved changed radically. She thought she was ugly, worthless, and unable to "hold onto" a man. She hated her boyfriend and saw him as a cruel liar and betrayer. She felt helpless and furious at the betrayal by her sister. The sister seemed to be gloating about what had happened, and this hurt the patient even more. The woman wanted to hurt her boyfriend and her sister, make them both feel guilty, and ruin their lives. At the same time, she blamed herself for what had happened. After being treated with psychotherapy, the woman was still angry but had developed a more realistic view of the situation. She believed that she had been naive and blinded by her need to be loved. She also became aware, for the first time, of an intense rivalry with her sister. She still felt hurt but not worthless, and stopped blaming herself. She still cared for her boyfriend but now saw him as impulsive, self-centered, and disloyal. Although she was still furious at her sister and her boyfriend, she no longer saw a reason to hurt herself. She realized that they had had the affair because of their own problems and conflicts and not because of her inadequacies. ◄||

Helping patients identify and understand the change in object relations prior to, during, and after a suicidal or violent event is a powerful intervention. Patients who are unable to do this psychological work with the physician may be helped to understand changes in their feelings by having a session with their significant others present.

Cognitive-Educational Interventions

Many of these principles have been incorporated into the treatment approach for suicidal and violent patients. Patients may be taught a problem-solving strategy that focuses on a selective past history (Table 11–6) and steps they can take to resolve a crisis situation (see above, Stressors).

➡ For example, a 55-year-old woman became suicidal while she was trying to sell the home she had

TABLE 11–6. Cognitive-Educational Crisis Resolution Strategy

1. Recognize the early warning signs of a crisis.
2. Talk over the problem with a crisis practitioner or a trusted friend.
3. Discuss painful feelings and emotions.
4. Identify the specific area of life that is most affected by the crisis.
5. Identify the stressors over the past 6 weeks, and develop a timeline.
6. Decide who in the support network can help or hurt.
7. Formulate the crisis.
8. Obtain information that would help in crisis resolution.
9. Make a specific plan based on new information or feelings.
10. Implement the plan for resolution of one of the causes of the crisis.
11. Assess the results.
12. If the resolution has been successful, implement a plan for the resolution of the second cause of the crisis.
13. Try again, or get help at any point.

lived in for 15 years. Her son, who had been living with her, was planning to move out and live by himself. During the month of October, the woman became suicidal. The crisis treatment uncovered significant losses during previous Octobers (i.e., the loss of her health when she became ill with emphysema and the deaths of her father, mother, and husband). This knowledge helped the woman to understand her pain, and she was able to grieve and resolve her anguish. ◄||

New Coping Strategies

Patients can also learn to recognize their normal **coping style,** understand the current malfunction, and develop new or more successful strategies (Table 11–7). ➡ For example, a middle-aged man responded to job stress by continually asking his boss for assistance. This coping style was successful for a time and even resulted in the patient's receiving several promotions. When his boss became ill, the temporary boss expected the patient to be more self-sufficient and was annoyed by his constant questions. The patient became unable to function at work, was anxious and irritable at home, picked fights with his wife, and became depressed and suicidal. His psychiatrist suggested that his suicidal helplessness was related to his excessive reliance on his boss, which was reminiscent of his dependence on his mother. The patient agreed with this interpretation. Once he understood the problems and limitations of his old coping skill, he was able to develop a new one that increased his self-reliance at work. He realized that he could probably get help from the computer information service and the library at work. Once he felt more confident, he was able to discuss his work problems with his wife instead of fighting with her ◄||

Some patients, usually those with severe personality disorders (e.g., borderline pathology) or other long-standing psychiatric disorders, threaten suicide or violence on a daily basis. In such cases, the physician must attempt to discover the problem that the patient is trying to solve and suggest a more adaptive coping style.

Family Therapy

Family therapy can be extremely effective in treating suicidal or violent symptoms because they so often arise within the context of a transaction between two family members. It is often necessary to treat the entire family because other members may have the capacity to break the pathological interaction. Family therapy for suicidal and violent patients usually combines psychoeducational, strategic, and structural approaches.

Psychoeducational family therapy focuses on risk factors, the psychiatric illness that produced the symptoms, the role of substance abuse, and suicide and violence prevention. Families can learn how to

TABLE 11-7.   Coping Styles

Typical coping styles

Intuitive style: Using the imagination, feelings, and perceptions

Logical or rational style: Using careful reasoning, logic, and deductive reasoning

Controlling style: Controlling the self, other persons, or information to gain power

Trial-and-error style: Trying a solution and modifying it if it is not successful

Help-seeking style: Asking other persons for help

Informational style: Gathering information before making a decision

Wait-and-see style: Allowing time or circumstances to determine the outcome of a problem

Action-oriented style: Taking action immediately to rectify a problem

Contemplative style: Quietly thinking over a problem before acting

Spiritual style: Leaving a problem in God's hands

Emotional style: Expressing emotions, such as tears, anger, or fear

Pathological coping styles

Manipulative style: Using a variety of styles to get one's own way without concern for other persons

Suicidal style: Using the threat of suicide to solve a problem

Violent style: Using the threat of violence or acting violently to establish control

Impulsive style: Responding unpredictably according to impulse without anticipating possible outcomes

Random or chaotic style: Unproductive, extreme form of trial-and-error style or impulsive style, often seen in prolonged psychotic states

Antisocial or dishonest style: Lying, cheating, stealing, or other antisocial behaviors

Reproduced, with permission, from Feinstein, R. E., Carey, L. Crisis intervention in office practice. *In* Textbook of Family Practice, 5th ed, Rakel, R. E., ed., Philadelphia, W. B. Saunders Co, 1995.

recognize early danger signs, when to hospitalize a patient, how to administer medication, and when and how to involve an outside agency or call the physician. Crisis intervention can sometimes be integrated with these family therapy approaches.

Strategic family therapy usually addresses pathological patterns of communication. Family members may have extreme difficulty in listening to each other, expressing their feelings, interpreting messages, and negotiating disagreements. Family members are helped to strengthen these skills in order to resolve the underlying problem that may have caused the suicidal or violent symptoms. ⟹ In therapy sessions, an adolescent was unable to tell her parents why she kept trying to kill herself. Interventions geared toward breaking the pathological style of communication in the family enabled her to reveal that an uncle had been sexually abusing her. The incest was the family problem underlying her suicidal symptoms. ⟸

Structural family therapy focuses on the organization of the family into subgroups, e.g., of parents and children, the roles of the different members, and family rules. In a well-functioning family, the parents provide the organization and jointly make rules and set goals for the children. In a dysfunctional family, one or both parents may be impaired in some way, and this may result in chaotic role definitions, incon-

sistent rules, vague goals, and the need for the children to function as surrogate parents.

Radical changes in the organization of a family (e.g., a divorced parent's remarriage) can also produce violent or suicidal symptoms in a family member. ⟹ A 24-year-old man who lived with his mother and two younger sisters threatened his mother with violence when his new stepfather moved into the house. Intervention helped the patient express his anger about the new marriage, discuss his loyalty to his father, develop a new relationship with his stepfather, and assume a different role with his mother and siblings. Once the patient realized that his stepfather could take care of his mother and siblings, he felt free to develop a relationship with a girlfriend and prepare to move out of the house. ⟸

PSYCHOPHARMACOLOGICAL TREATMENT

The long-term pharmacological treatment of suicidal and violent symptoms is not yet specific. Recent interest has focused on medications such as the selective serotonin reuptake inhibitors (SSRIs) and buspirone, which may increase the serotonin levels in the cerebrospinal fluid. Disorders, such as mood disorders and personality disorders, that may be producing or aggravating suicidal or violent symptoms can also be treated. For example, suicidal patients who are depressed are usually given an antidepressant, and violent patients who have a seizure disorder may be given an anticonvulsant such as carbamazepine or valproic acid.

Antidepressants

Because suicidal symptoms are commonly associated with a depressed mood, an antidepressant drug is most often prescribed. The newer antidepressants, which are often used as first-line treatments, include the selective serotonin reuptake inhibitors (SSRIs), such as fluoxetine, sertraline, and paroxetine. Some case reports had suggested that certain SSRIs may elicit suicidal symptoms, but ongoing research has not substantiated this observation.

The clinical efficacy of conventional tricyclic antidepressants such as imipramine or desipramine is well established. The tricyclic drugs are also thought to be effective for suicidal symptoms that are not related to depression, although this has not been proved. Monoamine oxidase inhibitors are also effective in treating associated depression or panic disorder.

Because SSRIs regulate the serotonergic system, they have also been used to treat violent symptoms. Case reports have suggested efficacy, but definitive studies have not been completed.

Antipsychotics

When suicidal or violent behaviors emerge as part of a psychosis, antipsychotic agents are commonly used to resolve command auditory hallucinations, delusions, or a thought disorder. The same drugs, in lower dosages, may be given to patients with severe personality disorders in whom violent or suicidal symptoms are associated with transient breaks in reality. Patients must be monitored for therapeutic response and side effects.

Mood Stabilizers and Anticonvulsants

Lithium and anticonvulsants (e.g., carbamazepine, valproic acid) relieve suicidal or violent symptoms in several ways. They are used in the primary treatment of mood disorders, such as manic excitement or irritability, and also as a means of decreasing the impulsivity associated with personality disorders and impulse control disorders. They are also used as a secondary treatment for suicidal or violent symptoms. Patients must be monitored regularly for therapeutic blood levels, efficacy, and side effects.

In addition, anticonvulsants can be extremely effective against aggression that is related to partial complex seizures. These drugs may also be helpful in violent patients with traumatic brain injury, dementia, intermittent explosive disorder, or nonspecific abnormalities on electroencephalography. Carbamazepine is most commonly used, but valproic acid may also be given.

Anxiolytics

The **benzodiazepines** have limited use in treating suicidal symptoms. They are usually contraindicated as primary drug therapy in depressed suicidal patients because they may cause a depressed mood to worsen or may induce disinhibition, which may exacerbate impulsive behaviors. Benzodiazepines such as lorazepam are sometimes given in combination with antidepressant medication. Recent reports suggest that patients who have a primary panic disorder are more likely to attempt suicide. Treatment of the panic disorder with a benzodiazepine and an antidepressant may decrease the potential for suicide (see Chapter 6, Anxiety Disorders). The benzodiazepines usually have no place in the long-term primary management of violence, because they may exacerbate impulsivity.

Buspirone is a distinctive antianxiety agent that has been reported to increase serotonin levels, although this has not been proved. Some psychopharmacologists have reported an initial increase in violent symptoms followed by a decrease.

Propranolol

Propranolol is a beta-blocker that is probably helpful in the management of aggression associated with traumatic brain injury, Alzheimer's disease, and multi-infarct dementia. It may also be helpful in nonpsychotic intermittent explosive disorders. At higher than standard doses, propranolol begins to take effect in 4–6 weeks, although the full benefits may not be felt for months.

TREATMENT OF CHRONIC SUICIDALITY AND VIOLENCE

Some patients develop a lifelong daily pattern of violence or suicidality (e.g., the man who constantly abuses his wife and threatens his family, the psychotic individual who does not respond to medication, or the woman with a severe personality disorder who controls others by repeatedly threatening to hurt herself). The treatment of such patients is geared toward the underlying severe personality disorder or refractory psychosis. If treatment is possible at all, it is usually long term and multimodal. Individual psychotherapy, cognitive-behavior therapy, family therapy, or psychopharmacological treatment may be used in inpatient hospital settings or outpatient psychiatric settings, or in some combination of the two. Treatment sometimes lasts for several years when patients are in an institution such as a long-term psychiatric facility, group home, halfway house, or prison.

LEGAL ISSUES

The most difficult legal and clinical considerations for the physician who treats suicidal or violent patients are decisions regarding commitment or involuntary hospitalization, patients' right to confidentiality, and the duty to warn other people who may be harmed by the patients. State laws regarding these issues vary somewhat, but the basic concepts underlying them are similar.

Commitment or Involuntary Hospitalization

Patients can be involuntarily hospitalized if a physician or a court of law determines that they have a mental disorder and are dangerous to themselves or other persons. In practical terms, this means that a patient can be "committed" if the patient has a psychiatric disorder and has attempted or threatened suicide or violence. Many states have broadened the definition of *dangerous* to include "individuals whose mental illness has so impaired their judgment that they cannot recognize the need for psychiatric treatment." This law usually applies to chronically psychotic patients with illnesses such as schizophrenia or bipolar disorder who may be unable to perform even the basic functions of life, such as feeding themselves, getting medical treatment, or finding a warm place to stay when it is cold outside.

In most states, any physician can involuntarily detain a patient in an emergency room or admit a patient to a psychiatric facility. If it is medically necessary to save the life of the patient or another person, the patient can be held against his or her will for several weeks. This is not a punitive measure but rather an effort to provide essential emergency psychiatric treatment. A patient who has been committed usually protests at first but, in time, usually comes to appreciate the psychiatric treatment.

A patient who has been committed retains all of his or her civil rights, including the right to manage daily affairs (e.g., make decisions regarding finances or health care, vote in government elections). The patient has the right to retain a lawyer experienced in mental health issues at no charge and may request a court hearing if he or she disagrees with the need for commitment. A patient can be retained in a hospital for several weeks until a court hearing is held regarding the patient's situation. The hearing is usually scheduled as soon as possible. The judge must decide whether to release the patient or continue the commitment.

After several days of involuntary acute hospital treatment, most patients no longer pose an immediate danger and may be released. This may create a conflict for the physician, who may be required to discharge a patient before treatment has been completed.

The Patient's Right to Confidentiality

Generally speaking, the physician is required to maintain the confidence of all communications with the patient concerning psychiatric records and treatment. Significant exceptions to this rule exist, however, for a suicidal or violent patient.

In some cases, a patient may not want to reveal suicidal or violent feelings or intentions until he or she has asked the physician whether the conversations will be kept completely confidential. This question should alert the physician to the probable suicidal or violent intent of the patient, who is trying to use legal maneuvering to extract a promise that the physician will not reveal his or her intentions to family members or friends. A wise physician might respond, "Our communications are usually confidential, unless there is a danger to you or someone else. Under those circumstances, I cannot keep your intentions a secret." This response is reassuring to most patients, and it frees the physician to take whatever steps are necessary to prevent the loss of life, including disclosure of the patient's intentions to anyone who might need to know. In most states, the law recognizes that protecting the lives of the patient or other people takes precedence over confidentiality.

The Duty to Warn Persons Who May Be Harmed by the Patient

Physicians are usually exempt from confidentiality requirements when they become aware that a patient is likely to commit violence or homicide. State laws vary widely, but the **Tarasoff** decision has become a national standard for clinical practice (*Tarasoff v. Regents of University of California*, 17 Cal.3d 425,

131 Cal. Rptr. 14, 551 P2d 334 [1974]). Tatania Tarasoff was murdered by a former lover, who had confided his intention to a University of California therapist. The court found the university and the therapist guilty of a failure to warn Tarasoff or her family that her life was in danger. This case was the precedent for the therapist's duty to warn a potential victim of life-threatening danger from a homicidal patient.

A 1976 ruling broadened the options. According to this decision, a physician may warn potential victims but is not required to do so if he or she "uses reasonable care to protect the intended victim against danger." **Reasonable care** means that a physician must try to prevent the violence by taking action such as hospitalizing a violent patient or prescribing outpatient hospital treatment, crisis intervention, or other intensive outpatient treatments. The physician can warn all intended victims and suggest that the victims obtain an order of protection. A homicidal patient can be committed or involuntarily hospitalized or treated vigorously in a day hospital with psychotherapy or drug therapy, or both. These interventions should be specifically designed to decrease the potential for violence. According to the law, "Protective privilege ends where the public peril begins."

References Cited

Caplan, G. Loss, stress, and mental health. Community Mental Health Journal 26: 27–48, 1990.

Feinstein, R. E., L. Carey. Crisis intervention in office practice. *In* Textbook of Family Practice, 5th ed, Rakel, R. E., ed. Philadelphia, W. B. Saunders Co., 1995.

Feinstein, R. E., R. Plutchik. Violence and suicide risk assessment. Comprehensive Psychiatry 31(4): 337–343, 1990.

Selected Readings

Feinstein, R. E., Vanderberg, S. Personality disorders in office practice. *In* Textbook of Family Practice, 5th ed, Rakel, R. E., ed. Philadelphia, W. B. Saunders Co., 1995.

Havens, L. L. Recognition of suicidal risks through the psychologic examination. New England Journal of Medicine 276: 210–215, 1967.

Jacobs, D. Evaluation and management of the violent patient in emergency settings. *In* Emergency Psychiatry. Soreff, S. M., ed. Psychiatric Clinics of North America 6(2): 261–269, 1993.

Lindemann, E. Symptomatology and management of acute grief. American Journal of Psychiatry 47: 14–25, 1944.

Plutchik, E. H. M. Pragg, H. R. Conte. Correlates of suicide and violence risk III: A two stage model of countervailing forces. Psychiatry Research 22:215–255, 1989.

Pragg, H.M., H. R. Plutchik, A. Apter. Violence and Suicidality: Perspectives in Clinical and Psychobiological Research. New York, Brunner and Mazels, 1990.

Roy, A. Suicide. *In* Comprehensive Textbook of Psychiatry. 5th ed., Vol. 1. Kaplan H. I., and B. J. Sadock, eds. Baltimore, Williams & Wilkins, 1989.

CHAPTER TWELVE

PSYCHOLOGICAL FACTORS

AFFECTING MEDICAL CONDITIONS

EVE CALIGOR, MD

By understanding the psychological challenges faced by patients who are medically ill, physicians can help their patients cope with and adapt to physical illnesses and to the treatments and life-style modifications prescribed for them. In order to do so, those who practice medicine must pay attention to the human aspects of their patients—their emotions, behaviors, and relationships. A psychodynamic approach to the practice of medicine helps physicians integrate knowledge of human emotion and behavior into their day-to-day medical management of patients. Chronic illness, chronic pain, and HIV are three conditions in which psychological factors play a particularly important role.

The DSM-IV focuses attention on the interplay of psychological and behavioral factors with medical illness under the diagnostic category Psychological Factors Affecting Medical Condition. This diagnostic category covers conditions or problems that may require clinical attention but that do not necessarily imply the presence of a psychiatric disorder. Thus, while psychological and behavioral factors may play a powerful role in a given patient's medical condition, this does not mean that the patient has a psychiatric illness. Indeed, psychological and behavioral factors affect the physical conditions of typical medical patients—i.e., those who do *not* suffer from psychiatric disorders—in many different ways. In the DSM-IV, the diagnosis of Psychological Factors Affecting Medical Condition is made on Axis I and is accompanied by a medical diagnosis, which is coded on Axis III. The diagnostic criteria for Psychological Factors Affecting Medical Condition are described in Box 12–1.

PSYCHOLOGICAL REACTIONS TO PHYSICAL ILLNESS

All patients with physical illness experience psychological reactions to being ill. The reactions a patient has will vary according to the nature of the illness and the nature of the patient. Relevant aspects of the illness include its severity, chronicity, and the site and nature of the symptoms. Relevant patient characteristics include age, level of maturity, character style, previous experience with illness, and social supports.

A person's psychological reactions to being ill and the ability to cope with illness are extremely powerful factors. Psychological reactions and the ability to cope play an enormous role in determining a person's general well-being and quality of life during an illness, often an even more important role than the nature of the illness itself. This is particularly true in the case of chronic illness. In addition, how a person is able to cope has a powerful effect on medical course and outcome. Some responses to illness are adaptive. These reactions help the patient tolerate being sick and can make it easier for the patient to be compliant with treatment, procedures, and life-style modifications. Other reactions may be highly maladaptive and can cause the patient enormous distress and will often interfere with management and compliance.

Each person has an individual and very personal reaction to an illness. On the one hand, the reaction reflects some combination of the individual's personality traits and characteristic coping mechanisms and, on the other hand, certain general or typically human psychological reactions to and ways of coping with physical illness. Reactions reflecting personality traits can be viewed from the perspective of the patient as an individual who has a distinct character style that interacts in specific ways with the psychological stresses posed by physical illness. Reactions reflecting general psychological responses to illness can be viewed from the perspective of what it means to be ill to most people and the common ways in which they respond to the particular psychological challenges presented by physical illness.

General Psychological Responses to Physical Illness

Regression, denial, anxiety, depression, and anger are general responses to illness that are common to all human beings and originate in the various

BOX 12–1. DSM-IV Diagnostic Criteria for Psychological Factors Affecting a General Medical Condition

The DSM-IV organizes the various psychological and behavioral factors that affect medical conditions into six subcategories: mental disorders, psychological symptoms, personality traits or coping styles, maladaptive health behaviors, stress-related physiological responses, and other or unspecified factors affecting a medical condition.

Mental Disorder Affecting Medical Condition

This category applies to medically ill patients who have a coexisting mental disorder that adversely affects, in a wide variety of ways, the course or treatment of their medical conditions. For example, a middle-aged man suffering from chronic paranoid schizophrenia and insulin-dependent diabetes developed paranoid delusions about his insulin injections and refused to administer them. An elderly widow convalescing from an acute myocardial infarction developed major depression. An alcoholic businessman with peptic ulcer disease continued to drink heavily. A recent amputee with borderline personality disorder so infuriated staff members in his rehabilitation unit that they did not want to work with him.

The physician's approach to a patient who suffers from both a psychiatric disorder and a medical condition is, to a large extent, dictated by the patient's psychiatric diagnosis. Psychotropic medications must be prescribed with care because a patient with a medical illness frequently requires lower dosages, may be more sensitive than a medically healthy patient to side effects, and is likely to be taking medication for the medical condition, which increases the possibility of adverse drug interactions. "Start low and go slow" is the general rule of thumb when prescribing psychotropic medication for a medically ill patient.

Psychological Symptoms Affecting Medical Condition

Patients with Psychological Symptoms Affecting Medical Condition have psychological or psychiatric symptoms that do not meet the criteria for an Axis I disorder but that do significantly affect the course or treatment of their medical illness. Even when symptoms such as anxiety and depressed mood do not indicate the presence of a psychiatric disorder, they become problems that require treatment when they interfere with a patient's recovery. For example, one young man with chronic asthma found that his respiratory distress was exacerbated by anxiety. In another instance, an elderly patient became demoralized and apathetic following surgery; consequently, she was slow in getting out of bed and increasing her level of activity, which delayed her recovery. Another example is maladaptive regression in a hospitalized patient who alienates the nursing staff with constant, excessive demands for attention and care.

Personality Traits or Coping Style Affecting Medical Condition

Personality traits, or character style, refers to a person's characteristic way of interpreting and responding to what happens to them, and their characteristic way of trying to maintain their psychological equilibrium in the face of stressful situations. Personality Traits or Coping Style Affecting Medical Condition applies to patients whose character styles or ways of coping adversely affect their medical conditions. In the same way that many of the symptoms classified under Psychological Symptoms Affecting Medical Condition can be viewed as subsyndromal Axis I disorders, many of the personality traits referred to in this category may represent subsyndromal Axis II disorders. Examples of personality traits that might adversely affect a patient's medical condition include the hostile "Type A" personality, which is thought to be a risk factor for coronary artery disease, and the rigidly controlling patient who gets into power struggles with medical staff during an acute hospitalization. Examples of coping styles that might require clinical attention include pathological denial in the patient who discovers she has a breast mass and assures herself that "it's a cyst" without contacting a physician and maladaptive regression in the hospitalized patient who alienates the nursing staff with constant and excessive demands for attention and care.

Maladaptive Health Behaviors Affecting Medical Condition

The diagnosis Maladaptive Health Behaviors Affecting Medical Condition should be used when high-risk behaviors are adversely affecting a person's health or the course of a medical illness. Common and all-too-familiar examples include the patient with hypertension and coronary artery disease who continues to smoke cigarettes, fails to lose his paunch or to exercise, and consumes a high-fat, high-salt diet; the patient with pulmonary disease who smokes, the patient with valvular heart disease from recurrent endocarditis who continues to use intravenous drugs and shares dirty needles; and the patient with diabetes who is obese and refuses to regulate her diet. We will cover general management strategies relevant to such patients in our section on Compliance.

Stress-Related Physiological Response Affecting Medical Condition

Stress-Related Physiological Response Affecting Medical Condition should be invoked when psychosocial stressors appear to be causally related to the onset or exacerbation of patients' general medical conditions. In these clinical situations, patients' psychological state of feeling "stress" is directly affecting their physiological state.

Examples of clinically significant stress-related physiological responses include the investment banker with a previously well-controlled ventricular arrhythmia that developed into ventricular fibrillation when the stock market collapsed, the young man with quiescent eczema who suffered an acute flare-up during the first months of his medical internship, the diabetic patient whose blood glucose levels went "out of control" after she was fired from her job, and the college student with genital herpes who predictably experienced outbreaks of herpetic lesions during examination periods. The diagnosis of Stress-Related Physiological Response Affecting Medical Condition should not be used in situations where psychosocial stressors appear to be affecting a patient's general medical condition by influencing the patient's behavior (e.g., if the diabetic patient referred to above responds to her stressful state by eating an excessive amount of cookies), and Maladapative Health Behaviors Affecting Medical Condition should be used instead. It is often difficult to make such distinctions.

Other or Unspecified Factors Affecting Medical Condition

Other or Unspecified Factors Affecting Medical Condition is a residual category that should be used when psychological or behavioral factors are affecting the course of a general medical condition, but none of the specified subtypes apply. This category can be used, for example, in the case in which a patient refuses needed medical treatment on the basis of religious or cultural beliefs.

meanings that people attribute to physical illness, the fears typically raised by being ill, and the mechanisms commonly used to cope with the illness.

Regression

Clinical Features

Regression is a nearly universal psychological reaction to being ill in which people revert to more **childlike ways of thinking and behaving.** Regression helps patients to temporarily put aside worries about their job and family responsibilities and to allow themselves to be examined, poked, and prodded during hospitalization.

During the acute phases of an illness, some degree of regression is adaptive. **Adaptive regression** reduces the psychological stress of illness and hospitalization by making it easier for the patient to assume a dependent role and relate positively to physicians, nurses, and other caretakers. Regressed patients are likely to idealize their physicians, viewing them as powerful, good, all-knowing persons who always have the patient's best interests in mind. The **idealization** of caretakers provides powerful protection against anxiety and worry for patients, who must put their physical and emotional well-being into the hands of strangers.

➡ For example, a 50-year-old woman was admitted to the hospital with a mild heart attack. She was usually a domineering matriarch who ran her household and her family real estate business by barking out orders and attacking anyone who tried to give her advice. Her internist and her family feared that her hospitalization would be nightmarish and that she would be a truly "impossible" patient. However, to everyone's amazement, she was a model patient in the critical care unit. She followed the physicians' orders for getting bed rest, receiving oxygen by nasal cannula, and taking intravenous medications; cooperated with diagnostic procedures; and interacted pleasantly with the nursing staff when they helped her use the bedpan and wash and dress herself. This patient regressed from her usual domineering attitude to a more childlike, passive demeanor, in which she unquestioningly put her faith in her caretakers, assuming that they knew best, and followed their instructions. ⬅

While a moderate amount of regression can be adaptive, regression can become maladaptive when it takes a more extreme or long-lasting form. Extreme regression in patients can produce whiny, **oppositional,** and demanding behavior during hospitalization. Such patients may refuse to undergo necessary procedures or comply with treatment, or they may become excessively **passive** and unwilling, or even unable, to do anything for themselves. ➡ The woman described in the case above, for instance, spent her entire hospital stay in bed, even after she was transferred out of the critical care unit, refusing to participate in cardiac rehabilitation. She constantly called on nurses and visiting relatives to help her with even the smallest requests. ⬅ Physicians, nurses, and family members tend to be alienated by this kind of demanding regressive behavior. Their withdrawal may further escalate patients' demands for gratification of their dependency needs.

Excessive or unduly prolonged regression can become especially problematic once the acute phase of an illness has passed and it is time for patients to take more responsibility for their care and their lives. Patients who have recovered from an acute illness and patients who have become medically stable while still suffering from a chronic illness may fail to leave the sick role behind, remaining passive and disabled and refusing to comply with further medical treatment. Their regressed role may have become so gratifying or, conversely, so demoralizing that they lose their motivation to recover. Even after they have been discharged from the hospital, they may continue to behave in a regressive manner, failing to resume their usual activities or responsibilities and relying on family members to take care of their needs. Such patients often do not comply with outpatient follow-up treatment, participate in ongoing medical care, or follow recommendations for outpatient rehabilitation.

➡ After being released from the hospital, the patient in the case above continued to be demanding and passive, doing nothing for herself and insisting that her family wait on her. She refused to take walks or otherwise increase her tolerance for exercise, as her physicians had recommended, and would not resume her usual household or business responsibilities. ⬅

Interview and Management

If regression is interfering with a patient's cooperation with medical recommendations or recovery from illness or both, either during hospitalization or after discharge, intervention is necessary. The first step is for the physician to **explore** the reasons for, and meanings of, the behaviors with the patient. (See Interviewing and Management Guidelines box.) This discussion can begin by the physician's commenting on the patient's behavior and inquiring about it: "I notice that you are relying very heavily on the nursing staff. For example, you are still asking for assistance when you go to the bathroom. Are you feeling afraid to do more on your own?" The regressive behavior may remit in some patients after their conscious fears have been alleviated by **education** and **reassurance.** ➡ In one case, a cardiac patient believed that her overly active, bossy, "take-charge" life-style caused her heart attack and was therefore fearful of increasing her activity or relinquishing her newfound passivity. Her physician discussed these concerns with her and assured her that they were unfounded or, at least, highly exaggerated. The physician then counselled her on how to avoid undue physical and psychological stress while behaving more like her usual self, and he encouraged her to gradually take on more responsibility and become more active. Each step along the way, the patient had the opportunity to address her fears and concerns with her physician. ⬅

Interviewing and Management Guidelines

- Do not underestimate the power of the physician-patient relationship. Some of the strongest "medicines" available are taking time to talk with the patient and showing your concern for him or her.
- Do not assume that you know what it means to a given patient to be ill. This is a personal matter that involves both psychological and practical issues. Make it a goal to learn about this from the patient.
  - Ask the patient how he or she is coping with the illness.
  - Ask specifically about practical problems resulting from the illness, such as family, financial, and job-related problems.
  - Inquire specifically about emotional effects, including anxiety and depression, and the use of alcohol, tranquilizers, or other substances. Introduce these subjects by saying that these are common feelings and behaviors in patients who are trying to cope with medical illness.
  - Ask about stress that may have preceded the onset of the medical problems or may be a result of being ill. The most common stressors are family problems, including illness and death, financial problems, and problems with employment. Inquire about each of these areas.
- Always meet with the patient's family members as well as with the patient. The family is a crucial source of information for the physician and a valuable source of support for the patient.
- Offer support to the family by meeting with them periodically and inviting them to call you if they feel the need.
- When prescribing a treatment or life-style modification, assume out loud that compliance will be a problem. Invite the patient to work out a strategy with you for approaching this challenge. Involving the family in the discussion of the treatment plan can improve compliance.
- When a patient is asking for advice or reassurance that you cannot honestly offer, remember that it may be reassuring and therapeutic to simply inquire about and listen to the patient's feelings.
- Remain aware of your own reactions to the patient, particularly when the patient is suffering from a chronic illness.

If discussion and reassurance fail, the physician may find it useful to **set limits** or create a **behavioral contract.** Ongoing individual work with the patient and meetings with the patient's family are usually helpful, because the physician can correct interactions with family members that reinforce the patient's regressive behaviors. If a maladaptively regressed patient is in the hospital, the physician should work with the nursing staff to help them kindly, but firmly, set incrementally more demanding limits on the patient's behavior or institute behavioral contracts.

Denial

Clinical Features

Denial is an unconscious psychological defense mechanism in which the existence or significance of a painful or frightening situation is kept out of the patient's conscious awareness. It is a way of **warding off feelings of anxiety or depression** until they can be dealt with more comfortably. Some degree of denial is an extremely common reaction to medical illness. For example, a patient in the critical care unit who had had an extensive, acute transmural myocardial infarction was convinced that her physicians would discover that she was merely suffering from indigestion.

A moderate degree of denial need not be a problem and can even be helpful, especially if the patient is denying the seriousness of or emotional reactions to the illness rather than the existence of the illness. Denial can be especially adaptive during the acute phase of an illness because it can mitigate severe anxiety, panic, or despair and can help the patient maintain a calm, hopeful attitude. For the patient who develops chronic medical problems, relatively mild denial may help to maintain hope and ward off depression.

Although some degree of denial can be adaptive and helpful, more extreme denial can pose serious problems. For example, a patient who had a festering skin cancer postponed visiting a dermatologist because he was sure that it was nothing serious and subsequently refused potentially curative surgery for the same reason. Thus, denial in the acute phase of an illness can lead to a **delay** in seeking treatment and to **refusal** of necessary interventions or diagnostic tests. In chronically ill patients, maladaptive denial often causes the patient to refuse to take medications or make necessary life-style modifications.

Interview and Management

When denial is of mild to moderate proportions and does not interfere with the management of the illness, physicians should generally respect patients' needs to defend themselves in this way. The physician should follow the patient's lead, indicating his or her availability to discuss matters with the patient but not pressuring the patient to do so.

For the patient whose denial is interfering with treatment or is maladaptive in other ways (e.g., prevents the patient with a potentially life-threatening illness from writing a will), a more active approach is needed. Rather than resorting to direct confrontation, the physician should "chip away" gradually at the denial by introducing **new information** to the patient about the illness or the management decision that must be made. After presenting one piece of information, the physician should watch for the patient's reaction to and retention of the material before introducing the next piece of information. In this way, the physician can diagnose feelings of anxiety or depression underlying the denial and help the patient deal with these feelings as soon as they arise.

More pressing situations in which the patient's denial is leading to frankly dangerous or life-threatening behavior (e.g., refusal of necessary treatments) require that the physician challenge the patient's defenses by confronting the denial. Patients often react to such a **confrontation** with powerful feelings of anger, anxiety, panic, or depression. Some patients react by threatening to leave the hospital against medical advice or becoming suicidal. Other patients rapidly slip back into even more rigid denial, sometimes of psychotic proportions, which is often accompanied by enormous hostility and even threatening behavior.

These reactions present serious management problems and should be treated as a potential emergency. Physicians and staff members should maintain a calm but firm attitude toward such patients, and family members, if available, should be enlisted to help calm the patient and perhaps even convince the patient to comply with necessary treatments. In the case of psychotic denial, the patient may lack the capacity to give informed consent, in which case the family may be able to help with decision-making.

In emergency situations, ensuring the safety of the patient, the staff, and other patients takes the highest priority. If the patient is threatening to leave or to commit suicidal or violent acts, **one-on-one supervision** and, if necessary, the involvement of the hospital security staff, should be arranged immediately. Low dosages of antipsychotic medications may improve the patient's impulse control and help the patient to feel calmer, less threatened, and less hostile.

Anxiety

Clinical Features

Being ill stimulates many fears, and most medically ill patients suffer from some degree of anxiety at some point during the course of their illness. Anxiety is essentially an **alarm reaction** that warns an individual of incipient danger. Cognitive manifestations of anxiety include fear, worry, and ruminations. Somatic symptoms include palpitations, sweating, dizziness, shortness of breath, hyperventilation, tremulousness, and mild agitation. (It goes without saying that one must rule out a physical cause for these symptoms before attributing them to anxiety; see Chapter 6, Anxiety Disorders.)

Anxiety is most common and is, indeed, to be expected during the early phases of an illness. Some medical patients continue to be anxious and fearful on a chronic basis. A mild degree of anxiety may be adaptive because it keeps patients alert to potential dangers that they may encounter and may therefore enhance compliance with treatment.

Moderate to severe anxiety in medically ill patients can pose a significant problem. In the acute setting, extreme anxiety in patients can interfere with their ability to absorb information, follow instructions, or cooperate with necessary diagnostic procedures and therapeutic interventions. In some illnesses, anxiety can even pose a direct physiological risk. In a patient who has had an acute heart attack, extreme anxiety and agitation can increase the cardiac work load and the risk of arrhythmia. In a patient who is having an asthma attack, feelings of panic can result in hyperventilation and intensify respiratory distress. Excess anxiety and fearfulness in chronically ill or convalescing patients can interfere with rehabilitation and recovery and lead to unnecessary chronic invalidism.

Interview and Management

The first step in managing anxiety is for the physician to clarify with patients the **specific content** of their fears. Common sources of anxiety include fears of death, long-term disability, or dependence on others; concerns about changes in relationships with family members or about the loss of their love and approval; worries about losing the ability to maintain professional and social roles; and fears of losing control of bodily functions or of all aspects of life in the future.

Once the worries have been identified, the physician can plan appropriate interventions. Anxious patients are commonly confused about what has happened to them medically or about the significance of these events. Patients may be worrying about concerns that are unrealistic. For example, many patients assume incorrectly that a diagnosis of cancer means that they are terminally ill; that a diagnosis of heart failure means that the heart has permanently "failed"; that a diagnosis of HIV infection means that they can never again hug their loved ones; or that a diagnosis of uncomplicated myocardial infarction means that they will be unable to return to work or resume normal sexual relations with a spouse. In many cases, physicians can reduce a patient's anxiety by simply correcting distortions, giving more **accurate information,** and providing realistic reassurance.

Patients may also have reasonable, well-founded fears about their medical status. These patients benefit from realistic **reassurance** that emphasizes the range of available treatments. It may be even more important for physicians to let anxious patients know that they will "stick by" them through the ups and downs that lie ahead. The physician's positive attitude, calm demeanor, ongoing concern, and availability are powerful antidotes. For example, a physician might say to a patient who has been recently diagnosed with breast cancer, "I understand that being told you have breast cancer can be very frightening. Let me assure you that we have excellent treatments available. I will go over the options with you in detail and will help you make decisions at each step along the way."

If the interventions of exploration, clarification, education, and reassurance are unsuccessful and the patient continues to suffer from moderate to severe anxiety, the judicious use of **benzodiazepines** on a short-term basis (i.e., for several days to several weeks) may be indicated. Lorezapam is often a good choice for medically ill patients because it has no active metabolites, has a medium-long half-life, and generally does not cause rebound anxiety when the dosage begins to wear off, as do the shorter-acting benzodiazepines. When benzodiazepines are discontinued, the dosage should be tapered rather than abruptly stopped. If, after a few weeks, a patient is unable to stop taking the medication or continues to be significantly disabled by anxiety, it may mean that the patient is unable to cope with the anxiety generated by being ill. A complete psychiatric evaluation is warranted at this point, with the goals of more fully clarifying the sources of the anxiety, both conscious and unconscious; making a thorough search for physical factors, especially medications, that may be exacerbating the anxiety; and making a more accurate diagnosis. Such an evaluation paves the way for a comprehensive treatment plan.

Depression

Clinical Features

Whereas anxiety is essentially an alarm reaction that warns an individual of incipient danger, depression is an emotional response to a catastrophe that the individual believes has already occurred. This catastrophe is commonly experienced as a loss, for which the depressed person feels in some way responsible.

It should not be surprising that depressive thoughts and feelings are common psychological reactions to physical illness. Becoming ill is usually experienced as **a loss.** In fact, when people become ill, they experience many different kinds of losses, ranging from the loss, at least transiently, of certain physical abilities to the loss of bodily integrity to the loss of organs or limbs. **Feelings of loss of control** are virtually universal among hospitalized patients, who must adhere to routines and find that many crucial decisions are being made for them. Most patients find that they cannot do some of the things that they have always done and that have been an important part of their identities (e.g., fulfilling family roles, taking care of professional responsibilities, and participating in recreational and social activities). Even if such changes are only temporary, they may be experienced as a loss. In the best of circumstances, all medical patients suffer an important loss—the loss of their sense of being healthy.

Although transient depressed thoughts and feelings are common in medically ill patients, full-blown **major depression** is not. Though it is easy to err in either direction, depression tends to be underdiagnosed in medically ill patients. This error occurs, in part, because of the commonly held misconception that it is "normal" for people who are physically ill to be depressed. Major depression in medically ill patients is not normal and must be aggressively identified and treated.

Interview and Management

Distinguishing between a normal and to-be-expected depressive or grief reaction and a major depression in a medically ill patient can be difficult. The difficulty is compounded by the tendency of the neurovegetative symptoms of depression (including anorexia, fatigue, insomnia, and constipation) to overlap with the symptoms of many common medical illnesses and the side effects of many commonly prescribed medications. To identify symptoms as depressive, the following guidelines may be helpful. Medically ill patients who are suffering from major depression are more likely than are patients who are merely feeling "blue" or demoralized to

- lack interest in their medical management,
- have a personal or family history of affective disorder,
- lack reactivity of mood and have symptoms that are likely to be more pervasive and long-lasting,
- describe an inability to enjoy anything, and
- suffer from a profound sense of being "bad" or guilty and from a total sense of hopelessness and helplessness that may be accompanied by thoughts of committing suicide.

Undiagnosed major depression in medically ill patients can lead to **noncompliance** with treatment and a poor medical outcome. Patients tend to withdraw into themselves and become passive and uncommunicative. They may feel apathetic about their care and often relinquish decision-making responsibilities to others. They may eat poorly and lose weight, further compromising their medical condition. For some depressed, medically ill patients, certain behaviors (e.g., not taking medications, not communicating with physicians) reflect an unarticulated wish to be dead. Such patients should be considered to have suicidal ideation and should be evaluated and treated accordingly (see Chapter 11, Suicide and Violence).

For medically ill patients who are having depressive symptoms but are not suffering from a major depression, the physician should explain that some depressed feelings are not uncommon in people who are ill and that, for many people, feelings of depression are a way of coming to terms with what is happening to them and are often transient. The physician should keep in mind that patients often feel guilty or angry at themselves, believing that they have brought on the illness. A patient might believe, for example, that a malignant tumor has been caused by "too much stress" or "not getting enough sleep." Such concerns should be sought out and addressed. The physician might say, "Most people have a theory about how or why they have become ill. What are your ideas about why this has happened?"

The approach to patients with depressive symptoms is essentially the same as that outlined above for anxious patients. Interventions should begin with **clarifying** what is depressing the patient. **Correcting distortions** and offering support and appropriate **reassurance** come next. The physician should not be too cheerful or tell the patient to "pull yourself up by your bootstraps," because either of these attitudes will quickly alienate the depressed patient. Instead, a sympathetic but professional attitude and an air of quiet optimism are more helpful. The physician might say, for example, "I know it's tough to live with torticollis and that the pain sometimes makes it really hard to get through the day. Fortunately, there is good news. Your disease does not seem to be progressing, and there are many available treatments that we haven't even tried yet. Also, let me assure you that most people find the first months the most difficult. After that, things tend to get easier."

If these first-line interventions fail and the patient remains consistently depressed for several weeks or demonstrates suicidal thoughts or behavior, the diagnosis of a major depression should be reconsidered. Such patients require a **complete psychiatric evaluation,** including a detailed personal and family history of mood disorders, and a complete workup for **general medical causes** of depression. It should be kept in mind that many commonly used medications and certain medical illnesses may cause mood disorders (see Chapter 5, Cognitive and Mental Disorders Due to General Medical Conditions).

Medically ill patients who are suffering from a major depression usually require a combination of **medication** and **psychotherapy.** Currently, the **selective serotonin reuptake inhibitors** (SSRIs) are the antidepressants of choice for medically ill patients. The common anticholinergic side effects of the tricyclic antidepressants (TCAs), which include blurred vision, dry mouth, sinus tachycardia, constipation, urinary retention, and memory dysfunction, are generally not a problem with the SSRIs. Unlike the TCAs, the SSRIs are not usually associated with electrocardiographic changes or orthostatic hypotension. While the SSRIs do have side effects (most commonly, nausea, diarrhea, or loose stools; insomnia; and sexual dysfunction), they tend to be relatively mild, are often transient, and are generally well tolerated by medically ill depressed patients.

Anger

Clinical Features

Many patients experience anger about being ill, but some patients become enraged and, in an effort to feel less helpless, guilty, or afraid, lash out at the people around them. These patients can become **hostile, suspicious,** and **accusatory** toward family members and the medical staff and get into power struggles and instigate arguments, even with their physicians. ➡ For instance, a patient who developed a painful duodenal ulcer repeatedly lashed out at his wife for nagging him and causing him "stress." Unfortunately, the result of this behavior was to alienate his wife just at the time he most needed and wanted comfort and reassurance from her. A more extreme example with more serious sequelae is the patient who was hospitalized following a myocardial infarction and believed that the complications were

caused by medications inappropriately prescribed by his intern. This patient refused all medications and went into a rage whenever the intern attempted to enter his room or examine him. ◀▥

In extreme cases, an angry, paranoid patient may become frankly delusional and believe, for example, that medications are poisoned or that a nurse is maliciously refusing to follow physicians' orders. When evaluating someone who has become extremely angry or paranoid during hospitalization or any phase of a physical illness, the physician must remember that the patient's reactions may not be entirely psychological. The patient may be suffering from a mental disorder due to a general medical condition (see Chapter 5, Cognitive and Mental Disorders Due to General Medical Conditions) or a substance-related disorder (see Chapter 7, Alcohol and Substance Abuse).

The most common causes of anger, irritability, and suspiciousness in medically ill patients are **medications** and **substances of abuse.** For example, an alcoholic, antisocial homeless man who has been hospitalized and is being treated with steroids is a time bomb waiting to explode. A frail elderly patient, especially one who is taking multiple medications or has mild impairment of baseline cognitive functioning, is also vulnerable. In addition, the physiological effects of many **medical and neurological illnesses** can cause patients to become angry and paranoid, as can a host of metabolic abnormalities and deficiency states. The common general medical causes of severe anger and suspiciousness, as well as delusions, are listed in Table 12–1. Because many patients who become paranoid are suffering from delirium or dementia, careful evaluation for these disorders is necessary (see Chapter 5, Cognitive and Mental Disorders Due to General Medical Conditions).

Certain groups of patients are at especially high risk for paranoid reactions. Included are **elderly patients,** patients who suffer from **depression** or **cognitive impairment,** and those who have a prior history of **psychotic illness.** Patients with **severe personality disorders,** including paranoid, borderline, narcissistic, antisocial, schizotypal, and schizoid personality disorders, are also at risk for becoming angry, hostile, paranoid, or delusional when they are under stress, including the stress of illness and hospitalization. In addition, patients in these high-risk groups may be more sensitive than the average patient to the effects of the physiological factors listed above. For example, even a urinary tract infection, if it occurs in a frail elderly patient who is dealing with the cognitive and psychological stresses of hospitalization, can cause paranoid ideation.

Interview and Management

The first priority for managing an angry patient is to **prevent the patient from hurting** himself or herself or caretakers. It is best to **minimize conflicts** and help the patient feel in control of what is happening. The physician should try to circumvent power struggles and capitulate to the patient's demands (e.g., for a change in a primary nurse) when-

TABLE 12–1. Causes of Anger, Suspiciousness, or Delusional Syndromes

Medications
  Anticholinergic medications*
  Antidepressants
  Antihistamines
  Antiparkinsonian medications*
    (e.g., L-dopa, bromocriptine, amantadine)
  Chemotherapeutic agents (e.g., cyclosporine, procarbazine)
  Corticosteroids and ACTH*
  Digitalis
  Isoniazid
  Muscle relaxants
  Nonsteroidal anti-inflammatory agents
  Opiates (e.g., meperidine, pentazocine)
  Sympathicomimetics
Substances of abuse
  Alcohol**
  Amphetamine
  Anabolic steroids
  Cannabis
  Cocaine
  Hallucinogens
  Inhalants
  Phencyclidine
  Sedative-hypnotics**
Endocrine and metabolic disorders
  Cushing's syndrome
  Hepatic encephalopathy
  Hypercalcemia
  Hypercapnia
  Hyperthyroidism
  Hypocalcemia
  Hypoglycemia
  Hypothyroidism
  Hypoxemia
  Paraneoplastic syndrome
  Porphyria
Neurological disorders
  Central nervous system malignant disease (primary and
    metastatic)
  Cortical dementia (early manifestation)
  HIV infection (AIDS encephalopathy)
  Infection (e.g., viral encephalopathy)
  Multiple sclerosis
  Porphyria
  Stroke
  Subarachnoid hemorrhage
  Subcortical dementia (e.g., Huntington's disease)
  Temporal lobe epilepsy
  Trauma (e.g., postconcussion syndrome)
Connective tissue disorders
  Systemic lupus erythematosus (lupus cerebritis)
  Temporal arteritis
Deficiency states and toxins
  Folate deficiency
  Niacin deficiency
  Heavy metal poisoning (e.g., lead poisoning)
  Vitamin B_{12} deficiency

*Especially likely to cause suspiciousness.
**Withdrawal syndromes can also cause anger, suspiciousness, or
  delusions.

ever possible. If confrontation is necessary, physicians should **acknowledge the patient's concerns and anger** but not argue about whether the behavior is reasonable. It may be helpful to ask family members to be present when the physician meets with the patient.

Patients who are frankly delusional should be managed like any patient with an acute psychosis (see Chapter 4, Schizophrenia and Other Psychotic Disorders). Acute interventions include **adequate supervision, physical restraint,** if necessary, and **antipsychotic drugs.**

Individual Personality Traits in Physical Illness

The ways in which a person responds to and ultimately copes with or fails to cope with a physical illness are powerfully affected by his or her personality traits. Personality traits are a person's characteristic and automatic self-protective mechanisms, which tend to become exaggerated in stressful situations such as physical illness. Personality traits are not typically pathological. However, sometimes, such as during an illness, personality traits may become so exaggerated that the patient may appear to have a personality disorder. This is in part because many of the diagnostic criteria for the DSM-IV personality disorders are exaggerated versions of normal personality traits. The distinction between a personality disorder and a gross and transient exaggeration of normal character traits is, at times, difficult to make in the medical setting. Sometimes the distinction can only be made over time. See Chapter 8, Personality Disorders, for interviewing techniques and more detailed treatment of individual personality disorders.

By assessing a patient's character style, the physician will gain a greater understanding of how being ill is affecting this particular person as well as useful clues for patient management. Following this strategy can be enormously beneficial: The relationship between patient and medical staff will be enhanced, hospitalization and treatment will proceed more smoothly, compliance with treatment will be improved, and the patient will be subject to less distress and will cope more effectively with the illness.

Kahana and Bibring (1964) developed a useful schema for assessing patients' personality traits in the medical setting, classifying personality traits or character styles under seven general categories: dependent, controlled, self-dramatizing, long-suffering, suspicious, superior, and aloof. A modified version of this schema, along with suggestions for management approaches, is described below.

Dependent Personality Traits

Clinical Features

People with dependent personality traits have a **fear of abandonment** and of being alone and frequently harbor **unrealistic expectations of boundless care.** In part, because their expectations are too unrealistic to ever be completely met, they are often disappointed and frustrated by others, particularly caretakers. Frequently, dependent people come to anticipate repeated disappointment and frustration, which only compounds their feelings of anger and depression. Patients with prominent dependent personality traits tend to be **demanding** and, at times, impulsive. In the medical setting, these patients seem to need special attention and limitless time and care from the staff. These are the patients who infuriate the nursing staff by "leaning" on the call button and who are often avoided during rounds because they won't let the staff "get out the door."

Interview and Management

For hospitalized patients, routine nursing and medical care provide a fair amount of dependency gratification, and for some dependent patients, this routine care may be enough to satisfy their expectations. The staff can enhance the beneficial effects such care has on the psychological equilibrium of a dependent patient by communicating, either implicitly or explicitly, their willingness to provide care and by acknowledging the patient's need for reassurance and anxiety about being alone. Even something as simple as the physician's saying, "I understand that it is difficult for you to be in the hospital, away from your family," can provide psychological support.

For the patient who has more extreme needs and demands excessive amounts of time from physicians and nurses, **gentle limit-setting** can be helpful. Before limits are set, they should be explained clearly and expressed in a way that shows the staff's general concern for the patient. For example, the physician might say, "I understand that it is difficult for you to be alone here in the hospital, and I have asked the nurses to check on you every half hour. On your end, I ask that you refrain from using the call button unless there is an emergency. I am concerned that if you continue to ring the nurses as frequently as you have been, they might be slow to respond if there were an emergency." Another helpful strategy is to offer the patient some kind of **token compensation** in exchange for necessary restrictions, such as a special diet or friendly "tips" about parking for hospital visitors. Dependent patients usually do well when interactions with the staff are relatively predictable and **consistent.** Physician visits with both hospitalized patients and outpatients should take place at a prearranged time, last for the expected amount of time, and be conducted in a relatively structured manner.

Controlled Personality Traits

Clinical Features

Patients with controlled, or compulsive, personality traits tend to be **self-disciplined, orderly, and conscientious.** They are frequently "sticklers" for details. These patients need to feel that they have as much information as possible about their circumstances and that they are **in control** of what is happening to them. In moderation, controlled traits can result in a "model" patient. However, these traits often become exaggerated, which can lead to problems. For instance, an overly controlled patient who had a myocardial infarction insisted on doing her regular morning exercise routine on the floor next to her bed in the coronary care unit only two days after the infarction.

Patients with compulsive personality traits can become highly **oppositional,** for example, insisting

that they know best and should be in charge of their own management. Other patients with these traits become paralyzed by **indecision.** When they are anxious or under stress, people with controlled personality traits rely heavily on routine, and, as patients, they tend to closely monitor all staff activities. Any perceived break in the routine (e.g., if a medication is not given at its scheduled time or if the physician is late in getting to the office to see them) may be a cause for anxiety, scathing disapproval, and criticism.

Interview and Management

Management strategies for patients with compulsive personality traits should be designed to give these patients as much actual and symbolic control over what is happening to them as possible. They should be provided, in advance, with thorough, logical **explanations** and instructions of all medical procedures and interventions, even the details of hospital routines such as bathing. Test results should be delivered promptly, even when reporting that a routine blood test was normal. Patients with compulsive personality traits respond well to active **participation in their own care** and should be invited to help plan the treatment and management of their condition. For example, patients can be taught to change their own dressings, monitor and chart their urine output, or obtain their blood glucose levels and calculate their insulin requirements.

Finally, patients with compulsive personality traits are gratified by the medical staff's taking note of their exacting standards and high level of understanding. A comment such as, "I can see that you are a highly intelligent and discerning person. Am I right to assume that you will want to be promptly informed about all test results?" is often a more effective anxiolytic than Valium for these patients.

Self-Dramatizing Personality Traits

Clinical Features

Self-dramatizing patients tend to be charming, imaginative, seductive, and emotionally engaging. They talk about themselves, their experiences, and their symptoms in an exaggerated and dramatic style that is typically lacking in detail. They have an accentuated need to be considered attractive or admired for some outstanding quality, especially by people in positions of authority, such as physicians. In the medical setting, these patients are often interesting to talk with initially and gratifying to care for, but they can become somewhat demanding over time. Their **need to feel "special"** easily leads to their feeling slighted when they do not receive the attention they desire. Self-dramatizing patients may invite **undue familiarity** with the medical staff by presenting themselves in a manner that is charming, seductive, or "defenseless." Female patients may dress up and put on makeup before the physician visits them on rounds. Typical male patients may need to demonstrate their manliness by making grossly inappropriate sexual comments to female physicians and nurses or by bragging to everyone about their professional or athletic successes. Self-dramatizing patients often respond to the stresses of illness by **denying the seriousness** of their condition and, instead, using it to obtain **special attention and sympathy.**

Interview and Management

To effectively manage medical patients with self-dramatizing personality traits, the staff must carefully straddle the line between being too reserved and being too familiar in response to the patient's need for attention and admiration. If invitations of familiarity are received with too much reserve, patients may feel painfully rebuffed. On the other hand, the slightest friendly comment can cause the self-dramatizing patient to "fall into" an emotional overinvolvement with a caretaker, which inevitably leads to the patient's disappointment, hurt, and anger. The best approach for a physician is to communicate interest and concern in a professional manner and help the patient feel important and admired only in ways that are appropriate to a physician-patient relationship, e.g., by spending time listening to the patient's concerns and explaining test results or by commenting favorably on the devotion shown by family and friends.

Long-Suffering Personality Traits

Clinical Features

Long-suffering patients usually have a lifelong history of suffering, whether caused by illness, failed relationships, or other adversities or failures. They typically have been involved in **self-sacrificing relationships** and often perceive themselves as burdens to others. They are inclined to disregard their own discomfort, live in the service of others, and appear to be modest and humble, although they may display their suffering in an exhibitionistic manner. These people want love and acceptance but feel that they do not deserve it. Thus, their suffering becomes a way to punish themselves and, at the same time, to maintain their self-esteem by getting the attention and love they crave. When they become ill, people with long-suffering personality traits respond by viewing their condition as a much-deserved punishment and as a legitimate way to gain attention and love; they almost seem to enjoy their suffering and complaining. Beneath the self-flagellation and complaints of these patients are implicit demands for attention and control. It is as if the patient were saying, "See how I suffer. You have to love me and take care of me because I suffer so."

Long-suffering patients may be perplexing at first. They complain and appear to request sympathy, yet they systematically and emphatically **reject all reassurance and encouragement.** The physician may offer advice or point out improvements, but the patient may counter by demonstrating how the advice is useless and the improvements illusory. Then the patient complains even more pitiably. This type of interaction usually leaves the medical staff feeling frustrated and irritated.

Interview and Management

Successful management of the long-suffering patient is predicated on understanding that the patient wants to be told that the suffering is appreciated and does not want to be told that the suffering will end. In order to convey this message, the physician must spend a reasonable amount of time listening to the patient's complaints and **acknowledging the patient's suffering** with comments such as "It's very tough having to be hooked up to an IV day and night" or "Chest tubes are very painful." Doing so will gratify the patient and leave him or her feeling that the physician is appreciative and understanding. Reassuring or encouraging comments to the effect that things are going well or will be better are best skipped or at least greatly abbreviated. In recommending treatment or diagnostic tests, it is best to frame the recommendation in terms of its potential benefit to others. One might recommend hip replacement surgery to a long-suffering grandmother by saying, "This is a major operation, and there is a demanding recovery period. Nevertheless, I am recommending that you consider hip replacement because it would allow you to resume babysitting for your grandchildren. I understand that your daughter really counts on your help."

Suspicious Personality Traits

Clinical Features

Suspicious patients are mistrustful of others, always ready to assume that they have been wronged, grossly oversensitive to slights, and find criticism or malevolence where none exists. More than anything else, however, suspicious patients **fear becoming vulnerable** to others, which they assume will result in their being taken advantage of or hurt. Having a physical illness, with all its implications for actual and imagined dependency on others, is clearly a crisis for suspicious patients. Being in a medical setting heightens their suspiciousness, causing them to assume that the worst possible scenarios are taking place. They might, for example, suspect the staff of being negligent in caring for them; medical personnel of concealing important information from them; or the hospital of exploiting them by hospitalizing them in order to supply medical students with patients "to practice on," to conduct research, or simply to make money. As their suspicions and anxiety grow, so does the likelihood that such patients will lash out at those around them with angry accusations and criticisms.

Interview and Management

It is most important that these patients receive **detailed information** about the nature of their condition and all plans to treat it, including the potential risks and benefits attendant to proposed medical interventions. It is almost inevitable that these patients will feel they have been slighted or mistreated in some way, and they will complain to their physicians about their experiences. Physicians should respond to patients' reports with calm, courteous, but not overly friendly, concern. The best course of action physicians can take is not to try to dispel or dispute patients' suspicious thoughts, which may only reinforce them, but rather to **acknowledge their concerns** by making a statement such as, "I see that you have little confidence in our staff or in myself. I can appreciate that this puts you in a very uncomfortable position." The way is then paved for enlisting patients' cooperation by suggesting that, for the time being, they tolerate the unpleasant situation.

Superior Personality Traits

Clinical Features

Patients with superior personality traits are typically self-important, self-centered, and condescending to others. This attitude may be superficially cloaked in a patronizing "humility." In the medical setting, these patients often insist on being taken care of by the most important specialists or the chief of the medical service. They often idealize a few "special" staff members but are rude and depreciative toward others. Superior patients behave as if they are **entitled to special treatment.** They expect their requests and needs to be automatically met and believe that hospital rules or routines do not apply to them.

Interview and Management

The management of superior patients involves understanding that their grandiosity protects them from a fragile sense of self-esteem and a horror of having to depend upon others. These patients are most comfortable and supported when they feel that they are being appreciated as people with special attributes and achievements. To this end, it is helpful to behave in a **particularly respectful manner** with superior patients and to inquire about their professions or other accomplishments. To most effectively take care of these patients, the medical staff should **emphasize their own expertise** and demonstrate self-confidence. This attitude is usually reassuring to patients with superior personality traits, because they need to believe that they are receiving "the best." If this approach fails, the patient's deprecation should be met without defensiveness. If the patient is complaining about being taken care of by the house staff, it is often worthwhile to invite the participation of a senior consultant or ward attending.

Aloof Personality Traits

Clinical Features

People with aloof personality traits are unemotional, remote, reserved, and reclusive. They appear to be distant and uninvolved with other people and everyday life. In the medical setting, these patients tend to keep to themselves. They typically limit contact with the medical staff to a bare minimum, rarely asking questions and frequently avoiding eye contact. Their attitude toward their illness may be one of apparent detachment. They seem equally uninterested in and unaffected by hospital routines. They may appear to be odd or eccentric (e.g., preoccupied with certain dietary habits or religious concerns).

Interview and Management

In managing these patients, the physician must respect and accept their intense need for privacy and interpersonal distance. These needs are usually intensified during illness and hospitalization. It is not helpful to be overly friendly or warm or attempt to draw out the patient; such behavior may be experienced by the patient as an intrusive demand and can lead to even further withdrawal. It is best to maintain an **attitude of tempered interest** and consideration, without requesting that the patient reciprocate. A common mistake is to respond too respectfully to the aloof patient's need for privacy (e.g., by skipping the patient's room on rounds, not asking necessary questions about the medical history and symptoms, or omitting parts of the physical examination). It is important to spend enough time with the patient to provide adequate medical care.

PSYCHOLOGICAL FACTORS AFFECTING COMPLIANCE

Clinical Features

One of the most powerful influences that psychological factors have on the course of a patient's medical illness is the effect they have upon whether or not a patient follows medical advice. Compliance with medical advice becomes an issue when medications are prescribed, tests are indicated, or ongoing treatment or follow-up is needed. Compliance is also an important factor when a patient must modify high-risk behaviors, such as smoking cigarettes, that pose a serious threat to health.

Although physicians and patients tend to assume that compliance with medical advice is the rule, it is probably more commonly the exception to the rule. About 50% of patients with chronic illness and up to 90% of patients with acute illness do not take their medications as prescribed. Compliance with taking medications tends to be particularly low when the patient does not have symptoms of a disease (e.g., antihypertensive or prophylactic medications). Perhaps most important in terms of overall health costs, compliance tends to be exceedingly low with a physician's recommendations for modifying risk factors (e.g., stopping smoking permanently, losing weight and maintaining the weight loss).

While certain patients are at higher risk for not complying with medical treatment than others, no one is immune (not even physicians and medical students). Surprisingly, there is no way to predict who will follow medical advice. Among the groups of patients who are at especially **high risk for poor compliance** with medication are those patients who do not know why a particular medication is being prescribed. Other patients do not know how they should take a medication, so it is not surprising that they do not take it as prescribed. Patients who do not know in advance what side effects can be expected are also less likely to be compliant. Others at risk are patients who cannot afford medications, those who have cultural or religious biases against taking medications, and those whose families are opposed to the use of medications. Patients with psychiatric disorders due to general medical conditions and primary psychiatric disorders, including psychotic, depressive, and anxiety disorders, may also be especially vulnerable to noncompliance. Patients with maladaptive emotional and psychological reactions to illness, such as extreme denial, regression, depression, and anger, can also be at risk.

Interview and Management

While individual circumstances and patient characteristics require specific interventions, some general treatment strategies can improve the compliance of many patients. The first strategy is the physician's placement of compliance high on the list of clinical problems to be addressed with all patients receiving treatment. Patients should be informed that poor compliance is extremely common and that they must work with the physician to combat this almost inevitable intrusion into treatment.

When first prescribing a medication for a patient, the physician might say, "I am going to give you a medication that will help control your blood pressure. Controlling your blood pressure will lower your long-term risk of having a stroke or developing heart disease. This kind of medication needs to be taken daily. Believe it or not, even though it may not sound hard, many people find it difficult to take a pill every day on a long-term basis, especially when the problem being treated does not cause any symptoms." Such an introduction will make it easier for the patient to answer honestly when the physician inquires about compliance. The physician might go on to say, "Tell me your thoughts about starting medication, and then let's talk about how we can make it as easy as possible for you to take it reliably."

During follow-up visits, the physician should praise favorable results and **explore any compliance problems** with the patient without reprimanding the patient or making moral judgments. The physician might say, "I can see from the number of pills still in the bottle that you've been finding it difficult to take your medication regularly every day. As I mentioned when you started the medicine, this is a very common problem. Let's talk about why you are having difficulty."

The medication and the recommendations given the patient about taking it also affect compliance. The regimen should be made as **simple** as possible. The dosage **schedule** should be organized around the patient's daily activities; taking the medication at meals or bedtime may be the easiest schedule. If possible, the medication should need to be taken only once or, at most, twice a day. With more frequent dosages, patient compliance lessens precipitously. Possible **side effects** should also be anticipated and discussed with the patient.

When prescribing, the physician should write down and give to the patient the medication's brand name and its generic name, along with the indications, expected benefits, and length of time it will take before any benefits are felt. Writing out dosage schedules clearly and going over them with the patient is extremely important. For those who are taking numerous medications, the physician should suggest that the patient make a chart and use a pill box. Before the patient leaves the office with a new prescription, the physician should check again to make sure that the patient understands how to take the medication and that the patient's questions about it have all been answered. It is helpful to review information about medications when a family member is present. The support and participation of family members who understand the benefits of the patient's medications can play a significant role in improving compliance.

Patients are more likely to comply if the physician-patient relationship is positive. In fact, this **therapeutic alliance** may be the most powerful and reliable factor affecting compliance. Regularly scheduled appointments for monitoring compliance and progress are helpful, and patients should be encouraged to call with questions or concerns about their illness or its treatment. Physicians should foster a **collaborative atmosphere** between themselves and their patients. Patients who are actively involved in making decisions about their treatment are more likely to comply with it. If there is a choice of treatments, the options should be reviewed with the patient, and the one that is most desirable (e.g., on the basis of side effects or cost) to the patient should be chosen. If medications need to be evaluated over time or dosages need to be titrated, the patient should be involved in the process. For example, the patient who is starting a new medication for prophylaxis of migraine headaches should be asked to keep a log of symptoms (e.g., frequency, severity, and duration of headaches) and side effects and to review the log with the physician at the next visit. This information then becomes part of the process in which the physician and the patient decide together about whether the patient is taking the right medication and the most effective dosage.

PSYCHOSOCIAL STRESS AFFECTING A MEDICAL CONDITION

Clinical Features

In both the medical and the popular literature, discussions of psychological factors affecting medical condition, or the relationship between the mind and body in physical illness, frequently are based on the concept of stress. Everyone knows what it feels like to be "stressed," but the term *stress* is frequently used in a confusing, poorly defined fashion. **Stress** is best defined as the internal emotional reaction, or distress, that a person experiences in response to a given situation or condition, which is the **stressor.** To refer to a given set of conditions as stressful implies that the individual's capacity to cope comfortably with and adapt to these conditions has been surpassed.

According to this definition, stress is subjective. What constitutes stress is defined not only by the stressor but also by the person who is being stressed. This approach means that what is stressful for one person may not be particularly stressful for another. Whether an event is experienced as stressful is determined both by the meaning of the stressor to the individual and by his or her ability to cope. These factors, in turn, are affected by the individual's personality, life circumstances, and social supports. For example, a hysterectomy may be extremely stressful for a chronically lonely young woman who was looking forward to having a family, but the operation might not pose much of an emotional challenge to a postmenopausal woman who is happily married and has teenage children.

Sometimes, the factors that determine whether an event is experienced as stressful are purely psychological and may not even be apparent unless the physician knows the patient and understands his or her psychological makeup. For example, a fiercely independent person who is laid off from a job may find it extremely stressful to be unable to work and to have to collect unemployment compensation, whereas someone who is dependent and passive may find unemployment not at all stressful and even a relief. The person's attitude may make all the difference; being laid off from work might be extremely stressful for a pessimist but might not pose much of a psychological obstacle to an optimist who is convinced that he or she will easily find another job. The attitude of the person's spouse or family toward the layoff will also affect how stressful the experience is for the person.

Increased life stress has been associated with the onset and exacerbation of numerous medical problems, although the exact mechanisms that link stress and disease are extremely complex and incompletely understood. In considering the relationship between stress and illness, it is crucial to keep in mind that physical illness is, itself, stressful and may set in motion a vicious circle: Life stressors leave an individual vulnerable to illness; illness generates even greater stress; and greater stress leaves the individual even more physically vulnerable. Thus, it is important for physicians to understand patients' psychological reactions to physical illness and to do all they can to help patients cope.

Illness often introduces new stressful conditions into patients' lives, as well. Social supports appear to buffer the effects of stress: A person with solid social supports is less vulnerable to the emotional and physical sequelae of stressful life events, including medical illness, than is the socially isolated individual. Unfortunately, illness can sometimes disrupt the lives even of patients who have solid social supports (e.g., marital tensions are relatively common when one spouse is ill; losing a job because of illness frequently means losing a valuable social network at the same time; and physical illness may cause the patient to withdraw socially). Such disruption leaves the patient more vulnerable to the stresses of physical illness.

In thinking about the mechanisms by which stress affects a person's health, it is important to keep in mind that not all stress-related medical problems are stress-related physiological responses. **Stress-related physiological responses** are the direct result of psychological stress and distress on a person's physiology and physical health. These responses are not behaviors resulting from stress.

For example, a patient with hypertension and atherosclerotic heart disease had been asymptomatic with medical management. His wife of 30 years left him, and during the next 6 months, he developed angina. Before his physician assumed that the stressful marital separation was physiologically related to the angina, she took a careful history in which it was revealed that since the patient's wife left him, he had been smoking more, drinking alcohol, and using drugs to self-medicate his distress. He had gained weight and stopped exercising. He had stopped taking his medications. He had a recurrence of high blood pressure, but this had not been detected because he postponed his regular checkup. Any combination of these factors could account for the angina.

In the DSM-IV, this patient's problematic behaviors would be coded under maladaptive health behaviors affecting medical condition (see Box 12–1). When alcohol, nicotine, or drug use is the primary problem, the dual diagnoses of substance-related disorder and of mental disorder affecting medical condition should be used, both of which are coded on Axis I. The diagnosis of stress-related physiological response affecting a medical condition would be used for this patient if, for example, he had prominent dependent personality traits and if the loss of his wife had left him feeling overwhelmingly anxious. The autonomic arousal accompanying chronic high levels of anxiety may be contributing to his cardiac decompensation by affecting the heart rate, blood pressure, and myocardial conduction system and blood supply.

Interview

When interviewing a patient suffering from a general medical condition, it is important to take into account the role of stress. The first stress to consider is the illness itself. After taking the history, the physician should explore with the patient **how stressful the illness has been** for the patient and the patient's family. Asking a question such as "How are you coping with all of this?" gently invites the patient to open up a bit. The extent to which the illness is causing secondary problems for the patient (e.g., family tensions, financial or job-related problems) should be clarified. These factors may place additional pressures on the patient and the family, making it harder for all of them to cope with the illness.

The next step is to carefully assess the role that psychosocial stressors have played in causing the patient's medical problems. The physician should inquire about **recent life changes or stresses** that are temporally related to the onset or worsening of the condition. Asking specific questions about **financial problems, job-related problems, marriage, and family matters** is helpful. Other recent illnesses in the family or problems with children may also be significant. Most stressful life situations fit into one of these categories, and asking about each one specifically in an open-ended way will help patients to talk about them. Patients may not have regarded these situations as stressful until the physician inquires about them. The physician might ask, "How have things been going for you on the job?" If the patient proceeds to talk about massive layoffs, the physician might comment, "That must be very stressful for you." Most patients will "pick up the ball" and either concur or state that they had not really thought about it. The patient may say, "Now that you mention it, things have been pretty tense lately."

When a patient's medical condition has deteriorated during a period of psychosocial stress, it is important to carefully evaluate the mechanisms by which the stressors have affected the medical condition. The nature of the stressors should be clarified in detail, as well as the ways in which the patient has or has not been able to cope with them. The physician should ask about **symptoms of anxiety and depression** and should tactfully inquire about **maladaptive health behaviors** that may be reactions to stress. It can be helpful to say something like, "You've been under an awful lot of stress over the past few months. Many people in this type of situation resort to trying to comfort themselves with alcohol. Have you found yourself drinking more recently?" or "Typically, people take their medications less reliably during stressful periods. Have you found anything like this happening to you?" Questions framed in this way make it clear that such maladaptive behavior is common and that the physician is accustomed to hearing about it. These questions also communicate an attitude of tolerance on the part of the physician. This approach will make it easier for the patient to be honest about behaviors of which the patient is ashamed or about fears that the physician will disapprove of the patient.

It is important to ask the same questions of someone in the **patient's family.** People close to the patient may be able to provide information that the patient is unaware of or reluctant to reveal. One has to make the mistake of forgetting to speak with family members only once to remember to do so forever after. Consider again the patient with angina, discussed above, whose wife had left him. It would be common for the physician to assume that such a patient had "broken through" his previous medication regimen. The solution, based on this assumption, would be to increase the dosages of old medications or to add new medications, only to have the patient develop side effects and perhaps even toxicity. At this point, the physician might receive a phone call from the patient's daughter, to say that she suspects that the patient stopped taking his medication when his wife left the house.

As a final illustration of the importance of a careful, thorough evaluation of the role of stress in a general medical condition, consider a patient in her late forties with long-standing multiple sclerosis who suffered an acute exacerbation of her disease nine months after the death of her husband. Any of a number of factors may have an effect on this patient, and all of them should be considered in the differential diagnosis. The patient might be suffering from a stress-related physiological response to having lost her husband, which affected her immune system and resulted in increased autoimmune activity and an exacerbation of her symptoms. She might be reacting to the loss of her husband by not taking her maintenance medication as often as she should have been or by taking a "devil may care" attitude about her health. Her husband may have been responsible for making sure she took her medication as prescribed. The patient's increased fatigue, weakness, and mental slowing might be, in part, symptoms of depression. In order to determine which of these possibilities was the basic problem, the physician asked careful questions in a concerned, tolerant, open fashion (i.e., in the manner described above). The results of this inquiry, along with appropriate physical findings and laboratory tests, helped the physician make a DSM-IV diagnosis and put together a treatment plan.

It is extremely common for patients who become ill to describe having recently been under a lot of stress. As has been outlined above, it is important to clarify what role stress may have played in the medical condition. It is also important to understand that stress may *not* have played a significant role, even if the patient currently feels stressed or believes that the medical problems are stress-related. It is a common belief in the United States that too much stress is "bad." People tend to take it for granted that stress can cause ill health and exacerbate preexisting medical problems. Many patients and their families overestimate the role of stress in illness. Physicians should be alert to this possibility because patients and their families may suffer unnecessary feelings of guilt or self-blame for their illnesses and may have painful feelings of personal failure or responsibility when their illnesses flare up or recur. The role of stress in the course of an illness varies, depending on the disease, the patient's biological vulnerability to disease, and the patient's psychological and physiological vulnerability to stressful events.

Management

An accurate assessment of the role of stress in an illness will determine which medical and psychosocial interventions should be made. Careful assessment can spare the patient unnecessary diagnostic procedures and trials of medications, as well as unnecessary self-blame. Consider again the woman with multiple sclerosis, discussed above. Increasing the dosage of steroids for this patient would not have improved her health if the exacerbation was caused by decreased compliance with her maintenance medications. If the exacerbation was due to stress-related changes in the patient's immune system, interventions aimed at helping her to cope better might have reduced the total dosage of steroids required to control her symptoms. If she was depressed, treating her medical disease but ignoring her depression would not have been a successful approach. ◂▦

If none of these factors seem to be a major issue (e.g., if the patient has many social supports, is financially secure, and appears to be coping well but is nonetheless blaming herself for "letting stress get the better of me"), a different approach is needed. The treatment for the unnecessary guilt and self-blame is a combination of **education** and **reassurance.** A physician is in a powerful position in this regard, and just a few helpful words of explanation and encouragement can make an enormous difference to patients who are painfully and inaccurately blaming themselves for not taking proper care. One might say to these patients, "Believe it or not, people tend to overestimate the role of stress in this kind of situation. You are coping very well with the loss of your husband, and it may be that stress is not even playing a significant role in this exacerbation. It may have happened anyway, regardless of what was going on in your life. This may just be an unfortunate coincidence. It leaves you with an awful lot on your plate right now, but, as I said, I am impressed with how well you are handling everything." Patients in this situation are usually relieved to hear that the physician does not blame them for having become ill and does not expect them to blame themselves. Most patients will feel supported by the physician's favorable comments on their ability to cope.

PSYCHOLOGICAL ASPECTS OF CHRONIC ILLNESS
Clinical Features

Learning to live with a chronic physical illness presents a psychological challenge for patients and their families. Most people rise to this challenge and are able to adapt after a period of time, although there are always some ups and downs in the process. Sound medical management, including an ongoing relationship with a physician who provides information, guidance, and psychological support, facilitates the adaptation. Patients who are unable to make the adjustment to chronic illness may suffer many serious consequences. If a patient is having unusual difficulty in making the adjustment to a chronic illness, the physician should make it a primary focus of management to help the patient cope and adapt successfully.

Patients who are unable to adapt are at high risk for chronic problems with compliance, which may take the form of underuse or overuse of medications. These patients may delay seeking treatment during exacerbations, which may result in unnecessary hospitalizations and periods of acute illness. They may be too quick to panic when their symptoms change,

which may lead to overuse of medical services, especially the emergency room. Such patients may resort to "doctor shopping," which can interfere with the development of an ongoing relationship with one medical practitioner.

All of these factors make it likely that patients who are having difficulty adapting to chronic illness will be subjected to unnecessary diagnostic procedures, which can bring potential complications. Because of problems with motivation, patients who are having difficulty adapting to chronic illness are usually poor candidates for physical and vocational rehabilitation programs; they are more likely than other patients to suffer from impaired self-esteem, depression, and anxiety. Greater-than-usual tensions at home and disruption of family life are common. The multiple medical and psychosocial complications faced by such patients are illustrated by the following case.

▸ A 55-year-old married man, who was a veteran, suffered from chronic obstructive pulmonary disease. This patient's poor adjustment to his illness had numerous unfortunate sequellae, including overuse of bronchodilators, which led to drug tolerance and side effects of chronic anxiety and nausea; delay in seeking out of medical attention during infectious exacerbations, resulting in preventable hospitalizations; unnecessary restriction of physical activity, leading to deconditioning and increased functional disability; frequent changes in physicians, resulting in unnecessary procedures and blood tests and interfering with the development of a relationship with a physician who has also had an opportunity to get to know the patient's family; accepting Social Security Insurance rather than taking on the challenge of vocational rehabilitation; marital discord due to his wife's efforts to enforce compliance and more reasonable behavior in general; and problems with depression and alcohol abuse, which became increasingly severe as the patient's physical and psychological condition steadily deteriorated. ◂▦

In the course of adapting to chronic illness, patients must make many changes. The exact nature of these changes varies according to the illness, its severity and course, and the patient's psychology and personality, phase of life, previous experience with illness, and social responsibilities and supports. Some of the changes are external changes in daily routines and activities, and others are internal changes in the patient's view of himself or herself in relation to the world. External changes can be as minor as having to remember to take an antihypertensive agent daily or as major as having to give up a profession or the ability to ambulate independently. Internal changes may range from having to accept an increased awareness of a physical vulnerability to losing aspects of the self that have been important sources of self-esteem or a sense of identity. Patients must find new ways to define who they are and experience themselves as valuable.

When first given the diagnosis of a chronic illness, many people have a hard time fully appreciating what they have been told. There is usually a period of shock or denial, when the patient may feel that "the whole thing just doesn't seem real." Patients usually assume that the problem will resolve or that a cure can be found. When this fails to happen, many patients visit specialists and seek out traditional or nontraditional treatments in the hope of finding a cure. Over time, as these efforts fail to resolve the problem, many patients feel worried, anxious, and fearful and develop seemingly hypochondriacal preoccupations about their medical problems. Patients may also feel angry, guilty, demoralized, and depressed. Most patients will go through many, if not all, of these emotions at some point in the course of adjusting to a chronic illness.

In order to adapt successfully to chronic illness, patients must shift their focus away from trying to eradicate the illness and toward trying to live with it. This is a fundamental change in goals. Rather than looking for a cure, the emphasis is now placed on **adapting** to the illness and on minimizing disabilities and psychosocial complications. The shift involves a change in the patient's frame of reference from a more familiar perspective based on acute illness to a perspective that is more suitable for chronic illness.

The initial process is often experienced as "giving up hope" and can be painful. Over time, most patients come to see things from a more positive, active perspective, viewing themselves as involved in a challenging struggle to live with the illness. The patient who continues to feel hopeless and "down" over an extended period of time is the exception and may be suffering from depression. It is not "normal" for someone with medical problems to develop a major depression, and affective illness in chronically medically ill patients should be aggressively diagnosed and treated.

A 48-year-old disabled fireman, who lived with his wife and 17-year-old daughter, had been in good health until he injured his back four years earlier by falling backward in a broken lounge chair. This injury led to chronic low back pain that was not relieved by repeated spinal fusions. Conservative medical management had been recommended, including nonsteroidal anti-inflammatory medication, physical therapy, and exercise. Because he was still faring poorly four years after the initial injury, he was referred for psychiatric consultation. When the psychiatrist first saw him, the patient's mood was extremely depressed. He said that he was in constant pain, which preoccupied him day and night. He complained of insomnia and was unable to concentrate. He was extremely anxious and spent most of his waking hours ruminating about his financial concerns. His appetite was poor, but because he was inactive and ate mostly snack foods, the patient had gained 30 pounds since his injury. He spent most of his time in the ground-floor den, which he had made into his bedroom, lying on the couch and watching television. He had not complied with recommendations for physical therapy and exercise, and he rarely left the house. The patient had left his job as a fireman and

was receiving temporary disability compensation. He felt inferior to his wife, who was now bringing in more money than he was, and he revealed that he had always thought of his wife, who was a senior vice president at a computer company, as more intelligent than he. He had thought of himself as "handy" because he took care of the house and maintained the cars. Now that he was earning less money and was unable to take care of the house or the cars, he felt deprived of his customary role in the household. This change left him feeling useless and unnecessary. The patient felt that he was a burden to his wife and daughter.

The patient's predominant reactions to developing chronic pain were to become depressed and anxious and to regress. He was unable to cope effectively with his physical symptoms and with the psychosocial changes that followed. Most disturbing to him were his concerns about his financial future and the changes in his role in the family. He was left feeling helpless, useless, inferior, and unable to cope and adapt; he was spiraling downward.

Interview

When interviewing a patient who is suffering from a chronic illness, it is important to find out how the illness has affected the patient's life. Specific questions should be asked about the impact the illness may have had on the patient's **job, finances, family roles and responsibilities, sex life, recreational activities, and social life.** The physician may begin by asking, "Have you been able to continue to work?" If the patient answers affirmatively, the physician should ask for more detailed information, such as, "How hard has it been for you to continue working?" "Have you had to make any changes on the job because of your illness, or have there been any problems?" "Has this made things tight for you financially?" The physician should inquire about how the patient and the family are coping with the changes that illness brings. Specific questions should be asked about problems with demoralization, depression, anxiety, and substance abuse. The physician might introduce these topics by saying to the patient, "Often, when people are trying to adapt to a chronic illness, they go through painful periods of feeling demoralized or even depressed. Other people become very anxious. What has your experience been?" After exploring this topic with the patient, the physician can go on to say, "It's also very common for people who are trying to cope with chronic illness to turn to alcohol or sedatives for relief. Have you found any of these things happening to you?"

Asking specific questions will bring to light problems that many patients will not volunteer without an invitation and can identify areas in which helpful interventions can be made. The disabled fireman described above confided, in response to a question from the physician, that he and his wife had not had sexual relations in several years. In fact, he believed that his wife was repulsed by any physical contact with him. ⬅ Physical therapy, vocational counseling, treatment for depression and anxiety, or marital and individual counseling can help the patient who is having trouble adapting. Asking patients about their lives and their difficulties is, in and of itself, a therapeutic intervention. For most patients, the opportunity to talk with a trusted physician about their problems and concerns and to receive support and guidance is a powerful and highly valued "medicine."

Patients usually have a theory, often unfounded, about why they developed their illness and frequently believe that they are responsible for it. Patients may believe that they have become ill because they subjected themselves to too much stress, did not eat right, or did something bad for which they are being punished. Some patients blame their spouse, if there are marital problems, or their job, if it is stressful. It can be helpful to discuss these beliefs in order to **correct distortions** and alleviate unnecessary fear, guilt, and blame. Failure to do so can cause enormous distress and even depression, as well as unnecessary marital or vocational disruption.

It is useful for the physician to ask patients if they know other people who have the same illness. Patients often base their expectations for themselves on what they have seen happen to others. These expectations tend to be particularly powerful when a patient develops the same illness that has affected a parent or sibling. Similarly, patients who become ill at an age at which a deceased parent or sibling became ill or died generally assume that they, too, have been dealt a death sentence. Most patients will not bring up these topics unless they are asked about them. If they are encouraged to talk about such matters, most patients will experience enormous relief.

Patients with high-risk behaviors (e.g., smoking cigarettes or eating a high cholesterol diet) often feel particularly self-critical when they become ill. A common error on the part of physicians is to shy away from discussing such matters. Physicians often fear, incorrectly, that talking about these concerns will only make the situation more painful for the patient. This concern reflects the misfounded belief frequently held by physicians that they have little to offer patients who are struggling with realistic regret and self-blame. If a patient has a chronic progressive illness, such as Parkinson's disease, and is worried about progressive deterioration, physicians may sidestep the patient's desires to discuss the fears. Here again, physicians may feel that they have nothing to offer and that talking about a painful inevitability will only make matters worse. This is not necessarily true. Many patients feel much better after they have **shared their realistic regrets** with an empathetic, supportive physician. One might say something as simple as, "Parkinson's can be a tough disease to live with. Sometimes people go through periods of feeling down or worrying about the future. How has it been for you?"

Physicians play a critical role in helping their patients make a successful adaptation to chronic illness. In order to do so, physicians must deal with their own feelings about chronic illness. Many people become physicians in order to "help" and "cure" other people. They often share patients' expectations that physicians should be able to "fix" things. Such expectations on the part of physicians can lead to feelings of frustration and dissatisfaction when they are dealing with patients with a chronic illness. These feelings, in turn, can cause physicians to unduly blame themselves or patients or even to inadvertently push the patient out of treatment.

Management

There are many things physicians can do to help patients adapt to chronic illness. First, patients need to be **educated** about their illness, and, whenever possible, given **responsibility** for day-to-day management decisions. For example, patients who have diabetes can check their urine or serum glucose and adjust their insulin dosages accordingly. Patients with asthma can titrate the precise frequency of inhalers. Patients should be helped to anticipate the predictable fluctuations in their symptoms and taught how to distinguish these fluctuations from an exacerbation that requires medical intervention. Patients with coronary artery disease and angina can be taught to respond to an episode of angina by relaxing and taking nitroglycerin instead of panicking, rushing to the emergency room, or continuing to exert themselves. They can be helped to understand that, while occasional anginal episodes are likely, an increase or change in the typical pattern may be a warning sign of a problem that requires immediate medical attention.

In addition to education and guidance, patients suffering from chronic illness need **emotional support.** A positive relationship with a physician who is sympathetic and available makes a big difference. The physician should get to know the patient's family members because they can often provide information or raise concerns that the patient will not and because they are likely to need the guidance and support of the physician as much as the patient does. It is easy to underestimate the powerful and positive effect of physician-patient and physician-family relationships on helping patients cope with and adapt to chronic illness.

⬅ The case of the fireman with low back pain described above can be used to illustrate the management of a patient who is having difficulty adapting to chronic illness. The patient had been referred to a psychiatrist, who recommended the addition of short-term psychotherapy on a weekly basis for several months, along with an antidepressant and an anxiolytic, to the patient's regimen of nonsteroidal anti-inflammatory agents. In psychotherapy, the patient discussed his feelings of inferiority and related them to the recent changes in his role in the family. He and the psychiatrist also discussed, in concrete terms, what he might do to establish a new set of roles for himself. The patient decided to begin taking care of the bills and household paperwork and to cook the family's dinner. The psychiatrist encouraged him to pursue more intensive physical therapy and regular workouts and pointed out that losing weight and being fit and more active would help him to feel better about himself.

The psychiatrist also met with the patient and his wife several times and helped them to clear up misunderstandings that existed between them. The patient's wife was able to tell her husband that he was only imagining that she was recoiling from physical contact with him and that, in fact, she longed for physical affection. She assured him that she was comfortable with being the major breadwinner for the time being and was getting satisfaction from being able to do this for her family. The psychiatrist made suggestions to help the couple learn to communicate more openly with each other. She also recommended that they engage in more affectionate physical contact, without pressuring them to resume specifically sexual activities. At the same time, the psychiatrist discussed the logistics of how to have sexual relations without putting stress on the patient's back. This concern weighed heavily on the patient and, as it turned out, even more so on his wife. It had been part of the reason why they had stopped having sex.

Over the course of the next few months, the patient's depression gradually remitted. His previous good spirits returned, and he slowly began to regain his self-esteem. He was able to sleep and concentrate and discovered that by losing weight and exercising regularly he could increase his range of activities. He resumed his habit of maintaining the family cars and moved out of his den and back into the second-floor bedroom to sleep with his wife. He was on the road to adapting to his chronic illness. ◄▬

PSYCHOLOGICAL ASPECTS OF CHRONIC PAIN

Living with chronic pain and its sequelae can be tremendously challenging, both for patients and their families. Treating patients who suffer from chronic pain can also be extremely challenging for physicians and other health care providers. The group of patients that falls under the umbrella of chronic pain is a highly heterogeneous one, including patients of all ages who suffer from many different physical and psychiatric problems and whose psychosocial supports and stressors vary enormously. Examples include an elderly widower who is socially isolated and dependent on alcohol and who suffers from rheumatoid arthritis; a 40-year-old fireman, who is married and the father of four, who strained his back and now suffers from chronic low back pain; an unemployed young woman with chronic pelvic pain of undetermined etiology; and a 50-year-old married businesswoman suffering from a painful diabetic neuropathy. These people have many more differences than similarities. What they do share is the challenge of adapting to life with chronic pain.

Most experts consider a pain syndrome to be chronic if it has lasted for 6 months or longer. Chronic pain syndromes are subclassified as malig-

nant or benign, according to whether or not they are due to a malignant disease. The psychological issues involved and the management strategies employed are often different for benign and malignant chronic pain syndromes. The DSM-IV classification of chronic pain is presented in Box 12–2. (See also Table 10–5, DSM-IV Criteria for Pain Disorder.)

Clinical Features

Malignant chronic pain is pain due to cancer or its treatment. The two main causes are direct tumor invasion with compression of tissue (usually bone or nerve tissue) and treatments for cancer, including chemotherapy, irradiation, and surgery, which frequently lead to painful destruction of nerve fibers in peripheral pain pathways. Patients' responses to malignant pain have much to do with their attitude toward their illness. Especially in preterminal patients, the population of cancer patients for whom pain is most often a problem, pain serves as a constant reminder of a life-threatening illness. Approaches to the treatment of chronic malignant pain emphasize physical and psychological comfort and, as much as possible, **relief of pain.** Narcotics are used freely and liberally and are limited only by side effects. There is little emphasis on avoiding tolerance to, dependence on, or addiction to narcotics. Cancer patients are encouraged to speak up forcefully when they are in pain, and family members are encouraged to listen. These complaints are considered a call for action. New pain may indicate progression of the disease, which requires evaluation, and new or increased pain is always an indication for the titration of narcotic regimens.

Benign chronic pain can be caused by many medical conditions, including degenerative spinal disease, trigeminal and postherpetic neuralgias, diabetic neuropathy, arthritis, chronic headache, myofascial syndrome, reflex sympathetic dystrophy, and ischemia. Patients are usually preoccupied with their pain, feel that it has become the focus of their lives, and are in great distress. In most cases, patients have suffered significant psychosocial disruption, including depression, anxiety, substance abuse, marital problems, and difficulties at work, as a result of their pain.

The basic management approach for chronic benign pain is different from that for malignant pain. For chronic benign pain, **pain relief is deemphasized,** the use of narcotics is discouraged, and patients and their families are taught not to talk about or focus on the pain. Instead, the emphasis is on increased activity and return of function.

▬► The fireman with low back pain described above exemplifies many aspects of what can happen to patients with chronic pain before they get the help they need. At the time that he presented to the psychiatric consultant, the patient was totally preoccupied with his pain, had given up all his usual activities, was not working, and was virtually housebound. He was anxious and depressed, alienated from his

BOX 12–2.   Chronic Pain Disorders

In the DSM-IV, patients with chronic pain are classified under pain disorder associated with psychological factors, pain disorder associated with both psychological factors and a general medical condition, or pain disorder associated with a general medical condition. The first two entities are subtypes of pain disorder, which is listed under somatoform disorders and coded on Axis I. Pain disorder associated with a general medical condition is treated as a medical condition and is coded on Axis III. All of these diagnoses apply to patients who present with pain and who have suffered clinically significant distress or psychosocial impairment as a result of pain. The three diagnoses differ in the relative weight given to psychological factors in the onset, severity, and course of the pain syndrome.

The diagnosis of **pain disorder associated with psychological factors** should be used if psychological factors appear to have a major role in the onset, severity, or course of the pain. Frequently, no physical lesion or medical condition can be found to explain the patient's complaints in these cases. If a general medical condition does exist, it does not appear to be playing a major role in the pain-related complaints. This diagnosis implies that a somatoform disorder is present (see Chapter 10, Somatoform and Factitious Disorders) (i.e., that the patient's experience of pain is based more on mental factors than medical factors).

Pain disorder associated with psychological factors was the diagnosis for a 31-year-old housewife who was in good health but who developed abdominal pain after her alcoholic father died of appendicitis. Complete medical and gynecological evaluations were unremarkable. The patient was treated with psychotherapy, which focused on her feelings about her father's death. Her pain gradually resolved over a 9-month period. It recurred, transiently, 2 years later, when her older sister was diagnosed with colon cancer.

At the other end of the spectrum is the diagnosis of **pain disorder associated with a general medical condition.** It should be used when the psychological factors are not playing a significant role in the onset, severity, or course of the pain. For such a patient, the pain syndrome is not considered to be a mental disorder. It is treated as a medical disorder and coded on Axis III.

Pain disorder associated with a general medical condition was present in an otherwise healthy elderly man who suffered from postherpetic neuralgia. He presented to his internist with a complaint of severe pain. Though in distress, he had worked hard to maintain, as best he could, his previously active lifestyle. He had abstained from alcohol and sedatives and had been self-medicating his pain with double-strength acetaminophen tablets.

The diagnosis of **pain disorder associated with both psychological factors and a general medical condition** applies to the overwhelming majority of patients suffering from chronic pain. A general medical condition is present that can at least partially account for the severity, exacerbation, or maintenance of the pain. The disabled fireman described above was given the diagnoses of pain disorder associated with both psychological factors and a general medical condition plus major depressive disorder, single episode.

---

wife and daughter, felt terrible about himself, and was hopeless and fearful about his future. ◀▥

While this patient fared better than most, his experience illustrates how patients with chronic pain typically find themselves locked into a vicious circle of steady psychosocial deterioration and intensification of pain. Caught in this trap, patients tend to become increasingly depressed and preoccupied with their pain, as the rest of their lives become progressively disrupted. Patients may lose their jobs, be at odds with friends and loved ones, and give up all hobbies and interests. Pain can become the focus of the patient's world. Life can be reduced to a series of visits to medical specialists, looking for a "cure." Or patients may become virtually housebound, doing little except focusing on pain and medications.

The etiology of chronic pain is complex and, for many patients, involves an interaction between medical and psychosocial factors. Once a patient has developed a chronic pain syndrome, psychosocial factors play a major role in the course of the syndrome in a variety of ways. Different people have different pain thresholds, and a person's pain threshold will vary over time, depending on the person's mood, level of anxiety or fatigue, use of drugs and alcohol, prior experience with pain, and other factors. Patients who cope well are likely to experience less pain. Patients who are unable to cope and adapt are at risk for many secondary psychosocial problems that can intensify pain, interfere with treatment compliance, and make it even more difficult to cope. Depression and **substance abuse** often become prob-

lems. The most common substances of abuse are prescription narcotics, but abuse of alcohol and benzodiazepines is also quite common in chronic pain patients. Full-blown **major depression** is common. In fact, the presence of depressive symptoms at some point in the course of chronic pain is nearly universal. **Secondary social problems,** such as family tensions and breakups, loss of social supports, vocational difficulties, and financial problems, commonly result from chronic pain. This type of psychosocial disruption often makes it more difficult for patients to comply with medical management and adapt to chronic pain.

Another way that psychological factors can play a role in chronic pain is by providing **secondary gain** (see Box 12–3). A patient might enjoy getting solicitous attention from family, friends, and physicians; might be relieved to have fewer demands made on him or her at work; or might discover that he or she is eligible for medical disability and can afford to stay home with young children. Factors of secondary gain will interfere with a patient's motivation to make a full adjustment to the pain syndrome, because the gratifications or gains provided by being sick or disabled can outweigh, in the patient's mind, the gratification of making a more successful adaptation.

Interview

All patients with chronic pain require a thorough medical and psychiatric evaluation. It is important for the physician to take a detailed history of the

---

BOX 12–3. Primary and Secondary Gain From Being Ill

Primary gain and secondary gain are terms that were introduced by Sigmund Freud and that remain highly relevant to medical practice today. Primary gain is a situation in which unconscious psychological factors play a role in causing an illness or a symptom. The physical symptoms are psychologically determined and are seen as a response to an unconscious conflict. For example, patients with conversion symptoms express unconscious desires, fears, and conflicts in physical symptoms (see Chapter 10, Somatoform and Factitious Disorders).

A young man who is right-handed develops a functional paralysis of his right arm after having an argument with his father. Though the young man loves his father and feels he should be respectful toward him, he is also very angry. Deep down, he has fantasies of striking his father and severely injuring him, perhaps even killing him. These thoughts are unacceptable or "conflictual" to the young man because they are in conflict both with his love for his father and with his own internal code of good behavior. Because of their unacceptable or conflictual nature, the fantasies remain unconscious, repressed, and out of his awareness. Instead, the young man develops a functional paralysis of his arm, as if to ensure his unconscious mind that he is incapable of hitting his father, while at the same time he punishes himself for his unacceptable unconscious impulses by weakening himself. All of this goes on outside of the young man's awareness. When he presents to the emergency room, he truly will not know why his arm has become paralyzed.

Secondary gain refers to the benefits a patient is able to glean from an illness or a symptom. These benefits or gains are considered "secondary" because they develop after the illness or symptom presents and because they are not part of the etiology of the condition. Secondary gain can powerfully affect the course of a medical condition by interfering, more or less directly, with the patient's motivation to make a rapid or full recovery.

Examples of secondary gain from illness include the "taken-for-granted" homemaker who gets extra attention and affection from her husband and children when she develops viral pneumonia, the "stretched-too-thin" business executive who obtains a sanctioned reprieve from her professional and family responsibilities during medical hospitalization for acute appendicitis, and the "at-the-end-of-my-rope" paralegal who is working at two jobs and who receives workers' compensation benefits after a freak accident in his work place leaves him with a concussion.

It can be helpful to think of the secondary gain of medical illness in terms of patients' efforts to cope by getting what they can out of the situation they find themselves in. This approach implies that secondary gain is not the cause of illness, avoiding the customary confusion that to talk about secondary gain is to say that the medical condition is "psychogenic." This approach also avoids the accusatory tone frequently used when it is recognized that factors of secondary gain are playing a powerful role in the course of a patient's medical condition.

While, by definition, secondary gain is never the cause of physical illness, in many circumstances it can interfere with recovery from and adaptation to illness, in both the acute and chronic setting. As a result, while patients are largely unaware of the role that secondary gain may be playing in their illness, it is the job of the treating psychiatrist or general practitioner to identify these factors. In this extremely common clinical situation, it is the physician's goal to be aware of and try to minimize internal resistances on the patient's part that conflict with his or her motivation to make the fullest possible recovery. The need for this type of intervention should be assessed in all patients suffering from physical illness.

---

quality of the pain and the functional and psychosocial impairment that it causes. Patients should also be asked about past and present symptoms of depression and about abuse of narcotics, benzodiazepines, alcohol, and other substances. This inquiry is best prefaced by explaining that these are routine complications of chronic pain. The physician might say, "Many people suffering from chronic pain turn to narcotics, tranquilizers, or alcohol to help them get by. What has your experience been?"

Patients with chronic pain often do not appear to be in pain and do not have the signs of autonomic arousal characteristic of patients with acute pain. These factors can lead the physician (and others) to believe mistakenly that the pain is not "real" and to assume that the patient is malingering or suffering from a primary psychiatric disorder. Many chronic pain patients are sensitive about this and enter the physician-patient relationship with a chip on their shoulder. When interviewing chronic pain patients, physicians should emphasize that they understand that the patient's pain is genuine. The physician may say, "I know that many people with chronic pain have the experience of being told that their pain isn't real or that it's 'all in their heads.' I want to assure you that I know your pain is very real, as is your suffering."

Management

Patients and physicians must have realistic expectations about the treatment of chronic pain. Otherwise, both are likely to become frustrated and disappointed. The physician should tell the patient that he or she understands the magnitude of the problem and the difficulties of treatment. It is helpful to mix **encouragement** with **tempered expectations.** Patients can be helped to anticipate a positive outcome but should also know that the work will proceed slowly and the gains will be hard-won. After consulting with the fireman described above for the first time, the psychiatrist said, "I am confident that I can help you get back on your feet. But you have to expect that things will improve slowly and at the price of a fair amount of hard work and perseverance on your part. If you are able to accept this, you will be successful."

Patients should be educated about the role of psychological factors in the exacerbation of pain and the need to include these factors in the treatment plan. They should be helped to understand that secondary depression and substance abuse are common complications that must be treated. It is extremely important to emphasize that attending to psychological factors does not mean that the patient is weak or that the pain is not real. Over time, it will be necessary to help the patient make the transition from looking for a cure to managing with and adapting to a chronic problem.

Most patients with chronic pain require years, if not a lifetime, of treatment. As a result, most physicians try, if at all possible, to avoid prescribing narcotics for these patients because they inevitably develop tolerance to narcotics with extended use and require increased dosages over time. Many treatment programs begin with discontinuation of narcotics and other substances. Tricyclic antidepressants (TCAs) are frequently prescribed instead, along with nonsteroidal anti-inflammatory agents. Anticonvulsants are sometimes prescribed because they appear to be especially effective for neuralgia, such as postherpetic or trigeminal neuralgia.

The use of **antidepressants** as analgesics is often a cause for confusion for patients and physicians. It may be unclear whether pain or depression is being treated. It has been clearly demonstrated that TCAs have analgesic effects that are independent of their antidepressant properties and that they can be effective in a wide variety of pain syndromes. Chronic pain patients who are not depressed are still able to benefit from the analgesic effects of antidepressants. TCAs tend to be particularly effective in the management of neuropathic pain, headache, facial pain, and arthritis. It is important to emphasize that the medication is being used as an analgesic, not as an antidepressant. Otherwise, the patient may feel misunderstood and even insulted, thinking that the physician secretly believes that the patient is depressed or that the pain is "all in the patient's head."

Confusion often exists about which antidepressants are most effective as analgesics and which dosages should be used. Many of the early studies focused on amitriptyline, but it has now been established that desipramine is equally effective. Clomipramine has also been widely and successfully used, and most, if not all, of the other TCAs are effective, as well. For many patients, particularly elderly or medically ill patients, desipramine and nortriptyline are better tolerated than amitriptyline and the other TCAs because both are much less sedating and have much less anticholinergic effect. (Desipramine has the least anticholinergic effect of all the TCAs, and nortriptyline causes the least amount of orthostatic hypotension.)

In selecting an antidepressant to use as an analgesic, the physician might want to choose among desipramine, nortriptyline, imipramine, or amitriptyline, according to the side effect profile. The efficacy of the selective serotonin reuptake inhibitors (SSRIs) in the treatment of chronic pain remains equivocal. SSRIs are generally not used as first-line medications for analgesia in the treatment of chronic pain. For at least some patients, antidepressant medications are effective as analgesics at approximately half of the standard antidepressant dosage, but other patients may require the full antidepressant dose.

➦ The psychiatrist prescribed a TCA for the fireman with low back pain described above, both to treat depression and to provide analgesia. The psychiatrist opted for desipramine, taken at bedtime and gradually increased to full antidepressant doses. The psychiatrist also prescribed low dosages of the benzodiazepine lorazepam on a short-term basis to reduce the patient's anxiety and help him sleep at night.

The patient's self-esteem began to return as his depression resolved and as he began to be more active and take on more responsibility. As he and his wife began to communicate more directly, she was better able to provide emotional support and help him adjust to his chronic pain. When he started to feel better, his motivation to comply with physical therapy and exercise increased greatly, and he undertook an ambitious exercise program. Exercise and antidepressants for analgesia made his pain more bearable and contributed to his overall adjustment to his condition. By taking a biopsychosocial approach and addressing the patient's difficulties from as many angles as possible, the psychiatrist was able to help him successfully cope with and ultimately adapt to his physical condition and the psychosocial changes it brought.

It became clear, in the course of the patient's treatment, that secondary gain had contributed to his difficulty in adapting to his chronic back pain. In the end, the patient did not return to the fire department, even though he was offered a desk job. He opted, instead, for long-term disability. When it became apparent that he would not be returning to his job, the patient, in fact, felt quite relieved. Over time, he acknowledged that in recent years he had become progressively disenchanted with the fire department and unhappy in his job. He had very much wanted to move to another less expensive, less hectic region of the country but had felt obliged to remain with the fire department until he reached retirement. Perhaps most important to the patient, his daughter was about to begin college, and he did not want her to move far away to attend school.

Leaving the fire department and being on disability meant that the patient could afford to sell his house and relocate his family to a small southern town that afforded the less harried, less expensive life-style for which he had been yearning. The move also enabled his daughter to attend the college of her choice and still live at home. This outcome is an example of secondary gain. The patient was able to take advantage of the opportunity afforded by his back injury and pain and to get out of a situation in which he felt trapped, namely, a job that he wanted to leave and that deprived him of the freedom to relocate with his daughter. That the patient obtained such benefits from his illness in no way implies that factors of secondary gain were the cause of his chronic pain or that he was malingering. Rather, the patient had a physical problem that, in the end, gave him certain advantages, or, to put it another way, he simply made the best of a bad situation. On the other hand, the difficulties the patient faced in adapting to his pain were increased by the role the pain played in offering the patient a way out of an oppressive situation.

If the patient had been told that he was eligible for long-term disability only for as long as he remained severely disabled, it probably would have been much more difficult for him to make the kind of physical and psychological progress that he did. If this had been the case, the physician would have done well to intervene, with the goal of minimizing the patient's internal resistance to making the fullest possible recovery. His dissatisfaction with his job and with the prospect of separating from his daughter would have to be addressed, which would entail exploring the aspects of these situations that were hard for him. Such a line of inquiry would probably lead to a new and deeper understanding of his feelings about his job and his daughter's leaving home. Such an understanding may in itself make a situation more acceptable to a patient; insight into a problem can be enough to reduce the gratification a patient obtains from being ill and can facilitate physical improvement and adaptation. In many cases, however, understanding is only the first step in the intervention. It is often also necessary to actively help patients to find practical solutions to their problems that do not rely on ongoing, severe physical and psychological disability.

Two years after he first met with the psychiatrist, the patient sent her a New Year's card to thank her and to say that he and his family were doing well. He wrote that he had come to see his back pain as a chronic disability that he could live with. He was no longer depressed or anxious but continued to take desipramine for analgesia. He expressed satisfaction in having been able to adjust to his pain physically and psychologically, and he reported that he was enjoying his new life.

Unfortunately, treatment does not always proceed so smoothly. It is worth noting that the patient in this case had a number of important factors working in his favor. He had always functioned well in the past. He had a good work history and a good history of close, long-lasting relationships with others. Though he had psychological conflicts around separation and masculinity, he had a healthy, well-integrated personality. He had a number of excellent social supports, including a loving wife and daughter who were willing to support him emotionally and financially for as long as he needed. He had been employed at the same job for 25 years and had excellent medical and disability benefits. Even at his lowest point, he did not develop problems with substance abuse, other than taking a little extra codeine.

When patients first develop a pain syndrome, they almost always take it for granted that the pain will go away (i.e., that it will either resolve on its own or that a cure will be found). Over time, as the pain does not improve, many patients become depressed and anxious. Preoccupation with the pain is common, and many patients appear to be hypochondriacal. During this phase, patients often visit many physicians. While the process described thus far could apply to a patient diagnosed with any chronic illness, chronic pain patients tend to have a particular experience as they go from physician to physician. Each new physician makes new promises and offers new hopes for relief, but, ultimately, all of these "fall through." This process happens over and over again, leading the patient to feel increasingly disappointed, frustrated, depressed, and angry.

The physician often has the same experience as the patient. There are initial feelings of optimism and hope of being able to succeed where previous physicians have failed, but these give way to feelings of increasing frustration and disappointment as all efforts fail to provide the patient with significant relief. It is not uncommon at this point for physicians to lose interest in the patient and to withdraw from the patient's care. The patient may experience this withdrawal as a painful rejection. Physicians may even respond to the situation by blaming the patient, becoming suspicious that the patient's pain is not "real" or that the patient "doesn't want to get well."

PSYCHOLOGICAL ASPECTS OF HIV INFECTION AND AIDS
Clinical Features

Human immunodeficiency virus (HIV) infection and acquired immunodeficiency syndrome (AIDS) can cause extremely powerful psychological reactions in patients, their families and support networks, their health care providers, and the population at large. All of these people are profoundly affected by HIV infection, though in different ways. Many factors contribute to the emotional reactions brought about by HIV-related disorders. HIV infection frequently ends in devastating physical deterioration; HIV tends to affect young people who are often in their prime; HIV infection is contagious; and the primary route of transmission is through sexual contact. The relative ineffectiveness of currently available measures for the prevention and treatment of HIV infection also plays a role. All of these factors touch people's deepest fears. Because the populations at highest risk include homosexual men, intravenous drug abusers, and prostitutes, some people's reactions are colored by biases against these groups.

When a person learns that he or she is infected with HIV, the person goes through many of the psychological and emotional reactions already discussed in this chapter. Shock and denial, often followed by anxiety and depression, are common. These reactions can be complicated by the patient's previous experiences with HIV infection and AIDS, especially the loss of close friends and lovers to the disease, and by feelings about having infected or been infected by loved ones. For men who are not open about their homosexuality, HIV infection can raise the issue of talking honestly about their sexuality with family and friends for the first time. This dilemma is particularly painful for the married homosexual or bisexual man and his family. As with other illnesses for which there are major behavioral risk factors, the initial reaction often includes guilt, remorse, and blaming of others.

With help from health care providers and a solid support network, many people with HIV infection are able to cope with the diagnosis and with physical symptoms as they develop. Initial distress gradually gives way to more successful methods of coping. Emotional ups and downs are common, with periods of successful adaptation interrupted by episodes of greater distress. The period of initial testing and diagnosis is always a particularly stressful time. Psychological distress and difficulty in coping are also common during periods of physical decline or the onset of new physical symptoms. Some HIV-positive individuals may feel overwhelmed when friends or lovers die of AIDS.

HIV-infected patients can be expected to feel overwhelmed at times, but it is not "normal" for them to develop a major psychiatric disorder. Despite the potentially catastrophic stresses presented by AIDS, most people are able to cope. Patients who are unable to cope or who present with psychiatric symptoms require aggressive evaluation and treatment.

Interview

When interviewing a patient with HIV infection or AIDS, the physician should be supportive and encouraging but not unrealistic or unduly cheerful. Optimism appropriate to the limits of the patient's medical condition should be encouraged. The emphasis should be on new treatments, improved longevity, and ongoing research. This perspective is especially appropriate with asymptomatic individuals, who often have many years of good physical health ahead of them before they become ill. Because patients may be concerned about being stigmatized or isolated, physicians must communicate in their attitudes and behavior that they neither fear nor blame the patient. Physicians should make it clear that they will stick by patients throughout the illness. This commitment is one of the most powerful forms of support that physicians can offer.

All patients need to be **educated** about their disease. It is crucial to be clear about how the virus spreads and give recommendations about safe sexual practices and the handling of bodily fluids. Patients and their families are at risk for being too cautious, as well as not cautious enough. For example, when one patient found out about his HIV status, he stopped having any physical contact with his wife, who was HIV-negative, opting even to sleep in a separate room. He felt desperately guilty about having contracted the virus, which he expressed by physically isolating himself. Both the patient and his wife

were relieved when, with reassurance and encouragement from their physician, they resumed safe physical contact.

Denial is often part of the coping strategy that people use in response to HIV infection. When denial appears to be adaptive, it should be supported. Some newly diagnosed HIV-positive individuals may become extremely health-conscious, believing that if they take good care of themselves, they can be able to "beat" the illness. While such behaviors may not have physical benefits, they may be helpful psychologically. This type of denial can make it easier for patients to cope and helps them to feel more optimistic and in control of what is happening to them. It can also be maladaptive because patients may be so convinced that a healthy life-style will protect them from becoming ill that they will refuse all conventional medical treatments. Maladaptive denial requires tactful, systematic intervention. In an ongoing physician-patient relationship, patients should be gradually encouraged to entertain the possibility that they may remain vulnerable to illness and that they may do well to cooperate with conventional treatments.

While denial is to be respected, there are times when a patient is interested in facing issues more directly and may want to air grief or fears with the physician. The physician should indicate a **readiness to listen** and directly encourage the patient to open up about what the patient is thinking and feeling. To the patient with AIDS who has been admitted to the hospital with pneumocystic pneumonia, one might say, "I get the impression that you're feeling worried about the road ahead. Do you think it would help to talk with me about it, maybe get some of it off your chest?" Reaching out to a patient in this way can be difficult. Sometimes it is harder for the physician to reach out than it is for the patient to open up because the feelings involved may be extremely painful, not only for the patient but also for the physician. The physician may simultaneously feel empathy for the patient's suffering and overwhelmed by the limitations of the medical treatments available. As in chronic illness, it is important not to underestimate the healing power for the patient of sharing painful emotions with a caring physician. Even when only a little reassurance can be honestly offered, simple acknowledgment of the painful situation and a willingness to listen to and sit with the patient can be enormously supportive.

For most patients, a **solid support network** is essential for coping with HIV infection, both emotionally and practically. The physician should be familiar with the supports available to the patient. Time should be set aside to meet with the patient's primary support persons to gain information, give advice, and help them to feel more supported. The patient's illness will generate powerful feelings in people close to the patient. Universal fears of physical deterioration, helplessness, and death will be superimposed on grief over the potential loss of a loved one and practical concerns about caring for the patient during the course of the illness. Caregivers may suffer from concerns, often unrealistic, about being infected during their contacts with the patient. HIV carries a stigma for some people, which can make it harder for them to be supportive. All of this can interfere with the optimal mobilization of support networks.

Many patients become involved in community-based organizations such as the Gay Men's Health Crisis. Such groups can provide emotional support formally through support groups and informally through involvement in projects and community services. Physicians should be familiar with the resources in their area and should encourage patients to take advantage of them.

Management

Although most patients are able to cope with HIV infection and AIDS, adjustment disorders are relatively common. Patients are vulnerable to the entire spectrum of psychiatric disorders, including affective, anxiety, and psychotic disorders. It is always necessary to do a workup to look for physical causes of a change in mental status. Physical or mental symptoms that appear to be due to psychological causes often prove to have an organic etiology.

Adjustment disorders usually respond well to **supportive psychotherapy.** Anxiolytic medications can be used as an adjunct when treating patients who are acutely anxious. In a supportive setting, the patient and therapist should work together to clarify the psychosocial factors contributing to the present psychological difficulties. Strategies for more effective coping should be developed. The goals of treatment are to enhance the patient's ability to cope by bolstering his or her defenses and shoring up social supports. Patients should be helped to feel more in control of themselves and their lives.

All major psychiatric disturbances, including mood, anxiety, and psychotic disorders, whether they are considered to have a general medical or psychological etiology, should be treated aggressively. In addition to treating any underlying medical conditions that appear to be contributing to the psychiatric symptoms, appropriate psychoactive medications should be used in conjunction with supportive counseling to target specific symptoms.

Current clinical practice favors the use of the **selective serotonin reuptake inhibitors** for depression in HIV-infected individuals. SSRIs have relatively few side effects, even in patients who may be physically and cognitively compromised. As patients become increasingly physically compromised, they usually require lower dosages of antidepressants. In terminally ill patients who are suffering from depression, **psychostimulants** are often used instead of conventional antidepressants. Psychostimulants have a rapid rate of onset and few side effects. For anxiety, the **shorter-acting benzodiazepines,** such as lorazepam, given at fairly low dosages, are the medications of choice for patients who are relatively physi-

cally healthy. In medically compromised patients, benzodiazepines may cause paradoxical agitation, behavioral disinhibition, confusion, intolerable sedation, or delirium. For these patients, relatively low dosages of high-potency antipsychotics are often better tolerated and more effective.

HIV-infected patients presenting with paranoid or psychotic symptoms should be treated with antipsychotic medications. **Antipsychotics** are also the medications of choice for patients with HIV-related dementia who present with agitation. It is especially important to rule out a potentially treatable physical etiology in HIV-positive patients presenting with paranoid or psychotic symptoms, as such symptoms are relatively common presentations of central nervous system disease in these patients.

Patients with HIV who are not suffering from an acute psychiatric disorder and who have relatively intact cognitive function may benefit from **insight-oriented psychotherapy.** Therapy usually focuses on helping patients grasp what the illness means to them; working through feelings of anger, guilt, and loss; and discussing concerns related to death and dying. This type of therapy typically relies more on interaction with the therapist and more direct support from the therapist than traditional insight-oriented psychotherapy.

Taking care of HIV-infected patients makes many demands on physicians and medical students. Fear of infection is common, especially when health care workers are first beginning to take care of these patients. A needle-stick can generate anxiety, depression, and resentment in health care providers. Caring for patients with HIV when they are sick is highly labor-intensive, and most patients ultimately die, despite all efforts. This prognosis can be extremely demoralizing for physicians, especially those working with large numbers of AIDS patients. Many HIV-infected patients are young. It is natural for medical students and the house staff to identify with such patients, which leads to sadness and even guilt when efforts to help the patient fail.

In order to defend against these painful feelings, physicians sometimes get angry at the HIV-infected patient and blame the patient for his or her illness. In this setting, the physician will often focus on the patient's participation in unsafe sexual practices, use of illicit drugs, or prostitution. The implication in this line of thinking is that "It's the patient's fault that he or she is suffering from this dread disease. Because this is so, I do not need to feel as sad and guilty about having so little to offer this patient, and I do not need to worry about the same thing happening to me." HIV-positive patients who are homosexuals, drug abusers, or prostitutes often stir up greater anger than patients with other illnesses who have participated in high-risk behaviors (e.g., cardiac patients who smoke cigarettes), which reflects the deep-seated, often unconscious biases against these groups held by many physicians.

In order to deal effectively with the emotional challenges of taking care of HIV-infected patients, physicians need to be honest with themselves. There is a tendency to feel that all negative or fearful feelings toward patients are unacceptable and should be kept secret. To the contrary, it is natural to have strong feelings about certain patients. It is extremely helpful to share these feelings with others, especially with colleagues and mentors. This type of discussion can serve as a source of emotional support for physicians who are caring for HIV-infected patients and mitigates feelings of isolation and demoralization. Open discussion also offers an opportunity for physicians to confront subtle biases that they may hold against certain groups of patients.

Taking certain practical steps will help health care providers feel more comfortable and less threatened by patients infected with HIV. Precautions for avoiding infection should be followed carefully and consistently with all patients. Occasionally, physicians who are trying to deny their feelings about taking care of HIV-positive patients will take a cavalier attitude and flaunt precautions. This behavior is a dangerous, ineffective way to deal with feelings of anxiety, guilt, and anger. If infection due to a needle-stick occurs, psychological counseling and education about the actual risks of infection under the circumstances can be helpful. If a health care provider suffers from a preoccupation about being exposed to HIV or develops hypochondriacal concerns, education and counseling are indicated.

Selected Readings

Cohen-Cole, S. A., C. Haupe. Diagnostic assessment of depression in the medically ill. *In* Stoudemire, A. S., and B. S. Fogel, eds. Principles of Medical Psychiatry. Orlando, Florida, Grune and Stratton, 1987.

Docherty, J. P., S. J. Fiester. The therapeutic alliance and compliance with psychopharmacology. *In* Hales, R. E., and A. J. Frances, eds. American Psychiatric Association Annual Review. Washington, D. C., American Psychiatric Press, 1985.

Fogel, B. S., C. Martin. Personality disorders in the medical setting. *In* Stoudemire, A. S., and B. S. Fogel, eds. Principles of Medical Psychiatry. Orlando, Florida, Grune and Stratton, 1987.

Geringer, E. S., T. A. Stern. Coping with medical illness: the impact of personality types. Psychosomatics 27:251–261, 1986.

Kahana, R. J., G. L. Bibring. Personality types in medical management. *In* Zinberg, N., ed. Psychiatry and Medical Practice in a General Hospital. New York, International Universities Press, 1964.

Irwin, M. R., H. Strausbaugh. Stress and immune changes in humans: a biopsychosocial model. *In* Gorman, J. M., and R. M. Kertzner, eds. Psychoimmunology Update. Washington, D. C., American Psychiatric Press, 1991.

Molnar, G., G. A. Fava. Intercurrent medical illness in the schizophrenic patient. *In* Stoudemire, A. S., and B. S. Fogel, eds. Principles of Medical Psychiatry. Orlando, Florida, Grune and Stratton, 1987.

Stoudemire, A. S., M. B. Moran, and B. S. Fogel. Psychopharmacology in the medically ill patient. *In* Schatzberg, A. F., and C. B. Nereroff, eds. The American Psychiatric Press Textbook of Psychopharmacology. Washington, D. C., American Psychiatric Press, 1995.

Stoudemire, A. S., T. L. Thompson. Medication noncompliance: systematic approaches to evaluation and intervention. General Hospital Psychiatry 5:233–239, 1983.

CHAPTER THIRTEEN

LIFE DEVELOPMENT

JONATHAN A. SLATER, MD
AND JANIS L. CUTLER, MD

Although psychiatrists are still a long way from being able to describe all of the functions of the human mind, they do understand some of the patterns of emotions, thoughts, and behaviors that occur throughout the life cycle as part of normal human development, as well as the impact of disruptive events experienced during the different developmental stages. These events may contribute to the production of psychiatric symptoms, which may appear at the time the events occur or at later stages of life. Being able to view individual patients and their problems within the context of their emotional development over their life span helps physicians understand the normal challenges that all patients face at different developmental stages, the disruptive experiences that can produce psychiatric disorders, and the treatments that can help them.

A nearly infinite number of tasks accompany the complex development of human beings. Of primary importance are the tasks pertaining to emotional, social, and cognitive function, gender identity, and sexuality at each stage of life.

The tasks naturally change as the individual passes through infancy, the toddler years, the preschool years, the latency years, adolescence, adulthood, and old age. The somewhat arbitrary and oversimplified divisions of the life cycle into childhood, adolescence, and adulthood are best understood as general stages that overlap with one another rather than as phases that have discrete beginnings and endings. For example, the transition into puberty usually occurs over 1–2 years and not instantaneously, as one might conclude from a schematic discussion. Just as the time of each stage overlaps and varies from person to person, so do the developmental categories, particularly those of social, emotional, and cognitive development. In order to understand the developmental vulnerabilities inherent in each stage that may affect a person's response to illness or give rise to psychiatric disorders, it is first necessary to know what the normal developmental progression of each stage is.

NORMAL AND ABNORMAL LIFE DEVELOPMENT
Approach to the Study of Development

In almost all medical schools, the first year's curriculum focuses on normal anatomy and physiology and later, in the second year, moves on to the study of pathology and pathophysiology. This sequence helps the student distinguish illness from health (i.e., make a diagnosis), predict the effects of diseases on patients, and suggest treatment strategies. In general medicine, for example, the student learns that in order to treat a patient with hypotension, he or she needs to know what level of cardiac output is necessary for normal cardiovascular functioning (i.e., for providing adequate oxygenation of essential organs). When a patient presents to the emergency room complaining of lightheadedness and has extremely low, barely detectable blood pressure, the physician must be able to recognize that this hypotensive patient is ill and that the immediate effect of hypotension is impaired oxygenation of vital organs, including the brain, which explains the initial complaint. The physician must also know that other effects, such as kidney damage, can be predicted if the hypotension is not immediately corrected. This knowledge allows the physician to appreciate the urgency of recommending the necessary treatment strategy, which would include giving intravenous fluids to increase the blood pressure.

In psychiatry, this approach is no less essential, although somewhat more complicated. Psychiatrists are not able to fully describe normal brain function even as it relates to basic behaviors. They also do not understand all of the determinants of an individual's emotional life or of such complex behaviors as falling in love, grieving, and developing and maintaining social relationships. However, they understand a great deal about patterns of normal mental functioning, particularly psychosocial patterns that occur throughout the life cycle. Just as other physicians must understand patterns of health and illness, psychiatrists must understand psychosocial patterns in order to recognize psychiatric illnesses, predict the effects of these illnesses, and suggest treatment strategies.

➡ For example, a previously bright, happy 17-year-old adolescent boy became withdrawn, moody, and uncommunicative with his parents after his girlfriend broke up with him. After several months, he confided to his school guidance counselor that he had become terrified that he was in danger because he heard voices of people he never saw telling him they were going to kill him. These auditory hallucinations are a sign of illness. Although his withdrawal may have been a normal reaction to losing his girlfriend, this psychotic symptom is not normal and indicates that a psychiatric disorder is present. The counselor referred the young man to a psychiatrist, who first made a diagnosis of a psychotic disorder and then drew on an understanding of the particular psychosocial issues that adolescents face. He realized that the young man would be especially concerned about being different from his friends because he desperately wanted their approval and about requiring help from his parents because he was in the throes of trying to separate from them. A comprehensive treatment approach would include supportive psychotherapy that addresses these issues, in addition to antipsychotic medication. ◀

➡ In another case, the new parents of twins (who were the products of in vitro fertilization) were thrilled that their years of financial and emotional sacrifice had finally resulted in beautiful, healthy babies, who were their first children. Three months after giving birth, the 29-year-old mother reluctantly divulged the following information in response to prodding from her obstetrician, who was concerned that she looked listless and weighed 10 pounds less than she had at the time of conception. The woman said that she had been constantly exhausted but unable to sleep despite having full-time live-in help with the babies, she had no appetite and could not force herself to eat, and, worst of all for her, she derived no pleasure from being with the babies and avoided picking them up because she was preoccupied with worries that she would harm them. The obstetrician realized that this pattern was more serious than the frequently observed "postpartum blues," which resolves with reassurance, and appropriately diagnosed a major depressive episode. The obstetrician understood that this new mother felt extremely guilty that she was not interested in these much-longed-for babies. Guilt was one aspect of the particular effect that depression was having on this woman at this specific point in her life cycle. The psychiatric treatment for her depression could not occur in a vacuum but would have to take into account her life situation and its meaning to her. A developmentally informed understanding would suggest that a brief hospitalization would relieve the mother of her moment-to-moment guilt about not caring for the babies. It would also be helpful to reframe her lack of interest as an *inability* to be interested because of her current psychiatrically ill state. ◀

Patterns of Development

Psychological development occurs at different rates during the various stages of life. From infancy through young adulthood, mental functioning is characterized by enormous change and progression, and major shifts in functioning can occur virtually overnight. Rapid progression in one area is associated with stress, and often causes regression, in another area. For example, a previously even-tempered 3-year-old might abruptly, and seemingly without effort, give up her diapers but then almost immediately become much more clinging and dependent, a phenomenon that can be quite confusing to unsuspecting parents.

Although abrupt discontinuities are characteristic of the development of children and adolescents, one continuous aspect of their behavior is supplied by their individual temperament (see Chapter 8, Personality Disorders). **Temperament,** which is generally considered to be inherited, is observable at birth in the way a person tends to behave. For example, an infant who has a tendency to become hyperaroused in response to novel stimuli may manifest this tendency in somewhat different ways at various developmental stages and even as a pathology at a later stage of life. Thus, a person who has behavioral inhibition as an infant may have intense stranger anxiety as a 1-year-old, school phobia as a 6-year-old, and a vulnerability to panic attacks as an adult. Other traits that are fairly continuous over developmental periods are intelligence, superior motor coordination, musical talent, and a predisposition to certain illnesses.

Adults tend to have more stable and persistent emotional lives than do children and adolescents. Shifts and adjustments usually occur gradually in adults and their development can be seen in slowly evolving patterns.

Effects of Stress and Trauma on Development

Everyone encounters periods throughout the life cycle of particular emotional vulnerability to certain stressful and traumatic events. When such events occur during vulnerable stages of childhood, they may profoundly affect the developmental course of that person's life. Physical illness and the loss of a parent are particularly severe stresses for most children and adolescents. For example, children who are hospitalized many times before age 4 years seem to have a higher incidence of emotional problems later in life. Repeated hospitalizations later in the course of development do not seem to have the same lasting effects.

Regression, which is the reappearance of behaviors and coping mechanisms that were used at a younger age, is a common response to stress for children as well as adults. Regression can occur in one or more areas of functioning. For example, a 5-year-old boy who had remained dry at night for over a year began wetting his bed when his parents separated but otherwise moved ahead in his daily life at school and with friends. Periods of developmental vulnerability may be associated with the first appearance of psychiatric disorders, which may be identified during childhood or later in life.

PSYCHODYNAMIC THEORY

The principles of psychodynamic theory provide a useful framework for understanding the tasks of normal developmental progression as well as the occurrence of psychiatric symptoms (see also the discussion of psychodynamics in Chapter 2, The Psychiatric Interview). Two basic principles of psychodynamic theory are that all human beings have unconscious thoughts, feelings, fantasies, and desires and that early experiences influence later emotional development.

The field of psychoanalysis was founded by **Sigmund Freud,** who was a neurologist by training, in an effort to relieve his patients of symptoms for which no physiological etiology could be identified. Freud's unified approach to the mind attempted to explain normal emotional development as well as psychopathology. He used two related hypothetical models of the mind: the topographical model and the structural model. The **topographical model** has three entities: the unconscious, the conscious, and the preconscious. A "repressive barrier" maintains a strict separation between the unconscious and the preconscious, but the boundary between the preconscious and the conscious is fluid. (One common example of this fluidity is the experience of having a word "on the tip of one's tongue" and then retrieving it into conscious awareness.) According to the topographical model, psychiatric symptoms are a "compromise solution" to an otherwise unresolvable conflict between unconscious wishes and desires (i.e., the pleasure principle) and conscious awareness of social and cultural limits on the gratification of those wishes and desires (i.e., the reality principle).

The **structural model** of the mind is also comprised of three entities, the id, ego, and superego, but it is more complex than the topographical model (see also Chapter 2, The Psychiatric Interview). The **id** represents the unconscious drives, particularly those of a sexual and aggressive nature; the **ego** modulates between the unconscious drives, the external world, and the superego; and the **superego** is the conscience (i.e., guilt) and the ego ideal (i.e., what one would like to become). In its modulating role, the ego functions both consciously and unconsciously, providing reality testing, memory, intelligence, language, and defense mechanisms. **Defense mechanisms** are unconscious mental "reframings" of perceptions and feelings to make them more palatable and less anxiety-provoking. For purposes of enhanced communication between physicians, defense mechanisms have been divided into various types (see Chapter 2, The Psychiatric Interview). These mechanisms are crucial to normal mental functioning, but they may also be maladaptive and contribute to the development of psychiatric symptoms and personality disorders (see Chapter 8, Personality Disorders). Much of child and adolescent psychosocial development can be understood in terms of the growing maturity and flexibility of the ego as it gains more control over sexual and aggressive impulses.

The **object relations** model has been described as an alternative view of the workings of the mind. Many psychiatrists view this model as complementary to the structural (ego psychology) model. The object relations approach conceptualizes psychic structures as the internalized characteristics of important people, or "objects," in an individual's life. *Object,* a much used, widely accepted but unfortunate, depersonalizing choice of words, is the psychiatric term for another person.

The following case illustrates how an object relations approach may be applied. ➡ The guilt-ridden, depressed mother of infant twins, who was described above, was experiencing a conflict between her ego ideal, which was to be a perfect, all-loving, nurturing mother, and her ego's perception of herself as a "bad" mother. This perception was distorted by a depressed mood, which is an impairment in one aspect of ego functioning. According to the object relations model, the guilt with which she was plagued can be associated with her internalized image of a harsh, critical parental figure and a perception of herself as an angry, needy child. Therefore, her aggressive wishes toward the infants were met with guilt and self-hatred. This approach does not deny the possibility of a biological basis for her depression, which may have been precipitated by the abrupt hormonal changes characteristic of the postpartum state. It is an additional perspective that helps both the physician and patient to understand the current emotional and cognitive experience of the patient and the ways in which her depression may have been perpetuated or exacerbated. ⬅ This approach is useful for a developmental perspective on normal mental functioning as well as on psychopathology.

INFANCY: BIRTH TO 12 MONTHS OF AGE
Developmental Progression
Attachment

The nature of the newborn infant's first task is social: to ensure the devoted attention of a loving caretaker. Infants seem to enter the world with the genetically determined ability to gain such attention, first by crying and later by using facial expressions, especially eye contact, to actively engage and hold the interest of others. Infants selectively attend to the human face and voice over other competing stimuli and are apparently biologically programmed for the interplay between themselves and caregivers.

Adults seem to respond instinctually to the infant's efforts, adjusting their voices and facial expressions to imitate those of the infant. As the infant be-

Chapter 13 Life Development 249

comes more alert and curious about his or her surroundings at approximately 2 months of age, parents perceive the infant as behaving "more like a baby." The infant's increased eye contact and vocalizations and, most importantly, **social smile** in response to a human face feel like a well-deserved reward to the parents for the sleepless nights and endless diapers. Infants keep their caretakers involved—in fact, captivated—by their developmental progression. Videorecording of infants and their caretakers has recently elucidated the remarkable subtlety and harmony of the early social interaction between parents and infant.

An impaired infant (e.g., an autistic infant who avoids eye contact) does not elicit the same degree of bonding from the caretaker. In the past, this lack of parental responsiveness was mistakenly seen as the cause of autism, but it is now recognized that autism is a primary neurological condition that has secondary effects on the parent-child relationship.

Affect Regulation

The infant has several specific needs that must be met by the caretaker. First, the infant requires physical sustenance in the form of nourishment, cleanliness, and warmth. The infant's emotional needs are at least as important. A crucial role of the caretaker is to modulate the intensity of the child's feelings. The caregiver's empathic responsiveness guides the child toward the appropriate emotional response and appropriate amplitude of response. The infant smiles, and the parent smiles back. A mother calms her infant's harsh cries with soft soliloquy and gentle stroking. In such ways, infants turn to their caregivers for the soothing that they are innately receptive to, facilitating their developing capacity for self-regulation.

The infant also follows the caretaker's cues to learn to identify emotions and associate them with specific types of experiences in an appropriate way. Emotional signals are used extensively in the infant-caregiver relationship. Consistent nurturing by an empathic caregiver allows the infant to develop trust in an environment in which emotional and physical needs are met. Adequate responsiveness by the caregiver is necessary for the child to develop what **Erik Erikson** has referred to as **basic trust,** a precursor to the development of a sense of identity and mastery (i.e., the feeling of being essentially "all right"). This reciprocal relationship also lays the groundwork for the development of empathy.

By the second half of the first year, infants seem to have realized that they can share their inner emotional experiences with others, and this is a significant revelation to them. The infant can share a focus of attention (i.e., the infant's eyes follow a pointing finger and look back at the adult for a facial cue to validate that he or she is looking at the correct location). The infant also begins to "read" the emotional signals of others in order to modify his or her behavior. The infant attempts to resolve situations of uncertainty, such as how to respond to an approaching stranger, by watching the caregiver's face for signs of happiness, interest, fear, or anger.

Object Permanence

The attainment of object permanence at approximately 8 months of age is a major cognitive achievement. When infants who are between the age of 5 and 7 months are presented with an object that is then removed or hidden, they will either cry or turn their attention to other things. Their world is one in which objects are constantly "appearing" and "disappearing," as if they never existed or no longer exist. Objects have no past and no future. Just a month later, however, a remarkable thing happens: Infants begin to search for an object in the spot where they saw it disappear. Out of sight is no longer out of mind.

Stranger Anxiety

The emotional reaction referred to as "stranger anxiety" is closely tied to these cognitive developments. Before the age of 7–9 months, infants may have reacted indiscriminately or "neutrally" to strangers, although they may have been able to recognize and perhaps smile more at familiar faces. Stranger anxiety is caused by the ability to recognize something that is unfamiliar and cannot be matched with memories that have now solidified in the infant's mind. Infants now may react with distress when their caregivers leave or a stranger approaches. At this point, babysitting becomes more difficult. Caregivers feel that they are quite special in the infant's life and that substitutions are not acceptable.

Developmental Vulnerabilities

Since the crucial task of the first year of life is the development and solidification of the attachment between infant and caretaker, this relationship is the most vulnerable area with regard to possible disruption by physical illness or psychopathology.

Physical Illness and Caretaking Relationships

The infant's physical growth is the earliest concrete sign for parents that they are adequately caring for their newborn infant. Parents eagerly await the physician's findings about changes in length and weight and how their infant compares with others on standard growth charts during early "well baby" visits. Common disruptions in growth, such as colds and other minor illnesses, can contribute to parental demoralization if physicians are not sensitive to these concerns. The physician-parent relationship is ideally one of reciprocal affective and cognitive attunement that can serve as a model for the parents' efforts at understanding and nurturing their infant. The physician preempts the parents' worries and helps promote their faith in their caretaking abilities, in much the same way that parents learn to recognize and respond to their infant's needs.

When infants become seriously ill, parents may have greater difficulty in reestablishing their sense of confidence in themselves and the infant. During a chronic illness, relationship patterns can become dramatically distorted. When parents do not believe in the vitality of their infant, they may treat the infant in a drastically altered manner. If the parents feel guilty, they may fail to set appropriate limits, such as letting the infant fuss for a few minutes when going to sleep. If the parents feel angry about their own helplessness, they may divert the anger toward the infant who engages in the normal bedtime fussing. When parents are able to nurse the infant through a medical crisis, whether minor or major, their confidence in the infant's ability to weather stress is renewed and the relationship is set back on course.

Illness can also have a disruptive effect on the parents' caretaking role. When hospitalization is required, medical personnel usually need to assume some of the parental nurturing tasks, and this interferes with the attachment between parents and infant. The following case illustrates the effect of impaired bonding on a severely ill infant, the physician's need to help parents develop a role in their infant's care, and the usefulness of developmental knowledge in assessing the relationship between caregivers and their infants.

➤ An infant who received a single-lung transplantation at 16 months of age had spent only 2 months at home before he was admitted to the hospital, where he spent the next 14 months. Following the transplantation, which was performed at a tertiary care medical center to which he had been transferred, the medical staff became concerned about the lack of time that his parents spent with him. It almost seemed as if they had "dropped him off" to have a transplantation. The infant was alone in his hospital room for long stretches of time, unlike many of the other children, whose parents literally hovered by their bedsides and never left. The staff wondered whether this behavior constituted neglect. After the infant was discharged to go home, it became apparent that the parents had been completely misjudged. They became model parents, "never skipping a beat," according to their pediatrician. In reviewing this infant's life history, one can see that these parents had never had the opportunity to bond with him, because he had been admitted to the hospital in an extremely compromised state so soon after birth. His mother had been completely overwhelmed and had not been given the chance to "feel like a mother." Also, she felt that she did not have a role in his care because, out of necessity, a multitude of nurses had cared for her infant. A follow-up meeting with this family when the child was 3 years old found a beaming father, who was proud of and loving toward his son, describing his toddler as "just like any other 3-year-old," except for some speech and language problems. ◄

Psychopathology

The developmental disorders observed in infants include **motor skills disorders,** in which activities requiring motor coordination, such as crawling or walking, are delayed; **communication disorders,** in which speech or expressive or receptive language is delayed; and **pervasive developmental disorders** (e.g., autism, Rett's syndrome, childhood disintegrative disorder, and Asperger's syndrome). These disorders are all associated with severe deficits in language and social functioning, except Asperger's syndrome, in which there are no significant delays in language development. All of the disorders except Rett's syndrome are characterized by a severely restricted range of interests and stereotyped, repetitive activities.

Autistic children may seem "different" to their parents from an early age (e.g., the infant may make less eye contact, smile less in response to the human face, or feel "stiff" when held). Flapping limbs or rocking behaviors may be seen. Parents may say that they find it difficult to bond with the infant and that the infant seems qualitatively different from their other children when they were the same age.

Children with these disorders have varying outcomes as adults. In children with communication or motor skills disorders, the final outcome depends on the severity of the disorder and its response to treatment. In children with pervasive developmental disorders, there are also varying degrees of severity. Intelligence seems to be an important prognostic factor. Some autistic individuals with high intelligence may be relatively self-sufficient as adults.

Disruption of the parent-infant bond due to parental impairment (e.g., depression in the mother) or loss can lead to a depressive response in the infant, which may be manifested by feeding and eating disorders or by reactive attachment disorder in infancy or early childhood. **Feeding disorders** include pica, rumination disorder, and feeding disorder of infancy or early childhood. Pica is the repeated ingestion of substances other than food, such as paint chips. Rumination disorder is the repeated regurgitation of food in the absence of a gastrointestinal disorder. Feeding disorder of infancy or early childhood is a failure to thrive for which there is no physiological explanation. Infants with this disorder usually begin to gain weight when they are admitted to the hospital.

Infants with **reactive attachment disorder** have a significant deficit in social relatedness and attachment behavior caused by pathological care, such as neglect or abuse. These infants tend to bond indiscriminately to strangers in the hospital and to lack normal stranger anxiety. Parental psychopathology is generally associated with a greater risk of psychiatric disorders in children.

In both feeding disorders and reactive attachment disorder, the degree of lasting damage to the infant depends on the duration of the problem, the nature of care after the disorder develops, and many other factors, including constitutional factors. Infants with reactive attachment disorder may develop problems in forming relationships and a propensity toward depression.

THE TODDLER YEARS: ONE TO THREE YEARS OF AGE

Developmental Progression

Toddlerhood begins around 12–13 months of age, when the infant begins to walk, or "toddle." This occasion marks a motoric discontinuity of remarkable proportions. Children are often elated by their ability to be mobile in this novel way and revel in their exploration of the world from this new vantage point.

Emergence of Autonomy

Whereas the task of the infant is to become attached to the caregiver, the task of the toddler is to become a socially detached, separate, autonomous being. This **separation individuation** process has been described in great detail by **Margaret Mahler** and generally begins with what she referred to as the **practicing** subphase, in which the child practices recently acquired skills with compulsive repetition. Whether from being asked to help the child climb up the slide 50 times or having to clean up a mess after the toddler insists on eating independently, even the most dedicated of parents can find these times to be trying.

During the "terrible twos," a term commonly used to describe this phase, the toddler can be experienced quite negatively by caregivers. It is helpful for caregivers to keep in mind that this contrary behavior is a necessary part of the child's establishment of his or her own autonomy. Just as the nature of the tasks that the child must master has changed from infancy, the caregivers' tasks have also shifted considerably. The caregiver must allow the toddler to explore the world and become independent but also protect the child from the perils of the real world.

Ambivalence

Both parents and children struggle with many conflicting emotions during the toddler years. Parents who are delighted to glimpse the growing, independent child may feel sadness at losing their adoring, compliant baby. Similarly, the toddler alternates between clinging to and pushing away caregivers. The child feels sadness at losing the caretakers and wants to "refuel" with them but also wants to be on his or her own. The child may so desperately want to be independent that the caregiver's help may be rejected even when it is needed. Mahler labeled this struggle the **rapprochement crisis.**

Tantrums may be precipitated in a toddler if the child becomes frustrated when attempting to comply with the plethora of adult demands and requests. These demands address every aspect of the child's daily life, including meals, dressing, toilet routines, and bedtime, and they come at a time when toddlers are beginning to see themselves as autonomous beings. Because pleasing their parents is quite important to toddlers, who thrive on parental love and approval, they may be quite afraid that an angry parent will abandon them or withdraw love.

Freud referred to this developmental phase as the **anal stage,** since this area of the body is symbolic of the child's growing mastery over his or her body and actions. Power struggles between caregiver and child may occur around toilet training. The child is faced with the choice of either complying with the caregiver's wishes and relinquishing this product, which the child still considers as part of himself or herself, or of withholding the feces. If the child is not able to experience the sense that he or she has a will to be exercised, a "precocious conscience" may develop that is inhibiting and controlling. Caregivers who are overly controlling or critical of a child in the "terrible twos" may set the stage for future problems.

Erikson's description of these children as struggling with a wish for "autonomy" and yet a tendency toward "shame and doubt" reflects the same issues that were identified by Freud and Mahler. Overly critical caregivers tend to make children feel **shameful** and insecure rather than confident and autonomous. Children must be able to feel that they will not lose caring by having a mind of their own. They must be encouraged and praised. Children who are shamed in their quest to begin exploring their autonomy may develop self-esteem problems.

Decentering and the Acquisition of Symbolic Thought

Jean Piaget, a psychologist who described the development of **cognitive** abilities, characterized toddlers as experiencing a "Copernican revolution" in the way they regard themselves in relation to the rest of the world. Initially, they see themselves in an "egocentric" way, as if all events were determined by their own thoughts and actions. During toddlerhood, a "decentering" process occurs, whereby children learn to see themselves as one of many objects in a world where there are laws of cause and effect.

Another major cognitive milestone that marks the second year of life is the appearance of symbolic function, or the understanding that one thing can represent another. Symbolic play is one aspect of this developmental progression; for example, a little girl may pretend to sleep, cuddling with her teddy bear and closing her eyes. Language is another important aspect of this symbolic capacity.

Internal Representations

One result of the interrelationship between the emotional and cognitive lines of development is that temper tantrums may lessen as the capacity for the verbal expression of desires increases. This effect has implications for language-impaired children, who may have more behavioral problems even as adults.

During the sensorimotor period of the first 2 years, an object can only have cognitive and emotional meaning when it is with the child. As the cognitive skills evolve, the child's ability to hold onto stable images of others also evolves. This development of **internal representations** (i.e., stable images of others that exist within the child's memory and have both cognitive and emotional components) reflects the inseparability of emotion and cognition. Before the cognitive functions of evocative memory, symbolic thinking, and language develop, objects essentially do not exist for the child unless the child can see them. If the object is absent, the mental image cannot be evoked. This instability of mental images of caregivers seems to contribute to the **separation anxiety** to which toddlers are particularly prone. A child cannot be comforted by the image of the mother when the child is separated from her if the child cannot first evoke a mental representation of her and understand that she has not just "disappeared."

Children of this age tend to experience other people and themselves as completely good or completely bad. They are unable to reconcile contradictory feelings toward the same person. The "good" loving mommy and the "bad" withholding one seem to be two different people. This instability makes angry feelings particularly frightening for them, since they tend to "project" the aggression and see the parent as completely malevolent.

Around the age of three years, the ability to integrate conflicting feelings about the same person improves dramatically. This developmental milestone is called **object constancy.** The child establishes stable internalized "object relationships," which are the child's composite memories of interactions with the prototypical object (e.g., the parent) and which are accompanied by a feeling. Toddlers may now more confidently allow significant others to come and go, since they are able to hold onto stable images of others in their minds. The mother with whom a child is affectionate at one moment and angry the next is recognized as one and the same person, and because the child is now able to tolerate this ambivalence, the child can trust further that the mother will return if she leaves his or her presence. This process occurs at age 24–36 months, and it is no coincidence that this is when many children enter nursery school.

More prolonged separations, as when parents go away for a long vacation, can be especially difficult for children age 2–3 years, especially if they are left with adults with whom they are unfamiliar. By age 3–3 1/2 years, most children are able to master such separations easily, although they are always vulnerable to regression and increased sensitivity during a stressful separation, such as hospitalization. While they are mastering the anxiety of separateness from caregivers, children tend to become attached to a **transitional object,** such as a stuffed animal or a special blanket, to serve as an intermediary that symbolically represents "mother." The ability to be comforted by a transitional object is one of the first steps in the use of symbols, and it further exemplifies the interplay between emotion and cognition.

Establishment of Gender Identity

Infantile sexuality was first noted by Freud. Self-stimulation of the genitals begins early and continues throughout the toddler years. This manual stimulation may be observed by parents during bathing and diapering. It clearly appears to be quite pleasurable to the child.

Gender identity, or the sense that one is a girl or a boy, is established by 18 months of age. Interestingly, this is the age at which the child is able to recognize herself or himself in a mirror. It is not uncommon for little boys and girls to notice the difference in their external genitalia. Some girls, particularly if they have male siblings, may think that something is missing, has disappeared, or may later grow. They may even initially express some regret at this. With appropriate sensitivity, the mother can explain over time that the girl also has special organs, the clitoris outside and vagina inside, and that she has other special parts of herself that, for instance, will one day allow her to have a baby.

From early on, parents and others (including peers, other adults, and the media) begin to shape the emerging gender identity according to the prevailing trends in a specific culture. Generally, 2- and 3-year-olds are preoccupied with imitating their parents and usually identify most strongly with the same-sex parent. This process is obviously affected by child-rearing practices in particular cultures. Sexual development, sexual identity, and gender role development, therefore, progress in interconnected ways.

Developmental Vulnerabilities

As during the first year of life, the main area of vulnerability in the toddler's emotional development is the caretaker-child relationship. However, whereas separations between infant and caretaker exert their most profound impact by disrupting the growing attachment, separations between toddlers and caretakers have a much more direct effect on the child. Sudden, prolonged separations of 2- and 3-year-olds from their mothers result in behaviors that resemble mourning (e.g., if the mother dies or if the child must be hospitalized, especially if parents are not allowed to "room in," so that there is no single consistent caregiver to substitute for the mother).

Response to Illness

Accepting the "sick role" involves the ability, in a sense, to regress and accept nurturant care, even for an adult. For a child, that need is tempered by the pride taken in newly acquired skills, such as feeding, going to the bathroom, dressing and undressing, and having ever-increasing bodily control. Therefore, illness and hospitalization, especially, present threats to the child's strivings toward autonomy and control.

A practical application of a developmental understanding is that toddlers should bring transitional objects with them when being admitted to the hospital. A sheet from the child's crib at home may be comforting because it surrounds the child with a familiar sight, smell, and texture. The young child's life is dominated by concrete sensations. Children sometimes revert to using a pacifier during a hospitalization. This temporary regression provides an additional transitional object. Sucking on the pacifier soothes the child during an overly stressful experience.

Transient Symptoms

Bedtime fears are frequent in toddlers and may be exacerbated by nightmares. Fears of monsters or robbers or of being alone are especially common. Until toddlers have mastered separation anxiety, they may be frequent visitors in their parents' bedroom, motivated by the need to reassure themselves that their parents are still there and close by in case they are needed. Problems in separating initially at "goodnight time" are often handled best with a story and a ritual, which are comforting to children in this agegroup. The parents should honor the toddler's requests for leaving a night light burning and having a particular door open (usually, the bedroom door) or closed (usually, the closet door). Phobias, particularly toward animals, may emerge but tend to pass. In most cases, with empathic parental responses, these fears and anxieties gradually diminish over the next year or two, as the child progresses emotionally and intellectually. Overall, toddlers' coping mechanisms are relatively newly acquired and unstable. Therefore, their reliance on such "external" means of comfort as people or transitional objects is greater. In addition, they are more likely to manifest anxiety in behaviors, such as increased oppositional or clinging behavior, moodiness, and sleep or appetite disturbances.

The child in this age-group also has a more vulnerable sense of physical security and may be quite upset by the inevitable cuts and scrapes. It is the age of the Band-Aid.

Psychopathology

The psychopathology that is first noticeable in the toddler years includes many of the diagnostic entities mentioned in infancy, including motor skills disorders, communication disorders, pervasive developmental disorders, and reactive attachment disorder. Mental retardation may also be first suspected in young children. Many of these disorders may become more evident as toddlers have greater contact with other children and differences become more noticeable, especially in social settings.

Hyperactivity, impulsivity, and heightened distractibility (compared with same-age peers) may also become apparent during the toddler years. Some children with these traits may later be diagnosed with attention-deficit/hyperactivity disorder.

The prognosis of these children depends on the severity of the psychopathology, as well as factors such as temperament, intelligence, parental and family psychopathology, socioeconomic status, and quality of relationships with caregivers. Such factors can be protective (e.g., a child with an easy temperament who is born to well-to-do, high-functioning parents) or may predispose the child to problems later in life (e.g., a difficult child with low intelligence who is born to a poor household with an abusive parent).

THE PRESCHOOL YEARS: THREE TO SIX YEARS OF AGE
Developmental Progression
The Autonomous Self and the Emergence of Morality

As a result of positive social interactions between child and caregiver, the child begins to understand the word "we," which is internalized by age 3 years to the point where it can be brought into new relationships with others. The child has the sense that caregivers are "with" him or her even when they are absent, so that there is an enhanced sense of mastery and control. Children begin to recall aloud or to themselves parental prohibitions (e.g., "Don't touch electrical outlets") and listen to these "inner voices." The emotional core that the child brings from the toddler years is continuous and acts as a template for future relationships.

This stage corresponds roughly to **Erikson's** age of **initiative versus guilt** or **Freud's phallic-oedipal stage.** Erikson thought that at this time, the child is more able to use initiative in actively exploring the world and has less of the defiant quality seen in the earlier toddler phase. The potential danger in this phase, according to Erikson, is that excessive guilt might result if the initiative is too infused with aggression (e.g., rage associated with extreme sibling rivalry). Consequently, the child may fear retaliation for aggressive fantasies (e.g., the castration complex).

In this stage, children must, in a sense, renounce the earlier feeling that they could be "master of the universe" and temper ambitions with reality. This process includes giving up the fantasy of possessing the opposite-sex parent. In order to resolve the Oedipus complex, children must bury many such infantile wishes in the unconscious under a shroud of repression, which permits the emergence of an unconscious internal agency (i.e., the superego) that observes and guides them and produces guilty feelings when they have done something "wrong." Children turn toward the same-sex parent and identify with them. In other words, the child seems to be realizing, "If you can't lick 'em, join 'em." This newly formed superego can be rather harsh, as seen in children's tendency to believe that illness is a punishment for misdeeds. ⟹ For example, a 5-year-old who was told that his heart was failing and that he would need to get a new one (i.e., have a transplantation) was heard to comment that he wished he had not been so naughty. He asked his parents, "If I promise to be good, would my heart get better?" ⟸

The evolution in thinking at age 3–6 years has been described as a "civilizing process." Children accept a more "modest" position in the universe and become more fully aware of the feelings and rights of others. Parental and social values are grasped, and a sense of morality develops. An "internal government" begins to take shape, and this development is accompanied by a sense of discipline.

Imaginative Play

As a number of social and cognitive developmental lines converge, the child can now play cooperatively with other children. The child is able to inhibit the impulse to be aggressive or selfish with play materials and, instead, uses them constructively through sharing. The make-believe play that is so much a part of the life of a preschooler is crucial for the later development of adult modes of thinking and relating emotionally to others, representing a continuous line of development. Play is thought by some to be a prototype for imagination in adults. If a child does not have the ability to play, the child's social and academic functioning will probably be impaired from an early age. Play can be viewed as a microcosm of the world, in which the child has enhanced control over events and outcomes. It can also be a means by which children anticipate future events and replay past events in order to diminish anxiety and enhance mastery. Imaginary playmates are quite common and should not be a cause for concern. To the contrary, significant early childhood psychopathology can be associated with the inability to play imaginatively.

Parental tasks include encouraging play by providing a physically and emotionally conducive atmosphere and facilitating social involvement by introducing the child to situations in which the child will be able to interact with other children. The child will learn about sharing and reciprocity, which are lessons that will be needed during the school years. The preschool years are a time for parents to help secure a base for their children, who will soon be leaving the nest to enter school. Encouragement, love, and guidance will all help to consolidate an early sense of self that is competent and confident. These years are often among those most fondly remembered by parents, as they observe their preschoolers becoming "little people" who can carry on animated conversations as language development flourishes and truly share activities with adults, such as going to the movies and playing board games.

The Evolution of Magical Thinking

By age 3 years, the child has reached the stage that Piaget described as a preoperational level of cognition, during which the child becomes aware of time as a continuum with a past, present, and future. Even though the child may refer to all past events as occurring "yesterday," this perspective is a major shift from the child's earlier sense of existing only in the moment. The world, however, is still a confusing place for the preschooler, who has not yet grasped more complicated issues of relative size and space, as well as cause and effect. The child will understand these concepts when he or she achieves the level of concrete operational thinking at about age 8 years. For instance, one 3-year-old who had to have repeated cardiac biopsies became fearful that too much of her heart would be removed, causing it to fall into her stomach. An example of an early form of causality, or "precausality," is seen in the 3-year-old girl who was asked why it was dark outside and answered that it was dark outside because it was nighttime.

A preschooler's world is still infused with a great deal of magic, which may, at times, blur the line between fantasy and reality, as the following bedtime incident involving a 5-year-old boy demonstrates. One night when a breeze from the window gently rattled the bedroom blinds, the boy jumped out of bed and ran out of the room. In the hallway, he laughed nervously, admitting that he had suddenly become worried that a monster was behind the blinds, even though he lived on the sixth floor and "knew" that there was "no such thing as monsters." He was reluctantly coaxed back into his room when his parents offered to accompany him over to the blinds to take a look. He was noticeably relieved to see that nothing was there.

Understanding this magical thinking is crucial to providing medical care for ill preschoolers. Children may believe that if they do not say anything about their symptoms, they will go away or they may believe that verbalizing concern over being ill may precipitate or worsen the process. A 5-year-old girl recovering from surgery to remove a medulloblastoma underreported her pain symptoms because she was afraid that if she complained about pain, she would have to undergo another invasive procedure, due to her association between the two. She actually undermedicated herself with patient-controlled anesthesia.

Evolution of Sexuality

Preschool children may exhibit aggressive and sexualized behavior toward parents or other children in their play, where strivings for mastery and competition are often seen. Children become quite interested in storytelling and fairy tales, which often reflect their own fantasies, such as wanting to be mommy or daddy. This fantasy may include a certain degree of "showing off," especially in a coy manner, as well as possessiveness of the same-sex parent.

Sexual behavior is not uncommon in preschoolers and may include a wide continuum of behaviors, including touching their own genitalia or perhaps those of others, an interest in looking at naked people, inquiring about sexual organs and acts, watching people on the toilet, expressing interest in pregnancy and birth, showing other children their genitalia, being interested in their own feces, "playing doctor," and putting things into their orifices or perhaps those of other children. These behaviors may indicate problems if they seem to preoccupy the child relative to other activities in life. "Sex play" is normal if it is carefree, occurs voluntarily between children who know each other and are of the same age and developmental level, and is limited in type and frequency. Many of these behaviors may continue into the young school-age years.

Developmental Vulnerabilities
Response to Illness

The regression that sometimes accompanies illness can be quite anxiety-provoking for the preschooler, who, like the toddler, is still striving to become independent. The unconscious fantasies that are typical of preschoolers, such as the fear of bodily mutilation as punishment, may exaggerate fears associated with surgery, because young children typically attribute external events to intrapsychic thoughts and feelings. With respect to surgery, unconscious fears and wishes often modulate a child's conscious worries. The normal developmental concerns of a 3- to 5-year-old include the **fear of bodily mutilation,** as well as the struggle with angry feelings when a parent will not allow the child to do as he or she pleases. For these reasons, a surgical procedure may be seen as the actualization of an intense fear, a punishment for being bad, or a retribution for angry feelings toward a parent.

An appreciation of the defense mechanisms used in childhood is crucial to understanding reactions to illness and devising appropriate intervention strategies. A child with cystic fibrosis who ties her stuffed animals down to give them injections and at the same time soothes them demonstrates regression, repression (of unconscious fears and wishes), identification with the aggressor, and transformation of passivity into activity. The child identifies with the more powerful physician, who is in control, but also empathizes with the helpless stuffed elephant, whom she soothes. Allowing the child to play out the procedure on a doll beforehand fosters both intellectual and emotional mastery. By acting this scenario out repeatedly, the child helps master the anxieties associated with treatment of her chronic illness and turns a passive experience into a more active one. Interventions designed to bolster this function would be supportive of the child's developing ego, which can easily be overwhelmed by anxiety. Interestingly, interventions aimed at helping to prepare the parents and allay their anxiety usually also decrease anxiety in the child because these interventions fortify the major supporting objects of the child (i.e., the parents) and this may prevent the "emotional contagion" sometimes seen between parent and child.

Psychopathology

Psychopathology in preschoolers includes the communication disorders discussed earlier. Entry into school often allows such problems to be identi-fied, because the child is in an environment of adults and children who are not familiar with his or her idiosyncratic means of expression. Hyperactive children may begin to clearly differentiate themselves from other children who are better able to tolerate the transition into more structured class settings. The diagnosis of **attention-deficit/hyperactivity disorder** requires that symptoms be present prior to age 7 years (see Table 13–1 for DSM-IV criteria).

Anxiety disorders may also manifest themselves at this age. These disorders tend to be somewhat tenacious and may traverse subsequent developmental levels. Children with significant separation anxiety in childhood may have difficulty with separations later in life (e.g., when they go to college). **Adjustment disorders,** which are by definition transient, may result from a specific event, such as an illness, parental divorce, move, or birth of a new sibling, and may be manifested in mood or behavioral changes. **Specific phobias** are often seen in this age group and may be directed at animals, naturally occurring phenomena such as storms, or specific situations such as riding in an elevator. The fear of specific situations may be a prototype for later development of panic disorder with agoraphobia. **Posttraumatic stress disorder** can be seen in preschool children. It may result from an acute event in which there is a sudden, brief exposure to a trauma (e.g., a schoolyard shooting) or from a chronic situation (e.g., chronic physical or sexual abuse of a child).

Selective mutism, in which the child will not speak in specific social situations but does not have a communication disorder, can also become evident. Children with selective mutism may be at higher risk for later developing symptoms of social phobia. The **elimination disorders** (i.e., encopresis, which is lack of bowel control in children who are at least 4 years of age, and enuresis, which is lack of bladder control in children who are at least 5 years of age) are also problems seen in this age-group.

THE LATENCY YEARS: SIX TO TEN YEARS OF AGE
Developmental Progression

The latency years are the middle childhood, or school-age, years. This period begins at age 6 years and ends with puberty. As their social world expands beyond the family to include friends and teachers, children of latency age find it easy to be physically apart from their parents. The tasks of latency include developing a sustained sense of mastery and competence, morality, and stable self-esteem.

Acquiring Competence

Erikson underscored the importance of social processes for children of elementary school age when he described this period as one in which children must either achieve "industry" or suffer from "inferiority." During this period, children leave the world of their parents and are taught the fundamen-

TABLE 13–1.   DSM-IV Diagnostic Criteria for Attention Deficit/Hyperactivity Disorder

A. Either (1) or (2):

   (1) six (or more) of the following symptoms of **inattention** have persisted for at least 6 months to a degree that is maladaptive and inconsistent with development level:

   Inattention

   (a) often fails to give close attention to details or makes careless mistakes in schoolwork, work, or other activities

   (b) often has difficulty sustaining attention in tasks or play activities

   (c) often does not seem to listen when spoken to directly

   (d) often does not follow through on instructions and fails to finish schoolwork, chores, or duties in the workplace (not due to oppositional behavior or failure to understand instructions)

   (e) often has difficulty organizing tasks and activities

   (f) often avoids, dislikes, or is reluctant to engage in tasks that require sustained mental effort (such as schoolwork or homework)

   (g) often loses things necessary for tasks or activities (e.g., toys, school assignments, pencils, books, or tools)

   (h) is often easily distracted by extraneous stimuli

   (i) is often forgetful in daily activities

   (2) six (or more) of the following symptoms of hyperactivity-impulsivity have persisted for at least 6 months to a degree that is maladaptive and inconsistent with developmental level:

   Hyperactivity

   (a) often fidgets with hands or feet or squirms in seat

   (b) often leaves seat in classroom or in other situations in which remaining seated is expected

   (c) often runs about or climbs excessively in situations in which it is inappropriate (in adolescents or adults, may be limited to subjective feelings of restlessness)

   (d) often has difficulty playing or engaging in leisure activities quietly

   (e) is often "on the go" or often acts as if "driven by a motor"

   (f) often talks excessively

   Impulsivity

   (g) often blurts out answers before questions have been completed

   (h) often has difficulty awaiting turn

   (i) often interrupts or intrudes on others (e.g., butts into conversations or games)

B. Some hyperactive-impulsive or inattentive symptoms that caused impairment were present before age 7 years.

C. Some impairment from the symptoms is present in two or more settings (e.g., at school [or work] and at home).

D. There must be clear evidence of clinically significant impairment in social, academic, or occupational functioning.

E. The symptoms do not occur exclusively during the course of a Pervasive Developmental Disorder, Schizophrenia, or other Psychotic Disorder and are not better accounted for by another mental disorder (e.g., Mood Disorder, Anxiety Disorder, Dissociative Disorder, or a Personality Disorder).

Code based on type:

   Attention-Deficit/Hyperactivity Disorder, Combined Type: if both Criteria A1 and A2 are met for the past 6 months

   Attention-Deficit/Hyperactivity Disorder, Predominantly Inattentive Type: if Criterion A1 is met but Criterion A2 is not met for the past 6 months

   Attention-Deficit/Hyperactivity Disorder, Predominantly Hyperactive-Impulsive Type: if Criterion A2 is met but Criterion A1 is not met for the past 6 months

   Coding note: For individuals (especially adolescents and adults) who currently have symptoms that no longer meet full criteria, "In Partial Remission" should be specified.

tal skills that are prerequisite to becoming productive members of society, such as being literate and having a functional understanding of society.

As they watch their children go through this stage, parents must be protective but not intrusive, and so facilitate their children's continued socialization and development of morality, academic skills, and autonomy. A major determinant in the development of a sense of competence is the manner in which important people react to children's growing abilities and successes. Responses that "affirm" and "validate" these developing skills facilitate self-esteem. Through the encouragement and acknowledgment of their attempts at mastery, whether in schoolwork, athletics, or music, children come to recognize their talents as "real" and part of themselves. As a result of this process, the "exhibitionism" of preschool children is transformed into a sense of pride and mastery.

Hobbies, in particular, represent an intermediate step between play and work. Activities undertaken for pleasure, such as model building and stamp collecting, require realistic planning and preparation.

Evolving Coping Styles and Morality

While preschoolers are prone to being overwhelmed by stressful external events and manifest these feelings by withdrawal, fears, and other behavioral disturbances, latency-age children have an expanded repertoire of coping responses and defense mechanisms. They are, in a sense, more emotionally flexible and better able to take care of themselves. Essentially, latency is a time in which ego functions grow and consolidate, allowing children to tolerate frustration and delays in the gratification of their wishes and desires.

Temperamental characteristics, such as shyness, level of activity, persistence in approaching tasks, resilience, and quality of mood, follow children through the latency period and endure. Temperament may have important influences on achievement during this phase of life.

As children approach adolescence, their idealization of parental figures that characterized the preschool years is transformed into an appreciation of the values for which their parents stand. An intermediate stage in this transition is the idealization of other role models, such as sports heroes and teachers. Children also look to their peers for positive feedback and a sense of belonging. If they receive support and encouragement, their self-esteem becomes more stable and is less shaken by failures or disappointments. The need for both independence and attachments is satisfied by group affiliations, which is also the arena in which children must first perform or compete with others.

The conscience evolves during the latency period, developing more mature determinants, including empathy, internal guilt, and a concern for what is morally right. As children's social development progresses, their relationships become based on mutual respect. Although younger children follow rules handed down to them by authority figures, children between the ages of 7 and 8 years begin to see rules as agreements made between all interested parties that can be changed if a consensus is reached. At this point, justice becomes an operative force rather than an act of simple obedience. When a child truly identifies with parents or authority figures, rules are followed independently and without the need for external enforcement. However, even at this stage, ambivalence regarding parental figures mediates the child's following of rules (e.g., a child may be angry at his or her parents and disobey them but later feel guilty and become compliant). In this way, cognitive, social, emotional, and moral lines of development intertwine.

Reading, Writing, and Arithmetic

During the school-age years, children progress a great deal in the cognitive sphere. Piaget believed that the stage of **concrete operations** begins around age 7–8 years and concludes when children reach preadolescence, around age 11–12 years. He called the operations "concrete" because they involve thinking about physical objects as opposed to abstract thinking, such as hypothesizing. Examples of concrete operations include joining (e.g., mother and father together equal parents); ordering (i.e., the ability to arrange numbers in a sequence or objects in order of increasing size); conservation (i.e., the understanding that the properties of an object are not changed if its location or position is changed); and classification (i.e., the ability to arrange objects according to color or shape). Children also understand the concept of reversibility of operations, that operations have opposites (e.g., subtraction is the reverse operation of addition; separation is the opposite of joining). Latency-age children are able to understand the concept of numbers instead of only being able to recite them. The concepts of spatial measurement (e.g., the length of a line), time, and speed also fall into the category of concrete operations.

In one famous experiment involving the concept of conservation, children watched as an amount of liquid was poured from a beaker into either a taller, thinner container or a shorter, wider container, which caused the height of the water level to change. When asked whether the amount of water had changed, children of 4–5 years of age said that there was more water in the beaker with the higher water level. Children who had attained concrete operational thinking knew that the amount of water had not changed.

Gender Differentiation

A crucial aspect of the latency period is the further development of gender identity. Children's possessiveness toward and wish to become the spouse of the opposite-sex parent seem to lessen. They tend to turn to the same-sex parent and to identify and share in more culturally defined, gender-specific activities. The form of this identification depends on the specific sociocultural context.

Children usually prefer same-sex peers at this age, although their interest in opposite-sex children never disappears. Boys and girls seem to differentiate into opposing camps. Members of both sexes tend to join sex-specific groups and clubs. Sex-specific behaviors and tendencies are observed, and it remains unclear to what extent these differences can be attributed to inborn divergences or to cultural influences. In general, boys are drawn to aggressive play, especially play involving competitiveness and prowess, while girls seem to mature more quickly and use more diplomatic, less aggressive means of persuasion in their play. Girls often find boys overly controlling and militant. Boys tend to cluster in larger groups that are organized around a common interest or goal, while girls focus more on the interpersonal aspects of relationships, such as sharing confidences, interacting within smaller groups, and operating by consensus rather than dominance. It is important to recognize that not all boys and girls fit comfortably into these general patterns.

Sexual Curiosity and Modesty

Children are socialized about their sexuality through experiences with their parents. Cultural factors are, therefore, extremely important, because the values of the parents are passed down to the children. The parents' attitudes about sexuality and their bodies are revealed indirectly by the way in which they bathe, dress, change their children's diapers, and take them to the toilet. Parental reactions to nakedness, both with respect to their children and themselves, become part of the internalization process that molds children's attitudes toward sexuality and their own bodies. Children learn how to feel about their bodies from the direct and indirect lessons that their parents teach them in subtle but quite influential ways. They also learn about sexuality and physicality within a relationship by observing the way in which their parents interact with each other.

When children enter school, they begin to learn social etiquette. Their parents and older siblings inculcate a sense of sexual modesty in them. Standards for what is appropriate with regard to toileting or showing one's body are reinforced by teachers and classmates. By fourth or fifth grade, most children are extremely self-conscious about having their underwear show, let alone being seen naked, especially by the opposite sex. As adolescence approaches, children may be uncomfortable during physical examinations, and physicians should be sensitive to their need for privacy by exposing only the part of their body that is to be examined. Children often begin to exhibit increased modesty about their bodies in the presence of their parents and may prefer to take baths in private. At the same time, children's thoughts and their communications with peers reflect their preoccupation with sexual themes.

Freud initially dubbed this developmental phase the **latency** phase because he believed that during this time the sexual curiosity present in earlier childhood becomes dormant and is not reactivated until adolescence. Recent observations suggest that this is not completely true. Instead of being dormant, the sexual interests of latency-age children are concealed from adults.

Latency is a time for learning rules, particularly about sexual transgressions. Perhaps because of this, latency-age sexuality is somewhat obscured as the child's conscience, which can still be fairly severe at this time, dictates against these sexual wishes.

Developmental Vulnerabilities

Potential dangers during the latency phase of life are related to children's inability to successfully navigate the pressures to perform academically and socially. School can be a trying place for children of this age, especially if they feel incapable of meeting the expectations of parents and teachers or of competing with peers. For other children, accomplishments may become the only priority. When parents or coaches place too much emphasis on winning in sports rather than on having fun and building skills, children may suffer significant self-esteem problems and even depression if they feel they do not measure up.

Response to Illness

Physicians caring for latency-age children with serious medical illnesses can use their knowledge of developmental progressions to help the children adjust. Because these children are in the process of becoming increasingly competent and autonomous, they will appreciate receiving booklets and videotapes that explain the illness, anticipated procedures, and treatments. Their interest in peer groups can be turned to advantage by encouraging contact with other children who have similar illnesses.

Physicians and parents should not make the mistake, however, of assuming that latency-age children have the same understanding of illness that they have. Both regression and variable progress along cognitive or emotional lines can result in misunderstandings and worries. ➡ For example, a bright, mature 8-year-old boy surprised his parents with a remnant of magical thinking when he developed the flu during his first ice-skating expedition. He was convinced that the skating had made him sick, "like getting car sick," because he felt fine before he started skating, became progressively nauseated and weak while skating, and became febrile and vomited at home that evening. ⬅

Psychopathology

Children who have learning disabilities or attentional problems, such as **attention-deficit/hyperactivity disorder,** often first manifest problems when they enter school. If such problems are not addressed early, these children's self-esteem may be profoundly affected. When appropriate interventions are not made during this extremely sensitive period, children may deviate from the normal course of development and not acquire the skills and self-confidence necessary for entry into the occupational world. A subgroup of children with attention-deficit disorder has chronic symptoms that continue into adulthood. When substance abuse disorders, conduct disorder, or affective disorders complicate the clinical course of children with attention-deficit disorder, a greater propensity for chronic, more serious difficulties exists.

Anxiety disorders are also prevalent in children in the latency stage. Obsessive-compulsive disorder is especially likely to be first diagnosed in this age-group. Adjustment disorders, which can be associated with mood and behavioral changes as well as anxiety, can also occur (e.g., after a change to a new school). Symptoms of posttraumatic stress disorder may be seen, as noted in the section on preschool development; if they are not treated early, symptoms may become chronic and cross developmental periods.

Tic disorders may also be seen in this age range. In children with Tourette's syndrome, motor tics may appear at age 6–7 years and vocal tics at age 8–9 years. Obsessive-compulsive symptoms may develop later in individuals who are susceptible to both Tourette's syndrome and obsessive-compulsive disorder. Children with Tourette's syndrome often have associated behavioral problems with features of attention-deficit/hyperactivity disorder, which may cause more impairment than the tics. Simple tics are not uncommon in school-age boys, especially, and are usually transient. Even in Tourette's, the tics often fade by late adolescence or early adulthood.

Mood disorders are often first seen in the school-aged child. The prevalence of unipolar depression has recently been more fully appreciated. Early prototypes of bipolar disorder are also observed in children who may present with phenomena, however, that are different from those found in adults with bipolar disorder. The symptoms may resemble those of attention-deficit/hyperactivity disorder (i.e., impulsivity and distractibility) more than the symptoms seen in adults who have classic distinct mania. In general, extreme irritability, decreased need for sleep, or an *increase* in activity level in children are indicative of bipolar disorder. Serious mood disorders in childhood may be a marker for an increased risk of recurrent mood disorders later in life.

Communication disorders can present problems for the school-aged child because mastery of academic tasks is a developmental imperative. **Learning disorders,** which affect reading, mathematics, or writing, are often first diagnosed. Children with learning disorders or low intelligence seem to be at higher risk for developing psychiatric disorders later in life, including disruptive behavior and mood and anxiety disorders.

Psychotic disorders, such as schizophrenia, are extremely rare in childhood and may be misdiagnosed in a child who has a language or mood disorder because these disorders may result in idiosyncratic thought patterns that resemble those of psychosis.

ADOLESCENCE

Adolescence is a time of great change. It begins with puberty, the period of sexual maturation (in which the primary sex organs develop and become capable of reproduction) and the appearance of secondary sex characteristics (such as facial hair in boys and breast enlargement in girls). Girls usually mature 2 years earlier than boys, although there are "late developers" in both sexes. Late development may have profound consequences for adolescents' self-esteem because they place great importance on body image, comparison of themselves with peers, and sexual attractiveness.

Developmental Progression
Achieving Independence Through Groups

As they develop socially, children in early adolescence tend to identify with groups in order to deal with the anxieties associated with the lack of a coherent sense of individual identity. The teenager may form love relationships for the same reason (i.e., at the outset, the relationship is not so much sexual as an attempt to clarify the teenager's self-image by having it reflected by a partner).

The apparent lack of tolerance for difference is often seen in the cliques and prejudices of the adolescent (e.g., against skin color or other cultures). This intolerance can be another way in which adolescents try to protect themselves from the fear of not having a clear sense of who they are. All adults can remember the "in" crowds and the "outsiders" and how, as teenagers, they desperately tried to figure out what was "cool" and what was not with respect to attitude or dress. The unsettling feeling of not being quite sure of who one is or what one will become is soothed by being part of a group that is homogeneous in some respects (e.g., with regard to ideals and behavior, as well as enemies). One other task is to remain faithful. Tests of loyalty are not uncommon and may be intense.

Young adolescents usually rely on others for praise to help them feel good about themselves and may, therefore, be somewhat vulnerable to criticism and become angry with a person who has offended them. Parents are characteristically **de-idealized** in early adolescence, as adolescents come to see them more objectively. Adolescents need to give up their parents as sexual targets once again. This distancing may be associated with feelings of irritation and frustration with parents (i.e., almost as if the adolescent has been "let down" by the parents). Following this developmental task, the adolescent continues to want some person to idealize, which may manifest it-

self in the wish for a love relationship. Adolescents may also idealize other adults or the parents of friends, a process that may help young adolescents retain a sense of support as they separate and individuate from their own parents. These longings indicate that the adolescent has not traveled far from needing his or her parents; this becomes painfully evident in the face of stresses such as illness. Achieving autonomy becomes an all-important goal for the adolescent and may propel him or her into oppositional behavior, although this defiance tends to be mitigated by a continued need for parental support. These conflicting feelings often result in alterations between rebelliousness and neediness.

In the middle years of adolescence, the adolescent typically ventures out of the peer group to form a relationship with single others; this helps to further refine the sexual identity. The tasks of this phase include separating from the family, establishing intimate relationships, beginning to take responsibility for one's life, and learning to weather the feelings of anxiety or loneliness that may accompany this transition. It is generally not until late adolescence (age 18–22 years) that the peer group's influence recedes in relation to the importance of the significant other. Until then, the task of separating from parents and becoming autonomous is often worked out more in relationships with friends than with lovers because the peer setting is more acceptable for obtaining support and sharing experiences.

Consolidation of Identity and Growing Emotional Maturity

Identity consolidation involves the evolution of a new self-image that integrates physical and emotional changes and represents a constellation different from the self-image that existed during latency. Adolescents often feel that adults do not understand them, but in early adolescence they have not yet solidified their new identities and therefore look to their peers to help define themselves. This partially explains the intensity of fluctuating relationships with friends.

The **early adolescent** may be relatively unfocused and **confused about roles and expectations** in less structured settings. Early in puberty, young adolescents tend to experience more anxious or depressed feelings than they had during the latency years and may find it difficult to enjoy themselves. Because their sense of identity is evolving and unclear, young adolescents may have difficulty in trusting themselves or others. They may consider themselves incompetent and find others overly demanding and not emotionally available. Early adolescents often experience a sense of discontent and loneliness as they attempt to forge new social paths.

Parents continue to play an important role in the adolescent's life. Empathic and protective responses that continue to provide support but allow for independent growth can undoubtedly facilitate adjustment during this phase of life. The major psychological tasks of adolescence involve what has been referred to as the "second phase of separation-individuation," one goal of which is to achieve psychological autonomy from the parents. As in the toddler's phase of separation-individuation, parents must be able to tolerate the increasing disengagement of the adolescent.

The adolescent's de-idealization of the parents and the accompanying growing autonomy and emergence of sexual identity may cause a **mourning reaction in parents,** who may long for the latency years. The ability to work through their own adjustment is important to the adolescent's passage through these years. Pathological separation difficulties in the parents may predispose the adolescent to the same problems. Healthy parents are able to relish their adolescent's achievement without having their own self-esteem compromised and without trying to quash the process of separation.

Erikson referred to this stage as one of "identity versus role confusion," in which the adolescent must consider, in addition to the relatively rapid bodily transformations, a psychological "revolution" in the consolidation, integration, and growth of mental functioning. Erikson believed that the adolescent is searching for some of the continuity and sameness found in earlier developmental periods and looking for present-day meaning in the skills mastered earlier. Adolescents are also trying to find a place for themselves. A risk of role confusion becomes evident as the adolescent develops his or her sexual identity or tries to make decisions about a future occupation.

The age of 16–17 years has been regarded as the **midpoint of adolescence,** when much of the feeling of omnipotence present earlier becomes tempered by adulthood, which looms ahead. By this time, the adolescent has grown accustomed to the bodily changes that heralded puberty and tends to be less anxious about his or her body and more focused on the future. This adjustment usually takes about 2 years after the onset of puberty.

Adolescents in this age group tend to feel less anxious or depressed and are perhaps more trusting of others than during pubescence. They tend to identify with a more diverse group of mentors and idealized adults and appear more content and upbeat. On the other hand, middle adolescents often have feelings of arrogance, defiance, and superiority alternating with feelings of deflation, compliance, and inferiority. Their self-image is more coherent but still has a certain degree of instability, especially when their independence is challenged. Arguing with adults may be a way of trying to bolster their sense of autonomy from adults while allowing values to be incorporated in a manner that appears less dependent on authority figures. For similar reasons, middle adolescents typically have difficulty being appreciative to adults.

The **consolidation of identity** can be thought of as involving the late adolescent's increasing conception of his or her own perspective, in such a way that behavior and motivation become more consistent (e.g., future career plans and value systems are often embraced).

As adolescents make the journey into young adulthood, they must abandon some grandiose dreams and fantasies and begin to develop more realistic conceptions of possible future roles and accomplishments. Adolescents develop a more realistic assessment of their individual capabilities and opportunities, a process that has often been described as a second "decentering" process. Being able to test their abilities in the work place helps adolescents develop their autonomy.

The establishment of intimate relationships is another crucial milestone. Erikson thought that the establishment of a stable identity was a prerequisite to the development of intimate relationships. Obviously, if adolescents have not fully resolved issues involving separation from their parents, the establishment of intimate relationships with others may be affected.

Acquisition of Abstract Thought

Piaget's stage of **formal operational (abstract) thinking** between 12 and 16 years of age reflects further central nervous system maturation at this time. In adolescence, a "disconnection" from thought and objects, or "liberation of form from content," occurs so that the adolescent can hypothesize about things that have not yet happened or evaluate hypotheses in which he or she does not believe. The adolescent becomes able to use known truths to accurately predict unforeseen events through the process of reasoning; this process marks the onset of "hypothetico-deductive," or "formal," thought. This change in perspective is also crucial with respect to emotional and social development.

Adolescence is a time of philosophizing and of taking pleasure in ideas. Parental values remain quite important during this phase of life, but considerable thought and revision is given to the parents' value system as the adolescent evolves his or her own sense of identity and ethics.

The development of creativity manifests itself predominantly during adolescence, although prerequisites to the ability to initiate the creative process occur earlier during childhood. Much of the impetus for creativity may derive from feelings that accompany the separation from parents, growth of autonomy, and identity development that occur in adolescence. Creative endeavors probably help to consolidate the identity, as well as pave the way for creativity during adulthood.

Gender-Related Issues

The onset of menarche is a time of intense feeling for an adolescent girl, who may feel surprised or even hide the fact that it has occurred. If a girl is uninformed, she may be confused about what exactly has happened. The first ejaculation in boys may be similarly experienced. The first demonstrable evidence of reproductive function can stir up many conflicting feelings, which may include embarrassment, anxiety, or guilt, since this function had been "prohibited" during latency. Distorted perceptions about these experiences and bodily functions are extremely common at this age and complicate matters for the early adolescent.

The adolescent boy tends to be much more aware of primary sex characteristics than the adolescent girl is, because his genitals are more readily visible and because, traditionally, education about female genital anatomy has been poor. Adolescent boys are generally quite concerned about the size of their penises and will overtly or subtly make comparisons. They are fond of "dirty jokes" but are very little interested in direct sexual contact.

Young adolescent girls may have a variety of interests, ranging from the more "traditional" female roles to athletic pursuits. They often share sexual secrets with one or two close friends, and their friendships tend to be more intense. The social role for young adolescent girls has undergone a significant evolution as it has followed changing cultural and intellectual trends.

Most adolescent males place a premium value on muscular strength and athletic prowess. Smaller or unathletic boys may fear that they appear "feminine." Girls are generally not as interested in developing their muscles.

Some of the differences between the sexes may result from the boy's need, in a sense, to turn away from his "primary love object," which is his mother, in order to identify with his father and consolidate his sexual identity. The girl, on the other hand, can identify with her mother as part of this process. In Western culture, male independence is highly valued, and boys may have a more difficult time with relationships; intimacy with women may threaten this separation and therefore the boy's sense of gender identity.

Young women tend to define their identity in terms of relationships and caregiving roles as wife or mother, stressing empathy with others. Males tend to define themselves more by their individual achievements or occupations. The sense of morality in women also tends to be associated with beliefs about being sensitive in relationships with others, while men tend to derive a sense of morality from abstract concepts that stress independence and have much less emphasis on relationships.

Adolescence can be a developmental crisis for adolescent girls in Western culture because they may experience a conflict between making the needs of others within a relationship a priority and sacrificing their own needs and wishes. This conflict carries over into young adulthood, during which many women struggle with the conflicting roles of a professional life and a family life. Cultural values and sexual taboos further complicate development for adolescent girls as they try to come to terms with their own identities and balance traditional values with new expectations. The different issues in adolescent development for males and females may contribute to the higher incidence of depressive symptoms in adolescent women.

Sexual Development

Increased sexual thoughts or wishes and uneasiness with bodily changes may affect the young adolescent's behavior with his or her parents (e.g., a girl may no longer feel comfortable sitting on her father's lap). Adolescents may even have short-lived, conscious sexual fantasies about the opposite-sex parent and may "jokingly" make sexually inappropriate comments to them.

Young adolescents generally do not pursue sexual interests in an active way, although they may have many social contacts. Young adolescents are quite curious about sex, and peers are probably the main source of information. When parents are able to discuss sexuality and, especially, pregnancy with their teenagers, a lower incidence of precocious sexuality or premarital pregnancy seems to prevail. This type of discussion may be more the exception than the rule, however.

In the past 20 years, the proportion of adolescents who are sexually active has increased, although the increase varies widely by gender, ethnicity, and socioeconomic status. Overall, about one-third of boys and one-quarter of girls are sexually active by middle adolescence.

For boys, the first sexual experiences raise anxieties about performance and competition with peers, fears of intimacy, guilt, and concerns about impregnation. Adolescent girls have fears about pregnancy and the continuity of the relationship, guilt, and self-esteem issues. Mutual masturbation, homosexual experimentation, conflicts over bisexual urges, and appropriate protection against sexually transmitted diseases (including AIDS) are other relevant sexual issues for adolescent men and women.

Developmental Vulnerabilities
Response to Illness

Physical illness affects adolescents when it results in delayed physical or sexual maturation. This delay may be due to medications (e.g., chronic steroid use), genetic anomalies, or chronic illness (e.g., cystic fibrosis). The adjustment to chronic illness seems to be enhanced if the adolescent is able to accept that in some ways he or she will be "different." This is obviously particularly difficult in adolescence. ➡ In one case, a mother speaking to her 13-year-old daughter, who had had a heart transplantation, put this conflict succinctly: "It's a 50–50 thing. Yes, you're normal. But yes, you had a heart transplant. If you don't accept the fact you had a transplant and take your medicine, you can't be normal." ⬅ Psychological adjustment seems to be facilitated when adolescents take an active role in their recovery and maintenance, whether this involves physical therapy, medication, or other treatments. With proper education and support, most 12-year-olds are capable of taking their own medication. Taking a more active role reinforces the adolescent's strivings for autonomy and helps to counter the regression accompanying the stress of illness.

A "regressive pull" may exist in adolescent struggles against the need and wish to be taken care of. This conflict may be visibly acted out (e.g., when adolescents refuse to take medication as a way of exercising their autonomy but then have an exacerbation of their illness and must rely on others even more). **Regression** can also cause the adolescent to "retreat" to earlier modes of magical thinking. In general, however, adolescents are able to view illness with a more sophisticated perspective in which they see themselves and their behavior (e.g., compliance with prescribed medication) as playing a role in their recovery. In addition, adolescents are able to understand that different symptoms can be associated with the same illness, and the illness can be seen with a longitudinal view that includes different stages, including an onset, middle course, and ending. When the adolescent reaches the stage of formal operations, he or she has acquired an understanding of the inner processes and anatomy of the body, and causality is understood with respect to biological processes.

It is important to remember that physical illness can be used as a way of avoiding many of the conflicts of the adolescent's world, such as fear of the transition into adulthood, social and sexual anxieties, or family difficulties. Staying ill may provide adolescents with secondary gain by allowing them to avoid scenarios that cause anxiety or fear.

In adolescents, self-image is so dependent on body image that the physical manifestations of chronic illness can have devastating effects on self-esteem. ➡ For example, a 16-year-old girl had a relapse of a soft tissue sarcoma of the right leg but refused amputation because of the disfigurement. That she would probably die without the treatment meant nothing to her because she felt that she looked so abnormal that her life was "hopeless," anyway. ⬅

The connection between body image and self-esteem may also be affected as chronically ill adolescents measure their ideal image of themselves ("ego-ideal") against where they realistically stand or will stand with regard to interpersonal, educational, and occupational goals. The extent to which they feel they will live up to their own expectations and realize their ambitions may have a sobering and, perhaps, disastrous effect on their self-esteem. Low self-esteem, in turn, may cause physical symptoms to become worse.

The separation from friends during a hospitalization can be quite stressful for the adolescent, who craves these attachments. The separation from parents may also precipitate loneliness. The adolescent with a chronic illness has the reality of the illness superimposed on the sensitivity to feeling different or rejected common to this phase of life. As a result, self-esteem problems can be exacerbated, as the tendency to be moody is affected by real events that may have profound consequences on body image and the ability to feel "normal."

Psychopathology

The passage through adolescence is not the same for all persons. Recent studies of adolescents have disputed earlier notions that this was necessarily a tumultuous, unstable period. In fact, approximately 80% of adolescents function normally. An adolescent whose rebelliousness includes severe disturbances in conduct, mood, or drug abuse should not be dismissed as merely going through a stage. The adolescent in turmoil needs help.

In males, the main developmental vulnerability is that the cultural emphasis on "machismo" may lead to rebellious, self-destructive behavior that threatens connections; in females, the priority of maintaining connections may lead to the denial or suppression of autonomous needs.

ADULTHOOD*
Developmental Progression

Adult life begins when adolescence ends, which is usually in the early twenties. Many observers of adult development have divided adult life into a number of discrete phases according to age. This division seems somewhat arbitrary, however, since the age at which adults are preoccupied with their main developmental tasks can vary enormously.

Adult life is characterized somewhat more by stability than by change. However, various patterns of evolution occur throughout adulthood in each of the developmental lines discussed for children and adolescents (i.e., social, emotional, and cognitive function; gender-related issues; and sexuality). As in children, these changes may lead to psychological growth and maturity but may also result in conflict, regression, and psychiatric symptoms.

Gratification in Work and Love

The main social developmental tasks for adults take place in the realms of work and intimate relationships. The degree to which adults achieve fulfillment in these two areas varies widely.

A shift from play to work accompanies the developmental course from childhood into adulthood. Advanced schooling serves as an intermediate step, particularly college and postgraduate studies, including professional training. The transition to the "real" world of work is a major one. Adults who are able to negotiate this step well have completed adolescence with a secure sense of themselves as competent people and with the capacity to relate to others in a stable manner. Joining the work force requires making a commitment to a chosen career path. This step can cause anxiety for people who have concerns about separation and independence and for those who have difficulty in giving up the grandiose adolescent fantasy that anything is possi-

*The following sections were written by Janis L. Cutler, MD.

ble. Some avoid the step altogether by becoming "professional students" who are unable to complete graduation requirements (e.g., they may work on an endless dissertation) or rationalize that they need yet another degree.

Achieving a **successful work life** is one of the ultimate tests of an individual's ability to join society as a productive member. Work can be a source of much gratification in the financial, intellectual, and social realms, among others, and can contribute to personal growth. Like children of latency age, whose view of themselves as competent grows each time another task is mastered, adults can grow significantly in self-confidence with successful work experiences.

Failure in work may have devastating consequences. Work can be a source of much frustration and disappointment. Even individuals who were successful students can be vulnerable to injured self-esteem resulting from failures in work. ➡ A male attorney who had completed each aspect of his training with the highest honors at the best schools found that what had been strengths in his academic pursuits (i.e., attention to detail, willingness to put in long hours, and perfectionism) became liabilities at work. His inability to set priorities and cut corners left him exhausted, overwhelmed, and unable to keep up with the work load. Interpersonal difficulties surfaced, as well. He felt both intimidated by and contemptuous of authority figures, and these conflictual feelings left him unable to deal appropriately with his superiors. Instead, he veered between being overtly ingratiating and covertly aggressive. While silently complying with a partner's refusal of his request to take off a week after the birth of his first child, he expressed his resentment when he cavalierly encouraged law students spending the summer at the firm to give up law and go to medical school. As he became increasingly aware of his difficulties, his confidence in himself as a lawyer plummeted; this caused his work performance to deteriorate even further. ◀

For many adults, failure can occur at any transitional stage in a career. A promotion or job change that requires different strengths or abilities may suddenly bring to the forefront previously unrecognized areas of weakness or conflict. ➡ For instance, a bright, conscientious high school teacher, who inspired her students with her enthusiasm and intellectual curiosity, was rewarded with a promotion to an administrative position. In this position, she was plagued by disorganization and interpersonal conflicts that she was unable to resolve. ◀ This difficulty is an example of the "Peter principle," which is the tendency for society to keep promoting workers until they get to a level at which they cannot function fully. It can be the source of failure and loss of self-esteem for many adults, particularly in middle age. Some adults have conflicting responses to success, which may be partially related to unresolved oedipal guilt and competitive issues and which may result in self-sabotage to avoid success.

The establishment of **mature, committed, intimate love relationships** is the other key social developmental task in the transition from adolescence to adulthood. Commitment to a monogamous relationship requires that adults relinquish their fantasies of the "perfect" mate. Identity consolidation is essential, as well, including coming to terms with sexual orientation and values. Finally, the adult must have a capacity to tolerate closeness and dependence while preserving a sense of autonomy.

George Vaillant, a psychiatrist with a particular interest in development over the life cycle, thought that the achievement of a satisfactory career path can occur only if the adult has a capacity for intimacy. Whether or not this proposed developmental sequence always holds true, the ability to form an intimate, loving, sexually satisfying relationship is at the core of a gratifying adult life.

A major milestone for many adults is **parenthood.** Becoming a parent together with a loving partner can be a source of enormous fulfillment. Parenthood is also an opportunity for significant psychological growth and mastery. Adults have the satisfaction of providing their offspring with a childhood that is in some way an improvement over their own, not to mention the joy of seeing the world again through the wondrous eyes of a growing child.

Parenthood significantly changes the adult child's relationship with his or her own parents. New parents can enjoy sharing the experience with their own parents of raising offspring, gaining a better appreciation for the challenges and demands that their own parents met in raising them. If new parents feel insecure in their parental roles or in their separateness from their own parents, intergenerational conflict or overinvolvement may result.

Unplanned pregnancies and unwanted children can be the source of tremendous grief and stress. For all of the joy they can bring, children are, by their very nature, demanding of parents' time and energy. These demands, and the conflicts that they may exacerbate or reawaken, can be stressful even for the most emotionally mature, socially supported, and financially secure couples. For single parents or parents struggling with abusive or otherwise impaired partners, social isolation, or poverty, those demands may be overwhelming. Physicians should be aware that parenthood can be a time of particular stress and that parents under stress are at high risk for psychiatric disorders as well as child abuse.

As was discussed above, each phase of child development requires different parental responses. The parents of infants face the task of taking care of a completely helpless, dependent human being; this responsibility can often arouse intense fears and anxieties. The parents of toddlers and adolescents witness their children's struggles with sexual and aggressive impulses, as well as conflicting yearnings for dependence and autonomy. Just as a promotion or job change might highlight a previously unrecognized area of weakness in adults, the developmental transitions of children may precipitate crises in parents who lack the flexibility and coping skills to adjust their parenting style to their child's needs.

A significant minority of adults must come to terms with the realization that they will not have children, either because they have reproductive difficulties or because they lack a suitable partner. For professional women who delay child-bearing while they develop their careers, the failure to conceive can be particularly painful and may be accompanied by guilt and self-blame. The onset of menopause for these women can precipitate strong feelings of grief and loss. Supportive psychotherapy, whether it be individual, marital, or group therapy, can be quite useful in assisting people through this crisis. A healthy adjustment frequently involves redirecting the urge for what Erikson described as the "generativity" of middle age into activities other than parenthood that can serve a similar function and allow one to guide and mentor the next generation.

Emotional Maturity

Much of adult emotional development can be regarded as an evolution of ego strengths. A crucial aspect of ego functioning is the unconscious deployment of defense mechanisms to maintain emotional stability. Once most persons reach adulthood, they have the ability to use mature defenses (e.g., sublimation, humor, and altruism), which can be observed in emotionally mature behaviors, such as patience, flexibility, and responsibility; lack of impulsivity; and a significant capacity for empathy and acceptance of ambivalence in themselves and others.

Cognitive Awareness

In the realm of cognitive function, young adults have fully reached Piaget's stage of formal operational thinking, which permits **self-reflection.** Impairments in intellectual function or delays in cognitive development will obviously interfere with this process. In addition, the capacity for true creativity is achieved only during the adult years.

Aging involves a decline in certain cognitive capacities, especially memory and problem-solving abilities. At the same time, there seems to be an increased ability to conceptualize, put ideas into a context, and accept situations that may seem paradoxical. Some observers have, therefore, described a further stage of intellectual development beyond Piaget's stage of formal operations that is essentially characterized as being more practical.

As adult development progresses, major shifts in the **perception of time** occur. Children live in the present, without much ability to reflect on the past or anticipate the future. Adults can do both and begin to understand that their life trajectory does not involve unlimited time. Death becomes a more real phenomenon as adults experience the loss of friends and family and note their own physical deterioration.

Sexual Function and Dysfunction

Satisfactory sexual functioning is central to, and closely associated with, emotional and social well-being. Conflicts in this realm may involve the gender of one's sexual partner, the integration of sex with companionship, and inhibitions that may occur at any stage of the sexual experience, from desire to arousal to orgasm.

Sexual dysfunctions tend to have multiple causes. External relationship difficulties (e.g., disagreements over money) or internal emotional conflicts (e.g., excessive guilt or anxiety with regard to sexuality) may be a cause, as may be a history of sexual trauma or physiological abnormalities. The latter may be caused by medications or medical disorders, the most common of which are diabetes and cardiovascular disease. Psychiatric disorders, particularly depression, can be associated with a change in sexual functioning.

Physicians can play an important role in assessing their adult patients' sexual functioning. In screening for dysfunction, the physician should be aware that the diagnosis of physical causes can be a great relief for patients who are afraid to raise their concerns. In addition, education and information can be very helpful for many patients who do not have physical reasons for their difficulties. Because many adults have conflicts and worries with regard to sexuality, the physician's nonjudgmental attitude and acceptance of a wide range of sexual practices may be helpful in contributing to the patient's personal acceptance and improved functioning.

Premature ejaculation and **female orgasmic disorder** are two common sexual disorders that tend not to have an identifiable physical etiology (see Tables 13–2 and 13–3 for DSM-IV criteria). Behavioral therapy has been extremely effective for these disorders. Physicians should refer patients who are suffering from these problems and other sexual dysfunctions that do not respond to medical and educational interventions to therapists who are trained in appropriate techniques.

Developmental Vulnerabilities

The transition from late adolescence to adulthood can be accompanied by ambivalence because uncertainty about a career and the struggle to de-

---

**TABLE 13–2. DSM-IV Criteria
for Premature Ejaculation**

A. Persistent or recurrent ejaculation with minimal sexual stimulation before, on, or shortly after penetration and before the person wishes it. The clinician must take into account factors that affect duration of the excitement phase, such as age, novelty of the sexual partner or situation, and recent frequency of sexual activity.
B. The disturbance causes marked distress or interpersonal difficulty.
C. The premature ejaculation is not due exclusively to the direct effects of a substance (e.g., withdrawal from opioids).

TABLE 13–3. DSM-IV Criteria for Female Orgasmic Disorder

A. Persistent or recurrent delay in, or absence of, orgasm following a normal sexual excitement phase. Women exhibit wide variability in the type or intensity of stimulation that triggers orgasm. The diagnosis of Female Orgasmic Disorder should be based on the clinician's judgment that the woman's orgasmic capacity is less than would be reasonable for her age, sexual experience, and the adequacy of sexual stimulation she receives.

B. The disturbance causes marked distress or interpersonal difficulty.

C. The orgasmic dysfunction is not better accounted for by another Axis I disorder (except another Sexual Dysfunction) and is not due exclusively to the direct physiological effect of a substance (e.g., a drug of abuse, a medication) or a general medical condition.

velop intimate relationships often leave the late adolescent confused. Adolescents may mourn the many losses that are necessary as they make the transition into adulthood and may feel an emptiness in their lives that was once filled by their relationship with their parents. This provides a counterpoint to the eager anticipation of the freedoms that adults enjoy. Cultural and economic factors, such as a poor job market, can also affect this process and exacerbate the ambivalence and threats to identity.

Problems in this age-group result from conflicts about work, love, school, or family. Many of these conflicts cause short-term anxiety or depression, but more serious problems with work inhibition or depression also occur as perhaps biological vulnerability interfaces with environmental factors. Many of these symptoms may be acute or short-lived and may cause the late adolescent concern that is out of proportion to the actual severity of the problem. Chronic problems may develop in the late adolescent as earlier unresolved issues become extrapolated into a new developmental phase. A person who had separation problems as a toddler and who experienced difficulty in developing a sense of independence in early and middle adolescence may later find it difficult to leave home and attend school or to develop intimate relationships with others. If adequate coping skills have not been developed earlier, problems may develop as adolescents leave the home.

As life proceeds, significant stresses may be imposed by financial responsibilities, such as mortgages, shifts in the work place and marketplace, problems in interpersonal and marital relationships, and uncertainty about whether the chosen life path has been the correct one. These concerns can precipitate a "midlife crisis," which may be more accurately labeled a period of reflection, or reassessment, during which adults may wonder whether their life-style, job, and relationships are the ones that were most desired. These questions were first confronted in late adolescence and now appear again.

Response to Illness

As anyone who has huddled under the bedclothes with a cold and enjoyed being pampered well understands, adults who are physically ill frequently regress emotionally. Sick adults may use the adaptational strategies of childhood as illness makes them once again physically or emotionally dependent on caretakers. This dependence can also evoke strong childhood fears and wishes about such caretakers. Physicians will be much more successful in managing their relationships with their patients if they recognize these responses.

In many ways, the effective approaches described above for physically ill children and adolescents are also relevant, with modification, for adults (e.g., hospitalized adults may be comforted by such transitional objects as pictures of their loved ones, and they should be encouraged to bring these and other personal items to the hospital).

The degree of emotional regression and other responses to which adults are prone varies enormously, depending on the solidity and benevolence of previous development, the temperament of the person, and the severity of the stressor. Like children, adults respond to physical illness according to their present and past life situations. The meaning of a diagnosis of cancer is very different for a woman in her late thirties who was born with an anxious temperament, was sick as a child, and has just divorced than it is for a married man who is middle-aged, has never been ill, and is more inclined to deny feelings. The first patient might have a better appreciation of what it is like to be sick and be more compliant with medication regimens but may be so severely depressed and anxious that she is completely unable to function. The second patient might have angry outbursts at his wife and refuse to take certain medications but may be able to continue his work. (See Chapter 12, Psychological Factors Affecting Medical Conditions, for an extensive discussion of this topic.)

Psychopathology

Many psychiatric disorders appear initially during the period of young adulthood through the thirties, including the **mood disorders** (see Chapter 3) and the **anxiety disorders** (see Chapter 6). **Schizophrenia** typically begins in late adolescence but can also occur in the twenties (see Chapter 4). The manifestations of **personality disorders** and **eating disorders** are generally present by early adulthood, although patients may not present for treatment until years after the problem begins (see Chapter 8 and Chapter 9).

Throughout the life cycle, particular events and stages of life hold individual meaning for different people. Thus, there are many possible ways in which the environment can interact with an underlying vulnerability to produce psychiatric illness or to cause someone to seek help for a long-standing psychiatric problem. ⟹ For example, the lawyer referred to above sought psychiatric consultation at age 29 years, when his legal career was in jeopardy and he developed a major depressive episode. ◀ At the same time, events and life experiences that are stressful for some people are not stressful for others. This variability depends in part on previous experiences, areas of intrapsychic conflict, and sources of vulnerability.

Brain structures such as the locus coeruleus, which is a part of the brain stem that mediates arousal, anxiety, and fear, as well as certain pathological anxiety responses, undergo changes in enzyme capacity, decreases in the number of cells, and increases in neuromelanin, which is a pigment that accelerates cell loss throughout the adult years. This phenomenon may contribute to certain psychological changes during middle age, such as the "mellowing phenomenon" and the "burning out" of certain psychiatric illnesses (e.g., bulimia, panic attacks). Biological factors become enmeshed with environmental factors and the psychological response to aging in influencing the developmental course. The brain continues to be an adaptable, plastic structure throughout adulthood. The appearance and disappearance of dendrite structures and the release of neurotransmitters are modified by a person's daily experiences. Brain senescence and continued plasticity initiate development and change throughout the life cycle, even into old age, affecting not only the personality but also the development of psychiatric disorders.

OLD AGE
Developmental Progression

As adults approach old age, the stability that they have achieved over the preceding 40–50 years must, in some respects, give way to great change. At the same time, the range of individual approaches to a life phase is more varied during old age than during any other age. The age at which people become "old" may be as early as their late fifties or early sixties or as late as their seventies or eighties. Some people seem "old before their time," and others remain active, vigorous, and "youthful" into their eighties. These variations result from individual differences in people's capacity for adapting to and interpreting the psychosocial, cognitive, sexual, and physical changes that accompany old age.

Changing Relationships

One of the main changes for the elderly results from alterations in their social realm. The constellation of important people in the elderly individual's life changes for several reasons. First, since most people have retired from work by the time they are in their seventies, their circle of colleagues with whom they had had daily contact at work is virtually eliminated. While relationships with some of those people may be maintained, the former character of those interactions, which focused on joint goal-oriented, productive work, will never be the same. **Retirement** generally leaves the elderly more involved with and reliant on family and friends. For those who are financially secure, retirement allows them to spend their time as they wish, in leisure and pleasurable pursuits, charitable work or other activities aimed at benefiting society at large, or increased time with family and friends. This release from the constraints of a daily work routine can be liberating for some elderly persons, but it can also precipitate feelings of loss, guilt, anxiety, and purposelessness. Elderly people without adequate savings or retirement income are beset by an additional set of worries with regard to supporting themselves.

The passage of time is inevitably accompanied by the deaths of family members and friends. In earlier stages of adulthood, most people must grieve and work through the loss of their grandparents and, later, their parents. For the elderly, **death** becomes more commonplace and closer to home because many of those lost will be of similar age or even younger. These losses serve as reminders of one's own mortality, as well as sources of grief and survivor guilt. Death and illness inexorably whittles away at the social network that has been put into place over a lifetime. Even elderly persons who are resilient, flexible, and optimistically willing to reach out and develop new friends cannot easily replace intimate relationships that have spanned decades. Some losses, especially of a spouse or a child, are particularly difficult for the elderly to accept.

The social configuration of the elderly is also affected by their changing roles in relation to others. An elderly person is no longer a boss or supervisor, a family wage-earner, a head of a household of dependent children, or even, in some cases, a financially or physically independent, self-sufficient adult. Elderly men and women with children relinquish many of these roles to their middle-aged offspring, who are in their "prime." Those who are childless may worry about who will take care of them if and when they become unable to take care of themselves. The **shifting roles** can reawaken conflicting feelings about dependence and autonomy. Children may even come to represent powerful parental figures in the perceptions of the elderly. The capacity of middle-aged children to tolerate these changing roles can affect the adjustment of the elderly person. The following case illustrates the three major developmental issues faced by the elderly.

◀ A 74-year-old retired physician and mother of two nursed her husband through several years of declining health. He died several months before what would have been their fiftieth wedding anniversary. She had enjoyed a full, gratifying career; a strong, intimate marriage; and a close circle of friends. By the time she became a widow, however, many of her friends had died or were too ill to be active. Turning for companionship to her two daughters, who were both physicians with families, she became hurt and rejected when she found that their busy lives left them with little time to spend with her. In psychotherapy, she explored her fears that she had been a "bad mother" for "abandoning" her children to continue to practice medicine at a time when few women with young children worked outside of the home and that she was now being "punished" by their lack of interest in her. Her therapist helped her reframe her children's preoccupation with their own challenging careers and growing families as evidence that she had done a good job in raising successful, independent women, who had chosen to follow her career path. Through therapy, this woman realized that she had been a pioneer in many ways; this perspective allowed her to contemplate her life course with the sense of inner peace and satisfaction that Erikson referred to as integrity. ◀▥

Three of the many positive aspects of old age are the satisfaction of seeing one's children functioning as healthy, happy, and competent adults; the joy and gratification experienced from becoming a grandparent and great-grandparent; and the ability of some adults who found parenthood to be fraught with conflict and stress to enjoy being grandparents with much less ambivalence.

Gradual Decline

Physical and cognitive capacities continue to decline during old age. Elderly persons realize that life is finite and that more years have been lived than are left to live. This fact is often brought into stark relief when close friends and relatives die. The inevitable real losses, such as the deaths of loved ones, accompany these other symbolic role losses in stature and prominence.

In old age, reminiscence tends to become a more central feature of one's reflection on life. One may recall hopes that were never fulfilled, perhaps in a nostalgic way, and reflect on one's life course with a critical eye.

Sexuality in the Elderly

There is much variation in the degree to which the elderly remain sexually active. For some, sexuality remains an important part of life and of loving relationships. For others, sexual desire fades, perhaps because a partner is lost or because there is a decreased capacity for sexual gratification due to physical infirmity. For women, the decline in estrogen associated with menopause can cause a number of physical changes, such as an absence of vaginal lubrication during arousal, that may interfere with sexual functioning. Men as well as women must come to terms with the changing physical appearance of their own bodies and their partners' bodies.

As with younger adults, information and education can sometimes be quite helpful. Elderly men should be informed that they may very well retain the capacity to achieve orgasm even if they suffer from erectile dysfunction (the term *impotence* has come into disfavor with the medical establishment). Women should be made aware of the advantages of hormone replacement therapy in avoiding vaginal atrophy and dryness (as well as preventing osteoporosis and cardiovascular disease) and should also be counseled that one of the best ways to avoid these vaginal changes is to remain sexually active. Finally, it is crucial that physicians not assume that their elderly patients are sexually inactive. Such an assumption may not only be based on social prejudices but also on the age difference between the physician and the patient. The patient may be the same age as the physician's parents or grandparents, and the physician may prefer to think of persons of such an age as being uninterested in sex.

Developmental Vulnerabilities

Erikson theorized that elderly persons who are unable to achieve a sense of integrity are at risk for feeling "disgust" and despair. ▥▶ In contrast with the widowed physician described above, who derived satisfaction from the roles that she had played as a productive physician, loving wife, and nurturing mother, the man described below was unfortunately not able to achieve such self-acceptance. He was a 62-year-old divorced father with one child, who had worked for over 40 years as a window washer. His retirement, which was precipitated by increasing difficulties with his balance, represented a loss of the stable source of self-esteem in his life. He was an isolated, somewhat mistrustful man who had maintained a caring but emotionally distant relationship with his daughter, despite separating from her mother when she was only 3 years old. He had been a conscientious, steady worker who took great pride in a job well done. After retirement, he filled his days by listening to country and western music on the radio and watching sporting events on television. These pursuits left him feeling unproductive and despairing as to the lack of meaning or purpose in his life, and he complained that "there's no point any more." ◀▥

Response to Illness

As with children and adults, the elderly may have a whole range of responses to physical illness, which depend in large part on their psychological makeup, previous experiences with illness, and current developmental state. One of the challenges for physicians in caring for the elderly is understanding the needs and wishes of individual patients. It is crucial to avoid making assumptions about their fears or wishes with regard to death. As with the issue of sexuality, physicians should be wary of distortions resulting from the patient's resemblance to the physician's parents or grandparents. This caution is particularly important if a patient refuses further treatment. The physician should recommend a thorough psychiatric evaluation for such a patient rather than simply assume that the refusal makes sense for anyone in their seventies or eighties (see Chapter 14, Therapeutic Settings).

Psychopathology

The most prevalent psychiatric disorders in elderly persons are the cognitive disorders, particularly the dementias. It is a misperception that the elderly are more susceptible to mood and anxiety disorders than are middle-aged adults. Most psychiatric disorders appear by age 40–50 years. However, perhaps because of an increase in chronic medical illnesses and a lack of social supports, which are two risk factors for suicide, the incidence of suicide increases in the elderly.

As has been pointed out, the elderly are not immune from conflicts and psychic pain. Psychotherapy and carefully monitored pharmacotherapy, when indicated, can be extremely helpful. Old age is not a contraindication to adequate psychiatric treatment.

Selected Readings

Blos, P. On Adolescence. New York, Free Press, 1962.

Erikson, E. H. Childhood and Society. New York, W. W. Norton, 1950.

Freud, A. The concept of developmental lines. The Psychoanalytic Study of the Child 18:245–265, 1963.

Freud, S. Three essays on the theory of sexuality. The Standard Edition of the Complete Psychological Works of Sigmund Freud. London, Hogarth Press, 1905.

Gilligan, C., Hartman, H., and E. Kris. The genetic approach in psychoanalysis. The Psychoanalytic Study of the Child 1:11–30, 1945.

Lewis, M. (ed). Child and Adolescent Psychiatry: A Comprehensive Textbook. Baltimore, Maryland, Williams & Wilkins, 1991.

Mahler, M. S. On the first three subphases of the separation-individuation process. International Journal of Psychoanalysis 53:333–338, 1972.

Nemiroff, R. A., and C. A. Colarusso (editors). New Dimensions in Adult Development. New York, Basic Books, 1990.

Oldham, J. M., and R. S. Liebert (editors). The Middle Years: New Psychoanalytic Perspectives. New Haven, Connecticut, Yale University Press, 1989.

Tyson, P., and R. Tyson. Psychoanalytic Theories of Development. New Haven, Connecticut, Yale University Press, 1990.

Vaillant, G. E. The Wisdom of the Ego. Cambridge, Massachusetts, Harvard University Press, 1993.

Winnicott, D. W. Transitional objects and transitional phenomena: a study of the first not me possession. International Journal of Psychoanalysis 34:89–97, 1953.

TREATMENT

CHAPTER FOURTEEN

THERAPEUTIC SETTINGS

JANIS L. CUTLER, MD

Each of the settings in which psychiatric patients are seen—emergency rooms, inpatient units, outpatient clinics, and general hospitals—has distinct features. Just as physicians must modify their general approaches to interviewing and evaluating psychiatric patients in order to meet the needs of particular patients and specific disorders, they must also modify their focus to fit the setting in which they see each patient.

EMERGENCY ROOM

A physician working in an emergency room treats patients who are in crisis, whether the problem is a broken arm, chest pain, or a psychiatric symptom, such as psychosis or suicidal ideation. *In this setting, it is crucial to focus the initial evaluation on identifying the crisis.* While interviewing the patient, the physician must keep asking himself or herself, "Why is this patient here, in the emergency room, telling me this information, at this time?"

The following clinical situation demonstrates how the physician's focus should be modified by the emergency room setting. ➠ A woman with chronic thoughts about wanting to kill herself who has never made a suicide attempt has been monitoring this chronic problem with her psychiatrist and assessing with him any changes in ongoing outpatient treatment. When this patient suddenly appears in the emergency room, the physician must more seriously regard her potential to behave self-destructively. Until proved otherwise, the patient is in crisis. Even though she has not acted on her suicidal thoughts in the past, her status is now different in some, possibly dangerous, way, and this has caused her to come to the emergency room. ⬅

Assessment
Gathering Patient Information

First, it is important to ask patients how they came to be in the emergency room and to confirm their answers with the staff members who first saw and registered them. Patients who are in crisis frequently have poor insight into their conditions and poor judgment about their need for help. The more impaired patients are, the less reliable may be the information they provide. They are often not willing or

able to discuss their conditions and have not come to the emergency room voluntarily but were brought in by someone who noticed their bizarre behavior or was concerned about them. The emergency room physician should ask family members—and other persons connected to the patient's arrival at the emergency room—to share any information they have about the patient's present condition.

➠ For example, a 40-year-old man was brought to the emergency room by police officers, who had picked him up on a nearby bridge. The patient told the psychiatrist in the emergency room that he had been walking on the bridge "to calm my nerves" after an argument that evening with his estranged wife. He denied that he was depressed or had suicidal ideation. He appeared to be somewhat anxious but was able to sit quietly during the interview. When the psychiatrist tried to "step back" to see the complete picture, something did not fit. If, indeed, the patient had been out on the bridge only for a late evening walk, why did the police officers bother to question him and take him to the emergency room for further evaluation? The patient had no explanation for their concern. At this point in the interview, the physician could have taken the patient's history at face value, assumed that it was a slow night for the local police, and discharged the patient after giving him the phone number of the psychiatric clinic, in case he felt like speaking with someone about the stress of his marital difficulties or other problems. Instead, the physician remembered to consider the real possibility that any patient appearing in the emergency room is in crisis. The physician tracked down the police report and asked for details from the officers who had brought in the patient. The officers said that the patient had been halfway over the railing when they first saw him and had fought desperately with them to get over the side of the bridge. They finally had to handcuff him to the railing to prevent him from going off the bridge while they called for assistance. When the patient was confronted with these facts, he admitted that he had been despondent that night and convinced that he and his wife would never be reconciled. He had wanted to die then and still wanted to die but had denied having suicidal ideation when asked about it in the emergency room for fear that he would be admitted to the hospital. He did, in fact, require psychiatric hospitalization, during which he was successfully treated for a depressive episode complicated by alcohol and cocaine abuse. ◀▥

As this case illustrates, the consequences can be catastrophic if the physician does not adequately address the reason for a patient's visit to the emergency room. If this patient had been released from the emergency room, he would have been at high risk for another, perhaps successful, suicide attempt (see also Chapter 11, Suicide and Violence.)

Identifying Patient's Underlying Concerns

The near-suicide described above is an extreme example of how a patient's impaired insight and judgment can complicate assessment in the emergency room. Patients who present with physical complaints or underlying medical conditions can also represent a diagnostic challenge for emergency room physicians. Patients may describe only their physical complaints even though they also have concerns about their emotional state. Another obstacle to identifying underlying concerns is found in patients who come voluntarily to the emergency room and have some idea that they need psychiatric help but are not able to articulate that need clearly.

▥▶ A homeless man came to the emergency room complaining of a rash, which was barely visible. He launched into an elaborate description of how he was being poisoned and how the rash was just one early manifestation of the systemic poisoning that he believed would soon kill him. Although he was delusional (he had impaired reality testing regarding this set of beliefs) and had poor insight into the causes of his rash, he came to the emergency room because he felt that he needed help, not just with the rash but with the terrible fear that he was the target of a conspiracy to kill him. He responded with relief to the staff's empathy with his fear, and he agreed to be admitted as a psychiatric inpatient because he understood that this plan would help him to deal with his stress. ◀▥

In contrast to the above situation, a patient's initial presenting complaint may consist of psychiatric symptoms even though the underlying source of the crisis is actually a medical condition. Just as physical complaints may be manifestations of a psychiatric disorder, behavioral and emotional disturbances may be manifestations of a medical disorder. It is always important, therefore, to evaluate carefully the medical status of patients in the emergency room.

▥▶ In one case, a 33-year-old woman came to the emergency room accompanied by a friend. Although the patient's chief complaint was of nausea, her friend had brought her to the emergency room because she appeared to be excited and agitated, with rapid, pressured, loud speech. The triage nurse, focusing on the patient's behavior as well, noted that she was grandiose and irritable and decided to call the psychiatrist. The first clue that this was not a typical manic patient was the absence of any prior psychiatric history. On physical examination, the psychiatrist discovered a profoundly rigid abdomen, with rebound tenderness, indicating an acute abdomen. The patient underwent surgery and was found to have a perforated duodenal ulcer. In this case, the stress of an infection and probable metabolic derangements apparently caused the patient to become transiently manic. The patient's psychiatric diagnosis was mood disorder due to a general medical condition, with manic features. More importantly, the medical disorder was diagnosed and treated. ◀▥

Assessing Patient's Family and Support System

Another crucial variable to consider when assessing a patient in the emergency room is whether or not the patient's support system is in crisis and, if so, in what way the crisis relates to the patient. This process is a "two-way street": The patient's symptoms and difficulties may be putting stress on the support system and creating a crisis; or a failure or change in the support system may be adversely affecting the patient. Obviously, both problems can occur simultaneously.

The degree to which family members and significant others will tolerate disturbed behavior before they seek help varies. If the family has decided to send or bring the patient to the emergency room, the physician should find out what caused them to do so. They may be overreacting to behavior that is not particularly disturbed because they themselves have reached an intolerable level of stress or need help for psychiatric problems of their own.

▥▶ For example, a single mother brought her 16-year-old daughter to the emergency room for assessment of "out-of-control behavior" when the daughter's arguments with her overprotective, controlling mother escalated. As the evaluation proceeded, it became clear to the physician that the mother was depressed and in need of help, whereas the adolescent was not particularly "out of control."

On the other hand, the mother of a man in his late twenties with a long history of schizophrenia delayed taking him to the emergency room in spite of months of bizarre behavior in which he had isolated himself in his room, spoke to no one, huddled on the floor in a corner, and ate only rice. When he shaved off all the hair on his body, his mother insisted that he go to the emergency room. The staff believed that he could receive treatment on an outpatient basis because he did not seem particularly different, had never before required hospitalization, and was not overtly suicidal or homicidal, although he did have a thought disorder and delusions. A week later, the patient took an overdose of aspirin and was admitted to the intensive care unit. The emergency room staff had made two mistakes. Because of his history of chronic symptoms, they did not consider his presenting to the emergency room seriously enough, when, in fact, the mere act of appearing in an emergency room should have indicated that something significant had changed. The staff also had a false sense of security because they were unaware of the unusually high level of tolerance for bizarre behavior that his mother had and, therefore, assumed that she might be overreacting to her son's strange but not dangerous behavior. The patient's isolation and withdrawal reflected his almost constant auditory hallucinations and complete loss of reality testing. Although his mother used poor judgment in not seeking help earlier, her concern about his shaving off his hair was appropriate, because this behavior reflected a worsening of his poor impulse control in response to an increase in and intensification of his auditory hallucinations. ⬅

Making a Diagnosis

Although the process of evaluation in the emergency room is similar to that in other settings, there is a definite difference. In the emergency room, a greater emphasis is placed on identifying the crisis than on making a diagnosis. In crisis situations, assessing a patient's **impulse control, insight,** and **judgment** takes precedence over ascertaining whether, for example, the patient's grandiose delusions and auditory hallucinations are best explained by schizophrenia or schizoaffective disorder. The evaluation process is similar to that used in cases of acute abdomen, in which a decision about whether or not to operate takes precedence over diagnosing the specific cause prior to surgery. In the emergency room, the decision is whether or not the patient requires psychiatric admission, medication, or other immediate action to resolve the crisis. Certain diagnoses have important implications, however, and need to be considered carefully in the emergency room setting. For example, when patients have symptoms of depression or psychosis, and even though they may deny suicidal ideation, the diagnosis of a major depressive episode with psychotic features must be considered because of the increased risk of suicide associated with this disorder.

The time constraints of the emergency room and its chaotic, hectic atmosphere can make the performance of necessary tasks seem particularly stressful and difficult to physicians. Because they are faced with so many "emergencies" and are pressed for time, medical students and residents, especially, feel that they must sometimes cut corners and not follow the usual routine. Evaluations should be time-efficient, but important steps should not be overlooked. When time is short, the physician must be able to quickly identify and focus only on information that is essential to resolving the crisis at hand. Valuable time cannot be spent in obtaining detailed historical information that is not immediately relevant. Physicians who are unable to distinguish between essential and nonessential information while evaluating patients will find it difficult to function in an emergency room. Questions that must be answered in order to complete a full evaluation of any patient in an emergency room setting are listed in the Emergency Room Evaluation Box. A good general

---

Emergency Room Evaluation

- Why is the patient in the emergency room at this time?
- Who referred the patient (e.g., self, family, physician, police)?
- Did the patient arrive voluntarily or involuntarily?
- Is the patient's support system in crisis?
- How does the patient's family assess change?
- Is the patient a danger to himself or herself or to others?
- Is the patient psychotic?
- What is the patient's medical status?
- Is a psychiatric admission indicated?

---

plan of action is to at least consider all of the standard parts of an evaluation and then, in a systematic manner, decide which parts can be cut short.

Crisis Intervention

Much of the emergency room staff's work is assessment and triage, so that patients can be referred to inpatient units and outpatient clinics. A significant number of patients require **crisis intervention,** however, before they can be safely discharged for outpatient care. The basic goal of crisis intervention is to resolve the crisis by significantly altering some of the factors contributing to it. This modification usually takes place when the crisis situation mobilizes and effects a change in the patient's support system of family and friends. Whether or not the intervention will succeed is not clear until it is attempted; if it fails, hospitalization may be required. (A more detailed discussion of crisis intervention is included in Chapter 11, Suicide and Violence.)

➡ In one case, an 18-year-old girl was treated for an overdose of acetaminophen. The psychiatrist in the emergency room found her to be withdrawn and uncommunicative; she would reveal only that she had taken 20 acetaminophen tablets over the course of 6 hours to relieve a headache after she had had a fight with her boyfriend. Interviews with the boyfriend and family members disclosed that she tended to become depressed rather than confront people with whom she was angry. A session was held in the emergency room, first with the patient and her boyfriend, then with the patient and her mother, and finally with all three. The patient expressed disappointment with her boyfriend's recent lack of availability and frustration with what she perceived to be her mother's lack of appreciation of her. Both her boyfriend and her mother reassured her that they loved her and would continue to love her even if she got angry with them. The session was emotionally exhausting for everyone involved, but in the end, it gave the patient a sense of hope for the future. Had the patient remained withdrawn, hospitalization would have been required to further evaluate her potential for attempting suicide. Crisis intervention allowed her to be referred for outpatient treatment. ◀

INPATIENT UNITS

Inpatient treatment is indicated when crisis intervention in an emergency room or outpatient setting is not sufficient to stabilize a patient. It may also be indicated for evaluating patients who have been newly diagnosed with a severe psychiatric illness or for whom other treatment modalities seem ineffective. Some treatments are best provided on an inpatient basis because they require careful monitoring (e.g., the administration of electroconvulsive therapy or the prescription of a tricyclic antidepressant to an elderly patient with cardiac disease).

Inpatient units are located within general hospitals and in self-contained private and public psychiatric hospitals. Because insurance companies and managed care organizations have increasingly tried to minimize health care expenditures, inpatient treatment has been reserved for severely ill patients who are only allowed significantly reduced lengths of stay. Consequently, it is particularly important that the psychiatrist, at the time a patient is admitted, formulate clear-cut goals to be accomplished during the hospitalization. In formulating these goals, it is helpful to view the patient's hospitalization as a crisis intervention with a more prolonged time course. Not all of the patient's problems must be solved before he or she is discharged from the hospital; instead, *the patient and his or her support system must become sufficiently stabilized in order for outpatient treatment to proceed.*

The economic burden of hospitalization is not the only reason for making the stay as brief as possible. Hospitalization can be extremely disruptive for patients who are employed and have active family and social lives. For patients who function less well, do not work, or are socially isolated, admission to the hospital can be a regressive experience. Therefore, it is usually in the patient's best interests to return to life outside of the hospital as soon as he or she is able.

The Inpatient Unit Milieu

Because inpatient psychiatric units provide care 24 hours a day, they can provide special types of treatment. One unique aspect of such units is the **milieu,** which is a structured environment maintained by staff members with interdisciplinary training who work with patients toward therapeutic goals. The degree of stability and structure of the unit depends on the length of time patients usually stay on the unit (e.g., a few days, several weeks, or several months), whether the ward is locked or unlocked, and the types of patients the unit tends to treat (e.g., psychotic and manic patients as well as impulsive patients with personality disorders tend to con-

tribute to a more chaotic milieu, as is not the case with depressed patients).

The basic component of the milieu is a series of **group meetings** designed to facilitate communication among staff and patients. Throughout the week, patients participate in a variety of staff-supervised activities and discussion groups; once or twice a week, all of the staff and patients meet together for a community meeting. Staff members usually receive a daily ward report supplied by the nursing staff, as well as attend team rounds or conferences (usually from one to three times per week). Other meetings for the staff only may be weekly administrative meetings and educational activities, such as a journal club at which relevant scientific articles are presented and discussed.

For some patients, the crucial role of the milieu is to **prevent regression.** The ward routine, with its group activities and individual responsibilities, compels patients to function at their highest possible levels.

➡ A 41-year-old single woman, diagnosed with schizoaffective disorder, worked full-time as an office clerk despite chronic auditory hallucinations. During a brief hospitalization that was required to evaluate and address her intensifying psychotic symptoms, she was not permitted to become overly dependent and helpless. Instead, she was encouraged to continue "tuning out" the voices and ignoring her paranoid preoccupations, participate in groups, attend to her grooming needs, and socialize. Being kept in the hospital and out of her independent routine for any more time than necessary would only make her transition out of the hospital more difficult. ◀

Acute Symptom Control and Goal Modification

The extent to which a patient becomes involved in the activities of the unit (i.e., the frequency of involvement and the demands placed upon the patient) depends on the individual patient, his or her overall goals for the hospitalization, and how far along he or she is in achieving those goals at a given time during the course of treatment. The various members of the **interdisciplinary team** share their perspectives on the patient's progress and modify the treatment goals. The following case is one example of how a patient's needs can be met within the inpatient milieu.

➡ An acutely psychotic and manic 53-year-old attorney, who was married and the father of two children in college, was admitted after accruing significant financial debt and engaging in an extramarital affair, of which his wife of 25 years had become aware. Initially, the patient's grandiose delusions, racing thoughts, intrusiveness, and psychomotor agitation prevented him from participating in structured activities. The goal for the first week of hospitalization was to diminish the patient's agitation through medication and a reduction in sensory stimulation. The patient was not required to attend any groups, except the community meeting; he was allowed to leave that meeting after 15 minutes because he had become increasingly anxious and prevented others from speaking. He was expected to shower and groom himself, with supervision by the nursing staff. During the second week of treatment, as the acute signs and symptoms of his mania resolved, increased demands were placed on the patient. He was expected to attend the community meeting for its entire length of 30 minutes, as well as group arts-and-crafts and cooking sessions conducted by occupational therapists, an aerobics exercise session, and a current events discussion group conducted by recreational therapists. These groups allowed the patient to begin feeling competent again. They also challenged him because he had to remain focused on the task at hand and could not interfere with the group process.

Individual sessions with a psychiatrist were initially brief and aimed at assessing the patient's psychopathology, including impulse control, and developing and strengthening the therapeutic alliance. A social worker concurrently met with the patient's wife and children to obtain historical information, assess the patient's support system, and explore the impact his affair and financial indiscretions had had upon them.

The nursing staff, psychiatrist, occupational and recreational therapists, and social worker exchanged information about the patient's progress at the beginning of his third week of hospitalization. The psychiatrist's mental status examination indicated that the psychotic symptoms were no longer present, which was consistent with the nursing staff's observations that the patient was sleeping well and the occupational therapist's report that the patient was goal-directed and acting appropriately in group sessions. Everyone agreed that the acute manic episode had remitted.

The goals for the final week of hospitalization were then set and consisted of higher expectations for the patient's participation in unit activities and preparation for discharge from the unit. In addition to his previous activities, the number of individual and group therapy sessions was increased and therapy sessions with his family were instituted. The ramifications of his manic episode needed to be addressed within the supportive, structured atmosphere of the hospital to ensure that the patient could tolerate the stress of realizing the damage he had done to his personal and professional lives. In his final community meeting, the patient warmly thanked the staff for their help and summarized the gains that he had made. His insight and progress provided a useful perspective for other patients who had been admitted more recently. ◄═

Exploratory Psychotherapy

Patients who are less acutely symptomatic at the time of admission than, for example, the patient described above may be able to participate more actively in groups from the beginning of their hospitalization. Issues requiring a particular emphasis may be clear at the time of hospital admission and may indicate the need for more intensive individual and family work than other patients who only need more straightforward medication stabilization.

➡ For example, a 25-year-old single female sales manager, who had been undergoing outpatient treatment for depression, was admitted after taking an overdose of sertraline. A number of immediate stressors were identified, including the recent breakup of an intimate relationship with a man who had initially seemed to be very loving and committed but had abruptly withdrawn when the patient began reciprocating those feelings; pressure from an arbitrary and difficult-to-please supervisor at work; an argument with a judgmental, critical older brother; and feelings of hopelessness about her persistent depression despite a recent change in medication. Consultation with the woman's outpatient psychiatrist helped the team focus on the need for family assessment, which had been lacking thus far in her two-year course of treatment. Her parents, both physicians and the children of Japanese immigrants, had been superficially supportive of their daughter's treatment but had remained emotionally unavailable, despite her efforts to reach out to them. She felt isolated from her family and believed that her older brother, a married physician with a 2-year-old son, had a much closer relationship to the parents.

This patient's depressive symptoms were not severe enough to prevent her from participating in groups on the unit. In fact, she tended to put on a cheerful front and function "normally" at work and with friends and family. She hid her despair from herself and others until, one day, the intensity of her feelings overwhelmed her and led her to attempt suicide. This patient would have happily spent her days in the hospital discussing current events and completing cooking projects. However, the therapeutic goal set for her was more important: to discuss the events preceding her overdose and their meaning to her, as well as her feelings toward her family, ex-boyfriend, boss, and outpatient psychiatrist. Individual and group insight-oriented psychotherapy was essential for this patient, as was family therapy conducted jointly by her psychiatrist and a social worker. The nursing staff played an important role by encouraging the patient to socialize during her free time rather than read in her room. For this patient, the milieu served to confront her maladaptive defenses while it also provided support. It was a safe setting in which to confront the family's pattern of labeling her as the "sick" family member. Within 10 days, the patient was ready for discharge, felt hopeful about the future, and planned to continue outpatient therapy, which would include individual psychotherapy with medication adjustments, as well as family therapy. ◄═

OUTPATIENT SETTINGS

Generally, the physician has the luxury of getting to know a patient over a longer period of time in an outpatient setting than in the emergency room, consultation service for medical and surgical patients, and most psychiatric inpatient units. The physician working in an outpatient setting does not obtain the data on how the patient is doing that would be available from an inpatient unit's interdisciplinary team or 24-hour-a-day monitoring system or from the crisis assessment and frequent involvement of the patient's family in the emergency room setting. Rather, the clinician often relies on the patient to provide information on how he or she is doing outside their therapy sessions. Compliance with treatment recommendations is another major concern in this setting. Outpatient treatment makes use of several different treatment modalities and settings.

Day Programs

Day programs, or **partial hospitals,** provide the structure and support of an interdisciplinary team for patients who are able to live at home. Home may be a supervised or structured situation, such as a group home, supervised apartment, or halfway house. Patients attend day programs from two to five days a week and stay from two to eight hours a day. The activities are similar to those in inpatient units: psychoeducational and psychotherapy groups, occupational and recreational therapy activities, social skills training, and community meetings. A process similar to the inpatient interdisciplinary milieu (discussed above) tends to develop for patients who participate daily in this setting. Patients have individual psychotherapy or pharmacotherapy, or both, with the day program staff, physicians affiliated with the day program, or outside therapists.

Patients with a variety of psychiatric diagnoses, including schizophrenia, mood disorders, and severe personality disorders, can benefit from a day program, in which the average length of stay is 3 to 12 months, although some chronic patients attend for years. Many patients are referred to day programs to receive help in making the transition from inpatient hospitalization. For some patients, enrollment in a day program precludes the need for hospitalization. Day programs are linked with vocational rehabilitation programs, and volunteer jobs or skills training workshops are often the next step for patients completing day treatment.

Psychotherapy and Psychopharmacological Treatment

In addition to attending day programs, patients in outpatient treatment may have one or two psychotherapy sessions a week and an appointment for medication management once every two to four weeks. Patients may be seen in clinics that are located within general hospitals or psychiatric hospitals or that are free-standing, as well as by psychiatrists in private practice.

The duration of treatment varies a great deal from patient to patient. Patients with chronic conditions, such as schizophrenia or bipolar disorder, may require years of treatment, perhaps for the rest of their lives. Patients with personality disorders or other problems, such as relationship difficulties that do not necessarily meet the criteria for a personality disorder, may require at least two to three years of psychotherapy. Treatment for those with anxiety disorders and episodes of depression may be completed within six months to a year.

It is important for physicians to realize that many patients do not present with a single diagnosis or require just one type of treatment and that their needs and goals are likely to change over the course of their illness and over the course of their lives. Often, after their acute, or even chronic, episodes of mood or anxiety disorder resolve, many patients become interested in more exploratory forms of psychotherapy in order to become "stronger" emotionally by gaining a better understanding of the stressors that contributed to their illnesses, their inner emotional lives, and the ways in which their illnesses have affected their lives and relationships. Other patients may experience episodes of depression while undergoing psychotherapy for a personality disorder or other problem. To meet patients' changing needs, psychiatrists must be flexible in their approach, and, in fact, most regard their approach as an eclectic one capable of, for example, combining psychotherapy with pharmacotherapy as needed.

Setting Goals and Developing a Therapeutic Alliance

While the time frame may be prolonged in outpatient care, it is essential that the clinician formulate treatment goals with the patient at the beginning of treatment. Because of the patient's changing needs, these goals need to be reexamined from time to time; otherwise, the patient and the physician may drift along without a sense of purpose or may even have different goals in mind. In the following example, the psychiatrist's unstated agenda was at odds with the patient's agenda; as a result, the treatment alliance was nearly lost.

⟹ A 45-year-old married woman, who was a paralegal and the mother of two children, consulted a psychiatrist for help with her chronic insomnia, anhedonia, low energy, increased appetite, and significant weight gain. She described her feeling of frustration with the lack of intimacy in her marriage in general and her husband's lack of sexual interest in particular.

She agreed with the psychiatrist's diagnostic formulation of dysthymic disorder and with his treatment plan. She was to take fluoxetine for her dysthymia and participate in weekly psychotherapy sessions to gain a better understanding of how she dealt with stress. Initially, the treatment proceeded smoothly. The patient felt less depressed and was pleased to achieve an 8-pound weight loss in 10 weeks, which was accompanied by improved energy and uninterrupted, restful sleep. In psychotherapy, she and the psychiatrist focused increasingly on the patient's relationship with her husband. As the psychiatrist pointed out the patient's anger and disappointment with her husband, the patient began to confront her husband about his withdrawal. He abruptly moved out of their home. The patient felt devastated; she had never expected to lose him. The psychiatrist realized that she had become focused on goals that had not been made explicit to the patient (i.e., increasing the patient's autonomy and decreasing her reliance on this withdrawn, apparently chronically angry man, who refused a psychiatric evaluation for himself). Because these issues had not been explored, the psychiatrist had been unaware that, given the choice, the patient would have preferred to avoid confronting her husband if it meant risking losing him. Clearly, the patient might have recognized that risk herself. Because they had not discussed the treatment goals or the direction the therapy was taking since the first session, the patient blamed the loss of her husband on the therapy. The psychiatrist was able to salvage the therapeutic alliance and the treatment by reviewing the goals with the patient. The patient chose to look for fulfillment in areas of her life other than her marriage. She had resigned herself to a marriage that would probably continue to be far less than perfect. ◄■

As the above case illustrates, setting treatment goals is an important part of developing a **therapeutic alliance.** Such an alliance is particularly crucial with outpatients because it influences their willingness to comply with treatment.

Compliance

In outpatient settings, compliance cannot be encouraged through staff and peer pressure as it can be on inpatient units. Instead, compliance occurs only when patients believe that treatment will be helpful. When patients have limited contact with the clinic or psychiatrist, they must be able to hold onto this belief and continue to view the physician as helpful and caring. Especially for seriously ill patients, this task is a crucial first goal of treatment. Their ability to feel connected to the psychiatrist between sessions is closely linked with their compliance. The achievement of this connection is analogous to a child's gradual acquisition of object constancy (see Chapter 13, Life Development). This developmental perspective is helpful in devising strategies for maximizing compliance. For example, patients might be assigned "homework" that reminds them of their physicians and, thus, serves as a kind of transitional object.

Extremely compliant patients and noncompliant patients are quite distinctive, with the latter sometimes requiring hospitalization. Patients who consistently fail to follow physicians' instructions or miss scheduled appointments require careful evaluation. The differential diagnosis of extreme **noncompliance** includes memory problems or confusion, which may prevent patients from recalling instructions; psychosis, especially paranoid delusions about the treatment team; and demoralization that includes pessimism about the treatment and that may extend

to passive suicidal intentions. (See Chapter 12, Psychological Factors Affecting a Medical Condition, for a more detailed discussion.)

Perhaps more common, and in some ways more difficult to recognize and address, are the subtler forms of noncompliance. Unlike extreme noncompliance, the more subtle forms of noncompliance, as in the case below, are often related to the physician-patient relationship.

■► A 45-year-old woman with non–insulin-dependent diabetes mellitus and generalized anxiety disorder was undergoing supportive psychotherapy. She reported to her psychiatrist that she had not had an appointment with her internist in several months and was concerned because her urine contained glucose, according to the dipstick testing that she did at home. Her psychiatrist agreed that she should make an appointment with the internist as soon as possible. Over the ensuing weeks, the patient did not make the appointment, despite more and more insistent instructions from her psychiatrist to do so. As her psychiatrist became more concerned, the patient seemed paradoxically less worried about her physical health. After rethinking the situation, the psychiatrist decided to use a different approach. He did not bring the issue up; when the patient did, he pointed out to her that she seemed surprisingly unconcerned. The patient then became anxious and sad and told the psychiatrist how hurt she was that the internist had not called to find out what had happened to her. With her permission, the psychiatrist called the internist, who later called the patient to apologize for losing touch and to make an appointment, which the patient readily made and kept. ◄■

For some patients, clear instructions are enough. For others, being told what to do can escalate into a "power struggle," during which each party may become more determined to continue doing things their way. As the above case illustrates, once the patient's personality style and feelings about the physician-patient relationship are understood, simple interventions can make a big difference. This case also demonstrates the role that the physician's feelings can play in compliance difficulties. The psychiatrist had to examine his own rigid insistence that the patient was an adult and capable of scheduling an appointment herself. While routine gratification of patients' dependency needs can frequently be counterproductive, occasional gratification of the need to be taken care of can be quite helpful for patients. Like children who are struggling with conflicting wishes for independence and complete care, patients must gradually assume more responsibility for their actions, but this process should take place in the context of a caring, secure therapeutic relationship.

For patients requiring antipsychotic medications, a simple maneuver can be useful: the administration of long-acting intramuscular preparations of haloperidol and fluphenazine. Patients must be able to keep outpatient appointments and be willing to accept the injections, but, at the same time, they do not have to decide whether or not to take an oral medication once or twice every day. Those who are determined to be noncompliant will continue to be so, but patients who are at times ambivalent about their treatment will do well with this regimen.

Some states have passed legislation permitting courts to mandate outpatient treatment for patients whose noncompliance may have dangerous results. These commitment proceedings, which are similar to those conducted for inpatients, rely on the testimony of a psychiatrist and allow the patient to have legal representation (see Chapter 11, Suicide and Violence).

PSYCHIATRIC CONSULTATION AND LIAISON

In general hospitals, psychiatrists often serve two somewhat overlapping functions. As consultants, they evaluate patients at the request of a primary treating physician; as liaison psychiatrists, they provide support and advice to medical personnel, primarily attending and resident physicians and nurses, about the management of patients, but do not necessarily perform formal interviews or evaluations of patients. In performing these functions, the psychiatrist is confronted with a system of interpersonal relationships that is more complicated than that found in other psychiatric settings (i.e., it is not just a simple physician-patient interaction). One of the first tasks of the psychiatrist is to find out who is requesting the consultation. Common indications for psychiatric consultations include the patient who wishes to leave the hospital prematurely, refuses to cooperate with treatment, exhibits agitation, appears depressed, or is the focus of staff hostility or dis-

agreement. Three basic types of consultations are summarized in Figure 14–1.

Requested by Patient

In the most straightforward cases, a hospitalized patient asks a physician to recommend a psychiatrist or the physician suggests that a psychiatric referral would be appropriate and the patient agrees to it.

➠ For example, a 29-year-old attorney with multiple sclerosis felt that she needed some additional help in adjusting to her chronic condition, which had been diagnosed eight months prior to hospital admission. She had been attending a support group for people with multiple sclerosis, which she found useful, but was becoming increasingly discouraged as she realized the extent to which her life was being affected. She had previously been an active, energetic person who particularly enjoyed dancing with her friends and swimming. Her persistent double vision was making it difficult for her to function in her position at a busy law firm, and weakness in her lower extremities was constricting her social life. The psychiatric consultant noted that the patient had the neurovegetative signs and symptoms (i.e., anorexia, low energy, poor concentration, and anhedonia) that are consistent with a major depressive episode and that are not generally associated with multiple sclerosis or the regimen of steroids she was currently taking. Together, the consultant and patient devised the following treatment plan: The patient would begin taking sertraline, an antidepressant chosen for its minimal possible side effects, and would see the psychiatrist in weekly outpatient sessions to manage the

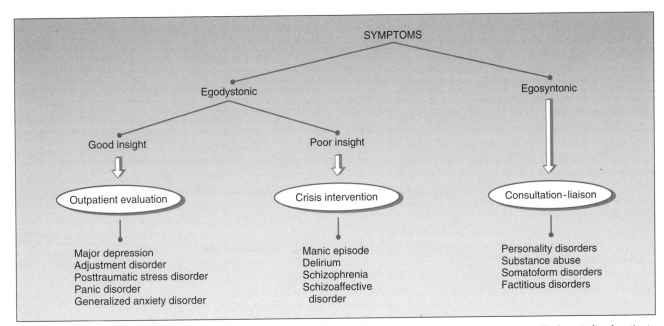

FIGURE 14–1. Type of consultation required for various disorders. The evaluation of medically and surgically hospitalized patients with egodystonic psychiatric symptoms and good insight is most similar to a psychiatric assessment conducted on an outpatient basis. Patients with egodystonic symptoms and poor insight require a crisis intervention that is similar to the approach taken in the emergency room. Patients with egosyntonic symptoms, regardless of their insight, require a consultation-liaison approach that takes into account the complex system of interpersonal relationships.

medication and engage in supportive psychotherapy. The psychotherapy would aim at strengthening her adaptive defense mechanisms, particularly as her depression resolved. Contact between the psychiatrist and the referring neurologist was relatively brief. The neurologist appreciated the consultant's diagnostic input. ◄

Even this relatively straightforward case demonstrates the complexity of evaluating patients with concurrent medical illnesses, when one must carefully rule out underlying etiologies associated with the medical condition (for a detailed discussion of this issue, see Chapter 5, Cognitive and Mental Disorders Due to General Medical Conditions). The complex interpersonal issues characteristic of the following types of cases, however, were absent.

Requested by Medical Team

A medical team may request a psychiatric consultation for a patient with a medical condition who also has a psychiatric syndrome that may prevent the patient from following through with medical treatment. Although the source of the referral in such cases is clear, the psychiatrist's task is still challenging because the patient has no interest in seeing a psychiatrist. The situation is similar to an emergency room evaluation of a patient who has been brought involuntarily to the hospital. As in the following case, these consultations frequently involve patients with agitated behavior and symptoms of psychosis.

◄ A 27-year-old single man, who had resided in a homeless shelter for two years, was admitted to the hospital with a persistent productive cough, pleuritic chest pain, shaking chills, and night sweats. Sputum examination confirmed a diagnosis of active tuberculosis. The patient had been partially treated for tuberculosis about six months earlier but had become noncompliant with treatment. He now required a six-month course of triple-drug therapy. After just one week in the hospital, he insisted that he was ready for discharge and that all he needed was "lots of fresh air." He was becoming increasingly reluctant to take his medications and follow respiratory isolation procedures. On the day the psychiatrist was called, he had become loud and threatening. A security officer stood outside the door as the psychiatrist interviewed the patient. The psychiatrist quietly and calmly empathized with the patient's frustration at being "cooped up" in the hospital. The patient proceeded to describe his understanding of his difficulties, which was that he had not been eating well and so had become "run down." The psychiatrist gently explained the medical team's assessment and asked if the patient thought that it was "possible that an infection could account for" how he had been feeling. The patient replied, "No way." This denial indicated that his reality testing was impaired, as did his insistence that several staff members on the floor were "out to get" him and were using a special set of signals to communicate with each other. His mental sta-

tus examination also revealed that he had significant loosening of associations and inappropriate affect and that his cognitive function was concrete but otherwise intact. The psychiatrist prescribed haloperidol and prophylactic benztropine, which the patient reluctantly took after the psychiatrist assured him that the medications would help him cope with the terrible stresses imposed on him by the hospitalization. The psychiatrist carefully avoided disagreeing directly with the patient's assessment of his medical condition; instead, he encouraged him to follow his internist's directions, so that he could "build up [his] strength and get out of the hospital as soon as possible." An attendant was assigned to watch the patient around the clock to prevent him from surreptitiously eloping (i.e., leaving the hospital), but he did not attempt to do so. After the patient began taking haloperidol daily, he became calmer, less paranoid, and had better insight into his medical condition. He allowed the staff to contact his mother, with whom he had not spoken in two years. Her description of her son's pattern of deteriorating functioning was consistent with chronic schizophrenia (i.e., several years of isolated, bizarre behavior after dropping out of college, including complaints that the KGB had an elaborate plot to control him). After he had been in the hospital for five weeks, he was discharged to live with his mother and receive outpatient medical and psychiatric follow-up care, including haloperidol decanoate injections. ◄

This case illustrates some of the ethical and public health issues that can arise for psychiatrists when they participate in a consultation-liaison service. Apparently, during his first hospitalization for tuberculosis, the patient's mental status abnormalities were not recognized, and he was never seen by a psychiatrist. When he was discharged, he posed a significant public health hazard if his psychosis and lack of insight into his condition were as extreme then as they later became. One could have easily predicted that he would stop taking his antituberculosis medications and that the disease would recur, possibly as a drug-resistant strain but certainly as a contagious disease. During the current hospitalization, if the patient had refused antipsychotics and had insisted on signing out of the hospital "against medical advice," the psychiatrist, in order to have him committed for the remainder of his treatment, would have testified in court that the patient's insight and judgment were severely impaired. The judge would have rendered a decision about the patient's competency (i.e., his ability to make a rational decision about his medical care). Such cases present complex ethical and public health questions. One common misconception regarding the psychiatrist's role is that he or she can make decisions about the patient's "competence." Such decisions are, by definition, legal ones. The psychiatrist can only describe the patient's mental status examination, including the patient's ability to understand the illness and the consequences of the options that are available to the patient.

Requested to Resolve Conflict

A psychiatric consultation that is requested to resolve a conflict between a patient and the health care providers is, in some ways, the most difficult to perform. It may not be immediately clear where the main intervention should be directed (i.e., how much of the problem lies within the patient and how much within "the system," including the responses that the patient is eliciting from the medical staff). A number of factors may be involved, including the patient's psychopathology and personality style; the staff's reactions to the patient, which may be related to the patient's medical illness, psychiatric illness, or personality style; and the staff's reactions to each other as they work with the patient. To suggest that the staff is playing a role in the perceived need for a consultation is not to imply that the staff needs psychiatric treatment or is being unprofessional. As the following cases illustrate, patients can evoke particular **responses in caregivers** that contribute to a "system malfunction."

➡ A 22-year-old man presented to the emergency room with "the worst headache of my life." His physical examination was normal, except for meningismus (pain and difficulty in moving his chin toward his chest), and he did not have a fever. These data and his history suggested the possibility of a subarachnoid hemorrhage, which frequently can be detected on CT scanning but may require a lumbar puncture for a definitive diagnosis. The patient adamantly refused to undergo a lumbar puncture. A psychiatric consultation was requested to assess his "competency." The patient was lying quietly on a stretcher when the consultant approached him. The patient calmly reviewed his symptoms and his own conclusion that this was "just a bad headache" that would soon be gone. He could not consider the possibility that it might be something serious, and he desperately wanted an analgesic stronger than the acetaminophen that he had been given. The patient was willing to have a CT scan but continued to refuse a lumbar puncture, which seemed like a dangerous, frightening procedure to him. It quickly became clear that this patient was using denial to deal with the fear that there was something seriously wrong with him. The more he was pressured to have the lumbar puncture, the more frightened he became and the more adamantly he refused to acknowledge the real risks involved in not allowing the lumbar puncture.

The house staff had other issues with regard to this patient, who they saw as "unreasonable." He made them anxious and angry for a number of reasons: He was about the same age as many of the staff, had become ill very suddenly, was uninterested in their "scientific" explanations, and was extremely anxious. Their emotional reactions made it difficult for them to be objective and see the entire clinical picture, including the risks and benefits of the various options available to the patient. It barely occurred to them that the CT scan might be sufficient to make the diagnosis, that the patient could be admitted for observation even if a definitive diagnosis were not made immediately, or that a "middle position" regarding treatment could be taken that would keep the patient calm (in fact, this is an important part of the treatment for a subarachnoid hemorrhage).

The psychiatric consultant intervened to help the house staff maintain their self-esteem as competent health care providers, even though they were taking a less-than-optimal course of action with this patient. From a medical and legal perspective, the issue of competence may have been relevant for this patient. Pursuing a lumbar puncture against his wishes would have ultimately not been therapeutic, however, because it would have raised his anxiety level and his blood pressure, putting him at risk for more deleterious consequences. ◄

This scenario is quite common. Patients who elicit strong reactions in their physicians are the most likely patients to require consultations because the physicians need help in dealing with their reactions to them. Patients with personality disorders and substance abuse disorders often fall into this category.

As mentioned above, liaison psychiatrists may work with a medical team on an ongoing basis to help avert crises. This process helps the staff deal with their reactions by allowing them to "ventilate" and by providing them with another perspective on potentially difficult situations.

A detailed discussion of the psychiatric treatment of patients in the medical setting is beyond the scope of this book. Once a psychiatric condition has been identified in a hospitalized medical or surgical patient, treatment must be provided within the context of the entire medical team. Treatment approaches can include medication and various psychotherapeutic modalities, including behavioral interventions and short-term focused dynamic psychotherapy.

APPROACH TO PATIENTS WHO DO NOT SPEAK ENGLISH

A final issue to consider is how to evaluate and treat a patient whose first language is not English. Such patients are encountered in all of the treatment settings discussed above, and the problem of communicating with them has particular implications for psychiatrists, who rely on observations of patients' thought patterns and on discussion with them about the intimate details of their personal lives.

An **experienced translator** is crucial for obtaining accurate information about the patient's history and mental status, including thought process and thought content. Family members and friends are extremely unreliable as translators. In addition to the obvious fact that patients may feel inhibited about fully disclosing their symptoms and concerns in the presence of a family member, other pitfalls exist as well. The family member may be reluctant to translate the interviewer's questions or the patient's responses accurately, particularly when they concern self-destructive thoughts and psychotic symptoms. The family member may also try to present the patient's responses as being more organized and coherent than they actually are. These distortions may be conscious or unconscious. An inexperienced translator may make the same errors, but there is generally less motivation to do so.

It is possible to perform an empathic, sensitive interview that is diagnostically and therapeutically useful despite the use of a translator. A few guidelines can be quite helpful. The interviewer should make eye contact with the patient, not the translator, and the translator should sit off to the side. This arrangement will encourage the patient to focus on the physician. The physician should encourage the translator to maintain the give-and-take flow of the interview but to interrupt if necessary to explain areas of confusion or difficulties in fully conveying the patient's meaning. The interviewer should use his or her usual body language, including hand gestures, to express himself or herself, as well as an expressive tone of voice. Much emotional content can be conveyed through body language, eye contact, and voice. Along the same lines, the interviewer should pay careful attention to making observations of those nonverbal signals in the patient.

Selected Readings

Gabbard, G. O. Psychodynamic Psychiatry in Clinical Practice: The DSM-IV Edition. Washington, D. C. American Psychiatric Press, Inc., 1994.

Gerson, S., and E. Bassuk. Psychiatric emergencies: an overview. American Journal of Psychiatry 137:1–11, 1980.

Groves, J. E. Taking care of the hateful patient. New England Journal of Medicine 298:883–887, 1978.

Main, T. F. The ailment. British Journal of Medical Psychology 30:129–145, 1957.

Meyer, E., and M. Mendelson. Psychiatric consultations with patients on medical and surgical wards: patterns and processes. Psychiatry 24:197–220, 1961.

Oldham, J. M., and L. M. Russakoff. Dynamic Therapy in Brief Hospitalization. Northvale, N. J. Jason Aronson, 1987.

Perry, S., and M. Viederman. Adaptation of residents to consultation-liaison psychiatry. I: Working with the physically ill. II: Working with the non-psychiatric staff. General Hospital Psychiatry 3:141–147 and 149–156, 1981.

CHAPTER FIFTEEN

PSYCHOTHERAPY

DAVID D. OLDS, MD

Psychotherapy is a powerful form of treatment that is effective for many patients. There are many types of psychotherapy, each with its own indications and contraindications, advantages and disadvantages. The nine major forms of therapy are cognitive therapy, interpersonal psychotherapy, behavior therapy, brief dynamic psychotherapy, psychoanalysis, psychoanalytically oriented psychotherapy, supportive psychotherapy, family therapy, and group therapy (Box 15–1 presents a brief history of the major psychotherapies). Determining which type of therapy is appropriate for a given patient is a complex process. (Figure 15–1 provides an oversimplified, although generally valid, depiction of this process.) In general, they all work by effecting a change, through meaningful interactions with a therapist, in the way a patient feels, thinks, and behaves.

Since the 1950s, the categories of disorders have become more clearly defined, which has led to the development of treatments that are specifically tailored to certain diagnoses. These therapies focus on the specific pathology of certain disorders: i.e., behavior therapy for anxiety; cognitive therapy for depression. For some patients with these disorders, one particular form of therapy may therefore be clearly indicated. Other patients may receive equal benefit from a number of different therapies. For example, any one of the several psychoanalytically based therapies, whose broader focus addresses the whole personality, can be equally effective for patients with more diffuse pathologies, such as the personality disorders. When the physician selects a form of therapy, the goal should be to provide patients with the shortest-term, least expensive, and most effective treatment. Because the more recently developed therapies tend to focus on special problems, they require much less time than the psychoanalytic therapies, and the physician should consider them first. For patients with complex disorders, however, the most economical, most effective therapy may be long-term psychoanalytic treatment.

Many therapists believe that their particular type of therapy is unique and even incompatible with other types. All therapies, however, work with the same entity, the human mind; a common thread that runs through all of them is the concept of **learning.** In attempting to change the way a patient feels, thinks, and behaves, each therapy begins by focusing on one or more of the four basic modes of learning: developmental, behavioral, internalizing, and semantic. The major apparent differences among the therapies have to do with the relative emphasis they place on the different modes of learning. The more specific, short-term therapies focus on a single mode of learning and produce similar results, while the longer, more generalized therapies, which are required for the most complex personality disorders, broaden the focus to encompass all of the modes of learning and also produce similar results despite the differences among their schools of thought.

Because learning takes place in the brain, where all of the different modes of learning are integrated with each other, the effects produced by modifying one mode of learning become generalized and have a rippling or spreading effect on the other modes of learning. The effects of the different types of therapy on the learning modes, and the ways in which these effects become generalized, are presented in Box 15–2. (The different mental functions and associated phenomena and pathology connected with the various modes of learning are presented in Table 15–1).

The idea of therapy as a form of learning that focuses on and emphasizes one particular mode of learning, which then generalizes into the other modes, is useful in explaining how the same results are achieved by therapies based on different theories. (In fact, the success of therapy seems to be related to the personality of the therapist rather than to the type of therapy; in other words, the most experienced, talented therapists get similar results no matter what theory they espouse.) This observation is not to denigrate psychological theories but to shed light on the purpose of having a theory, which is twofold: Theory provides organization for the therapist's thinking, and it provides a base of confidence from which the tremendous complexity of the human psyche can be addressed.

THE THERAPEUTIC PROCESS

The progression of a patient in therapy is subject to many variables, including the patient's motivation, amount of time and money that can be spent on therapy, the types of therapy available, the match between the personalities of the therapist and patient, and the therapist's level of experience. In gen-

BOX 15–1. History of Psychotherapy

Various forms of psychotherapy have been present at least as far back as Neolithic times. In such primitive cultures, some of which still exist, psychotherapy is not differentiated from the medicine practiced by shamans and indigenous healers. By the time of the Greek city-states, a physiological basis for medicine had been developed. Healers understood, to some degree, that there was a difference between mental and physical illness and that some physical diseases could be caused by psychological stress. For the most part, the healing arts of organized religion and the occult focused on a person's ailments, using prayers, nostrums, herbs, or magic, and did not clearly differentiate between mental and physical illnesses. In the nineteenth century, as medical science advanced and the physical and infectious bases for many medical illnesses were discovered, patients with severe mental illnesses (e.g., the psychoses and severe mood disorders) began to be treated separately in asylums, which were often warehouses and prisons in which insanity was treated with barbaric methods. In France, Philippe Pinel worked to change the conditions in mental asylums, so they gradually became more humane. For patients with less severe mental illnesses, who would later be called "neurotic" or "character-disordered," there was no officially recognized form of psychotherapy. People with emotional problems consulted priests, family physicians, or other types of practitioners, such as soothsayers, psychics, or palmists.

In 1885, Sigmund Freud (who was by then a successful neurologist) went to Paris to study with the renowned neurologist Jean Martin Charcot and to confront the apparent physical and neurological illnesses of grand hysterics. The symptoms could be brought on by psychic stresses, and they could be manipulated and sometimes cured by physicians who were skilled in hypnotic therapies. During the next phase of Freud's career, he explored this phenomenon. From it emerged the theory and practice of psychoanalysis, which is a profound psychological theory that has been the "parent" of most therapies that are practiced today.

It is important to note that psychotherapy has changed remarkably in the last few decades. There has been a revolution in psychiatry that is almost as profound as that which occurred in medicine when antibiotics were discovered. This transformation has taken place in two stages.

The largely supportive therapies of the nineteenth century provided the background for the first stage, which was the development of psychoanalysis and the psychoanalytic psychotherapies. The supportive therapies continue to be important and are widely used. Their purpose is to shore up the patient's temporarily or permanently inadequate defenses. But psychoanalysis provided the means to confront and change a person's defensive structure and, therefore, to *cure* the illness. Psychoanalysis and its "progeny" still form a major part of the theoretic basis for psychiatry.

Since the late 1950s, however, a second revolutionary phase has taken place, during which short-term, specialized techniques for individual, family, and group therapies have been developed and new psychopharmacological agents have become available. The focus of the therapies has become more specific because the diagnostic categories of psychiatric illnesses have become clearer. Many diagnostic categories have had treatments that have been tailored to fit them.

There are advantages in specialization, as there are in any field. A therapist who has more experience in treating one illness becomes an expert in that illness. There are also dangers, namely, that the specialists know more and more about less and less, and that they may lose sight of the broader picture of mental illness. Specific therapies for depression, anxiety disorders, and eating disorders have produced gratifying outcomes. The mixed and complex personality disorders (see Chapter 8) are treated with the specialty that is appropriate for them, that is, long-term psychoanalytic therapy or psychoanalysis. Consequently, the relatively specialized longer-duration treatments, including psychoanalysis, which are being increasingly combined with new, more specific medications, are yielding impressive results. In addition, during the past four decades, there has been a rapid growth in therapies devoted to systems of people (e.g., families and groups), which are based on different theoretical principles from those of the individual therapies.

Conducting research on the results of psychotherapies has always been difficult. For the long-term therapies, most research has been inconclusive because the therapeutic process is so complex and it is difficult to find and use matched controls. Even so, some studies have supported the validity of these treatments. Also, there are robust research findings that psychotherapy plus medication is a most effective treatment in disorders that have depression or anxiety as a major component. For the contemporary short-term therapies, research has become somewhat easier to conduct and has provided more acceptable validation. One striking finding is the overall effect of psychotherapy on the patient's general medical well-being, or, at least, on health expenditures. Several studies have shown that such expenditures decrease for patients who engage in psychotherapy; one such study showed a decrease of 33%. This effect points up the folly, in terms of economics and public health, of the current practice of medical insurance plans to deny or curtail coverage for psychotherapeutic treatments.

---

eral, however, all therapies follow the same progression and have a beginning, middle, and ending phase. In the beginning phase of therapy, the patient learns the particular requirements of the technique and how the therapist and the theory work.

The first therapeutic step, which takes place before therapy begins, occurs when the patient comes to the realization that he or she has been living in a precarious situation, which is characterized by mental anguish, anxiety, depression, or some other symptom. This realization typically takes place after a stressor has broken through the defensive system established by the personality and has upset the patient's usual equilibrium. At that time, the patient seeks help and, usually, through a referral from another professional, enters therapy.

At the beginning of therapy, the patient and physician enter into an explicit or implicit contract, in which both parties agree to meet certain expectations. The patient is expected to behave in ways that will allow the therapy to proceed (e.g., come to sessions, try to communicate openly, and pay bills). The therapist will also follow some **basic rules** (e.g., be reliable in keeping appointments, remain attentive, apply the therapeutic technique consistently, and follow the ethical code [Box 15–3]). The physician is required by the ethical code to be motivated by a desire to benefit the patient for the patient's sake and not by a desire to gratify his or her own professional self-image. Even in therapies in which manipulative therapeutic techniques are intentionally employed, e.g., hypnosis or behavior therapy, the therapist should not use them in an exploitative manner.

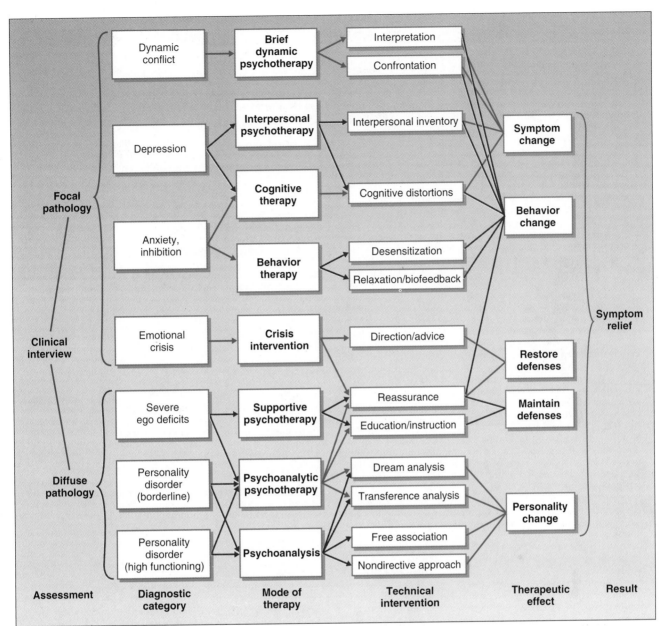

FIGURE 15–1. Matching patients with the appropriate form of therapy. This diagram summarizes how diagnostic categories might be matched with different types of therapy. It could be used as a kind of decision or flow chart, although it provides very loose guidelines. The determining factors include the diagnosis, but would also include the patient's motivation as well as the practicability and availability of particular kinds of therapy in the community.

All effective and ethical therapies share some basic characteristics. Several of these characteristics originated in psychoanalytic theory but are found in all forms of therapy, even those that are ostensibly unrelated or opposed to Freudian theory. **Transference** is a ubiquitous process that occurs in a variety of relationships, e.g., between student and teacher, patient and physician, client and attorney, and customer and car salesperson. It is the reactivation, in a later stage of life, of a person's feelings, attitudes, or behavior patterns that were first established in response to parents or other early caretaking figures. The feelings reactivated may be the awe and idealization that was felt for a beloved parent or the rage and disappointment felt for a par-

ent who was perceived as cruel or inadequate. Transference is usually unconscious and most often manifests itself as an emotional expectation that current relationships will be similar to those experienced in childhood. The **positive transference,** which usually becomes apparent in the first session or two, arises from an attribution of power and trustworthiness to the physician, and consists of hopeful expectations and a positive feeling toward the physician. The associated feeling of hope improves the patient's mood and ego capacities, which, in turn, further enhance hopeful expectations about therapy. If the initial improvement in the patient's mood provided by the positive transference is not sufficient or if the patient's underlying affective symptoms are of such a

BOX 15–2. Modes of Learning and Psychotherapy

Theories of how and why therapy works are many and complex. One theory explains the process in a simplified way by using a model based on learning, which is broadly defined as a change in computational ability. Four different modes of learning have been identified: developmental, behavioral, internalizing, and semantic.

Modes of Learning

Developmental, or maturational, learning refers to brain development and is learning at its most basic level. This developmental learning is the most "hard-wired" form of change in the brain because it is based on a kind of genetic "program" that is timed to proceed by steps during certain periods in an individual's life. Its unfolding is most obvious in infants, in whom dramatic changes, such as the development of certain reflexes, perceptual capacities, and affective responses, are seen to take place over days and weeks. The program itself may be faulty and lead to severe developmental defects, such as G6PD deficiency or Down's syndrome. In another scenario, the program may be within normal limits but still be influenced by the environment. It is now believed that the developmental schedule has evolved as an adaptation to what has been called an "average expectable environment." The genetic program can be disrupted when the environment deviates sharply from the rather broad range of normal limits, i.e., when parents are grossly neglectful, psychotic, or abusive.

The interaction between the genetic schedule and the environment leads to the development of a set of biological characteristics; it yields a brain with certain computational capacities, i.e., intelligence level and various sorts of "talents," and certain affective patterns, i.e., personality predispositions to cheerfulness, depression, anxiety, activity, passivity, and many more. These characteristics, once in place, tend to be stable, although in some cases, modest changes may occur throughout the life cycle. This developmental learning, or unfolding of the genetic program, in interaction with the environment, exists in all living beings; in the most primitive organisms, it is the only learning there is. It provides a fixed repertoire of responses to known stimuli. The interaction between inborn characteristics and environmental influence is extremely complex. But researchers have begun to tease this interaction apart and have observed instances in which environmental interaction leads to biological structure.

In **behavioral learning,** which is a slightly more advanced mode than developmental learning, events in life become related to affect, and the organism learns to avoid certain events and maximize other events because of their associated affects. For example, a baby learns that by crying it can get a change of diaper and become warm and dry and that when mother comes into the room feeding is imminent and hunger pangs will end. Such learning can also be quite sophisticated: An infant can learn that one set of footsteps means the parent who is impatient and rough, and the other sound of footsteps means the parent who is more warm and gentle. Or in later life, a person may generalize a humiliating experience in the classroom to a lifelong phobia of public speaking. In other words, behavioral learning is the association of two things, an event and a positive or negative feeling, which is the basis for learning cause and effect. Behavioral learning is what gets most animals through their lives. It does not require consciousness or language.

Among humans, and possibly some other primates, more advanced cortical hardware is required for two higher modes of learning: internalizing and semantic.

Internalizing arises from a growth in awareness of the people in one's world. The awareness developed is more than being able to distinguish among the people in the infant's world; a dog can distinguish the other dogs and the people in its world. In humans, awareness leads to the internalization of important figures; these internalizations build part of their self experience. In other words, people look and act like their parents not only because of their chromosomal inheritance but also because their internalization of the parents has become part of the way they think of themselves. This may be done on a conscious level: "I am patient just like my mother," or "I worry a lot, just like my father"; or it may occur on an unconscious level: A person who declared when he was 12 years old that he was nothing like his father discovers in his twenties that he is similar to his father in ways he would not have suspected.

The other main human mode of learning, **semantic learning,** is what is usually meant by "learning." It requires language, the verbal tool that makes the human species unique, and is the learning that takes place throughout all the years of schooling. Through this mode, an individual learns the basic elements of a culture and society—the laws of the land, the states of the union, and how to bake a cake.

Types of Therapy With Respect to Modes of Learning

Psychopharmacotherapy affects the biological roots of learning, particularly the biological foundations of affect and cognition. Medications may directly change the **affect** by

nature that therapy is not possible, the therapist might suggest a trial of medication. This intervention often enhances the initial transference and the patient's ability to engage in therapy.

For any therapy to be effective, the interaction between the therapist and patient must have a high emotional valence for the patient. Therapy is seldom beneficial when the patient is not engaged emotionally. Effective therapy also requires that the therapist be emotionally engaged and have an active attitude. Even in psychoanalytically based therapies, in which the therapist is to remain relatively "expectant," or quietly attentive, the therapist should be alert, exquisitely attuned to the patient, and engaged actively.

Countertransference is the therapist's neurotic response to the patient or to the patient's transference. It is, in fact, a transference from the therapist to the patient, who may resemble, or be misperceived as resembling, a person from the therapist's early life. ➧ For instance, a patient whose constant belittling resembles the behavior of the therapist's father is likely hitting a sore point and disrupting the therapist's self-confidence. The therapist may respond with anger or even depression and not know why, because countertransference, like transference, is usually unconscious. ➧ A well-trained therapist would not act on such feelings but, instead, would become aware of them and use them to learn something about the way in which the patient affects other people. When properly used, countertransference can be one of the most valuable elements of a therapeutic interaction.

In the **middle phase,** the therapeutic model is applied as the patient and therapist work through the patient's pathological symptoms and behaviors resetting the mood level or reducing anxiety levels. This effect may change the conditions for all of the other modes of learning. When the mood is improved, behavior therapy becomes easier because anxiety is decreased and optimism and empowerment are increased. The analytic and interpersonal therapies can become more effective because the therapeutic alliance improves and the positive transferential expectations are advanced. Cognitive therapy may be aided by the weakening of negative convictions that usually accompanies the improved mood. These phenomena are the basis for combining medication and verbal therapy.

Medications also affect the **cognitive** or **computational function** of the brain. The brain is a modular organ with many discrete functional agencies that cooperate in the activity of thinking. One or more of the areas serving these functions can be damaged or diminished. Disabilities caused by hereditary disorders, toxins, or other disorders may reduce the brain's capacity to comprehend, focus attention, resist distraction, perform abstractions, read, write, draw, and perform many other functions. Medications can help remedy these problems. In a patient with reduced computational abilities (e.g., attention deficit disorder), psychostimulants such as amphetamines or methylphenidate may be dramatically helpful. When antidepressants are given for mood or anxiety disorders, they often have a secondary effect of benefiting cognitive functions as well. When these functions are distorted by a thought disorder or hallucinations, the antipsychotics can help to restore ordered thinking. The effect of medication in improving computational abilities is similar to the effect antidepressants have, described above, of enhancing the other forms of learning.

Behavior therapy works primarily at the level of **behavioral learning**, usually with the aid of a method for reducing anxiety, such as medication or relaxation exercises. The previously learned conditioned responses are unlearned by disconnecting a feared situation from the affect associated with it. When this process is successful, there is an improvement in mood, interpersonal relations, and the general ability to cope.

Cognitive therapy works with negative expectations in the **semantic domain** that are expressed in language. The technique forces the irrational expectations into focus and confronts them with reason. This sequence feeds back into the affect system and improves the mood. The effect is to improve the quality of the internalized objects, reducing the harshness of self-criticism and the overly pessimistic expectations.

Interpersonal therapy operates in the domain of external objects, particularly loss of objects. When successful, this too elevates mood and improves behavioral expectations and the quality of internal objects.

Psychoanalytic therapies work primarily in the domains of **semantic learning** and **internalizing**, but may have effects in all four modes. The transference reveals the nature of the internal objects, which can be revised through cognitive understanding, new affect learning with the analyst, and new internalizations of the analyst. The therapy also reveals much about the cognitive patterns, negative expectations, and maxims that one lives by. The process leads to an improvement in internal object integration and the cognitive rules by which the patient lives. The regression takes the patient back to the mode of thinking that set up the patterns in the first place. In this way, the patient has an opportunity to revise some of the results of **developmental learning** in which the internalized objects took on their permanent qualities. In some patients, the conflict about internal objects leads to severe problems in self-esteem and, often, to a depressive affect, which may alternate with mania in bipolar patients. The moderation of the merciless self-criticism of a harsh internal parental object can itself relieve the depressive affect. The corrective emotional experience has behavioral ramifications: Guilt and anxiety about things that made the patient miserable may be relieved and some inhibitions may be reduced. In other words, the more intensive, long-term therapies have effects in all four realms of learning.

One important aspect of the psychoanalytic therapies, insight, is manifested primarily in the semantic realm and can be expressed in language. Although insight is in the semantic realm, the phenomena that the insightful patient describes may be in the other domains. The sense of self, one's internal objects, and one's identifications with significant people are in the internalizing mode and are usually unconscious. The role of insight is to describe the self, the similarity with parents, and the internal voices of the parents. Similarly, the lifelong patterns mentioned earlier are in the behavioral realm. They are unconscious chains of behavior that are sometimes described as "procedural" knowledge. Insight helps in understanding them when the patient can describe them in words (see Figure 15–2).

The **supportive** therapist, like the psychoanalyst, deals with all four learning domains but usually avoids regression and far-reaching changes. Supportive therapy tends to enact aspects of the transference instead of interpreting them. Therefore, the therapist is allied with the good internal object and accepts that role without interpretation. In performing the role of auxiliary ego, the therapist enhances self-esteem and confidence, which spreads into the general mood level and leads to more positive expectations.

and together set out to achieve the goals of the therapy. The goal of short-term focal therapies is to eliminate or reduce the intensity of the patient's symptom or discrete problem. Reaching this goal often produces generalized "ripple" effects, which provide more widespread benefits to the patient's personality. The more general goals for patients in longer-term therapies are to improve the functioning of the personality and achieve important life goals concerning, for example, work and family. In supportive therapy, restoring and maintaining the patient's best previous level of functioning is often the goal.

Corrective emotional experience, a concept involved in most therapies, refers to the new emotional experience the patient has when the expectation that the therapist will behave as his or her parents had is not met. Instead, the therapist responds as a therapist, which is usually different from the way the parents responded in the past. The patient often comes to therapy expecting to be criticized and shamed or, perhaps, adulated and seduced. The contrast between the patient's expectation and the therapist's actual behavior is a powerful force for change. By contradicting the expectations, the therapist's responses lead the patient to new internalizations and, ultimately, to a new concept of self.

After the patient has made satisfactory progress, the therapist initiates the ending phase of therapy and makes plans for termination. Depending on the length of therapy and the patient's degree of involvement in it, the termination of the therapeutic relationship—and the consequent prospect of facing the realities of life without the fantasy parent—can be a

TABLE 15–1. Learning Modes and Associated Pathology

Mode of Learning	Mental Function	Associated Phenomena and Pathology
Developmental	Cognitive capacities Talents Perception Integration	Cognitive deficits Dyslexia Dysgraphia Learning disorders Psychoses Dementias
	Affect patterns	Mood disorders Anxiety disorders

	Behavior patterns
	  Activity/passivity
	  Introvert/extrovert
		Personality traits
		  and disorders

Behavioral	Cause and effect	Anxiety disorders
		  (inhibitions,
		  phobias)

Internalizing	Incorporation
	Introjection
	Identification
	Formation of self
		Personality
		  disorders
		  (splitting,
		  dissociation)

Semantic	Language
	Thought
	Culture
	Rules, laws
		Depressive/manic
		  cognitions
		Other maladaptive
		  cognitions

wrenching and challenging experience. The experience of termination, however, can also be the most growth-promoting part of therapy because, as with most experiences of mourning, the self emerges more integrated and mature. During this **ending phase,** the therapeutic gains made by the patient are reevaluated, consolidated, stabilized, and placed in the context of the future when the patient is no longer seeing the therapist. The final goal is for patients to continue to learn on their own as they did in therapy. Patients are often able to do this and seem to have adopted the therapist's methods and ideals.

SHORT-TERM THERAPIES (NONDYNAMIC)

Two psychotherapies of fairly recent origin, cognitive therapy and interpersonal psychotherapy, were designed as short-term therapies for the treatment of depressive disorders.

⇒ A 50-year-old teacher, the married mother of two teen-aged children, had been a somewhat pessimistic person and a chronic worrier for most of her life. After her 18-year-old son left for college, she had begun to worry obsessively about him, telephoning him intrusively and badgering him about coming home to visit. She had become impatient with her pupils at the primary school where she taught and found that she had little energy, early morning insomnia, and a general feeling of being a "bad person." Her relationship with her husband was stable but had become distant and was punctuated with frequent bickering and mutual complaining. Her relationship with her daughter, which previously had

been very close and mutually dependent, had become more antagonistic and frequently erupted into screaming arguments.

An evaluator would probably diagnose a major depressive episode that is nonpsychotic with a reactive component that had been triggered by her son's leaving home and her daughter's fighting for more independence, which signaled the end of a life phase. A likely first choice of therapy for this patient would be either cognitive therapy or interpersonal therapy, the two short-term therapies that have demonstrated effectiveness in treating patients with mild-to-moderate depression. ⇐

COGNITIVE THERAPY

Cognitive therapy, which was developed by Aaron T. Beck and his colleagues, focuses very closely on the patient's cognitive processes and distortions. The theory underlying cognitive therapy is based on two principles: (1) Close correlations exist between a patient's habits, or patterns, of conscious thought and moods; and (2) certain habits of thought can cause and maintain a patient's depressed state. Behavior therapy techniques such as a directive approach and homework assignments are frequently used by cognitive therapists. Hybrid treatments called *cognitive-behavior therapies* combine elements from both cognitive and behavioral therapies.

The theory of cognitive therapy has been subjected to a considerable amount of research, which has demonstrated a regular correlation between negative thinking and depression, although such thinking has not definitively been shown to *cause* depression. The efficacy of cognitive therapy, which has also been heavily researched, appears to be higher than that of placebo in the treatment of patients with moderate depression and compares well with other forms of psychotherapy. Some studies have found it to be as effective as antidepressant medication.

Indications and Selection Criteria

Cognitive therapy is best suited for patients who suffer from a mild to a moderate degree of major depression, dysthymia, or depressed mood due to an adjustment disorder. This method is also suitable for patients who have anxiety disorders or severe major depression, bipolar disorder, or psychotic symptoms and who are simultaneously receiving appropriate medications.

Patients with severe substance abuse problems tend to be poor candidates for cognitive therapy. However, cognitive therapy can be used as an adjunct to rehabilitation in patients who demonstrate their seriousness about stopping substance abuse by regularly attending Alcoholics Anonymous or other 12-step programs or by admitting themselves to drug treatment programs. This method is often not appropriate for patients who are mired in destructive family or environmental situations, because such patients usually have far-reaching pathological syndromes that are supported by destructive

---

BOX 15–3. Ethics in Psychotherapy

Although ethical considerations are important in any medical interaction, they have special significance for the practice of psychiatry and psychotherapy. In general, the ethical issues in medicine involve the beneficial and wise use of authority by the physician, specifically, the physician's commitment to do good rather than harm and to treat patients with respect and dignity. A psychiatric patient is, in many ways, as vulnerable to the therapist's power and control as an unconscious surgical patient is to the actions of the surgeon. Two major areas of ethical issues relevant to psychotherapy are the right to privacy and confidentiality and the right to dignified, nonexploitative treatment.

Right to Confidentiality

The issue of confidentiality arises every day in the practice of psychiatry. Patients impart to therapists their most intimate thoughts and memories, which range from the embarrassing or shameful to the illegal. They must feel free to speak about these things in order for certain issues that are crucial for the therapy to be addressed. They must be able to trust that the therapist will not divulge information. The **patient's identity** must be protected by an impenetrable disguise, if the facts of the case are presented for teaching purposes or for publication in a professional journal.

An agonizing situation occurs when the therapist learns that the patient is abusing a child or contemplating assault or murder. In such cases, a therapist is allowed to and, in fact, may be required by law to break the patient's confidentiality in order to **protect the victim.**

Protecting the patients' privacy from **third-party payers** is another and increasingly frequent problem. Third-party payers may use information about patients to justify or ration a treatment or to disqualify applicants for insurance coverage. Another difficult situation is when patients voluntarily release information in the interests of pursuing a **lawsuit** or even in defending themselves in a **criminal case.** The physician may be in the delicate position of being required to release information that may later rebound to harm patients. In this area lie some of the most difficult decisions an ethical therapist may ever have to make.

Right to Nonexploitative Treatment

Exploitation is the most subtle and pervasive of the ethical issues. The therapist is in a dominant position with respect to the patient; he or she is a potent transference figure in whom the patient invests much of the great power and authority that parents have over children. The therapist must resist the constant temptation to take advantage of this power. The temptation is often a countertransference reaction in which the patient reminds the therapist of a disliked or seductive relative and the therapist is tempted to react as he or she would to that person. Or the patient may behave in a seductive manner, dress provocatively, or gratify the therapist in ways that could provoke a sexual response. The results of succumbing to this temptation are always disastrous even though the therapist may be able to rationalize that the actions are "for the patient's benefit." Much more subtle situations may also occur (e.g., when a therapist, motivated by his or her self-gratification rather than the patient's best interest, unconsciously pushes the patient into a certain career path or into a divorce). In this ethical arena, the best grounding and protection for therapists is obtained by undergoing intensive psychotherapy or analysis as part of their training.

The issue of exploitation arises when the therapist chooses a type of therapy for a patient. Therapists sometimes offer the brand of therapy they know best rather than the one the patient needs. Patients may also be exploited by institutional payers who restrict the length and intensity of therapy the patient receives purely for financial reasons.

A situation that combines a number of ethical issues is psychiatric research. As in all medical research, there are issues of avoiding damage to the patient. The possibility of exploitation may exist when a patient is motivated to become a research subject in order to please a therapist or for another reason that has been unconsciously induced by transference. Confidentiality becomes a problem when patient data are distributed via research reports, statistical summaries, or computer banks. All of these problems, which are usually overseen by institutional review boards, arise when the need for medical progress must be weighed against the potential benefit or harm to the research subjects. On the one hand, the risks of exploitation are real; on the other hand, the care that research subjects usually receive is excellent, sometimes above the average level of care for their community, simply because of the attention focused on their cases, which are supervised by a review board and research team.

---

family or environmental systems, against which any type of short-term therapy stands little chance of success.

Therapeutic Process

The goal of cognitive therapy is to help the patient achieve relief from and resolution of a **specific affective complaint,** which is usually depression. The technical goal is for the patient to more objectively observe all conscious self-denigrating thoughts and then change the content of these thoughts to reflect a more positive view of the self. The treatment is usually brief, consisting of one session a week for 15–30 weeks.

Cognitive therapy techniques require the therapist to take an **active and directive role** in helping the patient uncover **pathological patterns of thought** and develop ways to control them. To this end, the therapist asks the patient to complete homework assignments that usually involve recording in a journal his or her conscious thoughts and feelings in reaction to certain events.

Early in treatment, the therapist explains to the patient the nature of depression and the effects of pathological thoughts. In the first interview, the therapist usually elicits such thoughts from the patient and catalogues them. The following examples of this process pertain to the depressed mother described in the case above.

➡ The patient told the therapist, "My son never calls me. He has forgotten me." The therapist subsequently learned that the son calls once a week, and since that is not generally considered total abandonment, the patient's thought was labeled an **exaggeration,** or an example of negative thinking. The patient's next statement that "I've become totally useless to him" was an **overgeneralization.** "My husband used to be home on weekends when the kids were home. Now he plays golf all day Saturday. He obviously doesn't want to be with me." This might have been labeled a **selective abstraction,** or a negative conclusion based on inadequate information. ◄▦

When cataloguing pathological thoughts, the cognitive therapist should be careful not to label in a way that belittles the patient or suggests that the therapist thinks the patient is "just exaggerating." In order for an empathic mutual collaboration between the therapist and patient to be established, it is essential that both parties come to understand the patient's thinking. Therefore, the therapist should not automatically dismiss the patient's alleged distortions. ▦▶ For example, in the last statement made by the patient above, she may have touched on a potentially serious problem in her marriage. Her relationship with her husband could very well have genuine troubles and be foundering since the children left home. Another possibility is that the marriage may, in fact, be stable but the husband prefers playing golf with his friends to being at home with his wife when she is worrying and complaining. ◄▦

When the cooperative efforts of the patient and therapist are successful, the patient is able to notice depressive thoughts as they occur, view them somewhat more objectively, and question their validity. The patient's belief in the correctness of such perceptions then diminishes. Throughout the therapy, the cognitive therapist makes use of the positive transference, which gives the patient a sense of possibility, reduces the feeling of isolation, and empowers the patient to try new things and to believe that the firmly held, former convictions are reciprocally related to depression.

INTERPERSONAL PSYCHOTHERAPY

The depressed mother in the case above might also be an appropriate candidate for interpersonal psychotherapy. This form of therapy, which emerged from the interpersonal school of psychiatry of Harry Stack Sullivan and was further developed by Gerald Klerman, Myrna Weissman, and their colleagues, is a well-organized technique based on the theory that depression is a problem in interpersonal relations. According to interpersonal theory, depression is often correlated with events that occur in relation to other people. Depression not only contributes to the cause of interpersonal problems but also aggravates any preexisting difficulties a person is having in interpersonal relations. These difficulties then perpetuate the vicious circle by increasing the depression.

The therapist in interpersonal psychotherapy directs the patient to improve his or her communication and interpersonal skills and to develop more accurate perceptions of feelings. These changes enable the patient to engage in more fulfilling and pleasurable interpersonal interactions, which make the patient feel less helpless. The final ideal outcome of the therapy is the resolution of the patient's depression.

Research has shown interpersonal psychotherapy to be significantly more effective than therapies that are based on low-contact control relationships with a therapist, in which patients are seen once a month for a brief period of time. Interpersonal psychotherapy works well when combined with medication, proving to be as effective as amitriptyline alone, although amitriptyline seems to be somewhat more effective in maintaining the patient's euthymic state and preventing relapse. The combination of interpersonal therapy and amitriptyline is the most effective of all the therapies for improving patients' social relations and preventing the recurrence of depression. The success of this combination is linked to the medication's direct effect upon the patient's biological affect system, which causes a reduction in the vegetative signs of depression and leads to an improved mood. This improvement in mood is synergistic with the beneficial effects that interpersonal psychotherapy has on the patient's interpersonal skills and relationships.

Indications and Selection Criteria

Interpersonal psychotherapy is indicated for patients whose characteristics also make them good candidates for cognitive therapy. When both types of therapy are available, the evaluator is likely to choose interpersonal psychotherapy for a person whose primary concerns involve relationships, especially when bereavement or a significant life change is involved.

Therapeutic Process

Interpersonal therapy consists of 12–20 weekly sessions. In the initial interview, the therapist looks for recent crises or changes involving other people in the patient's life. Such problems fall into four general categories: (1) a **grief reaction** to the loss or death of a loved one; (2) an **interpersonal dispute** (e.g., a feud with a boss or a friend or some other major disagreement); (3) a **role transition** (e.g., graduation, retirement, or, as in the case above, a change in the parental role as the "nest" begins to empty); and (4) an **interpersonal deficit,** which is often a more chronic problem of insensitivity to others, inability to get along with others, or inability to form a relationship.

After first explaining the nature and usual course of depression, its damaging effects on a person's life and relations with others, and the rationale for inquiry into the patient's social world, the therapist then encourages the patient to describe in detail relationships and interactions with other people. Together, they explore the patient's interpersonal world and develop an **interpersonal inventory.** As the patient's story unfolds, a history of many interpersonal difficulties may emerge, including difficulties in communicating feelings, problems with understanding the mutual obligations in relationships, and a poor sense of what to expect from other people.

The therapist and patient examine what these interpersonal difficulties imply about the ways in which the patient affects other people.

The therapist encourages the patient to become aware of and express his or her feelings about other people. This focus on affect is part of the process by which the patient learns how to acknowledge feelings and how to more clearly express them in relationships. The therapist will conduct a **communication analysis** to remedy faulty communication skills, including the failure or refusal to communicate, which often contribute to interpersonal problems. In communication analysis, the interpersonal therapist approaches faulty communication in much the same way a cognitive therapist approaches cognitive distortions: by pointing them out to the patient when they occur and exploring ways in which they can be changed.

➠ This method worked well in the case of one patient who would usually complete the tasks his boss assigned him but would not inform his boss that he had done so. As a result, the boss would often be left wondering if the work had been done. The false impression that the patient gave was that he was unreliable and needed to be constantly supervised. In the sessions, the therapist discussed with the patient how the boss was likely to perceive him, and together the therapist and patient explored ways in which the patient could communicate better and role-played these techniques. ⬅⬛

As in cognitive therapy, the patient's establishment of a positive transference to an authority figure is one of the most effective features of interpersonal psychotherapy. During therapy, the therapist and patient collaborate in the investigation of the patient's problem areas, clarification of conflicts, and solution of problems. When a therapist's suggestion is resisted by the patient, the resistance is pointed out and the emotional reasons for it are explored. A patient may, for example, resist because he or she is afraid of making changes or feels that changes in personality style would threaten his or her relationships. Gaining insight into such fears is a major factor in the success of interpersonal therapy. When the patient uses such insight to make changes, the quality of his or her personal relations generally improves and causes an increase in the patient's self-esteem.

As mentioned above, the early phase of therapy is usually devoted to obtaining detailed descriptions of interactions within relationships, so that the therapist can obtain a full picture of the patient's interpersonal world. ➠ In the case discussed above, if the depressed mother were referred for interpersonal psychotherapy, her interpersonal inventory would focus on the relationships she has with each member of her family. The therapist would have her provide details of her interactions with her husband by asking, for instance, what happens when he comes home from work? The patient might answer that he hangs up his coat, puts his briefcase in the study, and looks for her. She is usually in the darkened bedroom in bed and responds to his inquiries with complaints about her day and their daughter's behavior, reiterating that their son has not called in 3 days and declaring that he must be in some sort of trouble. She asks why he has come home so late and doesn't he know she worries? She tells him that she had been worrying that he had been in an accident, mugged, or some other horrible thing. She launches into an invective about how he must not love her any more, saying, why should he? She is worthless and he must be looking for someone else. ⬅⬛ An interpersonal inventory would include many interactions like this.

Therapy then focuses on understanding these interactions and talking about possible ways to improve them. ➠ For example, the therapist might ask the patient how she thinks her husband feels about her tirade, and together they would speculate that he might find this unchanging pattern painful and guilt-provoking, and that it might eventually make him angry. He might very well not look forward to coming home, not because she is "worthless" but because her behavior causes him pain. The therapist might suggest that if the patient really feels depressed and hopeless and if the true source of her feeling of abandonment is her son's lack of communication, then she should acknowledge this to herself and discuss it with her husband in a nonaccusatory way. He might become more sympathetic with her feelings, and they could possibly have a more pleasant evening. The successful outcome of this work would be for the patient to understand her behavior and its underlying motivation, see beyond her set opinion that she is simply worthless, communicate better with her husband, and take action to alter this particular homecoming greeting. ⬅⬛

BEHAVIOR THERAPY

Behavior therapy grew out of the work of B.F. Skinner, who conceived of the mind in generally external terms, rejecting the notion of inner subjective experience and preferring to see the mind as behavior. His model was based on the reflexive learning that occurs in all animals, in which certain stimuli are followed by certain responses. He held that the entire repertoire of human behavior could be traced back to **conditioned responses** (i.e., learned reactions) from infancy to adulthood. Language, too, was thought to be an accumulation of conditioned reflexes favoring certain phonemes, pronunciations, and syntax. The radical behaviorists, such as Joseph Wolpe, thought that this is all there is to human cognition. This view dominated the thinking of academic research psychologists for several decades. In recent years, most behaviorists have accepted the existence of internal subjective experience, and behavior therapists have broadened their approach to accommodate this fact.

Behavior theory holds that all psychopathology arises from **inappropriate conditioning,** which mostly occurs in childhood, although it can occur later in life (e.g., a car accident might condition a person to fear driving a car). The conditioning model is based on the principle that one stimulus can replace another when the two stimuli occur close together in time. In Pavlov's famous experiment, food was presented to a dog at the same time that a bell was rung. Initially, only the food induced salivation in the dog. After a period of conditioning, however, the dog salivated when he heard the ringing bell. This phenomenon or process is known as **classical conditioning.** Another form of conditioning is **operant conditioning,** a typical example of which is the experiment with a caged pigeon which, while pecking randomly at the floor and walls of an enclosure, occasionally happens to peck and depress a small lever at one end of the cage. This movement releases a pellet of food into the bird's cage, and, eventually, the pigeon "learns" that to peck the lever is to be fed.

Most behavior therapy is built upon the process of classical conditioning. When applied to patients, this theory maintains that a person cannot be anxious and relaxed at the same time. Therefore, in order to eliminate the anxiety, behavior therapists attempt to replace the patient's anxious reaction with a more relaxed one.

➡ A 43-year-old architect came for a consultation because he had a fear of public speaking. For most of his career, he had been a talented assistant to senior architects. He had not been asked to make a presentation since he was a student in architecture school. In school, he made his presentations in a state of panic, getting through them with the help of diazepam. Recently, he had been promoted to the position of senior architect on a project, which required him to make a major presentation after two months. He was terrified.

He had a stable marriage, had two children, was in good physical health, and drank moderately. He had no history of mood swings, severe depression, mania, or thought disorder. He described experiencing anxiety on other occasions, such as when first being assigned to projects and when walking into a room full of colleagues.

It appeared that, for some reason, the architect had associated appearing in public with anxiety. He would express this as, "I'm afraid I'll mess up my speech. I'll forget what I plan to say. I'll be humiliated by making a fool of myself." The patient's less conscious fears might be expressed as, "I'll get angry and start smashing things" or "I'll wet my pants." The skilled behaviorist tries to uncover these deeper fears as well as the conscious fears that the patient first describes.

In the diagnostic formulation, the physician might conclude that the patient has a circumscribed phobic disorder (see Chapter 6, Anxiety Disorders) at a conscious level, which is manifested by anxiety and which would be best treated by behavior therapy. ◄

Indications and Selection Criteria

Behavior therapy is appropriate for patients who suffer from a **circumscribed disorder** that includes the symptoms of **anxiety.** This therapy works best in patients who do not have long-term, chronic problems that are likely to interfere with treatment (e.g., unstable relationships, obviously self-destructive and self-sabotaging patterns, substance abuse, severe depression, or psychosis).

Therapeutic Process

The goal of behavior therapy is to diminish the anxiety associated with a particular behavior that has inhibited or blocked the patient from engaging in that behavior. The treatment is most often short-term (4–20 once-weekly sessions). For the architect, the goal would be to weaken the association between a public appearance and his fears, and, because the dreaded presentation was coming up soon, twice-weekly sessions would be appropriate.

Behavior treatment is similar to cognitive therapy in its directive, informative, and focused approach to the patient's symptoms. Evaluation of the patient is of primary importance and requires that the therapist elicit from the patient his or her symptoms, the situations associated with them, and all possible associated fantasies. The therapist explores these aspects further by asking the patient to make a **list of feared situations** and rank order them. ➡ In the case above, the patient would put at the bottom of his list a presentation to a small group of friends and at the top a speech with no notes to an audience of a thousand. He might also construct a list of feared outcomes, which could include any scenario from momentarily forgetting and then remembering to going berserk and suffering complete degradation and humiliation. As the therapist and patient list these fears, they discuss the likelihood of their occurring, how terrible it would be if they really did occur, what would happen next, and so on. ◄

The second "arm" of behavior therapy is **learned relaxation,** for which there are several methods. One method consists of the therapist's leading the patient through a series of exercises designed to induce a relaxed state. In one set, for example, the patient is instructed to sit back in a recliner and, focusing on one group of muscles at a time, tense and then relax the muscles. By the end of the set, the patient usually feels more relaxed. The patient is often asked to practice this exercise two or three times a day. A variation of this method is to have the patient follow audiotaped relaxation instructions, provided by the therapist, several times a day.

In another relaxation technique, **biofeedback,** electrodes placed on a muscle group (usually on the patient's forehead) are connected to electromyographic equipment that registers the tension level in the muscles by different tones or by different positions on a meter. As the patient relaxes the muscles, the tone becomes lower in pitch or the meter shows the decrease. Biofeedback is a form of operant conditioning through which the patient begins to relax almost unconsciously and is rewarded by a corresponding change in tone or reading on the meter.

Systematic desensitization is a method that combines relaxation with the patient's hierarchy of fears. In this technique, the phobic situation is disconnected from the negative affect of anxiety. The patient, after having learned how to relax, is asked to imagine the items on his or her list of fears in ascending order. As each fear is imagined, the patient is instructed to deliberately relax and thereby counter the anxiety that usually accompanies the fantasy image. The goal is for the patient, after several sessions, to be able to relax while imagining the worst possible fear. Once the patient has made some progress in relaxing while fantasizing the phobic image, actual practice exercises are assigned. For example, the architect described above might practice by first giving a presentation to the therapist, then to some friends, and then to a professional group. As a result of the "in vitro" desensitization and the "in vivo" practice, his anxiety should diminish considerably. These exercises have the supplementary effect of getting the patient to take action, which by itself counters the helplessness the patient feels about his or her anxiety.

Other aspects of behavior therapy that contribute to its efficacy are the patient's establishment of a positive transference to a benign authority and the patient's and therapist's collaborative investigation into the areas producing the anxiety. Separating and listing these areas exposes and objectifies them. This process is similar to the listing of thought distortions in cognitive therapy, whereby the very act of listing the distortions helps to reduce their power. To help the patient separate an event from its associated severe anxiety, a form of classical conditioning is used in which relaxation and transference-induced confidence are substituted for the pathological fear.

As in cognitive and interpersonal treatment, a synergy exists between the effects of behavior therapy and the effects of the medication. Medications that may enhance the process of dissociating the anxiety from a feared situation can be combined with behavior therapy. Benzodiazepines or beta-adrenergic blocking agents, such as propranolol, inhibit the peripheral effects of anxiety, relieving the patient of, for example, the sweaty palms, hand tremors, dry mouth, and nausea that formerly accompanied public appearances. Pharmacological intervention may also relieve the actual symptoms that plague the patient during the event. Desensitization exercises are more effective than medication in ameliorating the anticipatory anxiety and terrifying fantasies that are experienced before the event.

Generalized benefits, or "ripple effects," can result from this highly focused therapy. ➡ For example, because the patient described above had resolved his public speaking problem through behavior therapy, his self-esteem was enhanced. His ability to speak in public with much less fear increased his general sense of confidence, which, in turn, rendered him more effective at work and more likely to be promoted, further improving his self-image. This benign circle is the opposite of the vicious circle that had been caused by his anxiety. ◀

THE PSYCHOANALYTIC THERAPIES

The therapies based on psychodynamics, the unconscious, and emotional conflict have their roots in the psychoanalytic theory of Sigmund Freud. Currently, the three types of psychoanalytically based therapy most likely to be encountered in an academic medical setting are brief dynamic psychotherapy, long-term psychoanalytic psychotherapy, and psychoanalysis. Supportive psychotherapy is often psychoanalytically informed, as well, although it need not be.

The psychoanalytic therapies originated from the theory that personality has unconscious as well as conscious elements. The unconscious elements are either hidden traumatic memories that are kept out of the patient's awareness (e.g., episodes of physical or sexual abuse or traumatic losses in childhood) or fantasies that represent conflicts over sexual and aggressive wishes (e.g., a man was incapable of participating in any competitive activities because of the feelings of guilt and inhibition of ambition caused by the hostile, aggressive feelings he had toward a younger brother during childhood). Unconscious elements are instrumental in determining behavior and can lead to neurotic symptoms and pathological personality traits.

Psychoanalytic theory traces maladaptive patterns to their childhood origins. At the heart of the system is the basic theoretical concept of the Oedipus complex, which Freud and the early psychoanalysts viewed as the primary conflict at the root of all neuroses. (The reference is to Sophocles's drama *Oedipus Rex,* in which the protagonist, Oedipus, unaware that he is the son of the king of Thebes, kills him in a chance encounter and subsequently marries the widowed Queen, whom he later discovers is his mother. His discovery of the horrifying nature of his crime and his subsequent guilt and need for expiation is the focus of the play.) The complex described by Freud refers to the dynamic *process* by which a child develops sexual longings for the parent of the opposite sex and feelings of jealousy toward and fierce competition with the parent of the same sex. In oedipal terms, successfully competing with the same-gender parent invites terrible retribution. In later life, this dynamic conflict may cause the person to have difficulties with sexual relationships, inhibitions or guilt about competition, and problems in relations with authorities.

Current psychoanalytic theory regards the oedipal conflict as only one of many patterns that have important psychopathological effects, which can be elucidated in psychoanalysis. Psychoanalytic theory no longer attempts to fit all patients into one or more basic complexes; instead, it focuses on the basic, personal, idiosyncratic, and particular schemas of each patient.

Of increasing importance in current psychoanalytic theory is the phenomenon of the **repetition compulsion,** which refers to a person's tendency to repeat patterns. It is common, for example, for an adult who has been abused in childhood to marry an abusive spouse and repeat the experience of childhood (direct repetition) or to become an abusive parent (identification). The pattern or identification that underlies the repetition is completely unconscious, and much work is needed for the person to see the pattern.

Insight is an improvement in the patient's understanding that may result from the therapeutic process. The gains in understanding usually relate to the causes of the patient's behavior, the particular attitudes and emotional responses that guide his or her life, the childhood events that may have influenced functioning, and the contingencies that may affect current behavior. In most patients, insight takes the form of pattern recognition, or a perception of the repetition compulsion. A patient who always sabotages his work when he is on the verge of success and "snatches failure out of the jaws of victory" is reenacting a specific pattern. The value of the psychoanalytic phenomenon of the transference lies in its ability to induce the patient to **reenact the pattern** in his or her relationship with the analyst. ➠ For example, a patient who was in the midst of describing or bragging about a recent success at work suddenly stopped and started to criticize himself because he feared that the analyst was "annoyed" with him. The analyst pointed out this sequence as an example of the patient's typical behavior pattern of needing to disavow success. To be useful, insight must have true emotional weight and the conviction born of an intense affect. ◄▦

For generally healthy patients with focal problems, psychoanalytic theory can be applied through brief dynamic psychotherapy in which the therapist, by confronting patients' defenses directly, can make the unconscious conscious. Patients with more diffuse personality problems require the more lengthy method of psychoanalysis in order to develop a transference neurosis, which can then be interpreted and resolved. Long-term psychoanalytically oriented psychotherapy, which is a more supportive technique that is sometimes combined with confrontive methods, is used with patients who have diffuse personality problems and some degree of cognitive deficit. With patients who have temporary or chronic serious cognitive defects, the therapist may use supportive psychotherapy to build up patients' defenses in order to help them achieve an optimal level of functioning.

BRIEF DYNAMIC PSYCHOTHERAPY

The goal of brief dynamic psychotherapy is for the patient to gain **emotional insight** into his or her **unconscious conflicts.** The theory and method are similar to those of Freud's earliest psychoanalytic treatments, which took months rather than years. One feature of this method, which is shared by all variations of brief psychodynamic therapies, is the importance of focusing on a problem while the patient is in a state of high **emotional intensity.** The pa-

tient must enter this intense state in order to prevent intellectualization and to break through to deep emotions, and thereby gain emotionally meaningful insights into the unconscious roots and supports of his or her problems. Different means are used by the various schools of brief dynamic psychotherapy to generate this intensity. David Malan, of the Tavistock Clinic in London, for instance, emphasized the importance of constant attention to the focus; James Mann, of Massachusetts General Hospital, makes strict use of the time limit; and Peter Sifneos and Habib Davanloo recommend a persistently confrontive style. This pursuit of the unconscious dynamic and conflict is the hallmark of psychoanalytic technique. With the possible exception of interpersonal psychotherapy, short-term nondynamic therapies do not place much importance on this pursuit.

This focus on unconscious conflicts is demonstrated in the following case. ➠ A 30-year-old associate in a successful middle-sized law firm complained of dissatisfaction with his work and difficulty in dealing with his superiors. He tended to be obsequious toward them but was also resentful and procrastinated in doing assigned work. This behavior had not threatened his job, but he realized that he had gradually disappointed the partners with whom he worked and that, ultimately, he might not be promoted to partnership in the firm. He had a stable relationship with a girlfriend, but with no definite plans for marriage. He had two good friends in whom he confided, one of whom he had known since high school. He described relations with his family as being warm and friendly, but it became clear during the interview that he felt his father was overly controlling, emotionally distant, and rather abrupt and awkward when relating to the patient and his younger sister. He was disappointed in his father and had a low-grade chronic anger toward him.

He said that he felt angry with himself for his self-sabotaging style at work. He intensely wanted to succeed and become an authority in his branch of the law. He said that he had never been seriously depressed or suicidal, did not suffer much from anxiety, and had no history of mood swings or substance abuse. He had not had the emotional crises at transition points, such as beginning school or going to college, that would suggest a major intolerance of separation.

By the end of the interview, the physician surmised that the patient's issue with authorities included anger at them and an apparent need to sabotage his relations with them and, consequently, his own prospects. From a psychodynamic viewpoint, the patient's fear of authority and apparent fear of competition with older men point to an oedipal focus. During the session, the physician suggested that the patient might be reacting to his senior partner with some of the feelings he had toward his father, noting that the patient, upon first entering the consulting room, had asked, "Where is the head-shrinking chair?" in a somewhat belligerent tone.

The physician wondered aloud if the hostile tone the patient used in greeting the therapist reflected his angry feelings for his father and that he might be reacting similarly, in an unconscious way, to his senior partner. The patient at first blushed and then said, "You caught me out! But it's true, I always expect somebody above me to put me down or push me around, so I guess I was expecting something like that from you."

The physician made a tentative diagnosis of a mild mixed personality disorder with obsessive and masochistic features and with a possible focus on the issue of the anger at authority figures and the fear of being punished for successfully competing with them. An appropriate treatment in this case would be brief psychodynamic therapy.

According to psychoanalytic theory, this patient has both a conscious and an unconscious set of motivations. The conscious set is his desire for a family and for success in his profession. His anger at his father and his fear of competing with him is the unconscious set. The latter motivation, which is derived from his fear of being punished if he were to successfully compete with his father, leads him to unconsciously arrange for his own failure. ⬛ When unconscious motives such as these are made conscious in a person who is otherwise relatively healthy, the contradictions become apparent and can then be resolved. The success of short-term therapy depends on the patient's ability to separate a focal problem from the rest of his or her personality and then, standing on the platform of a healthy personality, attack that one problem. The same formula works for the patient whose pathological area is more widespread or difficult, although a longer-term therapy is required because the only place on which the patient can stand is the platform of the therapeutic relationship itself.

Indications and Selection Criteria

Although the various schools differ somewhat in techniques and in the criteria used to select patients, brief dynamic psychotherapy is generally indicated for patients who have a relatively **discrete conflict** (some schools require that the conflict be at an oedipal level) that can become the focus of therapy. Patients should be **highly motivated, intelligent,** and reasonably **psychologically minded,** and should not be suffering from pathological dependence or chronic substance abuse, or have a history of psychosis or severe affective disorder. Patients who have a history of **good object relations** and who are not chronically isolated or untrusting make suitable candidates. A good prognostic sign is a patient's affective response to a **trial interpretation.** Brief dynamic psychotherapy would be appropriate for the patient above because he was able to feel, accept, and work with the therapist's interpretation that linked the patient's father, the senior partner in the law firm, and the therapist and did not abruptly withdraw, change the subject, or become paranoid or disorganized.

Therapeutic Process

The goal of brief dynamic psychotherapy is to resolve the patient's specific conflict through a brief treatment in which defenses are uncovered and psychodynamic interpretations that can lead to insight and change are presented. This process usually takes 15–20 sessions. The technique has been used successfully with patients who have more diffuse conflicts, chronic obsessional disorders, or borderline character structures, although the therapy for such patients requires 40–50 sessions.

In the opening phase of therapy, the focus is selected, the time limits set, and the developing transference, as well as the patient's resistance and defenses to the transference, are explored. In the middle phase, the patient's formerly positive transference may give way to disappointment in the therapist and in the perceived results of therapy. Negative transference issues that emerge must be interpreted. The emotional dynamics that maintain the patient's pathological symptoms come under repeated scrutiny and interpretation. In the final phase, the patient's resistance to termination is an issue and the patient's anger at the perceived abandonment and defenses against those feelings must be resolved. New symptoms may appear to justify the continuation of the therapy. By the end of a successful treatment, these issues will have been worked out in a rough fashion, and in the months after therapy has ended the patient can be expected to continue the process of working through them alone. Working through the termination is considered to be one of the most important aspects of the method.

Two major elements of brief dynamic psychotherapy are the focusing of therapy and the interpretive activity of the therapist. Adherence to the time-limited structure is another important element of the technique because the issue of termination pervades the entire therapy, and the reality of the separation provides a tension that furthers the work on the patient's focal conflict.

When a readily discernible conflict emerges, as in the case above, the patient and therapist agree to focus the therapy on this issue and do not attempt a broad exploration of the patient's life and personality. ➡ For the lawyer, the focus would be his relationships with authorities, including the passive-aggressive ways in which he expressed his anger at them, and his fear of being punished for success. The therapist would make it clear to him that even though he avoided direct confrontation by passive-aggressive means, his behavior was maladaptive enough to sabotage his prospects for success. ⬛

An important technique of brief dynamic psychotherapy is the **active engagement** of the therapist. (Transcripts of therapeutic sessions show some therapists to be so active that they talk as much or more than the patients, which is quite different from the behavior of therapists engaged in long-term therapies.) The active engagement does not include making suggestions, giving advice, or offering reassurance; instead, the therapist gently but persistently prods the patient about his or her defenses against being aware of feelings and points out similarities that exist between, for example, the patient's reactions to loved ones and to colleagues. The most highly regarded intervention in brief dynamic psychotherapy is the **TOP interpretation** (e.g., the "trial interpretation" mentioned above), which links the *t*ransference to the therapist, relations with contemporary *o*thers, and the *p*arents. The method is strictly psychodynamic in approach: The therapist does not wait expectantly for transference to develop; instead, every sign of transference is detected and its relationship to the patient's history is rapidly interpreted. This method brings out transference issues quickly although at a limited depth. For a deeper transference to develop, the more abstinent stance and frequent contact of a psychoanalyst is required. A deep, regressed transference, however, is neither necessary nor desirable for patients who require short-term therapy.

PSYCHOANALYSIS

➠ By the end of the first evaluation session with the lawyer described above, the therapist thought that the patient might be a candidate for short-term therapy, which would focus on his relationships with authorities, his problems stemming from his oedipal conflict, and his intensely hostile relationship with his father. However, the therapist was not completely certain about this plan and did the prudent thing, which was to ask the patient to return for a second interview before making a final determination.

In the second interview, the patient said that he had had a dream the night before in which he went to get a haircut, did not watch what the barber was doing, and suddenly realized that his hair had been cut much shorter than he wanted. He shouted at the barber and left in a rage. After telling the therapist about the dream, the patient seemed somewhat guarded in the session. He steered away from discussing his work problems and instead brought out issues concerning his girlfriend. It became clear that he had had serious problems relating to women since adolescence and had never really had a sexual love relationship. He had visited prostitutes several times but had been extremely anxious and unable to have an erection. He felt that he was unattractive to women, although he had reacted with arrogant aloofness when, occasionally, a woman had been interested in him. The physician pointed out that the patient had rejected these women because he felt they would reject him. The patient agreed that this was true. He had been able to confide in two male friends, one of whom was a friend of long standing. He revealed more about the level of his self-esteem, which was low and seemed to be defended by his general supercilious arrogance that many people found irritating and distancing. He said that he was mildly depressed most of the time. Occasionally, he went on a drinking binge, which might begin at a bar and then last for

several days. He normally drank one or two beers a day and did not feel that he was addicted to alcohol or impaired by drinking. He had no history of drug use, no suicidal depression, and no evidence of psychosis.

When the physician asked the patient about the dream, the patient at first said that he did not see much in it. When the therapist pointed out that the short haircut could relate to his feelings about having short-term therapy, which had been mentioned at the end of the previous session, the patient said, "Maybe." He then said that he did not see how his problems could be solved in a few months. The interviewer agreed. They discussed the possibility of psychoanalysis.

If, at this time, the patient appeared engaged in the treatment and did not reveal this deeper, chronic pathology, the physician could be confident that short-term dynamic therapy was the appropriate choice and would continue in that mode. The patient is intelligent and has good prospects but also demonstrates many diffuse personality problems. The deepest, most far-ranging changes were possible and desirable for him but, to achieve these changes, psychoanalysis would be required because it would go to the roots of his self-esteem and his deepest defenses. The hope would be that the patient would considerably improve his work style as well as his relationships and that his fears of women and sex and traits of aloofness and arrogance would also decrease (Figure 15–2). ⬅

Indications and Selection Criteria

Individuals with general problems in **adaptation** that are the result of **personality problems** and that do not respond to a focal treatment are good candidates for psychoanalysis. Their problems usually fit the pattern of a **mixed personality disorder** that has varying degrees of **narcissistic, masochistic, obsessional, histrionic, or avoidant features.** The patients most appropriate for psychoanalysis have a **high degree of motivation, intelligence, and psychological mindedness.** Practical factors such as time and money are often considerations, since the cost in both is high.

Psychoanalysis is not recommended for patients with a history of major substance abuse, psychosis, mania, or severe depression because the intense experience of analysis might aggravate such psychopathology. Other patients who are not appropriate for psychoanalysis are those who have a history of serious sociopathic behavior that would prevent them from being able to enter into a therapeutic contract or tolerate the inevitable frustrations involved; a history of paranoid features severe enough to make it impossible for the patient to establish a trusting alliance; or a history of severe narcissism, which would preclude any relationships other than superficial, exploitative ones.

These criteria must be somewhat flexible because analysis is frequently the only method that of-

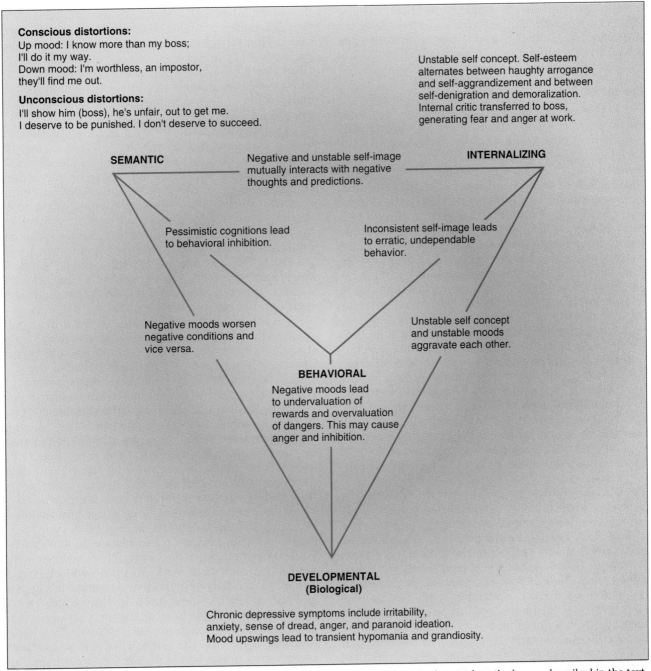

Conscious distortions:
Up mood: I know more than my boss;
I'll do it my way.
Down mood: I'm worthless, an impostor,
they'll find me out.

Unconscious distortions:
I'll show him (boss), he's unfair, out to get me.
I deserve to be punished. I don't deserve to succeed.

Unstable self concept. Self-esteem
alternates between haughty arrogance
and self-aggrandizement and between
self-denigration and demoralization.
Internal critic transferred to boss,
generating fear and anger at work.

SEMANTIC

Negative and unstable self-image
mutually interacts with negative
thoughts and predictions.

INTERNALIZING

Pessimistic cognitions lead
to behavioral inhibition.

Inconsistent self-image leads
to erratic, undependable
behavior.

Negative moods worsen
negative conditions and
vice versa.

Unstable self concept
and unstable moods
aggravate each other.

BEHAVIORAL
Negative moods lead
to undervaluation of
rewards and overvaluation
of dangers. This may cause
anger and inhibition.

DEVELOPMENTAL
(Biological)

Chronic depressive symptoms include irritability,
anxiety, sense of dread, anger, and paranoid ideation.
Mood upswings lead to transient hypomania and grandiosity.

FIGURE 15–2. For a patient with the diffuse pathology associated with personality disorders such as the lawyer described in the text, the problems in each learning mode aggravate those in the other modes. A long-term multimodal therapy (psychoanalytic psychotherapy or psychoanalysis) is often necessary to break this diffuse, self-perpetuating process.

fers any hope for being able to make major changes. In other words, although analysis will be extremely difficult for a patient, for example, whose narcissism makes a therapeutic relationship nearly impossible or who has a history of major self-destructive tendencies, any less inclusive techniques will not have much effect. In these cases, the therapist may modify the classical technique to fit the patient's needs.

Often the "best" cases for analysis are those patients who also meet the selection criteria for brief dynamic psychotherapy. The determining factor in choosing between the therapies would be a patient's

lack of focused, discrete symptoms and maladaptive behavior problems. Psychoanalysis is usually indicated for patients with diffuse, rather serious personality psychopathology who have enough ego strength to tolerate the process. Another indication for psychoanalysis is quite important: mental health professionals with psychological problems of varying degrees of severity who are motivated to learn more about themselves in order to become better therapists. The best way to understand how deeply therapy can probe and how it feels to give up a defense or achieve a profound insight is to experience it as a patient. For therapists, the best defense against potentially dangerous countertransferences is to understand their own deepest motivations and areas of vulnerability.

Therapeutic Process

Psychoanalysis requires 3–5 sessions per week for an extremely variable amount of time, ranging from 3 to 7 years. The classic method of psychoanalysis requires that the patient recline on a couch, have no visual contact with the analyst, and free associate. In **free association,** which is one of the main techniques employed in psychoanalysis, the analyst tells the patient to say "whatever comes to mind," explaining that any thoughts or feelings that the patient experiences during the session are of interest to the analyst. The patient is not expected to interact with the analyst in the usual conversational way but to begin speaking freely. Patients have varying abilities to do this. While some patients have no trouble pouring forth a cascade of thoughts, impressions, and feelings, others find it quite difficult to think, much less speak, freely and often are inhibited by their assumption that their thoughts are inappropriate or irrelevant. Most people fall within a middle category and have alternating periods of freedom and restraint. Psychoanalytic theory maintains that as patients speak more or less openly and without constraint, they will slowly reveal a narrative life story. Freely associating allows a person to wander down little-used byways, sometimes encountering forgotten, surprising memories.

Throughout the process of psychoanalysis, the analyst stands equally between the patient's **ego** (self interest), **superego** (conscience), and **id** (drives or biological needs). In this position, the analyst remains **neutral** with respect to the patient's behavior. Remaining neutral is one of the psychoanalyst's most difficult, but nonetheless essential, tasks. For example, when a patient is endangering his job by constantly getting into arguments at work, the analyst might feel angry at this self-sabotage and be tempted to strongly wish for the patient to stop the behavior. The neutral approach requires that the analyst avoid siding with the patient's ego or superego and, instead, continue interpreting what the behavior means to the patient. When the analyst is successful in accomplishing this, the change in behavior made by the patient will result from self-understanding and therefore be more permanent than if the change had been effected by the analyst's direct influence on the patient's behavior. (Of course, the analyst must intervene when the patient's behavior is truly life-endangering [e.g., driving extremely recklessly] or is threatening the therapeutic process itself [e.g., coming to sessions drunk].) The patient's ability to trust in the analyst's neutrality ultimately pays off in honesty and a willingness to reveal his or her deepest wishes, desires, and fears.

The analyst's role is to listen to the patient's discourse while, much of the time, silently absorbing the information that is emerging and allowing it to take an understandable shape in his or her own mind. This technique fosters the emergence of the patient's story in never-ending detail and ultimately allows both the patient and analyst to understand it. The classic techniques used in psychoanalysis are clarification, interpretation, defense analysis, and dream analysis.

Clarification is an attempt to help the patient flesh out and make clear what he or she is saying. To clarify, the therapist may elicit more details, ask about feelings, and clear up apparent misunderstandings or contradictions. ➡ For example, to a patient who said, "When I would get home from school, there was usually food or even a prepared snack in the fridge," the analyst responded by asking for more information: "You mean no one was home when you got home?" To which the patient replied, "Right. I never knew where my mother was, and I guess I felt I wasn't supposed to ask. Years later, I found out she had been having an affair." ⬅

An **interpretation** links together the various aspects of the patient's story. As was shown in the brief dynamic psychotherapy example above, the therapist reveals linkages and parallels between the patient's relationships in childhood, relationships in the present, and the transference relationship. ➡ For example, to a patient who makes the statement, "The last few sessions, I've been kind of dreading coming, feeling you were somehow angry at me. Then I came late and felt that was what made you angry. I couldn't even talk about it," the analyst would reply, "This has happened before with me. And it seems similar to those times when you thought your father was mad at you, and maybe he really was, but you avoided him, and that made it worse in the end. So you have developed this pattern of avoidance, which makes your superiors angry and probably interferes with your advancement at work. You feel I will be angry, and unconsciously you are trying to make me angry, and so you react to me as though I were angry." ⬅

Defense analysis is an important part of any analytic process. Throughout the treatment, the therapist will point out the ways in which the patient struggles to preserve his or her personality and its cherished defense mechanisms for fear of being overwhelmed by anxiety, humiliation, depression, or even a loss of the sense of self.

Resistance is the patient's attempt to maintain the emotional status quo, or "business as usual." Resistance may be manifested in defenses such as isolation of affect, intellectualization, or disavowal. The effect is to stall treatment and, when the resistance is very successful, cause the treatment to fail. The therapist must steadily, but gently, help the patient see through these defenses. In the process, the patient is expected to work through a transference neurosis.

➡ For example, a patient declares, "You are looking particularly well today. I was thinking how lucky I am to have you as my analyst." The analyst responds, "Could there be more to it? I am going away for 2 weeks, and yesterday you were speaking, in what you called 'general terms,' about how offensive it is when physicians keep people waiting or suddenly cancel appointments." The patient replies, "Huh . . . you know it's weird. Before I was thinking how great you are, I was in this rage about how you just go away whenever you want and I have no say in it. You know it really makes me mad."

In this vignette, the analyst has noticed and pointed out that the patient defends against his anger at the analyst by superimposing a more acceptable emotion, which, in this case, is idealization. The vignette also shows the value of the transference. Because of it, the patient finds the analyst's presence important enough to have strong feelings about it and to defend against these feelings in his characteristic way, which can then be examined. In this way, the transference is a kind of "laboratory" in which the patient's habitual personality style can be enacted and analyzed. ◄▦

Acting out is a potent mechanism of resistance. A patient in an intense transference relationship will develop strong feelings toward the analyst. These feelings may represent unconscious feelings from childhood, and there may be strong prohibitions to becoming conscious of them. The patient may take an action that substitutes for the unacceptable feeling and also obscures it. For instance, if a patient has unconscious anger at the therapist, the patient may miss sessions or frequently be late for them. Unconscious erotic feelings might be displaced to another person and result in an impulsive love affair. The interpretation of acting out is an important aspect of psychoanalytic therapy. As with transference, acting out occurs in all types of therapy (e.g., in behavior therapy, acting out may take the form of not doing homework assignments or not "having time" to do relaxation exercises).

In psychoanalysis, **dreams** and **dream analysis** are important. For Freud, the dream was the "royal road to the unconscious." The current view is that dreams represent a continuation of information processing during sleep. When a person wakes up from a dream and remembers it, it carries obvious remnants of the day's experience, called the "day residue." The narrative story of the dream, the "manifest content," may have deeper symbolic reference to basic themes in the patient's life, which is called the "latent content." The analyst listens carefully to dreams, often seeing the connection of the dream to the transference and to the patient's childhood experience.

▪➡ One example is the lawyer's "short haircut" dream, discussed above. He may have recently had, or thought of having, a haircut. He had probably also had, in the past, a haircut that he did not like. These feelings seem to have become symbolically connected to the interviewer through the association with the head, especially in view of his remark about the "head-shrinking chair." The evaluator picks up the connection between short hair and short-term therapy and notes the patient's feeling about the mode of treatment. Later in analysis, when early childhood issues are closer to the surface, the analyst might connect the hair cutting with fears of the father, of being belittled or castrated, or retaliated against by the father for the patient's success. Early in therapy, these deeper connections would probably not be mentioned, because they are so far from awareness that the patient would find them silly, or a "Freudian cliché." ◄▦ When used properly, dreams are an important source for finding out what lurks just below the surface of consciousness.

The increased frequency of 3–5 sessions per week provides increased continuity. The patient's mind becomes more and more focused on the analysis, and the patient has less time to reestablish the normal defenses. The purpose of the greater frequency, the lack of visual contact, and the relative silence of the analyst is to allow the patient to regress, sometimes to less mature and less rational modes of thinking. The transference, which was evident at the beginning, may intensify and become a complex neurotic relationship with the analyst.

This intense relationship is a **transference neurosis.** A transference neurosis is a complex transference that becomes a central feature of a person's thoughts and daily preoccupation. In the regressed state of analysis, the patient may return to the neurosis of childhood, the peculiar set of relationships with the parents. The result is a transfer of those feelings and attitudes onto the analyst. The patient may become preoccupied with questions such as, "Does the analyst like me or hate me?" The feelings may become erotic, so that the analyst fills the patient's sexual fantasies. Usually, this intense, necessarily distorted relationship remains in the office and does not seriously interfere with the patient's life outside. At times, however, it can become more overwhelming and may even reach psychotic proportions. The patient may sincerely believe that the analyst has malevolent or sexual intentions. When such distortions become too intense, the technique may have to be modified.

Working through is the process by which repeated confrontations with the transference, patterns of behavior, and turmoil of feelings generated in the analytic situation lead to insight and change. The interactions with the therapist are seen as the patient's typical reactions, and they become open for revision. Working through is probably the engine for change in all types of therapy. It is the process whereby the work of therapy leads to changes in the patient's life in the real world. This process is usually not a patient's sudden revelation of an infantile trauma, as is often portrayed in fictional accounts of psychoanalysis. The therapist must assist the patient in uncovering layers of memory and must repeatedly confront the patient's defenses against awareness and change. The repeated confrontations and interpretations help patients to understand their underlying motivations, enhance their ability to apply this understanding to different situations in life, and, eventually, enable them to change their self-concept and behavior.

➠ For example, a female patient who was obsessed with food and all aspects of eating always became depressed near the end of a meal, particularly the last meal of the day. She would look forward to it, but after a few bites, she would be unable to finish it. In the analysis of this phenomenon, its meaning became clear. Because the meal was nearly over, the patient was faced with the loss of eating in general, and for her, eating meant love and caring. The last meal of the day implied an end to eating for the whole night. In tracing this issue back to childhood, it became evident that the patient's mother, who was quite narcissistic and unable to relate empathically to the child, used food as a substitute for normal maternal love. The patient was reenacting this conflict every time she sat down to eat. She was hungry and needed food, but eating reenacted the enraging situation in which food had to stand for love. The revelation and elucidation of intimate, often unique, personal patterns such as this, frequently by way of their enactment in the transference, is an extremely important aspect of the psychoanalytic treatments. When the patient was confronted with the repetitive pattern of this scenario, she was eventually able to see that the pattern really existed. Her emotional response to food and to meals began to diminish. ◄▦

Modifications, which have been called "parameters of technique," are often temporary and may become unnecessary as the patient progresses. If the patient has lost touch with reality with respect to the analyst and this threatens to jeopardize the patient's marriage or job or the analytic process itself, a possible change might be to have the patient sit up and face the analyst. This change diminishes the more fantastic relationship in the patient's mind by providing the reality check of the analyst's visual presence. A reduction in the frequency of sessions might also reduce the intensity.

At times, the analyst may have to try to set limits. In general, if the analyst is to remain neutral, the patient's behavior cannot be too alarming. If a patient is having repeated traffic incidents while intoxicated or is abusing his or her children, the analyst cannot remain neutral and must intervene. When the analyst first becomes aware of the behavior, he or she asks for details, makes connections with events in the transference, and makes interpretations stressing these connections. This clarification and interpretation might reduce the patient's acting out, but it might not. The analyst then must depart from the usual mode of inquiring and interpreting and must make a more overt intervention, which might include reporting the behavior to the authorities. However, usually it is a request for a new contract: In order to continue the analysis, the patient will have to agree to give up the dangerous behavior.

The technical terms that have been defined here are associated with the "classical technique" of psychoanalysis. Another important trend in analytic method that has developed over the past decade is "intersubjectivity." Analysts have increasingly appreciated that any therapeutic relationship is a dyad and that there is a constant **mutual interplay** between the therapist and patient. The analyst cannot and should not be a purely neutral, "deadpan" figure. The patient's thoughts and feelings cannot merely be "distortions" projected onto a "mirrorlike" analyst. The analyst may start late, make errors in billing, express impatience, or forget facts. The analyst must take the patient's reactions to these events as serious information and not simply as misperceptions. In this trend, the two participants are seen as more equal and reciprocally interactive than in the classical model.

LONG-TERM PSYCHOANALYTIC PSYCHOTHERAPY

➠ By the end of the first evaluation session with the lawyer described above, the therapist was not completely certain as to whether short-term therapy would be the best choice, and so invited the patient to return.

The second interview, instead of suggesting that psychoanalysis was the appropriate treatment, could have gone in yet a third direction. Although in the initial interview, the patient seemed to be a possible candidate for brief therapy, in the second interview it became clear that he had not given an accurate or sufficiently detailed history. He had withheld the information that he had had three previous attempts at therapy. Each time, he would soon become argumentative and increasingly self-destructive and then quit in a rage. He had also failed to report that he was doing so badly at work that he was on a kind of probation, so that the next time he missed a deadline or had an argument with a partner, he would be fired. In the past, these disputes at work had often involved a loss of reality testing, a feeling that colleagues were plotting against him, and the conviction that his phone was being tapped. Furthermore, the girlfriend he mentioned at first was really an acquaintance with whom he talked occasionally on the phone but rarely saw. The relationship with this woman was the closest one he had to a trusting relationship. It also turned out that he rarely saw his parents and that the friends he mentioned didn't exist. After three sessions of brief therapy, he began to show more of his true style, becoming increasingly irritable over the therapist's attempts to get further information and make tentative interpretations. It soon became clear that the patient was "faking good" in an attempt to get help and to hoodwink an authority figure. By this time, he knew what therapists expected to see in a "healthy patient." Despite this turn of events, he expressed the wish to continue in therapy because he was terrified that he would soon lose his job and had some insight that he was compulsively working toward such a catastrophe.

The new information suggests that the patient has a borderline personality disorder with masochistic and paranoid features, which cannot be adequately treated in a brief therapy. He does not have the ego strength to tolerate the rigors of psychoanalysis. Thus, the best treatment for him is long-term psychoanalytic therapy. ◄▦

The goal of long-term psychoanalytic psychotherapy is to **integrate the patient's personality** through the combined use of supportive and interpretive techniques. ⇒ There is no clear-cut focus in the case of the above patient. The therapist has to engage him in the therapy and form a working alliance, limit his self-destructive behavior, and, eventually, help him work through a very ambivalent transference to a more healthy adaptation. At the least, this therapy can help the patient achieve a stable professional life, and it may also improve his life in the interpersonal sphere by helping him to become more trusting and capable of establishing a long-term relationship. ⇐

Indications and Selection Criteria

Many of the selection criteria for long-term psychoanalytic psychotherapy are negative ones that render a patient unsuitable for a brief therapy or psychoanalysis. Patients selected for this kind of treatment have multiple diffuse problems or a history of severe self-destructiveness or near psychosis. ⇒ The patient above has poor object relations: He has no close friends, is suspicious and isolated, and will probably "act out," possibly with serious consequences. He could lose his job, which would lead to a further sense of helplessness, persecution, and chaos in his life. The therapist will probably need to direct the patient and set limits on his behavior, and should expect strong resistance to exploration and interpretation.

There are some positive prognostic indicators for the success of this patient's therapy. He is highly motivated, even though it is mostly out of fear of losing his job, intelligent, has some ability to understand psychological issues, and can contemplate the possibility that his paranoid ideas may not be accurate. He is not currently psychotic, severely depressed, or suicidal and is not abusing alcohol or drugs. ⇐

Therapeutic Process

While the duration of psychoanalytic psychotherapy is generally several years, the exact length is difficult to predict at the outset. The frequency of sessions is 2–3 times per week. In long-term psychoanalytic psychotherapy, the therapist makes use of a slight positive transference to develop a therapeutic alliance. This alliance consists of a mutual feeling that the therapy can help the patient and that the therapist and patient can cooperate in the effort. The supportive alliance and the idealization of the therapist are allowed to empower the patient to be more self-confident and optimistic. The patient's defenses may be interpreted gently or even ignored, with the understanding that the patient's stability is fragile and that the defenses may be necessary to prevent further disorganization. Interpretations are usually directed at the patient's negatively oriented defenses and resistances to the therapy

process. The idealizing magical transference will probably not be interpreted until late in treatment.

Throughout treatment, the therapist will make clarifications, correct distorted perceptions of reality, and, at times, give advice, all of which will work to enhance the patient's coping abilities. The therapist's degree of activity may vary and, in general, the therapist is less talkative than he or she would be in brief therapy. Box 15–4 describes the two most prominent variations in long-term psychoanalytic psychotherapy: Jungian and Gestalt.

Medication is often used as an adjunct to the therapy, although the effects and benefits are not easy to predict. In patients who are significantly depressed or have chronic psychotic potential, medication may lead to an improvement in mood or a decrease in psychotic thinking that may strikingly enhance the alliance and therapeutic process.

Other Candidates for Long-Term Psychoanalytic Psychotherapy

Some people who might be appropriate candidates for psychoanalysis choose psychoanalytic psychotherapy because they cannot afford the time or the money required for psychoanalysis. Some people who might do well in a short-term therapy for a focal symptom have more ambitious goals and therefore elect a long-term treatment.

⇒ This choice can be illustrated by revising the case of the lawyer patient once again. This patient warrants treatment by psychoanalysis because his pervasive personality problems would benefit from such treatment and he has ego strengths that would allow him to tolerate it. The physician, who is analytically trained, discusses with him the possibility of psychoanalysis. The patient feels that such a time commitment would be overwhelming because each session lasts 45 minutes and it would take him an hour each way to travel between the physician's office and his workplace. His occupation prevents him from being absent for three hours during the day and it would be difficult for him to come on the two evenings a week that are available to him. He has no savings, and he could not afford to pay for four sessions a week on his present salary. He feels a good rapport with the physician and does not want to switch to a physician who would be more convenient because he still would not be able to afford psychoanalysis.

The physician feels that although psychoanalysis is preferable, psychotherapy twice a week would be very helpful and might achieve reasonable goals. ⇐ This choice is frequently made because, although analysis is the only method that has a chance of working for some patients, many patients will receive great benefit from either treatment and psychoanalytic psychotherapy may be the only choice available. The method of psychoanalytic psychotherapy differs from that of analysis in that the patient sits up during the sessions and there are two or three sessions a week. The therapeutic interac-

---

**BOX 15–4.   Variations of Long-Term
Psychoanalytic Psychotherapy**

Psychoanalysis has engendered many derivative
schools of therapy. In large urban centers, several of these
may be available. Many bear the names of early pioneers in
the field of psychoanalysis, such as Karen Horney, Alfred
Adler, Harry Stack Sullivan, and Wilhelm Reich. It would be
bewildering to try to introduce all of them here. There are
two, however, which have established themselves as widely
practiced variants and should be noted. These are Jungian
analysis and Gestalt therapy.

Jungian Analysis

Carl Jung was an early, close colleague of Freud. Jung
eventually separated himself from Freud and established
his own school of analysis in Zurich, Switzerland. At present, there are Jungian institutes in most large cities in the
United States. The philosophical difference in Jungian
analysis is its emphasis on archetypes, which are basic categories of thought. The archetypes are expressed in
mythology and religion (e.g., mythical representations of
the mother, father, teacher, hero). These same representations are present in the human psyche, and they determine
the shape and style of one's personality.

The analytic techniques are similar to those of the
Freudian system. In Jungian analysis, the sessions are usually twice a week for several years, but the couch is not
used. Less attention is given to the transference and more
attention to descriptions of the basic symbols in a person's
life and the personal style resulting from these symbols.
Dreams, fantasies, and artistic expression are of central importance because, according to Jungian theory, they reveal
the archetypal structures of the personality.

Gestalt Therapy

Fritz Perls, an analyst trained in Berlin in the late 1920s
and a student of Wilhelm Reich, developed an experience-
oriented therapy that is loosely based on the theories of
Gestalt psychology (see Hatcher and Himelstein, 1978).
This technique flourished in the 1950s and 1960s and was
based at the Esalin Institute in California. The technique is
confrontative and aimed especially at changing the intellectualization of defenses. One technique, "the empty chair,"
has the patient engage in a dialog with an absent person, often a parent. The patient takes both roles. This technique is
effective in eliciting the patient's inner models of parents,
caretakers, teachers, and siblings. The method can lead
rather directly to emotional uncovering. It is often used in
groups. With individuals, the therapy may be once or twice
a week for months to years.

This method is one of a number of systems that are
part of the "human potential movement." Their goals are
not usually expressed as psychotherapeutic but are seen
more as a way of releasing potential in people who may be
inhibited or in some way unfulfilled. These systems include
bioenergetic training (Alexander Lowen), hypnotherapy
(Milton Erikson), self-acceptance training (Richard Olney),
and primal scream therapy (Janov).

---

tion is usually more interactive and confrontative.
The method is similar to analysis in that the therapist tries to be nondirective, tends to listen, and in-
tervenes infrequently with clarifications and interpretations. The style of therapy varies considerably,
depending on the personal style of the therapist and
the perceived needs of the patient. Some patients
can talk about problems and even interpret some of

their own motivations without a great deal of activity on the part of the physician. Others are more passive and need the therapist to be actively involved
by frequently interjecting questions, confrontations,
and clarifications.

In some ways, psychoanalytic psychotherapy is
an intermediate form of therapy between psychoanalysis and short-term therapy. It is similar to analysis in its intensity, use of transference, long duration,
and far-reaching goals. It is like short-term therapy in
its use of face-to-face interactions, active dialog, and
directive interventions, which may limit the depth of
transference. An intense, deep transference, however, often does occur in psychoanalytic psychotherapy. With a well-motivated, self-directed patient, the
results may be similar to those obtained through
analysis. With a less motivated, less introspective
person, the increased intensity of psychoanalysis
might be necessary for success.

SUPPORTIVE PSYCHOTHERAPIES

Supportive psychotherapy is the oldest type
of therapy. The shamans of primitive cultures, the
priests of the Middle Ages, the general practitioners who talked to their patients, and the coaches
who said, "You can do it!" all provided a form of
supportive psychotherapy, the purpose of which
is to support the personality at its best level of
functioning. Because this functioning is largely accomplished by aiding the patient's personality
defenses, supportive therapy has been given
second-class status when compared with therapies that promote improvement and structural
change. The importance of supportive psychotherapy should not be underestimated, however,
because it may still be the most widely practiced
form of psychotherapy.

The therapies of the twentieth century developed from and made systematic use of specific
techniques from the repertoire of supportive therapy. For instance, pioneers in hypnosis and analysis distilled the magical power and omnipotence
attributed to the therapist into a positive transference, which became the keystone of therapy. The
inevitable disappointment in the idealized therapist became the equally important negative transference. The therapist's hortatory statement, "You
can do it. Maybe you could just start a conversation in the hall" (with the woman to whom you are
attracted but by whom you are intimidated), has
been appropriated by the behaviorist as the basic
form of "in vivo" desensitization. The encouraging
statement, "You are thinking very negatively. You
have no evidence that she hates you," is a presys-
tematic form of cognitive therapy. Interpersonal
psychotherapy uses many supportive techniques
in helping to improve interpersonal relationships.

Three main types of supportive psychotherapy are crisis intervention, therapy for long-term
medical problems, and therapy for severe ego
deficits.

CRISIS INTERVENTION

➠ The depressed woman, described above as being suitable for cognitive therapy, experienced a tragedy that changed her life drastically. Her son was killed in a car accident on his way to college. This tragedy meant that the patient was no longer experiencing a normal life developmental phase that had induced a depression. Instead, she was overwhelmed by one of the worst things that can happen to a person. She was naturally acutely distressed and beside herself with grief. As the weeks passed after the funeral, she was incapacitated, unable to concentrate, and unable to eat or sleep. She felt that her life was worthless and thought frequently of suicide, restrained only by thoughts of her husband and daughter who were still alive.

Although this patient needed help, she did not need and could not tolerate an open-ended exploration at that time. Supportive therapy was the most appropriate treatment for her. ⬅

The normal response to trauma or loss is a period of grief followed by a natural healing process, which may take months or years. In some cases, the trauma is so great and the patient so vulnerable that this process is prolonged. The goal of supportive psychotherapy is to speed up the process and ensure a better outcome for the patient. In the same way that a physician supports a patient with a physical trauma or a severe viral illness by maintaining vital physical functions until the body can heal itself, the therapist's support of the patient's temporarily weakened psychological defenses allows normal functioning to be regained more quickly.

Although restoration of normal function is the goal, patients frequently achieve more than that. By opening up their defenses and confronting, and emerging from, a severe existential crisis, the patient often experiences psychological maturation and growth. Through interpretations and reassurance, the therapist may take advantage of the opportunity to help the patient become even stronger than before.

The goal of supportive psychotherapy in this situation is to restore the patient's normal defenses and resolve his or her grief, insofar as this is possible.

Indications and Selection Criteria

Patients best suited for this type of supportive psychotherapy are those who are in **crisis situations**, which may involve a **loss, acute medical illness,** or **major trauma.** These patients may have previously been in good psychological health or have had varying degrees of pathological symptoms. The goal is to return them to their former level of adaptation.

Supportive psychotherapy is often more difficult for patients suffering from posttraumatic stress disorder, which occurs after a person has experienced an episode of emotional abuse, physical attack, or torture or lived through a disaster such as an earthquake or a flood, in which the person has not only undergone terrible physical ordeals but has lost all of his or her possessions, as well. These patients are frequently treated with medication and psychotherapy.

Therapeutic Process

Supportive psychotherapy lasts for an indefinite time, ranging from just a few sessions to many months. During a crisis, a patient tends to regress, and the supportive psychotherapist may have to accept, without interpretation, the patient's need to believe and unrealistically expect that the therapist's magical power can undo the tragedy. During the acute phase, instead of confronting the patient's intellectualization, rationalization, or denial, the therapist may encourage and support the patient's habitual defenses or, at least, let them be. The therapist's most important task is to maintain a warm, confident, supportive stance and provide a **holding environment** (i.e., a positive therapeutic alliance that offers a solid, reliable source of help).

In crisis intervention, the therapist responds empathically to the patient's feelings and demonstrates acceptance of the way the patient is reacting to the crisis. Although the therapist may counter exaggerated fears or excessive pessimism with encouraging doses of reality, this alternative perspective must be carefully presented. Patients usually experience tactless or unrealistic reassurances as evidence that the therapist does not understand their situation.

The supportive therapist does not employ the usual methods of increasing intensity and tension (e.g., through silence or confrontation) and should not set strict time limits on the therapy or adhere firmly to a specific focus.

As time goes by and the patient emerges from the acute phase, the therapist may bring up painful issues and interpretation becomes more useful. The therapist may then interpret the transference and ultimately confront the termination of the therapy.

Supportive Psychotherapy for Chronic Medical Problems

A variant of crisis intervention is helpful to many patients with problems of indefinite duration, the most common of which is **severe medical illness** (see Chapter 12, Psychological Factors Affecting Medical Conditions). Patients who poorly manage their severe diabetes, for example, or victims of treatable or terminal cancer can all benefit from the close support of an empathic, reliable physician who is skilled in knowing when to support and when to gently challenge patients' defenses.

The techniques and other aspects of this therapy are similar to those used in crisis intervention, although the length of treatment is indefinite (e.g., lasting until a terminally ill patient dies). Since therapy may continue for years, an intense, dependent transference can develop, which may go uninterpreted if it does not interfere with the patient's functioning outside of the treatment. The most sophisticated supportive therapists understand their patients' emotional dynamics and defenses and use this understanding to guide their support.

The psychodynamic life narrative developed by Viederman is one technique that has been effective in consultation-liaison work with medical patients and, in certain aspects, is similar to nonconfrontative forms of brief dynamic psychotherapy. The goal of this brief intervention, which attempts, in only a few sessions, to place the patient's illness into the context of his or her life and psychodynamics, is to return the patient to an even better than usual level of adaptation.

SUPPORTIVE PSYCHOTHERAPY FOR CHRONIC EGO DEFICITS

The goal of supportive psychotherapy for chronic ego deficits is to help the patient maintain the highest possible level of functioning and emotional well-being. The therapist supports the patient's defenses not only to sustain his or her psychological status quo but also to enable the patient to make striking gains and later be able to engage in a much more intensive, confrontive therapy. Like a surgeon's decision not to operate, the decision not to challenge the patient's defenses is a very important option in the therapist's repertoire of approaches.

Indications and Selection Criteria

While the goal of supportive psychotherapy for chronic ego deficits is the same as the goals of other forms of supportive therapy, the type of patient is different. Instead of a patient with a relatively healthy ego who has been afflicted by trauma or illness, the patient is a poorly functioning person who needs support just to survive, even in normal circumstances. Therefore, therapy usually continues for a long time, often for life.

Supportive psychotherapy helps patients with severe problems and thinking deficits who cannot really make use of the other forms of therapy. Patients with schizophrenia, paranoid delusions, poor reality testing, or the tendency to develop unmanageable psychotic transferences may be made worse in any type of intensive psychotherapy. Patients with poor impulse control, an inability to tolerate negative affects, or uncontrollable swings of affect cannot tolerate the negative feelings encountered in an intense, change-oriented therapy. They may become suicidally depressed or may quit therapy in a rage.

A patient who has severe problems with relationships, is suspicious and withdrawn, and has no friends will probably be suspicious and withdrawn and have severe problems in a therapeutic relationship that challenges his or her defenses or has any degree of intensity. A patient who is flat in affect and uninvolved will be frightened of anything more than a superficial, nonthreatening therapeutic relationship.

Some patients with cognitive deficits, who may have limited intelligence, low introspective ability, poverty of abstraction, and inability to communicate, will not be able to make use of more challenging therapies.

Therapeutic Process

All of the techniques described above are useful in supportive therapy for chronic ego deficits, and, as in the other two forms of supportive therapy, the key factor is the "auxiliary ego" role played by the therapist, who thinks out loud with and for the patient and makes up for the patient's temporary or chronic deficiencies in ego function. Some additions and modifications are often made to the above techniques.

One modification is the degree to which the therapist becomes involved and interacts with the patient, which must be individually determined. For the needy, self-hating, insecure patient, a high degree of involvement, empathy, and reassurance may be appropriate. For the schizoid, isolated person, it may be better for the therapist to keep a distance and simply take a stance of benign interest.

Suggestions from and **education** by the therapist, which may include giving advice on how to dress better or role-playing in preparation for a job interview, are often very important for these patients, who have not really learned to cope with life.

At times, confrontation and interpretation may be helpful and even necessary, especially when the therapist must deal with a negative transference or the loss of the therapeutic alliance. In some ways, supportive psychotherapy requires that the therapist have a richer repertoire of methods than is required by other treatments.

INTEGRATION OF PSYCHOTHERAPY AND PSYCHOPHARMACOLOGY

Combining medication with psychotherapy has become more common in recent years because medications and psychotherapy have both become more specialized with respect to certain diagnostic groups. Medications for certain disorders can now be chosen with more specificity (see Chapter 16, Psychopharmacology). In patients with mood disorders, the combination of therapy and medication is often more effective than either method alone. Medication may also make a great difference in patients with more complex personality disorders who are treated with psychoanalytically oriented therapies. Antidepressants, for example, are used to treat chronic mood disorder even in patients who are in psychoanalysis. The results may be an improved mood and an increased ability to participate in the therapeutic process. The analysis may proceed more rapidly and with greater long-term effects. Some patients may need medication for a limited period during the analysis and others may need it indefinitely. In supportive therapies, it is more common to use adjunctive medication than not to use it. In acute crisis interventions, an anxiolytic or a hypnotic drug is often given temporarily to reduce the unbearable anxiety and severe insomnia that patients usually experience. Medication is also frequently used in the treatment of patients with ego deficit disorders, for whom an antipsychotic drug may be prescribed to treat a thinking disorder and lithium or an antidepressant for a mood disorder.

Approach to Prescribing Medications

Some patients may refuse to consider medication as part of their treatment for personal or philosophical reasons. The therapy must then proceed without it. Even for those who reject medication, the therapist's having offered it may have a positive effect because it signifies that the therapist has heard the patient's complaint and taken it seriously. This perception alone may improve the therapeutic alliance and move the therapy forward, even though the treatment may not be optimal without the medication. On the other hand, the refusal of medication can be part of the patient's unconscious, possibly deadly, wish to defeat the therapy. When a patient is at risk for impulsive violence or suicide, the therapist may have to insist upon medication and refuse to engage in treatment without it.

Another response to the physician's suggestion of medication may be an enthusiastic welcome and hope for a magical cure. This attitude has its own set of problems. A patient who thinks, "Finally, now, we're doing something real" may suffer a crashing disillusionment when his or her high hopes are not fully realized and then think, "We've played the last card. If this didn't work, nothing will." It is important for the therapist to raise the subject in a tactful manner at the right time and to not promise too much. The idea should be presented in a somewhat optimistic way with the therapist pointing out that medication is an adjunctive treatment that could very well speed things up but is not a last resort.

Simultaneous Treatment by Two Therapists

In the past decade, psychiatry has become more of a medical specialty and psychotherapy more the province of nonmedical practitioners; it has therefore become common for two specialists to be involved in the treatment of a patient. This shift in roles has important implications.

The evaluation process that occurs prior to the referral for treatment must be conducted by someone with a firm knowledge of biological psychiatry and of the psychotherapies that are available in the patient's community. This psychiatric evaluation prevents referrals for inappropriate therapies, such as psychoanalysis for patients with Tourette's syndrome or for patients with bipolar disorder who are not taking medication. It also prevents medications from being given when it would be futile to do so (e.g., to a patient with a complex personality disor-

der who is seen only once a month for a 15-minute session). Mistakes have been made all too often because the evaluator did not know enough about diagnostic issues and indications for the range of psychiatric treatments.

The evaluator must be aware of the various types of available mental health practitioners. The evaluator may refer a patient to a therapist who is trained in analytic, cognitive, or other therapies; a pharmacologically trained psychiatrist; or a therapist who is trained in several modes. A therapist who does not use medication as part of his or her therapeutic armamentarium must develop a professional agenda that includes sharing treatment with a pharmacologically trained physician. The therapy is most effective when the two practitioners cooperate in a synergistic, noncompetitive manner.

The evaluator must consider several important issues when making a referral for dual treatment. Dual treatment has certain advantages, the main one being economic. Psychotherapy is very labor intensive, and therapists who are not medically trained tend to be less expensive. The pharmacological consultations with a psychiatrist, who usually charges a higher fee, are brief and infrequent (e.g., a 15-minute session once a month). Another advantage is that the therapist who is not distracted by having to deal with medications and their side effects can better focus on the psychotherapy.

There are also disadvantages to dual therapy. For many patients, treatment by a therapist who administers medication is more effective because any problems and side effects may be detected more quickly. Also, a physician is better equipped to manage the behavior of patients who use the medication to act out the feelings and fantasies they are experiencing in the transference. For example, a woman who was suffering from anxiety and depression lowered the dosage of her antidepressant because she was concerned that her physician was as untrustworthy as her alcoholic father. Certain patients with complex personality disorders, especially those who also have mood disorders, will do better with only one physician, if this option is available. Finally, medical training provides physicians with a sophisticated, integrated view of biological and psychological factors that many therapists may not have.

FAMILY THERAPY

Family therapy, which has undergone rapid development since the 1950s, includes the treatment of whole families, parts of families, and couples. The most obvious difference between this form of therapy and other therapies is that family therapy treats more than one person. Important changes in technique are required because the focus is not on an individual but a system of individuals and the communication patterns within the system.

➠ A year after her son's tragic accident, the mother described above was still attending supportive therapy once a month, which had been helpful, and she was no longer overtly depressed. Although still a worrier, she was able to function at work and had a somewhat better relationship with her husband. Her daughter, however, was even more troubled than before. Her grades had dropped, and she had joined a group of semidelinquent drug-abusing classmates. Recently, while she was drunk, she wrecked the family car but miraculously escaped injury. The parents realized that she might soon succeed in following her brother to destruction.

As a result of this family crisis, the father and daughter agreed to go with the patient to family therapy. Although brief individual psychotherapy might have helped the daughter to mourn her brother, she did not seem to have much motivation to seek therapy for herself and probably would not show up for appointments. More importantly, even if all three members of the family were engaged in individual therapy, certain problems in the family system would not be addressed.

The family went to the first appointment with an experienced family therapist, an elderly, avuncular man trained in the strategic method of family therapy. In the office, they found a circle of five chairs. It was natural for the daughter to sit next to her mother and for her father to sit opposite them with an empty chair on each side of him. The therapist said nothing directly about the seating arrangement but asked the daughter if she would please sit next to her father. She looked surprised but complied, and the therapist sat between her and her mother. The therapist perceived immediately that the mother and daughter were bonded and the father was isolated. He was not surprised to find out rapidly that the bond between mother and daughter was ambivalent and hostile and that the daughter's separation from her father was painful to both of them. The therapist had been well-briefed beforehand and knew that there was a fourth silent, but still present, member in the empty chair. He knew that there was some risk if he sat in a chair that would have been the son's and failed to address this fact. He said, "I've heard about the terrible tragedy in your family. I hope you are not offended if I have taken his seat." This acknowledgment immediately brought the family's mourning into the foreground, and for most of the session, the initial complaint about the "designated patient," the daughter, was forgotten. There were tearful memories of how the family missed the son, speculations about how nothing would ever be the same, and fears that the family would never recover, that tragedies like this often end in divorce, and so on. The patient felt that she "should be over" her grief but found that her wound had been reopened. The therapist pointed out that grief has no time limit, and the fact that she, and her parents, were still so stricken is a sign of their great love. This one session proved to be cathartic for the family.

Grief was not their only problem, however. The family dynamics were such that the mother, who had doted on her son, had been comparatively indifferent to the daughter, who did not feel that she could turn to her father and felt rejected by him, because he had always been emotionally isolated and unable to relate comfortably to her. As she had developed and become somewhat provocative at puberty, he had become more uneasy and withdrew further. She and her father were both isolated in the home where the mother and son were a team. The son's death had, among other things, upset this stable equilibrium. It had left the mother without her ally. She had wanted to turn to her husband for support, but he could not provide it and withdrew. The daughter, who had long been envious of her brother because he was her mother's favorite, felt extremely guilty about that envy. In mourning for her brother, she felt the need to cling to her mother, partly out of spite toward her father and despite her feeling that her mother did not really love her and would have been much less unhappy if she herself had died instead of her brother.

The daughter's bond with her mother included a great deal of rage, which she enacted in her delinquent, self-destructive behavior. This behavior got the attention of both parents and was, therefore, being perversely rewarded. This behavior also provided a focus for her mother's worry, which, in fact, helped relieve her mother's depression. It also forced the father to become closer to the mother as they dealt jointly with the daughter. Before her brother's death, the family situation had been a hard but stable compromise for the daughter. The family might have come apart even if her brother had not died and had merely left home for college. The tragedy of his death created a new equilibrium that was even more pathological than before.

By intuitively suggesting the seating arrangement, the therapist had effectively brought out the family's mourning and countered the prevailing family structure by separating the daughter from her mother and uniting her with her father. This arrangement gratified the daughter and made her a less reluctant participant although it angered the mother. But by placing himself next to the mother, the therapist had implicitly substituted himself for her son and the father, thus gratifying her. The father's isolation was at least confronted by having his daughter sit next to him.

During the ensuing months, the family met for 12 sessions, and the therapist, who knew how to manipulate the family structure to make it change, became a dominant force in the family.

Thus far, the story is really two stories, which represent the central interests of two major trends in family therapy: the **psychodynamic** approach and the **systems** approach (Table 15–2).

Psychodynamic Models

The psychodynamic model of family therapy incorporates the psychoanalytic principles of ego psychology and object relations and focuses on individual psychodynamics within the context of a family system and on the conflicts that have emerged. The family context includes the family's history, the inter-

TABLE 15–2.   Models of Family Therapy

Characteristics	Psychodynamic	Systems
Object	Individual within family	Family systems
Interest	Intrapsychic conflicts expressed within the family	Power relations between family members
Technique	Exploration and interpretation Family history Multigenerational analysis	Enactment of family patterns in the session Relabeling problems Paradoxical instructions Homework enactments
Goal	Insight leading to change in individual and family	Change in behavior with or without insight
Duration	Longer (months to years)	Shorter (weeks to months)

actions within the family, the process by which family members internalize one another, and the established patterns, based on these internalizations, of relating to each other. When a family does not provide for the needs of its members, it is "dysfunctional." The inner psychic struggles of family members result in pathological behavior patterns, which usually lead to conflict within the family.

The primary technique in the psychodynamic model of family therapy involves defining existing relationships within the **history of the family** and the **transferences** between its members. Transference is a very important concept in this form of therapy: A parent may see a child as being "just like" one of his or her parents or may feel and act like one of his or her own parents in dealing with the child. The therapist, whose role is analytic and inquisitive rather than active or manipulative, focuses more on understanding the family's history and interpreting that history than on examining current interactions.

One of the originators of the method, Nathan Ackerman, established an approach that powerfully challenges the defenses of family members in order to bring out their mutual transferences. Another important figure associated with the psychodynamic model of family therapy is Murray Bowen, who believes generational history is of key importance and that all living generations of a family should be interviewed to make the history as complete as possible.

Systems Theories

Systems theories of family therapy focus on the **current structural entities** within the family instead of the family history. These structures are either oedipal triangles involving two parents and one child or sibling triangles involving two children and one parent. Dyads occur as structural systems within the family as well, as does, of course, the family as a whole. In the family systems approach, the therapist attempts to (1) understand and describe to the family the **pathological patterns** in their relationships and (2) **manipulate** the family in order to thwart these pathological patterns.

Primary inspiration for this model is Gregory Bateson's biological theories, which emphasize the means of communication and homeostatic mechanisms that preserve the status quo in any system, including the family. Another leader in systems theory, Salvador Minuchin, developed a method called "structural family therapy." His technique has been particularly useful in eliciting and confronting the structural changes in a family that are caused by a member's psychosomatic illness. Another important school of systems theory takes the "strategic intervention" approach. Leading practitioners of this method are the hypnotist Milton Erickson and the communication theorist Jay Haley.

Therapeutic Process

Many therapists use both the psychodynamic model and systems theory in their approach to family therapy.

Psychodynamic Approach

➡ In contrast to the systems style that was used in the family therapy example above, a therapist taking a psychodynamic approach would have entered the session and sat in the customary chair. Sooner or later, the therapist would ask the family members to explain why they are sitting where they are, how they feel about it, and what they might like to change about it. A discussion of the family members' feelings toward each other and the ways in which they reflect certain transferences toward each other might then ensue. For example, the mother in the case above might say that she had felt very dependent on, and at the same time rejected by, her own mother and, fearing that she would do something similar to her daughter, she clung to her in an overwhelmingly intrusive way. ⬅ Although the psychodynamic approach concentrates more on interpretation than enactment and is less dramatic, it is often equally effective.

Systems Approach

➡ Some of the issues that a family therapist addresses are evident in the case described above. The therapist began with a strategic systems maneuver, manipulating the seating arrangement in order to enact a family pattern that would challenge the unspoken relationship patterns. By doing this, the therapist forced the family to talk about their relationships and, at the same time, to feel the forces that are at work within the family. This kind of intervention is an **enactment.** It may also be used as a homework assignment in which the family would be asked to sit at different positions at their dinner table. ⬅

Another technique is the **paradoxical instruction.** ➡ In the family described above, whenever the daughter tried to speak to her father, he withdrew and let the mother intercept the message. When this happened, the therapist would ask that the daughter address her father, the father remain silent, and the mother interrupt; in other words, he asks the family to act out their habitual pattern. ◂▬ This technique provides the family members with an immediate experience of a system of which they were unaware. Once seen, the pattern becomes more difficult and even embarrassing for them to continue.

Other techniques that the therapist employs are important early in the treatment, such as **relabeling the initial complaint,** which usually concerns the designated patient's behavior (e.g., the daughter's semidelinquent behavior). In the relabeling process, her behavior is described as part of the family system to which everyone contributes. Through this relabeling process, the family must come to an agreement about what exactly the family problem is and how the therapy will alleviate it.

GROUP THERAPY

Both group therapy and family therapy examine the interactions within a group of people, instead of focusing on the individual. Many of the same principles underlie both techniques, although the difference between group therapy and family therapy is a major one: The group in group therapy is composed of unrelated people whose history as a particular group is short and not of great concern (even though some groups exist for a period of several years and develop an identity and shared history of their own).

In group therapy, the important feature is the current interrelationships of the members. The goal of **psychoanalytically oriented group therapy** is to induce in the patient a greater understanding of how he or she perceives others and is perceived by others. The goals and techniques, which have a rationale similar to that of intensive individual therapy, often challenge defenses and produce insights. Some groups focus on current interaction between group members, while the more psychoanalytic groups use the transferences within the group to help recall childhood experiences. In either case, an important result is to induce in the patient a greater understanding of how he or she perceives others and is perceived by others.

As with family therapy, group therapy varies according to the therapist's underlying theory and personal style. But perhaps the most variable element in group therapy is the explicit purpose of each group. There are probably more different functional types of therapy in the group mode than in any other therapeutic modality. Groups serve many different purposes; for example, there are medical support groups, daily management groups for psychotic inpatients, and interactional outpatient groups that promote personality growth and change.

Specialized groups are made up of people with particular problems, such as eating disorders, phobias, sexual dysfunctions, drug and alcohol addic-

tions, and obsessive-compulsive disorders. The leaders and members of these groups are expert in dealing with a specific problem; particularly expert are those groups for the impulse disorders, such as drug abuse, in which all members of the group have had the same experiences and used the same rationalizations and defenses to perpetuate their disorders. They can often see through self-justifications that might fool a sympathetic individual therapist. The message "I have been there, too" that is expressed by the other members is a powerful engaging device that can get through to the most resistant patient.

Supportive groups for medical disorders include groups for diabetic, hypertensive, and cancer patients and for the relatives of such patients. **Supportive groups for psychiatric disorders** include daily groups for hospitalized patients, monthly groups for chronic patients who are taking psychotropic medications, and groups for other patients in need of supportive therapy. For these groups, the model is similar to that of supportive individual therapy, and the purpose is to maintain patients at their best possible level of functioning. In addition to receiving reassurance and advice and having a stable object to whom they can relate, patients gain the benefits derived from companionship and the feeling that a number of people are interested in their welfare.

▬▶ The daughter whose course of family therapy is described above participated in family therapy for 6 months. During that time, the interactions within her family improved considerably, and at the end of 6 months, the family made a decision, with which the therapist agreed, to end therapy. The therapist was well aware that the daughter still had problems, but sensed that her motivation to work them out in the presence of the family was coming to an end. She had found a way to live with her family. Next, she would need to learn how to separate from them as she approached young adulthood. She would clearly do better in another kind of therapy, without her family. In referring this patient for further treatment, the therapist considered two forms of therapy, individual psychoanalytically oriented therapy and group therapy, each of which had advantages and both of which were available in the community. Individual therapy would have the patient work through an intense transference in which she would react to the therapist in the same angry way she had reacted to her parents. The therapist would repeatedly interpret this pattern so that the patient would learn about her distorted expectations and then be able to change them. However, if the patient proved to be relatively unmotivated and antagonistic toward the parental figure/therapist, the interpretations might go unheeded. The therapist decided to send the patient to group therapy, having concluded that therapy in a group of peers with similar experiences would better serve her.

The group therapist was an experienced woman who had a reputation for working well with adolescents who are acting out their feelings. There were eight people in the group ranging in age from 16 to 22 years. Because of their similarity in age, the members tended to band together as siblings and developed a strong transference to the middle-aged therapist. This group experience was beneficial for the patient in a number of ways.

The patient soon realized that her age-mates had similar problems with their families. Some things that she had regarded as her own unique secrets were, in fact, universal issues that the members in the group talked about openly. Learning that some of the older members had worked through problems like hers and were becoming college students helped to reduce her feeling of hopelessness.

She acquired a lot of information, including answers to many questions that she had "always wanted to ask but was afraid to." In particular, she learned important information about birth control and about the hazards of drug abuse, which was imparted in ways that she could not have accepted from a parent.

She began to be genuinely concerned about other group members and realized that they were interested and concerned about her. This newly developed altruism led her out of her self-pitying self-preoccupation, so that she looked forward to the group meetings.

The group was very helpful in teaching her new techniques for socialization and letting her know that her sullen, pouty style was not the best way to win friends. She learned how to meet people, how to make small talk, and how to be less awkward in groups. Imitative behavior was important in helping her with socialization. She found herself imitating one of the more socially graceful women in the group and realized that this approach worked much better than her former style of relating to people.

As she became more comfortable in the group, she experienced a catharsis: She was able to express her feelings with less expectation of ridicule or criticism. She again went through the story of her brother's death, but this time, she felt a warm, empathic response, which became another step in her long mourning process. It was helpful to relive an experience in different contexts because each reexperience added something different. She did some work alone and some with her family. She felt that this reexperience in the group was a great new relief.

Corrective recapitulation of family experience is a form of transference that can be a powerful tool in a group. At first, the patient saw the therapist as a parent and tried to enlist support against her from her peers. Several members noticed this and pointed it out to her. One 20-year-old man reminded her of her brother, and she found herself reacting to him in the old familiar way. This response allowed her to reexperience her angry, competitive feelings toward her brother, which she had suppressed since his death. As always in the mourning process, it was important for her to bring these angry feelings to the surface.

Telling her story in the group and revealing her thoughts, feelings, and weaknesses generated a strong bond with the group. The patient gradually became more open to feedback from the group. At the same time, she brought her problems into an arena outside herself, which encouraged her to gain perspective on herself and a new objectivity. Through this **interpersonal learning,** she began to see her problems as less unspeakable than before. At the same time, she was able to take some personal responsibility for her problems and began to feel that her difficulties were not completely the fault of her parents. This realization, in turn, gave her a sense of empowerment to do something about her problems. ◀▦

Selected Readings

Basch, M.F. Understanding Psychotherapy: The Science behind the Art. New York, Basic Books, 1988.

Beck, A.T., et al. Cognitive Therapy of Depression. New York, Guilford Press, 1979.

Davanloo, H., ed. Short-Term Dynamic Psychotherapy. New York, Jason Aronson, 1980.

Hatcher, C., and P. Himmelstein. The Handbook of Gestalt Therapy. New York, Jason Aronson, 1978.

Kernberg, O. Borderline Conditions and Pathological Narcissism. New York, Jason Aronson, 1975.

Klerman, G.L., et al. Interpersonal Therapy of Depression. New York, Basic Books, 1984.

Malan, D.H. The Frontier of Brief Psychotherapy. New York, Plenum Press, 1976.

Mann, J. Time Limited Psychotherapy. Cambridge, Harvard University Press, 1973.

Sifneos, P.E. Short Term Psychotherapy and Emotional Crisis. Cambridge, Harvard University Press, 1972.

Viederman, M. The psychodynamic life narrative: a psychotherapeutic intervention useful in crisis situations. Psychiatry 46:236–246, 1983.

Yalom, I.D. The Theory and Practice of Group Psychotherapy. New York, Basic Books, 1985.

CHAPTER SIXTEEN

PSYCHOPHARMACOLOGY

L. MARK RUSSAKOFF, MD

Since the 1950s, drug treatment has played an increasingly important role in the therapy of psychiatric disorders. During the 1990s, a virtual explosion of new drugs that are safer for and better tolerated by patients has given physicians a much wider range of treatments from which to choose. Contrary to the spirit of the 1960s and some catchy advertising lines, however, there is not always better living through chemistry. Psychopharmacological intervention is only one component of an integrated treatment approach for psychiatric patients.

Some have referred to the introduction of modern psychopharmacological agents as the "second revolution" in psychiatry (with psychoanalytic influences being the first). These medications have been effective for many patients. Before they became available, psychiatric practice mainly took place in state hospitals and in outpatient psychotherapy sessions. Psychotic episodes frequently resulted in long-term hospitalizations. Electroconvulsive therapy (ECT) was the only treatment specifically effective for depression, regardless of the severity of the depression. When the new medications first became available, they were given to patients who were hospitalized. These patients recovered sooner and could be released sooner. As physicians became more comfortable with the medications, they used them for the initial treatment of many psychiatric disorders and, as a result, did not have to hospitalize patients as often. Box 16–1 provides a historical perspective of psychopharmacology.

GENERAL PRINCIPLES

Psychopharmacological medications are highly effective when they are used properly for specific conditions. This efficacy has been shown in double-blind, placebo-controlled trials. The medications are usually most effective when the patient taking them has a good ongoing relationship with a physician who can address the patient's concerns about taking the medications, and this often helps the patient to comply with the pharmacological regimen. For many people, realizing that something might be wrong with their mind and that part of the solution is taking a pill that will affect their mind is "a bitter pill to swallow." They still feel that psychiatric problems are evidence of moral weakness and that using "drugs" compounds the immorality. In recent years, this view has been somewhat ameliorated by the mounting evidence that psychiatric disorders are a result of chemical imbalances in the brain and that medications are a way of correcting the imbalances. Many patients, families, and physicians have found this concept to be useful and acceptable when they face the need for drug treatment.

Psychopharmacological treatment must be based on a careful, comprehensive psychiatric evaluation. Even if a patient has an anxiety or a mood disorder, for which medications are commonly used, the possible risks and benefits of treatment must be weighed. The milder anxiety and depressive disorders can be treated without medications and should be in patients who are uninterested in, are opposed to, or have contraindications to the medications. The more severe the Axis I disorder, the greater the likelihood that medications will play an important role in treatment. For the most severe disorders, treatment without medications (or ECT) may not only be ineffective but may constitute an unjustifiable denial of effective treatment.

All of the medications have side effects and risks. The more dangerous or incapacitating the illness, the more **side effects** the patient and physician may be willing to tolerate. Within categories of agents, there is a range of side effects and risks. When making a diagnostic assessment, the physician must also assess the patient's capacity to tolerate the various treatments. For instance, patients who have extreme preoccupations with their bodies may find it difficult to tolerate a medication that has many physical side effects. For example, many psychotropic agents cause weight gain, and if this would be intolerable, it may be possible to choose an agent that is less likely to cause this problem. If the patient is extremely agitated, many physicians choose an agent that has a sedating effect. If sexual functioning is crucial for the person's self-image, the physician might choose the agent that is least likely to disrupt sexual functioning. There are no perfect medications, and choosing the best one is always a matter of balancing the risks, benefits, and costs.

Medications that are prescribed but not taken are obviously ineffective. It has been estimated that half of all prescribed drugs are not taken. Because of

---

BOX 16–1. Historical Perspectives on Psychopharmacology

The era of modern psychopharmacology can be dated from the discovery of the antipsychotic effects of chlorpromazine in the early 1950s. Although the therapeutic effects of lithium carbonate were described earlier (1949), enthusiasm for this agent was dampened by the simultaneous finding that when lithium salts were used as a substitute for sodium chloride, death could ensue. It was not until decades later that lithium carbonate was commonly used.

Prior to the discovery of chlorpromazine, psychiatrists had few effective somatic interventions at their disposal. The most effective one was ECT. Sedatives were available, but, as is now known, they were effective only for short-term use and had a high addictive potential. Stimulants were available but had not played a prominent part in overall psychopharmacological treatments (except for attention-deficit disorder in children).

Chlorpromazine was important for several reasons. Most significantly, it was efficacious in schizophrenia, a disorder for which psychiatry had little specific to offer. Second, it was the agent that "proved" that a medication could have profound positive effects on the mental functioning of an individual. Although there was evidence that stimulants could improve performance, the dramatic efficacy of chlorpromazine in psychotic disorders shook the very premises of the different psychologically oriented schools in psychiatry. In fact, many of the original studies of antipsychotics were done to disprove their efficacy! Because of the resistance to the idea that chlorpromazine could be efficacious in a "functional" psychiatric disorder, the studies of its efficacy were made ever more rigorous. In the process, the problems inherent in the commonly used diagnostic system were clarified and many research scales were created to circumvent the limitations of the diagnostic system. Double-blind, placebo-controlled research designs assessed by independent raters who were trained with a reliable rating scale became the standard. All of these efforts demonstrated beyond a shadow of a doubt that these medications (for, in short order, the pharmaceutical firms had developed many variations of the successful phenothiazine compound) were effective.

The attempt to find yet another antipsychotic led to the discovery of the first TCA, imipramine. Imipramine did not improve the psychosis in schizophrenic patients but it did brighten their moods. Imipramine was not the first antidepressant discovered, however. That honor goes to the MAOI iproniazid. Iproniazid was introduced as an antituberculous medication. Physicians observed that the mood of patients who took this agent seemed to improve more than would be expected from the effects of the agent on the tuberculosis. Iproniazid was then tried in depressed patients and found to be effective. Other hydrazines were developed and tested, and the class of MAOIs was developed.

---

the many critical attitudes toward and meanings associated with psychotropic medications, **compliance** is often a problem. With many of these agents, there is a substantial lag between the time when treatment is initiated and the time when benefits are felt by the patient. For a while, the patient may experience only the side effects of the medication. The strength of the physician-patient relationship often sustains the patient during the period before the agent becomes effective. Another problem is that, with most of the medications, improvement occurs gradually (i.e., the changes occur almost imperceptibly on an hour to hour or day to day basis). (The antianxiety medications are an exception to this rule.) This improvement often causes patients to feel that they have gotten better on their own and to discount the effectiveness of or need for continued medication. This feeling must be explored, and the patient must be educated about how medications work and why they are necessary for continued treatment.

In addition to the moral factor, there are other common concerns about drug treatment for psychiatric disorders. Some patients see it as an act of control by the physician. This attitude should be addressed with patients by helping them see that they are the ones who can exercise control by deciding to take care of themselves. Psychotic patients may see the act of taking pills or receiving injections as having erotic or sexual meaning. With the more chronically ill patients, these concerns can sometimes be explored. With acutely ill patients, the physician's awareness that such distortions may occur can be helpful. These patients need to be reminded and reassured that they are being given medications and are not being asked to take part in sexual activities.

After a patient responds to a medication, it often needs to be continued for several months. During this time, patients may stop taking the medication because they feel better and do not understand the need for continuing it. If medications are discontinued too soon after the patient has returned to a baseline status, a relapse is likely to occur because the episode of illness has not truly ended. If the medication is discontinued too abruptly, there may be a recurrence (i.e., a new episode of illness). There must be a continuing dialog between the physician and patient to ensure that the patient understands the rationale for and need for continued treatment.

Psychiatrists are learning more and more about the recurrent nature of many psychiatric disorders. Data have also been accumulated on the role of **long-term treatment** with psychoactive medications. Most patients with schizophrenia and bipolar disorder must take medications for life. Many patients with recurrent depression find it advantageous to take an antidepressant on an ongoing basis. For the reasons discussed above, many patients are resistant to the idea of long-term treatment. They may make repeated attempts to surreptitiously or overtly discontinue the prescribed medications, and the inevitable relapses are often associated with shame and guilt. It is at this point that the physician-patient relationship is most crucial because it can provide a nonjudgmental atmosphere, support the need for continued medication, and ameliorate the narcissistic injury associated with treatment.

In recent years, there have been changes in prescribing patterns by psychiatrists. Previously, many believed that patients should be treated with a single agent. Now, however, multiple medications are being used, particularly in more complicated clinical situations. Although more than 60% of patients respond to the first antidepressant prescribed for them, the 40% who do not may need **augmentation strategies** (additional concomitant treatments). Of the 60% who initially respond to a single agent, some may relapse even though they continue taking the medication, and they may also be candidates for an augmentation strategy. This approach is no different in concept from the combination treatments used for hypertension, cardiac arrhythmias, or seizures. Unfortunately, a myth has been promoted that the "standard" treatment is a single medication. Equally unfortunately, some patients measure success or failure in terms of the number of medications needed and not the actual clinical improvement achieved. Physicians should not collude in such thinking. Patients should be given the fewest medications that are effective in the treatment of their conditions, but the ultimate focus of treatment should be on the outcome rather than the "pill count." Patients (especially, elderly patients) who need multiple medications are more likely to make errors in taking the medications and may need specific suggestions to help them with compliance (e.g., using containers to set up the pills to be taken for a day or a week).

ANTIPSYCHOTIC AGENTS

Antipsychotic agents were originally labeled major tranquilizers and neuroleptics. The **major tranquilizers** seemed to be uniquely effective for patients in agitated psychotic states, precisely the area where traditional tranquilizers had failed. The word major distinguished these tranquilizers from the older (minor) tranquilizers. The term major tranquilizer implied that these agents were simply more powerful tranquilizers and that they lacked any specific therapeutic efficacy other than tranquilization.

The label *neuroleptic* was suggested by the French discoverers of the first identified antipsychotic, chlorpromazine. The term *antipsychotic* is preferable for these agents because it more accurately describes their action and the reason they are prescribed. Physicians sometimes have told patients that their medications are neuroleptics in order to circumvent the issue that the patient suffers from a psychotic illness, but it is unclear whether this subterfuge is effective. Some patients who disagree with the physician's diagnosis take the prescribed medication anyway, and those who refuse to do so may not be convinced to take the medication if it is given another name.

Antipsychotics are derived from several classes of chemicals (Table 16–1). One of the main classes is phenothiazine, which is divided into three subclasses, the aliphatics, piperidines, and piperazines, depending on the substitution that occurs on the central ring of nitrogen. Chlorpromazine is derived from this class. The class of thioxanthenes differs from the phenothiazines in that the sulfur in the central ring is replaced by a carbon.

The originally available antipsychotics can be characterized by the following properties. They induce extrapyramidal side effects, raise prolactin levels, and are more effective against positive symptoms than negative symptoms of schizophrenia. The discovery that clozapine seems to be more effective than other antipsychotics, does not induce extrapyramidal side effects, does not raise prolactin levels in humans, and is effective against negative symptoms of schizophrenia led to it being described as atypical. The release of risperidone in 1994, designed with clozapine in mind, has led to the development of several atypical antipsychotics, which are characterized mostly by the low incidence of extrapyramidal side effects associated with them. These newer drugs are rapidly becoming the standard first-line treatment for patients with acute psychotic illness, especially when the costs of the drugs are not a primary consideration. At the present time, four of these drugs (clozapine, risperidone, olanzapine, quetiapine) have become available. These drugs will become important components of treatment if they prove to be well tolerated, do not induce extrapyramidal side effects (and thus, it is hoped, do not induce tardive dyskinesia), do not cause sexual dysfunction, and are effective in treating both the positive and negative symptoms of schizophrenia.

Indications and Contraindications

The primary indications for antipsychotics are **schizophreniform disorder, schizophrenia, schizoaffective disorder, mania and depression with psychotic features, delusional disorder,** and **psychoses associated with various medical conditions** (e.g., Alzheimer's dementia, vascular dementia) (see Chapter 3, Mood Disorders; Chapter 4, Schizophrenia and Other Psychotic Disorders; and Chapter 5, Cognitive and Mental Disorders Due to General Medical Conditions). It is not appropriate to think of these medications as "antischizophrenic" agents, because they are effective for all psychotic disorders. Low-dosage antipsychotic drugs are also used in borderline personality disorder (i.e., for refractory impulsivity or affective lability that does not respond to other medications) and in some paranoid and schizotypal personality disorders (see Chapter 8, Personality Disorders).

➡ In one case, a 26-year-old woman with borderline personality disorder had undergone various outpatient treatments since she had been 17 years old. She had tried several antidepressant agents but continued to be emotionally labile and dysphoric. Several hospitalizations had had no effect on her course, which was somewhat predictably unstable. Although she had never had delusions, hallucinations, or a thought disorder, her psychiatrist prescribed trifluoperazine, 2 mg orally three times daily. While taking this agent, she was able to attend therapy sessions and discuss events in her life without enacting her strong feelings. ⬅

Antipsychotics may be helpful in quieting extremely agitated people regardless of their diagnosis,

TABLE 16–1. Antipsychotics

Medications	Dosage Equivalence (mg)	Sedative Effects	Extrapyramidal Side Effects	Orthostatic Hypotension	Anticholinergic Effects
Chlorpromazine	100	Severe	Mild	Severe	Moderate
Thioridazine	100	Severe	Minimal	Severe	Severe
Fluphenazine	1–2	Minimal	Severe	Minimal	Minimal
Trifluoperazine	2.5–5	Mild	Moderate	Minimal	Minimal
Haloperidol	1–2	Minimal	Severe	Minimal	Minimal
Thiothixene	4	Mild	Moderate	Mild	Mild
Pimozide	0.4–2	Minimal	Severe	Minimal	Minimal
Molindone	10–25	Mild	Mild to moderate	Mild	None
Loxapine	15–25	Mild	Mild to moderate	Mild	Mild
Clozapine	50	Severe	None	Severe	Severe
Quetiapine	Unknown	Mild	None	Mild	Minimal
Risperidone	0.5–1 (?)	Minimal	<6 mg: None ≥6 mg: Minimal	Mild	None
Olanzapine	3(?)	Moderate	Akathisia: Moderate Dystonia: Minimal	Minimal	Mild

and this effect has sometimes led to misuse of these agents.

There are few substantial medical **contraindications** to antipsychotic agents. Patients who are allergic to a class of medications should not receive an agent from that class. If a psychotic patient is intoxicated, has taken an overdose, or is obtunded for any reason, he or she should not be started on antipsychotics until his or her status has returned to baseline. The rest of the contraindications are relative. In a patient with known liver disease (e.g., hepatitis, cirrhosis), it may be wise to avoid a medication such as chlorpromazine (which is known to irritate the liver in some cases) in favor of haloperidol (which is less likely to irritate the liver), unless there are specific reasons to use chlorpromazine that override the possibility of further aggravation of the liver disease. A history of agranulocytosis due to any cause excludes clozapine, since there is a much greater risk of that complication with clozapine than with other agents. Antipsychotics lower the seizure threshold but can be given to patients with seizure disorders if the patients are carefully monitored. These patients may need increased dosages of anticonvulsant medications. A history of extrapyramidal reactions (see Side Effects, below) to antipsychotics is not a contraindication to these agents. Some patients have severe, disabling extrapyramidal reactions, especially to high-potency antipsychotics. These especially sensitive patients can sometimes be treated successfully with lower-potency antipsychotics or may be candidates for newer atypical antipsychotics.

Evaluation

Before initiating treatment with an antipsychotic, the physician should take the patient's vital signs, including the pulse, blood pressure, and temperature; obtain a complete blood cell count; perform liver function tests; and record an electrocardiogram (ECG) if the patient has a history of cardiac disease or is over 40 years old. In emergencies, the medication can be initiated before these studies are performed if there are no clinical contraindications to the medication.

Treatment

The choice of an antipsychotic agent should be determined by the patient's specific needs, vulnerability to particular side effects, and history of response to and tolerance of **side effects** in general. Newer antipsychotics—risperidone, olanzapine, quetiapine, and several more that are likely to be on the market soon—cause fewer overall side effects but are much more expensive (with a cost of $8–$16 a day). They have rapidly become the medications of first choice for outpatient treatment and for inpatient treatment when it is anticipated that oral dosing will be sufficient. Currently, none are available in a parenteral form, so they are not used in emergencies as the sole treatment.

For aggressive individuals who require strong sedation, chlorpromazine is often the agent of choice. It is available for intramuscular injection or as an elixir. For patients with prominent features of psychosis but less agitation, a high-potency antipsychotic such as haloperidol or fluphenazine might be chosen. Both of these medications are available as pills, elixirs, short-acting intramuscular and long-acting intramuscular forms. The long-acting intramuscular dosage form is most useful when the patient is willing to accept the injections but otherwise would not be compliant with daily medication administration. If the physician would like to achieve more intermediate effects, an agent such as trifluoperazine or perphenazine might be chosen.

It has become common practice to treat all acutely ill patients with high-potency antipsychotics (such as haloperidol) and to supplement that treatment with parenteral lorazepam when greater sedation is required. The advantage of using a high-potency antipsychotic with lorazepam instead of chlorpromazine is that fewer side effects—orthostatic hypotension, constipation, dry mouth—develop.

If weight gain is a particular concern, some physicians choose molindone (see below). For a patient who has not responded well to adequate clinical trials of two agents, a course of treatment with clozapine is indicated. Clozapine is effective in patients who have not responded to or are intolerant of medications from at least two classes. It is the only antipsychotic that has demonstrated superiority for schizophrenic patients who are refractory to other treatments. There is hope that some of the newer atypical antipsychotics may possess this superior effectiveness without the risk of bone marrow suppression (see below).

The beneficial effects of the antipsychotics are delayed for about a week. Unfortunately, this is not true of the side effects. Early in the course of treatment, the observable effects are primarily sedation and other side effects. Dosage adjustments are often made on the basis of patient tolerance to the medication and its side effects and of statistical information about therapeutic dosage ranges.

Although many studies have been done to demonstrate the efficacy of the antipsychotics, there are many fewer data on the **proper dosage range.** The results of double-blind, placebo-controlled studies indicate that a minimum dosage of chlorpromazine of 600 mg/d is likely to be effective in most patients. The upper range of the dosage is set more by practice than by scientific evidence. Most psychiatrists use 600–1200 mg/d of chlorpromazine, or its equivalent, for antipsychotics of higher potency (see Table 16–1). Psychiatrists sometimes increase the dosage to sedate the patient. If greater sedative effect is needed and the upper limit of the range has been reached, a benzodiazepine can be added.

In the past, the traditional treatment for an acutely psychotic individual with uncomplicated schizophrenia and with no medical contraindications or special risks began with **chlorpromazine,** 50–150 mg, taken orally three times daily. If, after an initial 100-mg dose, the patient became calm but was not sedated, he or she would be given another dose of 100 mg. The doses were altered on the basis of the patient's therapeutic response to the medication and response to the side effects. The maximum total dosage for the first day was 450 mg. The dosage could be increased by 300 mg/d, up to 1200 mg/d, if needed.

The standard treatment has been a **high-potency antipsychotic** (e.g., haloperidol, fluphenazine). These medications are effective at dosages of 6–20 mg/d. A patient might be started on 2 mg, taken orally three times daily. This dosage may be increased incrementally up to a maximum of 20 mg/d, depending on patient response, and is eventually administered as a single dose at night over a 1-week period. With an extremely paranoid patient, the initial dose might be administered with an antiparkinsonian agent to try to prevent a dystonic reaction. For patients who are able to collaborate more directly in their treatment, especially if the initial dosages are low, an antiparkinsonian drug might not be administered prophylactically. The advantage of withholding prophylactic treatment is that some patients will not require it and can avoid taking another medication that has side effects (see below).

Risperidone was the first of the "designer-drug" atypical antipsychotics to reach the market. It is an effective antipsychotic at doses that do not provoke extrapyramidal side effects. Patients initially take 1 mg orally twice a day, which is increased to 3 mg, taken orally twice a day, depending on tolerance to side effects and clinical need. At 6 mg/d, risperidone produces no more extrapyramidal side effects than does placebo. At higher doses, it produces significant extrapyramidal side effects and its primary demonstrated advantage is lost. Because it is well tolerated and effective at low doses, it quickly became a first-line treatment. Similarly, olanzapine, started at 5–10 mg at bedtime and increased to 20 mg, if needed, is well tolerated and effective, with little propensity to produce extrapyramidal side effects. Because olanzapine is fairly sedating and long acting, it is administered at bedtime. Quetiapine can cause substantial orthostatic hypotension in the early titration phase, so it is started at a low dose, 25 mg, taken orally two times a day, and then built up by 50–100 mg/d to 300 mg/d. It does not cause extrapyramidal side effects even at higher doses, nor does it increase the prolactin level. There is a concern about ocular toxicity (see below).

Two antipsychotic agents are available in a **long-acting injectable form:** fluphenazine and haloperidol. There are two long-acting forms of fluphenazine (fluphenazine enanthate and fluphenazine decanoate) and one long-acting form of haloperidol (haloperidol decanoate). These agents can be given initially as oral agents; if well tolerated, they can then be administered intramuscularly. The advantages of the intramuscular method are that physicians know their patients are receiving the drug and patients do not have to remember to take the medication daily. Many of them will need oral adjunctive antiparkinsonian medication, however. For patients who have a history of noncompliance in taking medications, the long-acting preparations are a useful alternative. They are especially useful in populations in whom psychosis is associated with violent or self-destructive actions.

Fluphenazine enanthate is administered every 2 weeks; fluphenazine decanoate is administered every 3 weeks. Both agents may be administered subcutaneously (which is not recommended for haloperidol decanoate) or intramuscularly.

If a patient has been taking oral fluphenazine and is stable, the agent can be changed to fluphenazine enanthate or decanoate. Dosage conversion is calculated by assuming that fluphenazine hydrochloride, 12.5 mg/d, is the equivalent of 0.5 mL of the injectable form. Haloperidol decanoate may be administered intramuscularly every 4 weeks. It tends to be better tolerated than oral haloperidol hydrochloride. The dosage of haloperidol decanoate is 10–15 times the daily dosage of haloperidol hydrochloride, not to exceed 100 mg of haloperidol decanoate.

As was noted above, **clozapine** is a unique antipsychotic agent. It is often referred to as "atypical." It is the only antipsychotic agent with demonstrated evidence of superiority in schizophrenic patients who have not responded to other classes of antipsychotics (i.e., have been refractory to or are intolerant of them). Clozapine seems to cause improvement in the negative symptoms of schizophrenia, in contrast to the "typical" antipsychotics, which generally have no impact on that set of symptoms. Clozapine is also atypical in that it does not cause extrapyramidal symptoms, increased levels of prolactin, or tardive dyskinesia. Because of the significant risk of agranulocytosis with this agent, however, it is not used as a first-line medication. When it is being used, white blood cell counts must be done weekly. Because of frequent annoying side effects, clozapine is started at lower dosages, which are increased slowly.

Over the past 10 years, **combination therapy** with an antipsychotic and a benzodiazepine has become common. If a patient needs to be sedated and is given an increased dosage of an antipsychotic for this purpose, the patient receives more antipsychotic (i.e., antidopaminergic) "punch" than he or she needs. If a benzodiazepine is given, the patient will be sedated by it and will not receive the unnecessary antidopaminergic effects. The antipsychotic agent is targeted to the signs and symptoms of psychosis. The benzodiazepine is used to sedate the individual until the antipsychotic takes effect. In theory, this combination of agents should lower the amount of antipsychotic administered and also, it is hoped, should lower the risk of tardive dyskinesia (see below).

Side Effects
Extrapyramidal Symptoms

Extrapyramidal side effects consist of tremors, akinesia, rigidity, dystonias, dyskinesias, and akathisia. The first five symptoms are sometimes referred to as **pseudoparkinsonism,** and they tend to

be treatable with adjunctive agents. **Akathisia,** which is an inner sense of restlessness, can be extremely difficult to treat. All of the extrapyramidal symptoms are associated with a sense of dysphoria. It has been demonstrated that an acute dysphoric response to antipsychotic agents predicts poor compliance with continued treatment with the medications. Akathisia must be treated differently from the symptoms of pseudoparkinsonism. One may need to change the dosage of the antipsychotic or switch to another agent.

The **tremor** tends to be coarse. It may be so severe that it interferes with the ability to eat or smoke a cigarette. When **akinesia** is combined with the depressive affect produced by the antipsychotic, it may be mistaken for the psychomotor retardation of depression. However, this "depression" can be "cured" two hours after an antiparkinsonian agent is given. The **rigidity** is also likely to respond quickly to antiparkinsonian treatment.

The **acute dystonias** are most likely to appear within a couple of hours to days of initiating treatment with, raising the dosage of, or receiving an injection of the long-acting form of the antipsychotics. Patients should be warned that their muscles may tighten or stiffen from the medications, that such responses may be scary but are not dangerous, and that other medications can easily treat this side effect. If patients have not been told that their muscles may tighten without warning, they may become terrified. If they have delusions that they are being controlled by outside agents, such experiences may confirm their worst fears. Muscle groups that are especially sensitive are the eye, neck, and paraspinalis muscles. The eyes may turn upward and outward to one side, a phenomenon known as oculogyric crisis, which is not a medical crisis. Rarely, the back muscles stiffen, as in opisthotonos. The neck may turn to one side, as in torticollis, and there may be posturing with the arms.

With outpatients or extremely wary inpatients who are being treated with high-potency antipsychotics, many psychiatrists initiate prophylactic treatment for extrapyramidal side effects. The most common regimen is **benztropine mesylate** given in one to three doses. The amount is based on the dosage of the antipsychotic agent. If the patient is receiving haloperidol, 5 mg orally twice a day, the patient should also receive benztropine mesylate, 1 mg orally twice a day. With low-potency antipsychotics, such as chlorpromazine, many psychiatrists are less inclined to give prophylactic treatment for extrapyramidal side effects. With atypical antipsychotics, routine prophylactic treatment is not indicated.

If a patient is having an acute dystonic reaction, one can provide relief within minutes by administering **diphenhydramine,** 25 mg intravenously slowly over 1 minute. During treatment, the patient will "loosen up" dramatically in front of one's eyes. If the agent is administered intramuscularly, the dosage is usually increased to 50 mg. Benztropine mesylate, 1–2 mg, can also be administered intramuscularly. This approach has a much less dramatic effect; it takes about 15 minutes for relief to occur. Oral administration of antiparkinsonian agents is not likely to be efficacious for acute treatment, because the dystonia usually resolves on its own before the agent takes effect. It is reasonable to predict that a patient who has one dystonic reaction will have more, and such a patient should probably be treated prophylactically.

Tardive Dyskinesia

Tardive dyskinesia has been defined in the DSM-IV as "involuntary choreiform, athetoid, or rhythmic movements (lasting at least a few weeks) of the tongue, jaw, or extremities developing in association with the use of neuroleptic medication for at least a few months (may be for a shorter period of time in elderly persons)." Classic tardive dyskinesia affects the bucco-lingual-masticatory muscles, leading to fly-catcher's tongue, bonbon sign, grimaces, or chewing movements. "Flycatcher's tongue" refers to the tongue's darting in and out of the mouth. "Bonbon sign" is the pushing of the tongue against the cheek wall, so that it looks as though a piece of candy is pressed against the cheek. An early sign of tardive dyskinesia is wormlike movements of the tongue while it is at rest in the mouth.

Data on the correlates of tardive dyskinesia have affected prescribing habits. Because it has been shown that a history of extrapyramidal symptoms and treatment for such symptoms is associated with the development of tardive dyskinesia, some physicians initiate treatment at very low dosages in hopes of preventing extrapyramidal side effects. No studies have been done to prove the efficacy of this approach, but it is a rational one. This approach conflicts with the economic pressures to treat patients rapidly because it takes longer for an adequate dosage to be reached.

It has been suggested that tardive dyskinesia results from **chronic dopaminergic blockage,** which causes the postsynaptic dopamine receptors in some motor pathways to become hypersensitive to dopamine. Two observations are consistent with this hypothesis: (1) Increasing antipsychotic dosages masks tardive dyskinesia, and (2) the addition of dopaminergic agonists (e.g., methylphenidate) exacerbates the condition. Adding anticholinergic agents typically worsens the dyskinesias, perhaps by causing further disruption of the balance between dopamine and acetylcholine. Clonidine has been reported to reduce the dyskinesias in a subgroup of patients, and this suggests that an adrenergic mechanism is involved. In clinically diagnosed cases of tardive dyskinesia, only 50% of patients followed the pattern predicted by the postsynaptic dopamine hypersensitivity hypothesis when the patients were subjected to various pharmacological probes.

Tardive dyskinesia is believed to develop in about 20% of schizophrenic patients who are treated for years. In studies that have followed patients longitudinally, about 4% of patients taking antipsy-

chotics developed signs of tardive dyskinesia each year. Thus, the risk for long-term patients mounts over the course of treatment. Elderly patients seem to have a much higher risk of developing tardive dyskinesia early in their treatment. Patients with diabetes mellitus may be at especially high risk for this side effect. It has also been reported that patients with mood disorders are more at risk than schizophrenic patients.

When psychiatrists first began to focus their attention on tardive dyskinesia, they believed that the condition was inevitably progressive and irreversible. It is now known that only a minority of patients have a progressive course, and, in most patients who develop this disorder, it does not progress if patients are maintained on the same antipsychotic dosage. It has also been observed that if tardive dyskinesia is identified in the early stages, when abnormal movements are minimal and few areas are affected, and if the antipsychotic can be stopped, the dyskinesia is likely to remit. However, many patients who are treated with antipsychotic agents need long-term maintenance with the agents. There have been some reports of patients treated with clozapine in whom tardive dyskinesia has remitted over time.

It is hoped that newer atypical antipsychotics will have a lower risk of inducing tardive dyskinesia. Clozapine is the only antipsychotic agent that has been on the market for a significant period of time that is not associated with a substantial risk of tardive dyskinesia. Risperidone is so new that there has not been a great deal of experience with it even in other countries, so its long-term effects are unclear. Although it has some of the same properties as clozapine, it does cause extrapyramidal symptoms at high dosages and, therefore, could cause tardive dyskinesia. Some preliminary data suggest that risperidone reduces the risk of tardive dyskinesia by more than tenfold after one year of treatment compared with haloperidol. Olanzapine causes akathisia. Its specific risk for inducing tardive dyskinesia is unknown. Similarly, there are no study results regarding quetiapine.

All patients who take antipsychotic agents for more than a few months should be assessed regularly for the development of movement disorders. The most common assessment scale is the **Abnormal Involuntary Movement Scale (AIMS),** which consists of 10 items that measure involuntary movements of the face, mouth, jaw, tongue, upper and lower extremities, and trunk. The scale helps to identify the abnormal movements, their location, and their severity. Any patient who develops a movement disorder while undergoing treatment must be assessed for tardive dyskinesia. If it is present, the physician and patient must weigh the benefits of continuing the medication against the risks of discontinuing it. It is sometimes wise to refer the patient and family for a second opinion at this time, because in rare cases the movements can be disfiguring and disabling.

No known treatments for tardive dyskinesia exist. There have been some preliminary reports that vitamin E, 400 U four times a day, may lead to improvement. Current data suggest that the disorder runs a variable course that waxes and wanes and that it is, therefore, impossible to derive firm conclusions about treatment efficacy from small studies. As noted above, some patients with tardive dyskinesia who were treated with clozapine also had improvements in their movement disorders. No studies regarding the effects of the newer atypical antipsychotics on the course of tardive dyskinesia have been done to date.

Other Side Effects

Sedation

Sedation is a side effect of all the antipsychotics to varying degrees. Roughly speaking, the higher the dosage in milligrams, the more sedated the patient will be. The low-potency agents are more sedating than the high-potency agents. Agitated patients who have not slept for days may quickly go to sleep after taking one or two doses of the low-potency agents. Interestingly, the patients can be easily aroused to take the next dose but may then go back to sleep. Nonagitated patients who are given a highly sedating agent (e.g., chlorpromazine) may become too sleepy to participate in activities. Patients who are sensitive to sedation may find that even extra cups of coffee do not help. The sedative effects usually wear off within two weeks once a stable dosage is reached.

Anticholinergic Effects

Anticholinergic side effects are particularly significant in the low-potency antipsychotics. They include a dry mouth, blurred vision, constipation, difficulty in initiating urination, precipitation of **acute glaucomic crisis** in patients with narrow-angle glaucoma, and delirium (atropinelike psychosis). Once a stable dosage has been maintained for about two weeks, the dry mouth and blurred vision may disappear. Many patients, however, have persistent problems with a **dry mouth** (cotton mouth), which makes speaking difficult. Such patients may chew sugarfree gum to keep the mouth moist. If they use gum that contains sugar, they are at risk for developing serious dental caries. **Constipation** can often be treated by dietary adjustments. For patients who refuse to modify their diets or who do not have the option of choosing high-fiber foods, stool softeners or fiber supplements may be helpful. Men with benign prostatic hypertrophy may develop acute **urinary retention.** The peripheral manifestations of anticholinergic effects can be directly treated with bethanechol, a peripherally acting parasympathomimetic, 10–25 mg, taken orally two to three times a day. Higher dosages are often needed in young adults with significant side effects.

The atropinelike psychosis is more likely to be induced by high dosages of chlorpromazine or thioridazine, with or without anticholinergic agents. Excessive dosages of anticholinergic agents can also induce this **delirium.** The clinical picture is typically that of delirium or confusion, with visual hallucinations developing as the condition worsens. There is usually tachycardia, flushed facies, and widely dilated pupils. The mucous membranes are dry. In the past, some physicians have treated the syndrome with physostigmine, but this entails a serious risk of cardiac arrhythmias. In addition, physostigmine is short acting and, therefore, repeated doses are needed. The wisest course is to discontinue the probable offending anticholinergic medications, not use physostigmine, and watch until the delirium has cleared.

Hypotension

Orthostatic hypotension can occur with most of the antipsychotic medications. Chlorpromazine, thioridazine, and clozapine are the biggest offenders. Dosages of these drugs should be increased gradually because tolerance to the light-headedness develops over time. Quetiapine is started slowly because of the risk of hypotension.

Metabolic and Endocrine Effects

Weight gain is common with all of the antipsychotics, with the possible exception of molindone. (One study has indicated that molindone may cause the patient's weight to normalize; that is, underweight patients will gain weight and overweight patients will lose weight.) It is unclear what the mechanism of this weight gain is. Some have suggested that it results from a loss of satiety or pleasure from eating, a process that is believed to be mediated by dopamine; others have suggested that the weight gain is related to the antihistaminic effects of the antipsychotics.

All of the antipsychotic agents, with the exception of clozapine and quetiapine, cause disinhibition of the secretion of prolactin. Male patients may develop gynecomastia, and female patients may develop **galactorrhea.** Patients with these symptoms may be embarrassed to talk about them and may simply refuse to take their medications. Menstrual irregularities have been attributed to the medications.

Loss of sexual interest has been reported in both men and women. In males, **delayed ejaculation** may occur, particularly with thioridazine. **Retrograde ejaculation** (i.e., diversion of the ejaculate into the bladder instead of out of the penis) may also occur, especially with thioridazine. Patients who have previously had sexual delusions may become extremely agitated if this side effect develops and they have not been warned about it.

Hepatic Effects

An idiosyncratic **cholestatic jaundice** used to be common in patients treated with chlorpromazine. The liver enzymes rise dramatically, as in hepatitis. If this syndrome develops, the medication must be stopped. When the liver enzymes return to normal, another agent, such as haloperidol, should be chosen. Many patients may develop transient, **benign elevations** of the liver enzymes with other antipsychotics.

Dermatological Effects

Benign skin rashes are not uncommon with antipsychotics. Unlike with penicillin, the patient can usually continue to take the antipsychotic while the rash runs its course. The most common rash is **acneiform.** The phenothiazine antipsychotics commonly induce **photosensitivity.** If patients are exposed to the sun, they burn easily, as they are unable to detoxify free radicals in the skin. All patients taking antipsychotics should put on sunblock and wear a hat when they are outside. Patients can suffer significant burns if they are not warned about this side effect and instructed in how to avoid it.

Hematological Effects

Hematological effects are not common, except with clozapine. For chlorpromazine, the incidence of **agranulocytosis** is approximately 1 in 10,000 persons, and it typically develops within the first 3 months of treatment. The patient has signs of infection and is unable to mount a white blood cell defense. Because of the rarity of this side effect, routine monitoring of the white blood cell count is not indicated, except in patients taking clozapine. All patients should be instructed to report possible infections and their signs, such as sore throats and fevers.

Clozapine is unique in its therapeutic effects and its propensity to induce agranulocytosis. Clozapine induces agranulocytosis in approximately 1–2 in 100 persons, or 100 times more commonly than chlorpromazine. Patients who are treated with clozapine must have the white blood cell count checked weekly throughout treatment and for four weeks after discontinuation of the agent. If agranulocytosis develops, it usually has a toxic, progressive course. **Weekly white blood cell counts** will pick up the trend and can lead to timely discontinuation of the medication. Some rare patients suffer a precipitous decline in the white blood cell count that is missed by weekly testing.

Seizure Threshold Effects

All of the antipsychotics lower the seizure threshold. Chlorpromazine (especially when it is administered repeatedly and parenterally) and clozapine (especially in dosages over 600 mg/d) are associated with grand mal seizures. A more gradual increase in the dosage presumably lowers the risk for seizures.

Ophthalmological Effects

Retinitis pigmentosa has been a side effect of thioridazine treatment, usually only if the dosage exceeds 800 mg/d. As a result, this is the absolute maximum dosage for this medication. If a patient complains of dimming of vision, he or she should be referred immediately to an ophthalmologist for examination. Pigment accumulates in the retina, and this condition may progress to blindness. Lenticular opacities have occurred with long-term treatment by high doses of chlorpromazine. Animal studies have raised concern about this side effect from quetiapine, and periodic slit lamp examinations are recommended.

Neuroleptic Malignant Syndrome

Patients treated with antipsychotic agents may develop neuroleptic malignant syndrome, which is characterized by high fevers, rigidity, autonomic instability, and delirium. It can progress to death if untreated; before it was recognized, the mortality rate was sizeable. It is more likely to occur in hot weather, when the patient is dehydrated. The most critical features are **fever** (usually, >102°F) and parkinsonianlike stiffness. The **stiffness** does not quickly respond to antiparkinsonian medications. The fever can rise quickly to over 106°F, with associated rhabdomyolysis and acute renal failure. If neuroleptic malignant syndrome is suspected, the antipsychotic agent should be stopped immediately and the patient observed. Fluids should be pushed and a search for other causes of the fever initiated. In more severe cases, patients must be treated in the intensive care unit and placed on ice blankets. There are no specifically effective treatments, although bromocriptine and dantrolene sodium have been used.

Drug Interactions

Antipsychotics are metabolized by the **cytochrome P-450 system** and can interfere with the metabolism of other drugs that are administered concomitantly. There are case reports of patients in emergency rooms being given chlorpromazine and going into cardiovascular collapse. These events do not seem to be related to orthostatic hypotension, because repositioning of the patient has reportedly been ineffective. The most likely explanation is a toxic interaction between chlorpromazine and another ingested agent, such as alcohol or a barbiturate. Because of this problem, chlorpromazine is no longer used as widely in emergency rooms, especially when it is not known whether the patient has ingested other chemical substances. Haloperidol is more widely used because its effects on the blood pressure are usually minimal. When an antipsychotic is added to a patient's treatment regimen that includes medications that are sensitive to blood level changes, the respective parameters should be assessed, e.g., digoxin level, prothrombin times, and the like.

ANTIPARKINSONIAN AGENTS

Careful assessments of patients treated with high-potency antipsychotic agents have indicated that more than half suffer from some extrapyramidal side effects. Most patients are therefore given one of the many antiparkinsonian agents during treatment. There are three classes of these agents: anticholinergics, dopamine agonists, and miscellaneous agents.

Indications and Contraindications

Some patients can be weaned from an antiparkinsonian medication after they have been taking a stable dosage of an antipsychotic for about three months, but many will need concomitant treatment for as long as they take the antipsychotic.

The contraindications are for the specific classes (i.e., some patients cannot tolerate anticholinergic effects, others are sensitive to the hypertensive effects of dopaminergic agents, and so on).

Treatment

The anticholinergic compounds are the most widely used antiparkinsonian agents. This class includes trihexyphenidyl, procyclidine, diphenhydramine, benztropine mesylate, and biperiden. All of these agents may cause atropinelike psychoses at high dosages. **Trihexyphenidyl** was commonly used until it developed a reputation on the street as a good psychedelic agent and became widely abused. It must be administered in divided doses, up to 15 mg/d. **Procyclidine,** 15 mg/d, is also given in divided doses. **Diphenhydramine** tends to be quite sedating and is short acting. It is also used in divided doses, 25–50 mg, taken orally three to four times daily. Biperiden has never been widely used but is effective. The dosage is 2–6 mg/d. **Benztropine** is the most widely used of these agents. It is the longest-acting agent and can be administered once or twice a day, up to 8 mg/d, depending on the patient's comfort and convenience.

Amantadine is an indirect-acting dopaminergic agent. One might wonder about the advisability of administering a dopaminergic agonist for a problem caused by a dopaminergic antagonist. Nevertheless, it has been shown to be effective in the treatment of extrapyramidal side effects. Amantadine appears to selectively affect the dopaminergic pathways that are involved in these side effects, because there is not a significant loss of clinical antipsychotic efficacy. The advantage of amantadine is that it does not have anticholinergic effects. In situations in which anticholinergic effects are particularly problematic (e.g., severe constipation, benign prostatic hypertrophy), amantadine may work well.

Other agents have been used to treat various extrapyramidal side effects. Akathisia has responded to propranolol. Caffeine sodium benzoate administered intramuscularly can be used to treat acute dystonic reactions, as can diazepam. Benzodiazepines have been used to treat akathisia, especially after other agents have not been effective.

Side Effects

The anticholinergic agents cause preexisting anticholinergic symptoms to worsen (e.g., dry mouth, blurred vision, and constipation) (see Anticholinergic Effects, above). When high dosages of anticholinergics are given in combination with high dosages of antipsychotics that have substantial anticholinergic effects (e.g., chlorpromazine, thioridazine, clozapine), the risk of developing an atropinelike psychosis is increased.

ANTIDEPRESSANTS

From time immemorial, many agents have been reputed to improve people's moods. However, much of the "knowledge" collected has been misinforma-tion. Many people say they "drink to feel better," as though alcohol were an antidepressant and not merely a sedative. Alcohol is not only ineffective as an antidepressant but it can exacerbate depressive mood states. Clearly, the disinhibition that some people experience when they have been drinking alcohol is mistaken for a mood effect. On the other hand, some agents such as cocaine clearly can induce a feeling of euphoria.

True antidepressant medications do not provide a momentary lift but instead alleviate profound, debilitating, persistent states of depression. Stimulants were the first true antidepressant medications on the market. However, because they are not robustly effective in the most serious depressive syndromes and have a high risk for abuse, their role has been limited. It was not until the discovery of electroconvulsive therapy (ECT) that psychiatry had a truly effective treatment for serious depressive illness. The next specific discovery was the monoamine oxidase inhibitors (MAOIs). Their antidepressant effects were discovered in 1952. However, these medications were associated with serious side effects and toxicities; when the tricyclic antidepressant (TCA) imipramine was discovered in the late 1950s, the MAOIs fell into disuse. The recent discovery of newer antidepressant medications with minimal side effects and greater safety has led to an explosion in their use. At the same time, it is becoming clearer that medications previously classified as antidepressants have broader indications than depression alone.

SELECTIVE SEROTONIN REUPTAKE INHIBITORS

A new subgroup of agents, which has altered psychiatric practice, is the selective serotonin reuptake inhibitors (SSRIs). Fluoxetine, sertraline, and paroxetine (Table 16–2) are used for depression and fluroxamine has been labeled by the FDA for treatment of obsessive-compulsive disorder in adults and children. Paroxetine is also labeled for treatment of panic disorder.

SSRIs have fewer side effects than TCAs, and there are no dietary restrictions with them, as there are with MAOIs. Because patients tolerate SSRIs so well, they have been used in patients with fewer symptoms and in disorders for which medications had not previously been used.

Indications

The primary indications for SSRIs are **major depressive disorder, panic disorder,** and **obsessive-compulsive disorder.** In contrast to TCAs, which were studied mainly in inpatients, the SSRIs have been primarily studied in outpatients, leaving open the question of whether SSRIs are as effective as TCAs for melancholic (profound) depressions that often require hospital stays. At this time, the evidence is unclear. Anecdotal data suggest that fluoxetine, sertraline, and other SSRIs are also effective in the treatment of social phobia.

TABLE 16–2. Selective Serotonin Reuptake Inhibitors and Other Antidepressants

Medication	Daily Dosage (mg)	Side Effects
Selective Serotonin Reuptake Inhibitors		
Fluvoxamine*	100–300	Nausea, insomnia, somnolence, nervousness, sexual dysfunction, sweating.
Fluoxetine	20–80	Nausea, headache, akathisia, weight loss, diarrhea, insomnia, rash, sexual dysfunction.
Sertraline	50–200	Nausea, headache, akathisia, diarrhea, sexual dysfunction.
Paroxetine	20–50	Sedation, nausea, headache, akathisia, diarrhea, sexual dysfunction.
Serotonin and Noradrenergic Reuptake Inhibitors		
Mirtazapine	15–45	Somnolence, weight gain, dizziness, nausea, dry mouth, constipation.
Nefazodone	300–600	Asthenia, dry mouth, nausea, constipation, somnolence, dizziness, blurred vision.
Venlafaxine	75–375	Hypertension, akathisia, nausea.
Others		
Maprotiline	75–225	Seizures, rash.
Trazodone	200–600	Sedation, nausea, priapism.
Bupropion	300–450	Hypertension, seizures, nausea, insomnia.

*Labeled by FDA for treatment of obsessive-compulsive disorder, not depressive disorder.

Treatment

As is the case with all antidepressants, patients must take a therapeutic dose of an SSRI for at least **4 weeks** (and some have suggested 6 weeks) before one can conclude that they will not respond to the medication. The first SSRI marketed and the one that is most widely prescribed is **fluoxetine.** The dosage range is 20–80 mg/d, with 20–40 mg/d being the most common. Fluoxetine and its metabolite norfluoxetine have a long half-life of approximately 90 hours; this means that patients who are taking a relatively low daily dosage may improve even beyond the usual 4–6 weeks of treatment, so physicians should generally avoid the temptation to increase the dosage rapidly when there is no immediate observed effect.

For **sertraline,** the dosage is 50–200 mg/d. Initially, the 50-mg tablet can be broken in half and the patient can take 25 mg/d to see how well the medication is tolerated. The half-life is approximately 24 hours. Dosages can easily be changed on a biweekly basis and can be rapidly increased to 100 mg. If, after 2 weeks, there is no indication that the patient is responding to the medication, the dosage may be increased again, up to 200 mg/d. A similar schedule may be used with **paroxetine,** with 10 mg/d given initially and then a rapid increase in the dosage to 20–50 mg/d.

Fluvoxamine is labeled to treat obsessive-compulsive disorder. It is started at 50 mg at bedtime and increased to 100–300 mg/d in divided doses. Fluvoxamine is unusual in that its pharmacokinetics are nonlinear: A disproportionately greater blood level is achieved at high doses than would be predicted from lower dosage values.

Obsessive-compulsive disorder seems to respond to all of the SSRIs. The dosages are usually higher than those for depression, and the duration of treatment is longer. Whereas in depression, patients typically show improvement in 3–6 weeks, in obses-sive-compulsive disorder, it may take 12 weeks before one can conclude that the treatment regimen is effective or ineffective.

In panic disorder, initial dosage should be low (e.g., paroxetine, 10 mg; sertraline, 25 mg; fluoxetine, 10 mg); because all SSRIs and other antidepressants may cause an initial exacerbation of panic. After a week on the low dose, these patients may have a more rapid dosage increase.

Side Effects

Patients who take SSRIs complain primarily of nausea, headache, diarrhea, and restlessness or agitation. If the dosage is increased slowly, they may not experience these side effects. Patients who have initial complaints of anxiety (especially, panic disorder) may experience exacerbation of anxiety with ordinary dosages. Therefore, the starting dosage in extremely anxious patients and those who report being extremely sensitive to side effects should be as low as possible and increased only as the patient's tolerance is assessed.

The **agitation** associated with SSRIs has been compared to akathisia. Patients who develop this side effect may need adjunctive medication (e.g., a benzodiazepine, such as lorazepam or alprazolam) or a reduced dosage of the antidepressant. If the dosage is increased slowly, patients often do not experience this side effect. Many patients are subject to **nausea,** which can lead in more severe cases to vomiting. Again, starting with low dosages and increasing them slowly is likely to prevent this side effect. **Headaches** induced by these medications typically respond to acetaminophen. Patients who have a history of migraine headaches may have an exacerbation of or improvement in their difficulties.

Patients taking SSRIs often complain of anorgasmia and loss of libido. **Anorgasmia** may be difficult to treat. Cyproheptadine, 4–8 mg taken 1–2 hours before intercourse, may be effective. Others have tried bethanechol with varying degrees of success. There is no specific treatment for **loss of libido,** although some physicians have tried yohimbine and reported success. Reduced dosages of SSRIs may be helpful, but the therapeutic efficacy may be lost. A significant number of patients stop taking these medications because of sexual difficulties. The addition of bupropion, 75–100 mg/d, has sometimes reversed the sexual problems.

Patients with bipolar disorder who are given SSRIs (as well as all other antidepressants) are liable to switch to **mania** and begin rapid cycling. The switches to mania sometimes remit rapidly upon discontinuation of the antidepressant, but, at other times, the state may become autonomous. When this complication occurs, the patient is simply treated for mania.

With fluoxetine, some patients have reported significant **weight loss.** Weight gain has been anecdotally reported with all of the SSRIs.

Treatment with SSRIs does not involve a serious risk of inducing seizures. Overdoses of SSRIs seem to produce few severe effects. In contrast with TCAs, SSRI overdoses have been lethal only when SSRIs were taken in combination with other medications.

Patients taking fluoxetine may rarely develop a **rash.** If this occurs, patients should stop taking the medication because the rash has been associated with autoimmune vasculitis, which on rare occasions has been lethal.

TRICYCLIC ANTIDEPRESSANTS

Tricyclic antidepressants (TCAs) have been the mainstay for treatment of depressive illnesses for almost 30 years (Table 16–3). They were discovered in 1957 during pharmaceutical research for new antipsychotics. TCAs were found to have specific effects on depressive moods in a range of patients. Because they were effective in the treatment of depression, did not require dietary restrictions, and did not cause the organ toxicities that were observed with MAOIs, they quickly replaced MAOIs as the treatment of choice for depression. Three of the TCAs have defined plasma response curves that link the blood levels to therapeutic efficacy. Two of these, desipramine and nortriptyline, have reasonable side

effect profiles. In circumstances in which one wants to be certain that one has provided an adequate trial of an antidepressant and in which there are no specific contraindications to these agents, either one may be used. Most of them are now available generically and, therefore, may be less expensive than other agents. The major risk of TCAs is that overdoses are lethal. As little as a week's supply of the full dosage may be lethal in an adult.

Indications

The primary indication for TCAs is **major depressive disorder.** The more a depression is characterized by classic symptoms of **melancholia** (e.g., pervasive low mood, early morning awakening, loss of appetite, loss of energy, and decreased ability to function), the more likely the patient is to respond to these medications. Nonpsychotic melancholic depressions are specifically responsive to TCAs. Atypical depressions characterized by hyperphagia, hypersomnia, and mood reactivity may respond to TCAs but are more likely to respond to SSRIs or MAOIs. TCAs in combination with an antipsychotic agent are used for major depression with psychotic features. TCAs are also effective for the treatment and prophylaxis of **panic disorder.** Imipramine has been used to treat enuresis of childhood, probably primarily because of its anticholinergic effects. Clomipramine is the only TCA labeled for treatment of obsessive-compulsive disorder. It has been demonstrated to be superior to desipramine.

Treatment

The minimum therapeutic dosage of most TCAs is 150 mg, and the usual maximum dosage is 300 mg. The exceptions to this rule are nortriptyline, 50–150 mg; protriptyline, 15–60 mg; and amitriptyline and clomipramine, with an upper limit of 250 mg because of concerns about anticholinergic effects.

Treatment regimens depend on the specific medication used. Using imipramine as the prototypical TCA, treatment may be initiated with 25 mg, taken orally three times daily for approximately 3 days. Depending on the patient's ability to tolerate the medication, the dosage may be increased rapidly to a minimum of 150 mg/d. The dosage may be divided and given three times daily at first and then ulti-

TABLE 16–3. Tricyclic Antidepressants

Medication	Daily Dosage (mg)	Sedative Effect	Anticholinergic Effect	Orthostatic Hypotension	Plasma Response
Imipramine	150–300	Moderate	Moderate	Moderate	Linear
Amitriptyline	150–250	Severe	Severe	Moderate	Unknown
Doxepin	150–300	Severe	Moderate	Mild	Unknown
Clomipramine	150–250	Severe	Severe	Mild	Unknown
Desipramine	150–300	Mild	Minimal	Mild	Linear
Nortriptyline	50–150	Minimal	Mild	Minimal	Curvilinear
Protriptyline	15–60	Mild	Moderate	Mild	Unknown
Trimipramine	150–300	Severe	Severe	Minimal	Unknown

mately given as one dose at bedtime. For imipramine, desipramine, and nortriptyline, **blood levels** may be measured after the patient has been stable with the same dosage for a minimum of 5 days. For imipramine and desipramine, the **plasma response curve** has a **threshold effect.** For imipramine, the threshold is approximately 225 ng/mL, and for desipramine, it is 150 ng/mL. Blood levels that meet or exceed these thresholds are expected to be therapeutic. Blood levels over 500 ng/mL are likely to be toxic.

For nortriptyline, the relationship between the blood level and the therapeutic efficacy is **curvilinear.** Patients are less likely to respond if the blood level is below 50 ng/mL or above 150 ng/mL. With other medications, patients are likely to complain substantially of side effects if blood levels are higher than the therapeutic level, but with nortriptyline, patients often do not complain about side effects even if the blood level is over 150 ng/mL. The therapeutic efficacy is lost without other signs of toxicity becoming evident. Blood levels of other antidepressants can also be measured, but their significance is unclear, unless the blood level is 0 and the patient has not responded to the agent. If the diagnosis is highly ambiguous, it may be preferable to use medications for which blood levels are clearly related to therapeutic effects. For instance, when the diagnosis of depression is confounded by other conditions, whether medical or psychiatric, the effectiveness of antidepressant treatment can be verified by using one of the three medications for which there are blood level data. When a patient is taking an antidepressant without a known effective therapeutic range, it can be difficult to ascertain whether a patient's failure to respond is caused by an improper dosage or by a lack of efficacy of that medication for that patient.

In the treatment of panic disorder, dosage should begin with 10–25 mg; if tolerated, the dosage should be slowly increased until attacks are blocked.

Side Effects

Anticholinergic side effects are common with TCAs (see Antipsychotics, above). Amitriptyline and other tertiary amine TCAs are likely to cause significant degrees of **orthostatic hypotension,** which occurs once a particular threshold is reached and then does not tend to increase proportionally as the dosage is increased further. After 2 weeks, patients often will accommodate to this side effect and, although drops in blood pressure may continue, the patient is no longer symptomatic. Patients may need education about making sure that their fluid and salt intake is adequate. All patients should be warned that they may develop orthostatic hypotension and, therefore, must be careful when they rise from a supine or sitting position. This effect is likely to be especially severe in patients with preexisting cardiac disease. An increased heart rate of 10 beats per minute and even sinus **tachycardia** are not uncommon with TCA treatment. As noted in the evaluation section, below, TCAs have **quinidinelike effects** on cardiac conduction and may precipitate a complete heart block in patients with second-degree heart block. TCAs are contraindicated in patients who have had an acute myocardial infarction.

TCAs will lower the seizure threshold. Overdoses regularly cause seizures, and **seizures** occasionally occur even at therapeutic blood levels. With the tertiary amine TCAs, especially, **sedation** may be a problem. Sedative effects often wear off after 2 weeks. Patients taking TCAs who are given a local anesthetic that contains epinephrine (e.g., for dental surgery) may develop panic symptoms because the TCA may enhance the effects of epinephrine.

Weight gain is a common complication of TCAs. Some patients have an increased craving for sweets, and others may overeat because they are not aware of having an increased appetite. It has been helpful to refer some patients to weight control groups to help moderate their intake.

Effects on sexual functioning are fairly common, including **delayed ejaculation** and **anorgasmia.**

TCAs have substantial antihistaminic effects. Patients with peptic ulcer disease or seasonal allergies may benefit from these effects. On the other hand, physicians must be careful, since all of the TCAs will interact with other antihistamines that have been given for allergies or excess acid secretion.

OTHER ANTIDEPRESSANTS

Other than the MAOIs, which are discussed below, the remaining antidepressants come from several different classes and have defied simple biochemical classification (see Table 16–2). Some of the agents that were introduced early, such as maprotiline, did not seem to add significantly to the therapeutic armamentarium, because their side effect profiles and efficacies were comparable to those of TCAs. On the other hand, venlafaxine and bupropion have distinctive side effect profiles that have expanded the available options for depressed patients.

The chemical structure of bupropion is related to that of the stimulants, but its mechanism of action is unclear. Venlafaxine and nefazodone have both noradrenergic and serotoninergic reuptake inhibiting effects without the concomitant anticholinergic and antihistaminic effects of TCAs. Nefazodone also blocks the 5-HT2 receptor, which is believed to be involved in anxiety regulation. Although trazodone has selective effects on serotonin metabolism, its effects are different from those of the SSRIs and it has different chemical properties.

Indications

The primary indication for these antidepressants is major depressive disorder.

Bupropion stands out as one of the few antidepressants that is ineffective in the prophylaxis of panic. Anecdotal, unconfirmed reports suggest that it plays a specific role in the treatment of bipolar depression, with a lower risk for a switch to mania than TCAs or SSRIs.

Venlafaxine has been tried in some treatment-refractory populations and may have a specific indication for depressions unresponsive to either TCAs or SSRIs. It binds weakly to plasma proteins and, as would be consistent with this property, does not appear to cause many drug-to-drug interactions.

Although **trazodone** is an antidepressant, it appears to be more widely prescribed for its strong sedative effects as an adjunctive nonabusable hypnotic. Trazodone has been used to treat insomnia resulting from SSRIs and MAOIs.

Nefazodone was synthesized to improve on trazodone, and it tends to be associated with less problematic side effects (see below).

Mirtazapine has sedative properties and can be administered once a day.

Treatment

Bupropion treatment is complicated by the agent's ability to induce **seizures** when administered as a single high dose. Single doses should never exceed 150 mg, and the maximum daily dosage should be 450 mg. Patients are often started at 75 mg two to three times a day, with dosages then increased to a maximum of 450 mg/d. At the recommended dosage schedule, the risk of seizures is comparable to that of other agents.

Venlafaxine is started at 37.5 mg twice a day; the maximum dosage is 375 mg/d. Tolerance to side effects limits the rate of increase in dosage, with nausea and agitation being the most common problems. Since hypertension may occur, it is advisable to record the patient's baseline blood pressure and *check it weekly until the patient proves to be not subject to this side effect*. The minimum dosage is usually 150 mg, but some patients respond to lower dosages.

Trazodone is started at 100 mg twice a day. Dosages above 300–400 mg/d are frequently necessary, although they may be difficult to attain because of side effects, particularly **sedation.**

Nefazodone has a similar dosage range and a therapeutic level is generally easier to achieve.

Side Effects

As noted above, bupropion has a serious risk of inducing **seizures,** and patients taking venlafaxine have an increased incidence of **hypertension,** particularly at dosages at or above 225 mg/d. Both medications tend to be activating, with insomnia and agitation being two common side effects. Their negligible effects on sexual functioning and on weight are significant advantages of these medications over the SSRIs, TCAs, and MAOIs. Many patients find trazodone to be extremely **sedating.** Men are at risk of developing **priapism,** and trazodone is generally con-

traindicated as an antidepressant in male patients for this reason, although it seems to be safe at hypnotic dosages of 25–50 mg/d.

Overdoses of trazodone seem to have fewer adverse effects than those of the TCAs. Overdoses have been lethal only when trazodone was taken in combination with other medications.

Nefazodone is generally much more easily tolerated by patients than is trazodone. Priapism has not been reported as frequently with nefazodone (nefazodone is, therefore, not contraindicated in men), and it tends to be much less sedating than trazodone. Its overall advantages are that it does not interfere with sexual functioning and is not associated with sleep disturbance.

MONOAMINE OXIDASE INHIBITORS

The monoamine oxidase inhibitors (MAOIs) were the first specific antidepressant medications to be discovered. They were identified by physicians treating tuberculosis with iproniazid. Patients seemed to be unusually bright and active when they were taking this drug, and the mood change seemed to be more significant than one would expect from the therapeutic effects of the agent on the tuberculosis. Iproniazid was tried in depressed patients and found to be effective. One of the early complications of the antituberculosis medications was organ toxicity, specifically of the liver. Other compounds similar to iproniazid were also developed.

There are two primary classes of MAOIs, hydrazines and nonhydrazines. The hydrazines include phenelzine and isocarboxazid. Isocarboxazid was recently withdrawn from the market for economic reasons. The nonhydrazines include tranylcypromine and selegiline. These drugs act by irreversibly inhibiting the monoamine oxidase enzyme system. The hydrazines and selegiline have been called "suicide drugs" because they irreversibly bind to the enzyme system and are destroyed while they inactivate the system. Tranylcypromine also binds tightly to the enzyme system, but this action can be reversed to some degree after the agent has been discontinued for 3 days. Selegiline is labeled by the FDA for Parkinson's disease.

Indications

Although MAOIs have classically been considered antidepressants, newer data suggest that they have a broader spectrum of indications with special efficacy. Major depressive episodes characterized by hypersomnia, hyperphagia, and reactive mood (i.e, **atypical subtype**) are particularly responsive to MAOIs. Patients with **social phobia** have a selective response to MAOIs. MAOIs are also indicated for patients who have failed to respond to SSRIs and TCAs and for patients with panic disorder.

Treatment

Phenelzine is the best studied of the MAOIs. A reasonable clinical dosage is 45–90 mg/d. The medication may be given in a single dose in the morning or at night. Some patients find that taking the medication at night disrupts sleep, whereas others find that they become sedated by the medication and that taking it at night helps them go to sleep. There is no way to predict how a patient will react. Ordinarily, the medication may also be given in divided doses.

Tranylcypromine is a dextroamphetamine with hydroxyl groups cyclized onto the ring substitution. It is possible to measure amphetamine levels in the blood of patients who are taking this agent. **Tranylcypromine** tends to cause the patient to be more active and alert than do the hydrazine MAOIs and, therefore, it is given early in the morning or no later than noon rather than at bedtime. It also tends to have an earlier onset of action, which has been attributed to the amphetamine. The dosage is 30–60 mg/d.

Selegiline is labeled for the treatment of Parkinson's disease, but it is an effective antidepressant when prescribed at 40 mg/d. At that dose, the MAOI diet must be observed.

Side Effects

The primary side effects of MAOIs are **agitation** or **sedation, weight gain** (which is less of a problem with tranylcypromine), **hepatotoxicity** (with the hydrazines), and hypertensive crises. **Anorgasmia** has also been frequently reported in both men and women. Bethanechol or cyproheptadine can be safely used to try to combat this effect.

Orthostatic hypotension is common with all of the MAOIs and may limit their usefulness. The treatment involves drinking adequate fluids, eating additional salt, wearing support hose, and taking fludrocortisone.

MAOIs developed a reputation for being dangerous because of their potential to cause a **hypertensive crisis.** This syndrome is characterized by high blood pressure, tachycardia, fever, and confusion. It is precipitated by eating foods or ingesting medications that trigger a massive release of norepinephrine at the synapses that control blood pressure. Patients have had fatal strokes as a result of eating the "wrong" foods when taking MAOIs. Patients who are to be given an MAOI must go on a **special diet** that emphasizes fresh foods and eliminates all aged-protein foods, such as salami or pickled herring. The offending dietary substance is **tyramine,** which is a derivative of the amino acid tyrosine. As proteins in foods age, they cause more tyrosine to be converted to tyramine. Patients must start the diet at the same time that the MAOI is started and must stay on the diet for 2 weeks after the MAOI is discontinued.

Certain drugs of abuse and medications may also precipitate a hypertensive crisis, most notably indirect-acting **sympathomimetic amines,** such as cocaine and decongestants. The treatment for hypertensive crises may be phentolamine given intravenously, chlorpromazine given intramuscularly, or nifedipine given orally or parenterally.

Meperidine administration in patients taking MAOIs has been associated with two potentially fatal syndromes: respiratory depression, hypotension, and coma; or hyperexcitability and convulsions. The mechanism of these interactions is unclear, but it appears to be specific to meperidine, since other narcotics can be cautiously prescribed safely.

MAOIs cannot be administered with SSRIs because this combination causes a hypertensive, hyperpyrexic syndrome that is mediated by serotonin and is as dangerous as the tyramine reaction. If a patient has been taking an SSRI and the physician wants to switch to an MAOI, the patient must stop taking the SSRI for a period of time that is proportionate to the half-life of the SSRI. For fluoxetine, the "washout period" is a minimum of 5 weeks.

GENERAL CONSIDERATIONS IN USING ANTIDEPRESSANTS

Selecting an Antidepressant

If the patient clearly has a melancholic depression (see Chapter 3, Mood Disorders), TCAs are definitely effective. The secondary amines (desipramine and nortriptyline) have been tolerated well, even by the elderly. The more severe the depression, the stronger the indications for a TCA as the first choice of medication because the data on their efficacy in severe depressions are unambiguous and blood levels can be used to follow the treatment.

If patients have "atypical" depression (see Chapter 3, Mood Disorders), the physician must weigh the options of using an SSRI or MAOI. MAOIs are clearly effective in this condition, but they have dietary restrictions and side effects that are difficult to tolerate. SSRIs have fewer side effects. The first choice may be an SSRI, and an MAOI may be selected as a "backup" agent. If the depression more closely resembles dysthymia than melancholia, an SSRI should be chosen. If patients have social phobia in addition to a depressive disorder, an SSRI is preferred. Patients with panic disorder are likely to respond to all of the antidepressant medications with the exception of bupropion.

Discontinuing Treatment

Patients who are being treated for their first episode of depression should take the antidepressant for a **minimum of 6 months,** including at least 3 months during which they are asymptomatic. If patients have been asymptomatic for at least 3 of these months, the dosage is tapered and the agent is discontinued over a period of several weeks. Abrupt discontinuation of TCAs is associated with an extremely unpleasant **flulike syndrome.** ➠ A 70-year-old man was hospitalized for reevaluation of his antidepressant regimen, which included imipramine. He developed nausea and vomiting 2 days after admission. These symptoms prompted an extensive gastrointestinal workup, until it was noted that the imipramine had been stopped without tapering of the dosage. ⬛ The SSRIs seem to be associated with a withdrawal syndrome, as well.

If the 6-month period ends at a particularly sensitive time for a patient (e.g., an upcoming job change, marriage, or graduation), the decision to discontinue the medication should be delayed.

There is growing evidence that patients who have had previous episodes of depression should be maintained on antidepressants for long periods of time, perhaps for life. About half of patients with depression have recurrent episodes throughout their lives. Patients with frequent and recurring depressions (i.e., more than three episodes within a few years) are likely candidates for **maintenance treatment.** Patients obviously must make the decision, weighing the risks of recurrence against the side effects and costs of the medication. The physician should review with patients how they felt when depressed and whether they want to risk experiencing that state again. The physician should also review the specific warning signs of depression, which are the symptoms that patients have previously experienced. This will help patients who choose to discontinue the medication to know as early as possible when to return to treatment. Patients who have regularly become seriously suicidal when depressed should be strongly discouraged from discontinuing their medication. Unfortunately, for some patients, taking medication is a narcissistic "mortification," and they jump at the chance to discontinue it. These are the patients for whom taking medication is the ultimate insult and failure. If this reaction is recognized early, the physician should address this attitude, first through education and then through psychotherapeutic exploration of the meaning of taking medications, which is crucial for these patients.

Augmentation Strategies

As was noted above, up to 40% of patients with major depression will not respond to the first agent chosen, even if sufficient dosages are taken for up to a month. These patients can be approached in one of two ways: (1) The first drug can be continued for a longer period of time (e.g., 6 weeks) before it is declared a failure. (2) An augmentation strategy can be used whereby a second agent is added to the regimen to see if a full response can be elicited.

The best-researched augmentation strategy is the use of **lithium carbonate.** This medication may be effective even below the usual therapeutic range. A dosage of 300 mg two to three times a day is typical. If the patient does not respond within 2 weeks, the blood levels of lithium should be measured and titrated to 0.8–1.2 mEq/L. At relatively low blood levels, lithium is tolerated well. The most important adverse risk is weight gain.

If lithium augmentation is rejected or fails, there is no simple algorithm showing which strategy to choose next. **Triiodothyronine,** 25 μg/d, taken in the morning, can be used. Some have suggested that this strategy works best in overweight or marginally euthyroid individuals.

Another strategy is to add a **stimulant** (most commonly, dextroamphetamine, methylphenidate, or fenfluramine). The efficacy of stimulants may involve their propensity to increase the blood levels of the antidepressant, but they do seem also to have euphorigenic properties. (Medically ill and elderly patients seem to respond particularly well to the energizing effects of stimulants, which are sometimes used alone rather than as augmentation agents.) **Amphetamine** affects both the noradrenergic and dopaminergic systems. **Methylphenidate,** like cocaine, primarily affects the dopaminergic system. With all stimulants, the last dose may need to be taken no later than late afternoon to prevent interference with sleep. It is not uncommon for patients to take one dose early in the morning and two doses around lunchtime.

Anorexia, insomnia, and hypertension are the most common side effects of these medications. The dosage must often be reduced to treat the insomnia. The alternative of prescribing both an "upper" and a "downer" (i.e., a sleeping pill) is rarely indicated.

Recent anecdotal reports suggest that combinations of various antidepressants may be effective (e.g., an SSRI plus bupropion, or an SSRI plus a TCA). The TCA dosage may need to be reduced since SSRIs frequently increase the TCA level. SSRIs cannot be combined with MAOIs. There is a long history of combining amitriptyline with phenelzine, starting at low dosages and increasing them slowly to 150 mg of the former and 45 mg of the latter.

Evaluation and Contraindications

Before an antidepressant is prescribed, the diagnosis of depression must be certain. The many other conditions that may mimic depression should be ruled out. The differential diagnosis includes medical illnesses that may masquerade as psychiatric disorders, and this means most of the illnesses that can affect an individual (see Chapter 3, Mood Disorders; Chapter 5, Cognitive and Mental Disorders Due to General Medical Conditions; and Chapter 12, Psychological Factors Affecting Medical Conditions). Some conditions, such as hypothyroidism, are more commonly misdiagnosed as depression than others. **Thyroid function tests** should be part of the diagnostic workup for all patients with suspected depression.

TCAs cause slowing of cardiac conduction through the ventricles just as quinidine does. Patients with preexisting cardiac conduction defects are at risk for further slowing of conduction and asystole. An **ECG** should be performed prior to initiating TCA treatment in all patients over 40 years of age or in those who have a history of cardiac disease. Patients with any degree of heart block should be treated with TCAs only in close consultation with a cardiologist, if at all.

Because TCAs are metabolized extensively in the liver, **liver function** assessment is indicated. If selected, TCAs should be used in lower dosages in patients with active liver disease. Most of the TCAs have significant anticholinergic side effects. Patients with narrow-angle glaucoma may develop acute glaucomic crisis and blindness. All patients known or suspected of having glaucoma should be evaluated by an ophthalmologist before a TCA is considered. Men with prostatic hypertrophy are at risk for acute urinary retention.

There are no specific contraindications to the SSRIs other than allergy to a specific agent. SSRIs cannot be combined with MAOIs (see Side Effects, above).

Special care should be taken when administering bupropion to patients with eating disorders and seizure disorders. The caution about seizures extends to TCAs and maprotiline, as well.

Antidepressants are metabolized by the **cytochrome P-450 system** in the liver. The various medications differ in terms of substrate specificity for the enzymes or isoenzymes. These enzymes oxidize and hydroxylate the substrates. Depending on the enzymatic activity of the patient (i.e., individuals can be slow or rapid metabolizers) and on the activity of other medications that might inhibit or compete at the enzymatic sites, the blood levels and side effects of the antidepressants may vary considerably.

MOOD STABILIZERS (ANTIMANIC MEDICATIONS)

The first specific antimanic medication was lithium salt. It was discovered by J.F.C. Cade during his search for the etiology of excited psychoses. When the therapeutic blood level was defined and blood testing became widely available, lithium carbonate became the standard agent for the prophylaxis and treatment of mania.

Neurologists were the first to note that epileptic patients who were treated with carbamazepine seemed brighter and had a more stable mood than patients treated with other anticonvulsants. This effect was sufficiently prominent for it to be noted in various studies. Carbamazepine was tried in patients with unstable mood and found to be effective in dampening lability and treating mania. Carbamazepine is believed to interrupt a process of kindling that is fundamental to recurrent affective disorder. With the success of carbamazepine, valproic acid and clonazepam were also tried and found to be effective. As newer anticonvulsants such as gabapentin and lamotrigine have been introduced, psychiatrists are quickly using them in patients who either cannot tolerate standard mood stabilizers or whose conditions are refractory to them.

LITHIUM CARBONATE

Indications

The primary indication for lithium carbonate is the treatment and prophylaxis of **acute mania.** Patients who are mildly to moderately manic may be treated acutely with lithium carbonate alone or in combination with a benzodiazepine. Patients with severe mania, especially those with psychotic features, usually require adjunctive use of an antipsychotic.

Lithium carbonate is useful in the **prophylaxis** of both the manic and the depressive episodes of bipolar disorder. It is also effective for the prophylaxis of depression in patients with recurrent unipolar depression. It is sometimes, but not reliably, an effective treatment for depressive episodes that occur during the course of bipolar and depressive disorders.

Lithium carbonate has specific **antiaggressive** effects, particularly in states of affective or irritable aggression. Individuals with "short fuses" report that they can think before they act. This effect is not specific to any particular disorder. It occurs in many diagnostic categories, including personality disorders, developmental disabilities, and cognitive disorders. There are no data suggesting that lithium is effective in aggression that is purposeful and not impulsive (i.e., violent behavior carried out by criminals for gain).

Lithium carbonate has also been used to dampen **excessive emotionality** in patients with personality disorders. These patients exhibit labile mood (i.e., broad swings in mood that do not meet the criteria for depression or hypomania) and frequent irritability. This indication has not been widely studied, but data extrapolated from the treatment of mania and affective aggressivity indicate that lithium may be considered in patients who are unable or poorly able to participate in psychotherapeutic treatment. Physicians sometimes think of these states as "dilute" bipolar disorder.

Evaluation

A physically healthy patient with mild bipolar disorder (manic state) should undergo the workup described below, although some physicians draw blood for the necessary tests at the same time that they initiate treatment. It is impossible to make accurate predictions of what will happen in a given individual if one administers lithium and alters the fluid and electrolyte balance. Therefore, it is important to define the fluid and electrolyte status as well as the renal function before starting lithium.

The **blood electrolyte levels** should be determined. The renal status is assessed by the serum **BUN** and **creatinine** levels and a complete **urinalysis.** The urinalysis, including microscopic examination, ensures that a concomitant renal disease is not overlooked. Lithium carbonate has been administered to patients with renal insufficiency (including patients on dialysis), for whom blood level determinations are done more frequently.

Since electrolyte imbalances can seriously affect cardiac conduction, an **ECG** is also important, especially for adults who have reached the age of risk for cardiac disease.

Lithium carbonate leads to demargination of leukocytes from the endothelial walls and leukocytosis. A **complete blood count** not only helps to determine the hydration status but provides a baseline for the white blood cell count. The count occasionally rises to 20,000/mL solely because of lithium treatment.

Lithium interferes with iodination in the synthesis of thyroid hormone. The **thyroid status** should be ascertained before initiating the agent. Initially, thyroid-stimulating hormone (TSH), triiodothyronine (T3), and tetraiodothyronine (T4) levels should be determined. For long-term management, the TSH levels are followed every 6–12 months.

Although lithium carbonate has been reported to both increase and decrease the frequency of seizures in epileptic patients when administered at ordinary blood levels, it is not necessary to perform an EEG before starting lithium.

Treatment

Lithium carbonate is efficacious in the prophylaxis of mania at dosages of 600–1200 mg per day, which result in blood levels of 0.6–1.2 mEq/L. The specific **blood level** that is effective for a given person may vary, with some patients requiring levels as high as 1.5–1.8 mEq/L. In the acute treatment of mania, the target blood level is about 1 mEq/L. The limiting factor is often tolerance to side effects, especially nausea, but also diarrhea and tremor. Therefore, even though one might anticipate that a high dosage of lithium will be needed, the starting dose is often 300 mg, taken orally two or three times daily. Many patients complain of nausea if this initial dose is taken four times daily. The development of nausea has been linked to the gradient of lithium in the blood, so dividing the dosage is important.

The therapeutic effects of lithium are often not apparent until 10–14 days after treatment has begun (assuming that the dosages are increased to a therapeutic level). The half-life of lithium is about 24 hours in adults who have normal renal function. Blood levels do not become stable until a fixed dosage has been taken for 5 days. Because of the lag time before the therapeutic effects are felt and because of the pressure to discharge patients from the hospital quickly, one must monitor the blood levels carefully and adjust the dosage of lithium to achieve a therapeutic level. Patients are carefully examined for side effects because, unfortunately, there is no lag time before they develop. The dosage is increased as tolerance of side effects allows, until the targeted blood level is reached. It is important to know that the relationship between the increase of lithium blood levels with a particular adjustment in dosage changes over the dosage range. As luck would have it, this change in relationship occurs around the therapeutic blood level, so as one gets closer to the therapeutic level, one must be careful not to inadvertently overmedicate patients.

Side Effects

The initial common side effects of lithium include **nausea, diarrhea, tremor,** and a **metallic taste** in the mouth. Most of these effects, which are linked to the gradient of lithium in the blood, can be avoided or minimized if the dosage is increased slowly. Lithium interferes with the action of antidiuretic hormone, which leads to a **diabetes insipidus**–like condition in about 40% of patients that is reversible upon discontinuation of the lithium.

Lithium can produce various neurological symptoms, such as **ataxia, myoclonus,** and **delirium.** If there is concern about toxicity, the lithium blood level and electrolytes should be tested. Lithium overdose leads to coma, seizures, and death. In a small proportion of patients, a **neurotoxic condition** develops even at therapeutic levels, with confusion, delirium, and, often, myoclonus. **Seizures** frequently follow if the medication is not discontinued. If a patient taking lithium becomes confused, the agent should be stopped and the blood levels tested. If they are high (e.g., >2 mEq/L), neurotoxicity is confirmed; however, neurotoxicity is not excluded even if the level is within the range of normal (e.g., 0.7 mEq/L). Some researchers have suggested that schizophrenic patients are especially susceptible to lithium neurotoxicity, but this hypothesis has not been convincingly proved. Lithium levels are sensitive to electrolyte changes, including those induced by alterations in diet, and patients who dramatically vary their salt intake can have significantly varying blood levels and side effects.

Lithium interferes with the synthesis of thyroid hormone in the process of iodination. Long-term lithium carbonate is associated with the risks of goiter and **hypothyroidism.** If these conditions develop, they are treated simply with exogenous thyroid hormone.

Patients maintained on lithium commonly gain 15–20 pounds.

The **renal effects** of lithium have been a concern, especially since 1977, when it was reported that several patients who had been receiving long-term treatment had developed varying degrees of renal insufficiency. This finding has caused some physicians to avoid using lithium or to do extensive renal function testing in patients who do use it, to prevent liability. The current data suggest that carefully treated patients who do not have episodes of lithium toxicity do not have an increased risk for renal insufficiency. The significance of this finding is that physicians must educate patients about the importance of taking the correct dosage, having their lithium levels tested regularly, and avoiding factors that are likely to alter lithium levels (e.g., factors that affect the fluid and electrolyte balance, such as significant dehydration resulting from sports or beach activities, diarrhea, or vomiting). They should also be warned about possible drug interactions, particularly between lithium and the **nonsteroidal anti-inflammatory drugs** and **diuretics.**

ANTICONVULSANTS

Valproic acid and carbamazepine are anticonvulsants that are also effective in bipolar disorder. Divalproex sodium, which is the combination of valproic acid and disodium valproate, is labeled by the FDA for the acute treatment of patients with mania. Patients who cannot tolerate lithium carbonate can be treated with these drugs alone. Patients who do not respond to lithium carbonate may have these agents added to their medication regimen. There is evidence that mixed bipolar states as well as rapid cycling bipolar patients respond better to these anticonvulsants than to lithium. Preliminary studies suggest that gabapentin and lamotrigine may be effective alternatives for treatment-refractory patients.

Indications and Contraindications

Divalproex sodium is indicated for the treatment of acute mania. The primary indications in psychiatry for anticonvulsants are **refractory bipolar disorder** (mania), **rapid cycling bipolar disorder,** and **severe mood instability.** There is evidence of efficacy of carbamazepine for refractory recurrent unipolar disorder. Patients with **intermittent explosive disorder** are candidates for these agents.

Some physicians try these agents in all patients with a refractory excited disorder (i.e., volatile emotionality that does not respond to other interventions).

Evaluation

A preliminary workup would include a complete blood count, and **liver and kidney function tests.** When treating patients with intermittent explosive disorder, it is advisable to obtain a baseline EEG because these agents will alter subsequent EEGs. A baseline EEG is not necessary for mood disorder patients who do not have suspected EEG abnormalities.

With valproic acid, the physician should pay particular attention to the **platelet count,** because this agent can suppress production of platelets, which results in bleeding difficulties.

With carbamazepine, particular attention should be paid to the **white blood cell count,** since this drug regularly causes a reduction in white blood cell counts and frank leukopenia. Rarely, it can cause agranulocytosis or aplastic anemia. Carbamazepine may exacerbate cardiac conduction delays; therefore, an ECG should be obtained in patients for whom this is a concern.

Gabapentin is not metabolized by the liver but is excreted by the kidney, so renal function must be assessed.

Treatment

Divalproex sodium is much better tolerated than valproic acid alone. The initial dosage is 250 mg, two to three times a day, increased until blood levels of 50–125 µg/mL or toxicity develops. It is possible to use a loading dose strategy that permits achievement of therapeutic blood levels much more quickly and can reduce hospital length of stay with minimal toxicity.

Carbamazepine is often used in combination with other agents, such as lithium, an antipsychotic agent, or an antidepressant. Carbamazepine induces **hepatic microsomal enzymes.** The increased activity of the enzymes can reduce the blood levels of carbamazepine as well as those of other drugs metabolized by that system, such as antipsychotics, tricyclic antidepressants, and benzodiazepines. Therefore, finding the best dosage can be difficult, and it may be helpful to measure the blood levels of all drugs being taken. Patients may be started on carbamazepine, 200 mg, taken orally twice a day, with the dosage titrated up to about 1000 mg/d. Because carbamazepine induces its own metabolism, the blood level usually rises initially and then falls when the dosage becomes stable. Dosages must be adjusted in response to **blood levels** to ensure that adequate amounts reach the central nervous system. Unfortunately, there is no clear relationship between blood levels and therapeutic effects. Blood levels are helpful guides to attempt to minimize or confirm toxicity. Because there is a lag between the time that adequate blood levels are reached and the time that the therapeutic response is felt, the dosage can be titrated to 6–12 µg/mL or until toxic side effects develop. If a patient does not respond at the lower blood level and toxicity has not occurred, the dosage should be increased. As higher blood levels of the drug are reached, patients regularly complain of more side effects.

If the patient's illness is exacerbated during ongoing treatment with either valproic acid or carbamazepine, his or her blood level should be checked. (Blood level data are not available to guide treatment with gabapentin or lamotrigine.) Poor patient compliance or increased metabolism may result in decreased blood levels, and the patient's status may deteriorate. When the patient is deteriorating, the situation is urgent, and if there are no side effects or no worsening in side effects, blood levels can be drawn and the dosage increased empirically without waiting for the results. Because no close correlation exists between blood levels of these drugs and the clinical response, the dosage is ultimately based on the patient's tolerance of the agent and clinical response.

Gabapentin is started slowly at 300 mg at bed time the first day, 300 mg twice a day for the second day, and then 300 mg three times a day. The dosage can then be increased depending on patient tolerance and response up to 3600 mg/d in divided doses. Because of the short half-life of the agent, three times a day dosing is preferable. Tolerance to side effects limits the rate of possible increase.

Lamotrigine is started at a very low dosage, 25 mg/d for 2 weeks, and is then increased by 25 mg/2 weeks until a dosage of about 150 mg/d is achieved. This slow rate of increase is important to avoid dangerous skin reactions (see below). The effective dosage range appears to be between 150–500 mg/d, although a number of patients have responded at low doses.

Side Effects
Carbamazepine and Valproic Acid

Carbamazepine routinely causes a benign drop in the white blood cell count to 3000–4000/μL. On rare occasions, the patient may develop **agranulocytosis**. In most cases, the pattern is that of a "toxic" condition (i.e., a gradual decline in the white blood cell count). Monitoring the white blood cell count will usually indicate that trouble is about to develop in time to prevent it. Granulocyte counts of 1000/μL are adequate to fight infections in patients who are not immunocompromised. If the granulocyte count falls to 1500/μL, the medication should be discontinued and the white blood cell count followed daily.

There has been debate about how often the white blood cell counts should be monitored for signs of toxicity. Some authors have been particularly cautious, recommending weekly complete blood cell counts for up to 2 months, then biweekly counts, and then monthly counts. Clinical laboratories have appreciated the economic benefits of such caution, but most neurologists do not believe that the expense is justified. Monitoring is definitely helpful when the patient starts taking the medication and during the period in which one would anticipate alterations in the blood level due to the enzyme induction and increased metabolism described above. There is no convincing evidence showing that measuring the blood count every week for months is justified if there are no signs of toxicity. As was discussed already, many patients develop a benign leukopenia that does not progress to agranulocytosis. Obviously, if the white blood cell count drops, it should be followed to see whether it is a benign or toxic reduction. A reasonable compromise is to monitor the white blood cell count every 2 weeks when the agent is started and then, in the absence of toxicity, monitor it less frequently. For long-term, stable patients, it may be adequate to check the blood levels every 3 or 6 months, as well as the white blood cell counts and liver and kidney function.

Valproic acid is more likely to cause **bleeding** through interference with platelet functioning. As with carbamazepine, a baseline determination of the platelet count is needed but routine monitoring is not required. If a patient complains of easy bruising or if ecchymoses develop, the platelet count should be checked and the medication withheld. It is best to monitor the patient clinically and ask the patient to check himself or herself for bruises in the mirror before showering.

Carbamazepine often causes neurological side effects, especially **ataxia** and **diplopia**. Diplopia may occur at therapeutic levels but frequently is an early sign of toxicity. Ataxia may seriously interfere with the ability of the patient to continue the medication. Valproic acid may cause the same side effects but is less likely to do so.

As noted above, both agents can cause organ toxicities. The liver is the most likely site to be affected by either drug, and baseline testing of liver enzymes and bilirubin is therefore helpful. Carbamazepine may cause renal complications.

Patients should be advised that if they take carbamazepine or valproic acid for prolonged periods, it is unsafe to precipitously discontinue them. **Withdrawal seizures** may occur if the medications are abruptly stopped.

Lamotrigine and Gabapentin

Gabapentin is well tolerated but can cause significant fatigue, somnolence, dizziness, and ataxia early in treatment. Slowing the rate of increase can minimize these problems. Additionally, patients report nystagmus, blurred vision, and nervousness.

Lamotrigine causes skin rashes in 10% of patients. Ten percent of these patients go on to a severe, potentially life-threatening **rash**. The development of a rash during treatment with lamotrigine should prompt discontinuation of the drug. There are no characteristics of the rash that predict which rashes are dangerous and which are not. The rash is more common when the dosage is increased rapidly and when lamotrigine is administered with valproic acid. The development of systemic illness is not generally fulminant, so patients should be advised to check themselves daily for the development of a rash and report any suspicions immediately for medical evaluation. Lamotrigine is generally well tolerated but is associated with headaches, nausea, dizziness, ataxia, somnolence, diplopia, and blurred vision.

ANTIANXIETY AGENTS AND HYPNOTICS

Antianxiety agents and hypnotics are the oldest psychopharmacological agents. The sedating properties of alcohol have been known for millennia. In the early twentieth century, the barbiturates were developed. In the 1950s, new classes of antianxiety drugs were discovered, and their use became widespread. In the last decade, drugs with less addictive potential have been developed. More drugs will most likely be discovered that are safe, effective, and have few side effects.

The major classes of currently prescribed antianxiety and sedative drugs are the benzodiazepines, propanediol carbamates, and barbiturates. The benzodiazepines are the most widely prescribed because of their safety and efficacy (Table 16–4). Recently introduced medications (e.g., buspirone, zolpidem) may represent new important classes that are even safer and have lower addictive propensities.

Indications

The major indications for the antianxiety agents and hypnotics are short-term or time-limited treatment of **generalized anxiety disorder** or **primary insomnia** (not due to any other cause), prophylaxis of **panic attacks** (for which specific benzodiazepines are efficacious), and treatment of **agitation** (for inpatients) or **anxiety** from any cause. These medications

TABLE 16–4. Benzodiazepines

Medication	Dosage	Half-Life (hours)	Metabolites	Absorption
Anxiolytics				
Alprazolam	1 mg daily, divided	12–15	(Y)*	Moderate to rapid
Chlordiazepoxide	40 mg daily, divided	5–30	Y	Moderate
Clonazepam	1 mg daily, divided	30	N	Rapid
Clorazepate	30 mg daily, divided	30–100†	Y	Moderate
Diazepam	15 mg daily, divided	20–70†	Y	Rapid
Lorazepam	2 mg daily, divided	10–20	N	Moderate to rapid
Oxazepam	45 mg daily, divided	5–15	N	Slow
Hypnotics				
Estazolam	2 mg at bedtime	10–24	(Y)	Moderate
Flurazepam	30 mg at bedtime	50–150†	Y	Rapid
Quazepam	15 mg at bedtime	50–150†	Y	Rapid
Temazepam	30 mg at bedtime	10	N	Slow
Triazolam	0.25 mg at bedtime	2–3	(Y)	Rapid

*(Y) = active metabolites but of no known clinical consequence.
†Half-life of primary metabolite, not parent compound.

are also used for **withdrawal syndromes** associated with addiction to alcohol or other sedative drugs. The **benzodiazepines** and barbiturates are effective in calming anticipatory anxiety in situations that do not warrant a medical diagnosis. The benzodiazepines are widely prescribed and are clearly effective for anxiety disorders. The therapeutic dosage usually has few side effects and minimal toxicity, in contrast to that of the barbiturates and the propanediol carbamates. In addition, the benzodiazepines are fairly safe in overdose (when not taken in combination with alcohol or other medications), in contrast to older antianxiety agents and hypnotics.

Buspirone is an effective antianxiety agent that does not cause dependence or tolerance. Because buspirone is pharmacologically unrelated to the other sedative hypnotic agents, it does not affect the symptoms of withdrawal from those agents. The newly introduced imidazopyridine agent zolpidem represents a new class of hypnotic agents that allegedly is more purely hypnotic in its effects, has low addictive potential, and, like buspirone, does not provide cross-tolerance with other sedatives.

The recommended restrictions on antianxiety and hypnotic agents (i.e., that they be given only for short-term or acute treatment) stem from fears that they will be used inappropriately to avoid confronting life stresses. Physicians should generally limit the use of these medications to **short-term situations** in which the patient's functioning is demonstrably impaired. In more chronic situations, the patient should be referred for psychotherapy. Buspirone may have a special role in these patients because it is nonaddicting. A small minority of patients do clearly benefit from long-term treatment with antianxiety agents, but specific characteristics that differentiate them from people who would benefit only from short-term treatment have not been identified.

While many patients present to physicians complaining of **insomnia,** the symptom rarely occurs in isolation and is often the chief complaint of patients suffering from **anxiety** and **depressive disorders.** Treatment of the insomnia with a hypnotic medication will not address the underlying disorder. Thus, it is particularly important to rule out anxiety and depressive disorders before treating insomnia. **Psychotic disorders,** such as mania and schizophrenia, may be heralded by sleep-wake reversals that are experienced as insomnia, but this symptom should be treated with antipsychotic agents and lithium. Insomnia may be a side effect of various antidepressants.

It is important to make a careful diagnosis before treating anxiety and insomnia because these symptoms are a part of many syndromes. When a patient has anxiety symptoms associated with another primary psychiatric disorder, the anxiety symptoms often improve with treatment of the primary disorder. Many psychotropic agents have sedative effects (e.g., the TCAs); when they are used, specific adjunctive treatment of the anxiety symptoms is not necessary. In some circumstances, it may be useful to combine an antianxiety agent with an agent from a different class (e.g., an antipsychotic or antidepressant).

Patients with insomnia often complain of difficulty in falling asleep or staying asleep or of awakening too early in the morning. Difficulty in falling asleep is often due to anxious anticipation or anger. When sleep problems are related to extreme anger, the dosages needed to help patients sleep are often those that would cause obtundation. Clearly, in such circumstances, pharmacological treatment is not appropriate, and patients frequently need to be referred for psychotherapy.

The primary contraindication for antianxiety agents and hypnotics is a **history of substance abuse.** Most of these agents have a potential for abuse and may be addictive, especially when given in high dosages for a long period of time. Although buspirone and zolpidem do not seem to have addictive potential, they should be prescribed with caution because this claim has been made about many new agents as they have been introduced.

Treatment

All of the benzodiazepines are effective for the treatment of **generalized anxiety disorder.** The specific agent is chosen according to the **pattern of anxiety** that occurs during the course of a day and according to how well the patient is likely to tolerate the effects. Patients usually recognize the effects of rapidly absorbed medications. Some may react positively to them and feel relieved that help has arrived, whereas others may feel controlled by them. Patients may also be aware of the loss of effects of the shorter-acting medications. None of the agents is more efficacious than the others (see Table 16–4).

Patients with **chronic anxiety** or a **history of substance abuse** may be candidates for buspirone therapy. Unlike other antianxiety agents, buspirone is not effective immediately. Several days or weeks of treatment are required before the effects are felt. Patients may be impatient with this treatment if they are accustomed to the more rapid onset of effects from benzodiazepines. Patients should be reassured that the effects are slower but will appear and should be reminded that the medication has the benefit of being nonaddictive. Dosages must be increased gradually in order to prevent nausea.

Propanediol carbamates and barbiturates are effective only for up to 2 weeks of continuous treatment. For this reason, and because they are addictive, they should not be used if longer treatment is needed. These drugs are lethal in overdose. Psychiatrists rarely prescribe these drugs now that the safer and more efficacious agents are available.

Not all of the antianxiety agents are effective for the prophylaxis of panic symptoms. Patients who suffer from **panic disorder** may be treated with alprazolam, clonazepam, or lorazepam. Alprazolam has an intermediate duration of action, but its rapid absorption leads some patients to abuse it and others to insist on taking multiple doses daily. Although alprazolam can be used as the sole treatment for panic disorder, its potential for abuse is a concern. Many physicians initially prescribe a benzodiazepine and an antidepressant and tell the patient that the benzodiazepine will be discontinued in 2 weeks. After the dosage of the antidepressant has been increased sufficiently, the benzodiazepine is discontinued. Clonazepam is a long-acting agent. Patients may find clonazepam and lorazepam more sedating than alprazolam.

Diazepam, chlordiazepoxide, and lorazepam are available for parenteral use. Only lorazepam is well absorbed when given intramuscularly. Diazepam and chlordiazepoxide may be given slowly by intravenous injection. Both are likely to cause anterograde amnesia and sleep when so administered. This effect is capitalized on when diazepam is used for minor surgical procedures. There have been rare reports of respiratory arrest with intravenous injection.

Patients with liver disease (e.g., cirrhosis, chronic hepatitis) and elderly patients have less difficulty in metabolizing benzodiazepines that have hydroxyl groups (e.g., oxazepam, lorazepam, temazepam), because glucuronidation is preserved in these patients.

Patients who present with focused, discrete difficulties, such as anxiety about speaking or otherwise performing in public, may be candidates for treatment with a **beta-blocker.** These patients suffer from **performance anxiety,** which may be considered a mild form of social phobia. The more discrete the problem (e.g., talking at a particular group event) and the more the patient is concerned about the physical symptoms of anxiety (e.g., palpitations, tremor, perspiration), the more likely the patient is to respond to a single dose of a beta-blocker taken about 2 hours before the event. Patients report feeling alert and energized but do not have self-consciousness, trembling hands, or cold sweats.

Sleep disorders are addressed according to the difficulty with which the patient presents. For patients who have difficulty only in falling asleep, a short-acting, rapidly absorbed hypnotic is a rational choice (e.g., zolpidem, triazolam). For patients with trouble in staying asleep, a drug with a modest half-life and slow to moderate absorption is a logical choice (e.g., temazepam). For patients with trouble throughout the sleep cycle, a longer-acting agent is indicated.

Insomnia is not an uncommon side effect of the MAOIs and some of the SSRIs. It is often treated with the antidepressant trazodone (see Antidepressants, above).

Extremely agitated inpatients who are being treated for an Axis I disorder with a specific medication (e.g., an antipsychotic or antimanic agent) may require sedation. Lorazepam, 2 mg intramuscularly or orally, has been highly effective and well tolerated in these situations.

Side Effects

Patients tolerate the benzodiazepines well. The most common side effect is **daytime sedation,** which tends not to be as serious as with the barbiturates. Some patients may have ataxia or diplopia. All patients must be warned about driving or using equipment while taking these medications.

Rarely, patients may become **disinhibited,** particularly when taking diazepam, chlordiazepoxide, or clonazepam, and find themselves acting more aggressively than usual. This effect is not substantial with oxazepam or lorazepam. It seems to be more likely to happen with patients who have "anxiety-bound" anger (i.e., patients who are angry and resentful but are afraid to voice those feelings); such patients should probably not receive diazepam, chlordiazepoxide, or clonazepam.

Patients have reported being unable to remember events that follow ingestion of these medications. Drugs that are rapidly absorbed, cross the blood-brain barrier quickly, and are tightly bound to receptors are most likely to produce this effect. Elderly patients are more susceptible to **anterograde amnesia.** This effect has been most prominent with higher dosages or parenteral administration of these medications.

Patients who take buspirone or zolpidem occasionally complain of nausea, especially if the dosages are high. Patients taking buspirone have complained of headaches. Because buspirone binds to dopamine receptors, there is the theoretic risk of tardive dyskinesia. Patients undergoing long-term (>6 months) treatment with buspirone should be monitored for the development of abnormal movements.

ELECTROCONVULSIVE THERAPY

Electroconvulsive therapy (ECT) evolved from an "observation" that turned out to be erroneous. It had been noted that epileptic patients had a lower incidence of schizophrenia. This observation led to the hypothesis that having epilepsy might protect one from developing schizophrenia. As a result, some physicians attempted to induce seizures in patients as a way of treating schizophrenia. Early attempts were crude and involved injection or inhalation of various agents. The timing and duration of the seizures were unpredictable.

In 1938 in Italy, Bini and Cerletti used electrical currents to attempt to induce seizures in dogs. They discovered that when the stimulus was applied to the head, the mortality rate was zero and they could fairly reliably induce a seizure. In this way, ECT was "born."

ECT was widely used for many years. It was the only specifically and truly effective intervention available for the severe psychoses. Unfortunately, as its efficacy in severe states became apparent, its use was extended to patients with almost any psychiatric condition. There are reports of nearly all of the psychiatric disorders "responding" to a course of ECT.

Indications and Contraindications

The primary indication for ECT is severe major depression, especially in suicidal patients. Other indications are **major depression with psychotic features, mania** refractory to medications, **schizophrenia with catatonic features, excitement** or **severe depression** that does not respond to medications, and severe **obsessive-compulsive disorder** that has not responded to medications.

The primary contraindication for ECT is **increased intracranial pressure,** which is usually caused by brain tumors or severe hypertension. If ECT is used in the presence of increased intracranial pressure, the result may be herniation of the temporal lobe and death. Other contraindications are those related to anesthesia (e.g., recent myocardial infarction, pulmonary disease, severe kyphosis of the spine). The risks associated with anesthesia must be balanced against the risks of not treating the patient with ECT.

Evaluation

The workup for ECT requires a complete history and physical examination. The eye fundi must be examined for **papilledema.** Electroencephalography, CT scanning, or spinal radiography need not be performed routinely. They are indicated only if there is a specific need for them. An ECG should be obtained because the patient will be receiving atropine for anesthesia. Liver function tests should be done because hepatitis is a risk factor of anesthesia.

Treatment

ECT is often administered in a recovery suite. An anesthesiologist is often present, but the psychiatrist may choose to administer it. An intravenous line is established for the administration of medications. The patient's forehead is cleansed with alcohol swabs, and electrodes are strapped onto the patient's head for administering the electrical stimulus and monitoring the EEG. Atropine or glycopyrrolate is administered to prevent bradycardia or asystole during the seizure. An anesthetic or hypnotic agent (e.g., thiopental) is administered. After the patient falls asleep, the muscle relaxant succinylcholine is given to suppress the motor component of the seizure (i.e., tonic-clonic movements of the trunk and limbs); this is not necessary for efficacy but minimizes the risk of fractures. It is particularly important that patients with osteoporosis, who are at greater risk for fractures, be adequately relaxed. After the succinylcholine has taken full effect, and with the patient still unconscious, the electrical stimulus is applied.

Seizures lasting 30–90 seconds are effective. Seizures that persist after 2 minutes are terminated with diazepam given intravenously. Seizures can be assessed by the EEG recording or by the tonic-clonic movements of the toes. It has recently been determined that the stimulation level must be 150% of the threshold value for inducing a seizure in order for the seizure to be effective. As the amount of current used to induce a seizure increases, the severity of memory disturbance also increases. Therefore, efforts are made to provide stimulation as close as possible to the 150% level.

Side Effects

The most frequent complaint that patients have after ECT is **headache.** Even though succinylcholine has been given, the electrical stimulus causes tonic contraction of the jaw muscles and soreness. The headaches usually respond to acetaminophen.

When ECT is administered bilaterally, there is often **loss of memory** of events that occurred around the time of treatment. The impairment is likely to be **retrograde** and **anterograde** until the series of treatments is ended. Patients often cannot remember specifically what led to their hospitalization. For severely suicidal patients, this effect might be therapeutic, but some patients find it distressing. They need to be reassured of the limited nature of the disturbance. A small number of people complain of chronic and persistent memory troubles. They have the usual amnesia for events surrounding the course of ECT but also report more extensive difficulties.

When ECT is administered unilaterally to the nondominant hemisphere (almost always the right hemisphere), memory loss is much less frequently a problem. Unfortunately, there are some patients who do not respond at all to unilateral treatment. Patients who do respond need more treatments than those treated bilaterally.

Fractures of the vertebrae are rare now that patients are routinely given succinylcholine. Injuries of the teeth, which are less uncommon, can be prevented by using special bite blocks.

A massive surge of many different transmitters and hormones occurs during the seizure. Cardiac arrhythmias are not uncommon and should be monitored until they resolve, either spontaneously or with treatment. Transient hypertension secondary to ECT does not usually require treatment.

Selected Readings

American Psychiatric Association. Task Force on Electroconvulsive Therapy: The practice of electroconvulsive therapy: recommendations for treatment, training, and privileging. Washington, D. C., American Psychiatric Association, 1990.

Bloom, F. E., and D. J. Kupfer, eds. Psychopharmacology: The Fourth Generation of Progress. New York, Raven Press, 1995.

Borison, R. L., et al. Clinical overview of risperidone. In Meltzer, H. Y., ed. Novel Antipsychotic Drugs. New York, Raven Press, 1992.

Chouinard, G., et al. A Canadian multicenter placebo-controlled study of fixed doses of risperidone and haloperidol in the treatment of chronic schizophrenic patients. Journal of Clinical Psychopharmacology 13:25–40, 1993.

DeVane, C. L. Pharmacogenetics and drug metabolism of newer antidepressant agents. Journal of Clinical Psychiatry 55(12) (supplement):38–45, 1994.

Jacobson, S. J., et al. Prospective multicentre study of pregnancy outcome after lithium exposure during first trimester. Lancet 339:530–533, 1992.

Janicak, P. G., et al. Principles and Practice of Psychopharmacotherapy, 2nd ed. Baltimore, Williams & Wilkins, 1997.

Kane, J. M., and J. A. Lieberman, eds. Adverse Effects of Psychotropic Drugs. New York, Guilford Press, 1992.

Salzman, C. Clinical Geriatric Psychopharmacology, 3rd ed. Baltimore, Williams & Wilkins, 1997.

Schatzberg, A. F., and J. O. Cole. Manual of Clinical Psychopharmacology, 2nd ed. Washington, D. C., American Psychiatric Press, Inc., 1991.

Schatzberg, A. F., and C. B. Nemeroff, eds. The American Psychiatric Press Textbook of Psychopharmacology. Washington, D. C., American Psychiatric Press, Inc., 1995.

Index

Note: Page numbers in *italics* refer to illustrations; page numbers followed by (b) refer to boxed material; and page numbers followed by (t) refer to tables.

WITHDRAWN